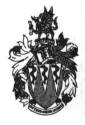

UNIVERSITY OF WALES
COLLEGE OF MEDICINE
CARDIFF

D0256810

PROCEEDINGS OF THE EUROPEAN DIALYSIS AND TRANSPLANT ASSOCIATION — EUROPEAN RENAL ASSOCIATION

PROCEEDINGS OF THE EUROPEAN DIALYSIS AND TRANSPLANT ASSOCIATION — EUROPEAN RENAL ASSOCIATION

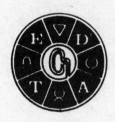

Twentieth Congress held in London, England, 1983

Editor
Alex M Davison

Associate Editor
Pierre J Guillou

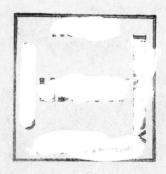

PITMAN

First Published 1983

Catalogue Number 21.0844.80

Pitman Publishing Ltd
128 Long Acre
London WC2E 9AN

Associated Companies
Pitman Publishing Pty Ltd, Melbourne
Pitman Publishing New Zealand Ltd, Wellington

ISBN 0-272-79769-3
ISSN 0308-9401

Printed and bound in Great Britain
at The Pitman Press, Bath

EUROPEAN DIALYSIS AND TRANSPLANT ASSOCIATION
EUROPEAN RENAL ASSOCIATION

OFFICERS AND MEMBERS OF THE COUNCIL
1983/1984

1984 CONGRESS

21st CONGRESS

OF

THE EUROPEAN DIALYSIS AND TRANSPLANT ASSOCIATION
EUROPEAN RENAL ASSOCIATION

FLORENCE
ITALY

23–26 September 1984

President of Congress
V Cambi

Secretary of Congress

Professor Mario Savi
Clinica Medica e Nefrologia
Università di Parma
Ospedale Maggiore
43100 Parma, Italy

Congress Secretariat

O.I.C., Via G Modena, 19
50121 Firenze, Italy

FOREWORD

The 20th annual Congress of the European Dialysis and Transplant Association (EDTA) – European Renal Association (ERA) was held in London from June 19th to 22nd 1983. The permanent record of the Congress is given in this volume.

It has been a great pleasure for all EDTA-ERA members to be in London for the 20th anniversary of our Association. The conception of EDTA (now EDTA-ERA), in fact, occurred in London. In September 1963, at the end of a symposium on Acute Renal Failure organised by Dr S Shaldon at the Royal Free Hospital, two English nephrologists, Dr S Shaldon and Dr D N S Kerr, and a Dutch nephrologist, Dr W Drukker, planned the creation of a Society which was called EDTA to report and record the treatment of uraemia by dialysis and transplantation. In twenty years our Association has grown considerably, the quality of the scientific Congresses has improved, more space has been given to clinical nephrology which is the basis for the prevention of the uraemic condition. The selection of two topics of nephrology for each Congress ('Hypertension' and 'Renal Stone Disease' in London), the help of experts as referees, the increased emphasis on poster sessions (in London a new model of poster sessions with limited slide presentation and discussion), the organisation of workshops, have all been successful measures for improving the quality and interest of our Congress.

The success of our recent policy is testified by the increased number of submitted abstracts which reached 600 in London (against 449 in Paris in 1981); the abstracts dealing with clinical nephrology reached 300 (against the 89 in Paris in 1981). For the first time in the history of the Association, the abstracts dealing with clinical nephrology exceeded those dealing with dialysis. For this success EDTA-ERA is grateful to the Presidents of National Societies of Nephrology for their important cooperation in suggesting topics of nephrology referees, lectures and lecturers.

I am pleased to express the appreciation of the Association and myself to all referees for the 20th Congress: Dr G Bianchi, Dr K Horky, Dr A F Lever, Dr P Meyer for 'Hypertension'; Dr A Fournier, Dr G H Nancollas, Dr C Y C Pak, Dr M Peacock for 'Renal Stone Disease'; Dr A D Barnes, Dr J Hors, Dr G Sirchia, Dr J J Van Rood for 'Transplant Immunology'.

Professor A Valek is leaving the Council. He has given a great contribution to Council activities in the past three years. I am grateful to him. I am pleased to acknowledge the continuous excellent activity of our Registration Committee and particularly to its chairman, Dr A J Wing. I am also grateful to Dr S T Boen, the Secretary-Treasurer, for his help in running the affairs of the Association.

I am finally happy to express the gratitude of myself, the Council, and of the whole Association to Professor D N S Kerr, President of the 20th Congress, and to the Congress Secretary Dr F J Goodwin for organising this successful Congress in London.

I acknowledge the excellent achievement of our Editor of these Proceedings, Dr A M Davison and Pitman Publishing Limited, our publisher: the publication of this volume is excellent as usual, but even more rapid than before, congratulations.

Vittorio E Andreucci
President of EDTA–European Renal Association

PREFACE

The Barbican centre in London was the venue for the 20th Congress of the European Dialysis and Transplant Association — European Renal Association. The Barbican provided excellent facilities for the Congress and lived up to its reputation — one Congressant described it as a highly sophisticated maze for city dwellers. It took some time to unravel the geography of the place but that in no way detracted from the excellence of the facilities and the lecture halls. An interesting feature was that all signposts to the Barbican Centre seemed to indicate the same distance, half a mile, and so one was frequently left with the sensation of going round in circles.

This year publication has been easier with the Congress being held in June. We are most grateful to the 75 per cent of authors who provided us with their manuscripts by the deadline date: the majority of the remainder arrived in the following week. It is interesting to us that those who were late last year were the same this year! Most authors have adhered to the requirements with respect to length and number of references but a few have been excessive. In these cases we have reduced the manuscript length and deleted all references in excess of ten. To do otherwise would be unfair to the very many authors who complied with the appropriate instructions. Two papers which appear in the programme do not appear in these Proceedings — both poster presentations and both from the United States of America. The authors failed to present their posters during the Congress and therefore cannot be included in this volume. In view of the large number of abstracts submitted and the small number accepted, this non-presentation of accepted material is to be deplored.

The Proceedings this year follow closely the pattern established over the past years. The author index has been restored as members have found this a valuable way of identifying papers they remember being presented by a particular author. I hope the addresses given are correct: all presenters were asked to check their address and that of their co-authors in the Editorial office during the Congress, but few availed themselves of this offer. The subject index again refers to the first page of the article, except in the case of the Registry Reports, Guest Lectures and discussion comments. This year we have tried, where possible, to reference the discussion comments and we hope we have found the appropriate references. In some cases these have proved impossible to find and therefore have been necessarily omitted.

It is a pleasure to record our thanks to Professor D N S Kerr and Dr F J Goodwin and the Organising Committee Members for the help given to the editorial staff. We are grateful to Mr Marcus Summersfield for his untiring efforts in providing the facilities we required, particularly with the recording of discussion sessions, which this year was performed to a high standard. The Editorial Office was organised again by Mrs Gillian Howard and we are most grateful to her for her many and varied efforts in making this volume possible. Mrs Betty Dickens and Mrs Vivienne Smith provided valuable secretarial help in typing the discussions during the Congress. Proof reading has been again undertaken speedily by Andrew Davison and we are grateful to him for his expertise. The rapid publication of this volume is due to the efforts of many and the introduction of a word processor for the compilation of the index. We are, however, particularly grateful to Mrs Betty Dickens and the staff of Pitman Publishing Ltd for their outstanding ability in completing their tasks within such a tight time schedule.

Alex M Davison
Editor EDTA-ERA Proceedings

Department of Renal Medicine
St James's University Hospital
Leeds LS9 7TF

Pierre J Guillou
Associate Editor

University Department of Surgery
St James's University Hospital
Leeds LS9 7TF

CONTENTS

xiii

PART I

STATISTICAL REPORTS

Chairmen: V E Andreucci
              D N S Kerr

COMBINED REPORT ON REGULAR DIALYSIS AND TRANSPLANTATION IN EUROPE, XIII, 1982

Members

M BROYER	Hôpital Necker Enfants Malades, Paris, France
F P BRUNNER	Departement für Innere Medizin, Universität Basel, Switzerland
H BRYNGER	Department of Surgery I, Sahlgrenska Sjukhuset, Göteborg, Sweden
R A DONCKERWOLCKE	Het Wilhelmina Kinderziekenhuis, University of Utrecht, Utrecht, Netherlands
C JACOBS	Centre Pasteur-Vallery-Radot, Paris, France
P KRAMER	Medizinische Universitätsklinik, Göttingen, Federal Republic of Germany
N H SELWOOD	UK Transplant, Bristol, United Kingdom
A J WING*	St Thomas' Hospital, London, United Kingdom

* Chairman

Research Fellows

S CHALLAH	Department of Community Medicine, St Thomas' Hospital, London, United Kingdom
N GRETZ	EDTA Registry, St Thomas' Hospital, London, United Kingdom and Klinikum Mannheim, University of Heidelberg, Federal Republic of Germany

CONTENTS

Acknowledgments

This work was supported by grants from the Governments or National Societies of Nephrology of Austria, Belgium, Bulgaria, Cyprus, Czechoslovakia, Denmark, Egypt, the Federal Republic of Germany, France, the German Democratic Republic, Greece, Iceland, Ireland, Israel, Italy, Luxembourg, the Netherlands, Norway, Sweden, Switzerland and the United Kingdom.

Generous grants were made by Asahi Medical GmbH, Bellco S.p.A., B Braun Melsungen AG, Cordis Dow B.V., Cobe Laboratories Inc, Enka AG, Extracorporeal Inc, Dr E Fresenius KG, Gambro AB, Hospal Ltd, Sorin Biomedica S.p.A., Travenol Laboratories Ltd.

The post of Research Fellow to the EDTA Registry, currently held by Dr Norbert Gretz, was funded by the National Kidney Research Fund, United Kingdom.

We acknowledge the support of UK Transplant, Bristol, United Kingdom.

We particularly thank those doctors and their staff who have completed questionnaires. Without their collaboration, this Report could not have been prepared.

Proc EDTA (1983) Vol 20

COMBINED REPORT ON REGULAR DIALYSIS AND TRANSPLANTATION IN EUROPE, XIII, 1982

A J Wing, M Broyer, F P Brunner, H Brynger, S Challah,
R A Donckerwolcke, N Gretz, C Jacobs, P Kramer, N H Selwood

Introduction

The twentieth meeting of the European Dialysis and Transplant Association was the nineteenth occasion on which the EDTA Registry reported. The Registry enjoyed an unrepeatable advantage of commencing its data collection at the very beginning of dialysis and transplantation in Europe. Between 1965 and 1970 separate reports on dialysis and transplantation were produced by Dr Drukker in Amsterdam and Dr Parsons in Leeds [1]. The Registry became

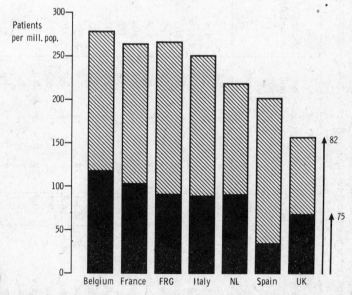

Figure 1. Patients per million population on 31 December 1975 and 1982 in countries with more than 2,500 patients alive on treatment on 31 December 1982

TABLE I. Summary of numbers of centres and of patients on haemodialysis on 31 December 1982, in each of 32 countries. Numbers on haemodialysis/haemofiltration are shown according to whether they were treated in hospital (including satellite centres and minimal care) or at home. Numbers on bicarbonate haemodialysis, haemofiltration and haemodiafiltration are a subset of those on haemodialysis/haemofiltration. Data from centre questionnaires supplemented by data collected by national Keymen from those centres which did not return centre questionnaires

Country	Pop in mill	CENTRES			Hospital haemodialysis	Home haemodialysis	Total	Per mill pop	Bicarbonate haemodialysis	Haemo-filtration	Haemo-diafiltration
		Known	Replied	Per mill pop of replies							
Algeria	18.3	3	1	0.1	17	3	20	1.1	0	0	0
Austria	7.5	24	24	3.2	899	62	961	128.1	32	28	9
Belgium	9.8	53	53	5.4	1,666	92	1,758	179.4	335	49	75
Bulgaria	9.0	30	29	3.2	803	23	826	91.8	0	28	20
Cyprus	0.6	2	2	3.3	89	0	89	148.3	0	0	34
Czechoslovakia	15.2	21	21	1.4	624	1	625	41.1	0	15	21
Denmark	5.1	12	12	2.4	406	98	504	98.8	5	5	20
Egypt	38.9	24	17	0.4	378	0	378	9.7	2	3	0
Fed Rep Germany	61.2	282	275	4.5	12,501	2,146	14,647	239.3	570	785	490
Finland	4.8	24	24	5.0	202	3	205	42.7	3	1	0
France	53.4	199	193	3.6	8,799	2,183	10,982	205.7	1,028	185	28
German Dem Rep	16.8	51	51	3.0	1,126	0	1,126	67.0	55	2	0
Greece	9.3	52	49	5.3	2,234	0	2,234	240.2	18	0	0
Hungary	10.7	10	9	0.8	180	0	180	16.8	0	0	54
Iceland	0.2	1	1	5.0	15	0	15	75.0	0	0	0
Ireland	3.3	4	4	1.2	117	35	152	46.1	0	0	0
Israel	3.8	26	26	6.8	861	62	923	242.9	77	0	11
Italy	56.8	361	251	4.4	9,798	1,555	11,353	199.9	1,138	201	274

TABLE I. *Continued*

Country	Pop in mill	CENTRES Known	Replied	Per mill pop of replies	Hospital haemodialysis	Home haemodialysis	Total	Per mill pop	Bicarbonate haemodialysis	Haemo-filtration	Haemo-diafiltration
Lebanon	2.7	7	3	1.1	77	0	77	28.5	0	0	50
Libya	2.9	3	2	0.7	83	0	83	28.6	0	0	5
Luxembourg	0.4	5	5	12.5	85	2	87	217.5	0	5	0
Netherlands	14.0	47	47	3.4	1,697	164	1,861	132.9	99	29	7
Norway	4.1	17	16	3.9	205	6	211	51.5	6	8	0
Poland	35.4	46	45	1.3	611	0	611	17.3	45	8	12
Portugal	9.8	22	15	1.5	551	0	551	56.2	0	0	0
Spain	37.0	175	170	4.6	6,893	360	7,253	196.0	176	89	254
Sweden	8.3	31	31	3.7	608	132	740	89.2	4	18	2
Switzerland	6.5	32	32	4.9	857	196	1,053	162.0	69	29	5
Tunisia	6.2	7	7	1.1	169	0	169	27.3	0	14	29
Turkey	44.2	15	15	0.3	263	0	263	6.0	78	12	35
United Kingdom	55.9	62	58	1.0	1,417	2,160	3,577	64.0	18	4	2
Yugoslavia	22.1	73	55	2.5	1,842	30	1,872	84.7	41	67	24
TOTAL REGISTRY	574.2	1,721	1,543	2.7	56,073	9,313	65,386	113.9	3,799	1,585	1,461

7

computerised in 1970 when it moved to Munich under the Chairmanship of Professor Gurland and at that time there were approximately 3,000 live patients. This number had increased ten-fold by the time the Registry moved to St Thomas' Hospital, London in 1976 [2]. This year's Reports were prepared from a computerised data base of over 141,000 registered patients, 87,000 of whom were alive on 31 December, 1982. Data from the individual patient records were augmented with information returned on the centre questionnaire.

Over three-quarters of patients (78%) were contributed by the seven big countries shown in Figure 1. Each of these countries had at least 2,500 patients alive on treatment at the end of 1982. On 31 December, 1975 Belgium treated 118 patients per million population, Italy 90 and Spain 35 [2]. By the 31 December, 1982 all seven countries had more than doubled their patient populations; there were over 14,000 patients in each of France, Federal Republic of Germany and Italy; Belgium treated 278 patients per million population and five of the other countries had over 200 patients per million population alive on treatment; the United Kingdom, however, reached only 157 per million population.

Seven patients who were still alive on 31 December, 1982 commenced treatment before 20 June, 1963 – 20 years before this year's Congress. The longest surviving transplant was a sibling graft carried out in France in June, 1959; the only one of these long survivors treated solely by haemodialysis was a British patient who commenced treatment in April, 1963. The longest UK survivor commenced treatment in October, 1961 in Scotland and survived for more than 20 years with a graft from his father received at the age of 12.

Demographic data from centre questionnaires

The EDTA Registry centre questionnaire was used to collect summary information from the centres. Table I and Table II show the numbers of patients recorded on haemodialysis and peritoneal dialysis in each of the countries reporting to the Registry. The number of centres which returned their centre questionnaire is also shown, but the information received from these centres has, in some countries, been augmented by direct enquiry through the national Keymen.

Table III and Table IV show the number of transplant operations performed in 1982 and of the total transplants and follow-up status of transplanted patients according to countries. This information has also been supplemented by direct enquiries via national Keymen and through the transplant registries with whom the EDTA Registry has established links.

Demographic data from patient questionnaires

Individual patient questionnaires provide the data base for analyses presented subsequently in this Report. The numbers of patients reported on individual questionnaires are shown according to country in Tables V and VI. Table V shows the stock of registered patients according to their mode of therapy on 31 December, 1982 and Table VI shows the numbers of new patients

TABLE II. Summary of numbers of patients on intermittent and continuous ambulatory peritoneal dialysis on 31 December 1982, in each of 32 countries. Numbers on continuous cycling peritoneal dialysis and on peritoneal dialysis combined with haemodialysis are subsets of the total on peritoneal dialysis. Data from centre questionnaires supplemented by data collected by national Keymen from those centres which did not return centre questionnaires

Country	Intermittent peritoneal dialysis	Continuous ambulatory PD	Total	Per million population	Continuous cycling PD (CCPD)	PD combined with HD
Algeria	0	6	6	0.3	0	0
Austria	1	16	17	2.3	1	0
Belgium	3	153	156	15.9	6	0
Bulgaria	0	0	0	0	0	0
Cyprus	0	0	0	0	0	0
Czechoslovakia	0	14	14	0.9	0	1
Denmark	56	106	162	31.8	2	1
Egypt	0	0	0	0	0	11
Fed Rep Germany	141	303	444	7.3	21	6
Finland	15	89	104	21.7	1	1
France	225	736	961	18.0	53	7
German Dem Rep	10	4	14	0.8	3	1
Greece	15	32	47	5.1	0	0
Hungary	14	3	17	1.6	1	3
Iceland	0	0	0	0	0	0
Ireland	2	32	34	10.3	0	1
Israel	59	65	124	32.6	3	4
Italy	152	909	1,061	18.7	52	11
Lebanon	0	0	0	0	0	0
Libya	2	0	2	0.7	0	1
Luxembourg	0	0	0	0	0	0
Netherlands	6	122	128	9.1	0	0
Norway	1	24	25	6.1	0	1
Poland	65	8	73	2.1	0	3
Portugal	1	3	4	0.4	0	0
Spain	529	347	876	23.7	15	13
Sweden	38	140	178	21.5	1	1
Switzerland	5	173	178	27.4	0	0
Tunisia	30	2	32	5.2	30	25
Turkey	71	15	86	2.0	1	37
United Kingdom	70	1,104	1,174	21.0	14	12
Yugoslavia	164	11	175	7.9	36	15
TOTAL REGISTRY	1,675	4,417	6,092	10.6	240	155

TABLE III. Summary of numbers of renal transplants performed during 1982 in each of 32 countries. Numbers of first grafts, patients aged less than 15 and foreign patients are subsets of total grafts. Data from centre questionnaires supplemented by data collected by national Keymen from those centres which did not return centre questionnaires

Country	TOTALS				CADAVER			LIVING DONOR		
	Cadaveric grafts	Living donor grafts	All grafts	Per million population	1st graft	Patients <15	Foreign patients	1st graft	Patients <15	Foreign patients
Algeria	0	0	0	0	0	0	0	0	0	0
Austria	147	15	162	21.6	128	5	72	15	0	0
Belgium	141	31	172	17.6	60	4	10	8	2	6
Bulgaria	1	0	1	0.1	1	0	0	0	0	0
Cyprus	0	0	0	0	0	0	0	0	0	0
Czechoslovakia	83	1	84	5.5	73	1	14	1	1	0
Denmark	105	6	111	21.8	29	1	0	3	0	0
Egypt	0	6	6	0.2	0	0	0	6	0	2
Fed Rep Germany	997	39	1,036	16.9	672	84	20	25	11	5
Finland	130	3	133	27.7	104	0	0	2	0	0
France	786	48	834	15.6	549	63	79	16	6	14
German Dem Rep	172	0	172	10.2	159	6	1	0	0	0
Greece	13	34	47	5.1	11	0	0	21	0	3
Hungary	40	2	42	3.9	39	1	0	2	1	0
Iceland	0	0	0	0	0	0	0	0	0	0
Ireland	52	10	62	18.8	43	1	0	10	1	0
Israel	76	22	98	25.8	51	5	0	21	4	3
Italy	214	17	231	4.1	177	5	0	9	2	0

TABLE III. *Continued*

Country	TOTALS				CADAVER			LIVING DONOR		
	Cadaveric grafts	Living donor grafts	All grafts	Per million population	1st graft	Patients <15	Foreign patients	1st graft	Patients <15	Foreign patients
Lebanon	0	0	0	0	0	0	0	0	0	0
Libya	0	0	0	0	0	0	0	0	0	0
Luxembourg	2	0	2	5.0	2	0	0	0	0	0
Netherlands	245	24	269	19.2	129	14	0	10	0	0
Norway	74	31	105	25.6	60	0	0	30	4	1
Poland	48	1	49	1.4	48	1	0	1	0	0
Portugal	26	0	26	2.7	26	0	0	0	0	0
Spain	321	46	367	9.9	254	10	0	32	2	1
Sweden	180	53	233	28.1	137	0	0	52	12	0
Switzerland	163	4	167	25.7	138	7	11	4	0	1
Tunisia	0	0	0	0	0	0	0	0	0	0
Turkey	7	38	45	1.0	7	0	0	38	0	2
United Kingdom	971	124	1,095	19.6	623	16	0	96	4	14
Yugoslavia	8	34	42	1.9	8	0	0	32	1	0
TOTAL REGISTRY	5,002	589	5,591	9.7	3,528	224	207	434	51	52

11

TABLE IV. Summary of numbers of renal transplants performed in all years and those still known to be functioning on 31 December 1982. Data from centre questionnaires supplemented by data collected by national Keymen from those centres which did not return centre questionnaires

Country	Total grafts performed all years	Functioning on 31 Dec 1982	Functioning in patients residing in foreign countries	Functioning and† followed-up in Reporting Centres
Algeria	0	0	0	0
Austria	1,069	344	108	207
Belgium	2,367	519	32	400
Bulgaria	18	9	0	8
Cyprus	0	0	0	0
Czechoslovakia	655	170	13	169
Denmark	1,541	369	0	308
Egypt	46	16	2	15
Fed Rep Germany	4,547	1,819	48	1,552
Finland	1,314	602	0	447
France	4,689	2,632	147	1,460
German Dem Rep	1,042	346	4	520
Greece	349	223	3	181
Hungary	185	9	0	105
Iceland	0	0	0	0
Ireland	458	199	3	146
Israel	577	226	5	161
Italy	1,207	526	0	583
Lebanon	1	1	0	0
Libya	0	0	0	26
Luxembourg	3	3	0	6
Netherlands	1,996	906	5	871
Norway	1,100	59	1	169
Poland	424	178	0	176
Portugal	54	33	0	46
Spain	1,575	835	6	830
Sweden	2,836	1,023	14	709
Switzerland	1,738	788	92	789
Tunisia	0	0	0	23
Turkey	232	104	2	129
United Kingdom	8,970	3,252	103	3,477
Yugoslavia	345	127	2	133
TOTAL REGISTRY	39,338	15,318	590	13,646

† In countries in which this number exceeds those "functioning on 31 Dec 1982" it must be presumed that more than one centre claimed responsibility for follow-up

12

and of deaths according to country. These two tables have been a regular feature of our reports.

Patient survival

Actuarial methods have been used to analyse mortality and survival of patients and grafts as well as treatment change rates. A theoretical example is shown in Figure 2. The period of observation (in the example given, six years) is divided into intervals which can be variable or constant (shown in the figure as one year). The number of patients dying in each interval is divided by the number

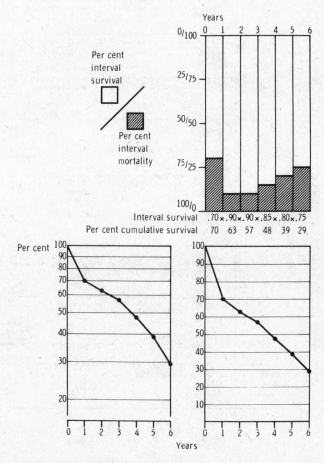

Figure 2. Calculation of cumulative survival rates: (top right panel) interval survival in each of six years, (lower left panel) semilogarithmic plot of cumulative survival, (lower right panel) arithmetic plot of cumulative survival

TABLE V. Registered patients known to be alive on 31 December, 1982, and those not yet updated in 32 countries. Data from individual patient questionnaires (including some late returns)*

Country	Centres replied	IPD	CAPD	on Haemodialysis/Haemofiltration				With func. trans.	Total	Per million pop.	OTHER REGISTERED PATIENTS		
				Hospital	Home	Total	% Home of total				Recovered	Lost to follow-up	Not† updated
Algeria	1	0	8	3	0	3	0	0	11	0.6	0	35	46
Austria	24	4	16	911	59	970	6.1	222	1,212	161.6	14	21	55
Belgium	50	2	129	1,556	112	1,668	6.7	711	2,510	256.1	42	38	79
Bulgaria	27	0	0	374	10	384	2.6	12	396	44.0	0	12	22
Cyprus	2	0	0	85	0	85	0	20	105	175.0	4	14	4
Czechoslovakia	21	0	12	645	1	646	0.2	173	831	54.7	8	5	17
Denmark	11	49	93	314	59	373	15.8	318	833	163.3	11	22	321
Egypt	17	1	0	343	2	345	0.6	9	355	9.1	6	69	53
Fed Rep Germany	247	109	193	10,255	1,801	12,056	14.9	1,607	13,965	228.2	156	363	1,848
Finland	24	10	63	155	3	158	1.9	249	480	100.0	7	8	339
France	189	176	567	7,782	1,690	9,472	17.8	1,640	11,855	222.0	120	321	1,764
German Dem Rep	51	6	5	1,014	0	1,014	0	375	1,400	83.3	7	13	102
Greece	36	4	1	752	3	755	0.4	175	935	100.5	18	106	384
Hungary	9	15	3	183	0	183	0	75	276	25.8	3	3	17
Iceland	1	0	0	14	0	14	0	7	21	105.0	0	0	1
Ireland	4	2	26	148	41	189	21.7	173	390	118.2	1	4	14
Israel	26	54	54	667	59	726	8.1	191	1,025	269.7	3	11	31
Italy	259	134	840	9,314	899	10,213	8.8	980	12,167	214.2	133	284	1,610

14

TABLE V. *Continued*

Country	Centres replied	PATIENTS ON TREATMENT AT 31 DECEMBER, 1982									OTHER REGISTERED PATIENTS		
		IPD	CAPD	on Haemodialysis/Haemofiltration				With func. trans.	Total	Per million pop.	Recovered	Lost to follow-up	Not† updated
				Hospital	Home	Total	% Home of total						
Lebanon	3	0	0	17	0	17	0	0	17	6.3	0	5	87
Libya	2	0	0	66	0	66	0	2	68	23.4	0	9	12
Luxembourg	5	0	0	69	2	71	2.8	4	75	187.5	0	0	0
Netherlands	43	1	87	1,521	150	1,671	9.0	754	2,513	179.5	53	49	463
Norway	16	0	23	211	5	216	2.3	464	703	171.5	19	15	41
Poland	35	27	6	414	12	426	2.8	134	593	16.8	4	20	61
Portugal	16	2	2	503	0	503	0	18	525	53.6	6	29	343
Spain	152	109	321	4,948	335	5,283	6.3	776	6,489	175.4	51	169	919
Sweden	31	34	120	560	127	687	18.5	836	1,677	202.0	39	17	70
Switzerland	32	3	167	805	194	999	19.4	619	1,788	275.1	28	33	37
Tunisia	7	0	0	104	0	104	0	1	105	16.9	1	0	32
Turkey	15	4	8	216	1	217	0.5	65	294	6.7	6	36	11
United Kingdom	50	70	855	1,103	1,716	2,819	60.9	3,126	6,870	122.9	61	125	1,655
Yugoslavia	50	8	8	1,524	17	1,541	1.1	123	1,680	76.0	21	69	324
TOTAL REGISTRY	1,456	824	3,607	46,576	7,298	53,874	13.6	13,859	72,164	125.7	822	1,905	10,762

† Patients known to be alive when last reported to the Registry but record not yet updated for 1982

15

TABLE VI. Registered patients who commenced treatment or died during 1982. Data from individual patient questionnaires (including some late returns)*

Country	Deaths in 1982 N	Per million population	New patients in 1982 N	Per million population
Algeria	3	0.2	14	0.8
Austria	166	22.1	286	38.1
Belgium	272	27.8	388	39.6
Bulgaria	45	5.0	168	18.7
Cyprus	15	25.0	28	46.7
Czechoslovakia	167	11.0	274	18.0
Denmark	105	20.6	137	26.9
Egypt	95	2.4	298	7.7
Fed Rep Germany	1,423	23.3	2,691	44.0
Finland	58	12.1	123	25.6
France	1,052	19.7	1,652	30.9
German Dem Rep	197	11.7	391	23.3
Greece	126	13.5	175	18.8
Hungary	43	4.0	82	7.7
Iceland	2	10.0	7	35.0
Ireland	24	7.3	64	19.4
Israel	124	32.6	221	58.2
Italy	1,023	18.0	1,922	33.8
Lebanon	1	0.4	11	4.1
Libya	7	2.4	27	9.3
Luxembourg	7	17.5	19	47.5
Netherlands	196	14.0	383	27.4
Norway	81	19.8	153	37.3
Poland	92	2.6	100	2.8
Portugal	31	3.2	387	39.5
Spain	405	10.9	1,211	32.7
Sweden	210	25.3	343	41.3
Switzerland	144	22.2	289	44.5
Tunisia	9	1.5	39	6.3
Turkey	74	1.7	199	4.5
United Kingdom	508	9.1	1,111	19.9
Yugoslavia	244	11.0	315	14.3
TOTAL REGISTRY	6,949	12.1	13,508	23.5

of patients at risk in each interval, resulting in the interval mortalities shown by the bottom portion of the bars in the upper right panel. Each interval survival, that is, one minus interval mortality, is then multiplied by the subsequent interval survival to calculate cumulative survival. The lower right panel shows the survival curve in arithmetic display. This allows one to recognise easily the proportion of the *initial* patient population which survives to a certain time. The semilogarithmic survival curve in the lower left panel allows one to recognise mortality of the initial population as well as interval mortality which is indicated by the slope of the curve. It is steepest in the first interval, where mortality is at its highest, stable in the second and third intervals and then becomes steeper as interval mortality increases. The semilogarithmic display reflects the way cumulative survival is calculated and allows visual comparison of the slopes and thus of interval mortality. It is for these reasons that we have preferentially shown survival curves semilogarithmically.

Figure 3 illustrates one of the problems of small numbers of cases. The five

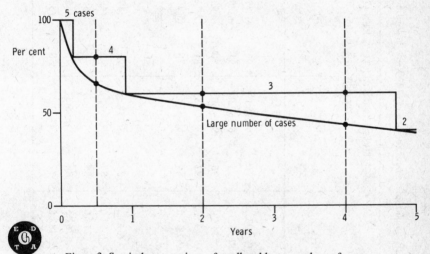

Figure 3. Survival: comparison of small and large numbers of cases

cases shown in stepwise fashion have exactly the same cumulative survival which results in a smooth curve when the number of cases is large. At six months, cumulative survival is 66 per cent, but four of the five cases are still alive which is 80 per cent. At two years the difference is small. At four years, due to the low interval mortality, none of the three cases will have died, indicating a falsely high cumulative survival of 60 per cent – the same as at one year – where a sufficiently large number of cases would have given the correct 43 per cent surviving. Therefore, one should not draw survival curves beyond the interval with the last death or where the number of patients at risk does not exceed 30 (or even more when the interval mortality is less than a few per cent).

17

TABLE VII. Patient survival after starting renal replacement therapy, 1979–1982, according to age group; non-diabetics and diabetics

Age group years	Sample size	MONTHS AFTER STARTING RENAL REPLACEMENT THERAPY – Per cent survival and number (N) at risk									
		3		6		12		24		36	
		%	(N)	%	(N)	%	(N)	%	(N)	%	(N)
NON-DIABETICS											
15 - 34	9,372	98	(9,108.5)	96	(8,498.0)	93	(7,774.0)	87	(5,784.5)	84	(2,946.5)
35 - 44	7,455	98	(7,252.5)	95	(6,782.0)	91	(6,205.5)	84	(4,619.0)	78	(2,347.5)
45 - 54	**	97	**	95	(9,797.0)	90	(8,939.5)	80	(6,619.0)	72	(3,292.5)
55 - 64	9,720	96	(9,430.5)	92	(8,570.5)	85	(7,723.5)	73	(5,604.5)	64	(2,636.5)
65+	7,210	92	(6,961.5)	86	(6,103.5)	76	(5,284.0)	60	(3,604.5)	47	(1,491.5)
DIABETICS											
15 - 34	633	96	(613.5)	88	(557.5)	77	(476.0)	59	(324.5)	50	(133.0)
35 - 44	674	92	(654.0)	84	(574.5)	73	(491.0)	56	(337.5)	47	(143.0)
45 - 54	796	94	(774.0)	85	(698.5)	71	(602.5)	53	(402.0)	40	(161.5)
55 - 64	793	93	(761.5)	86	(656.5)	70	(557.0)	50	(347.5)	37	(129.0)
65+	499	89	(483.0)	77	(409.0)	58	(331.0)	36	(200.5)	23	(70.00)

** = Number at risk greater than 10,000.0

18

Survival on renal replacement therapy (RRT) and hospital haemodialysis

Survival after starting renal replacement therapy between 1979 and 1982 irrespective of any changes in the modes of treatment is given in Table VII. The number of patients with any type of primary renal disease except diabetic nephropathy, who were at risk of dying during the third year varied between 1,500 in those aged 65 or older up to 3,300 in the age group 45–54. Three year survival decreased from 84 per cent in the age group 15–34 down to 47 per cent in the oldest age group. Mortality in diabetics was much higher, resulting in three year survival rates of 50 per cent in the youngest down to 23 per cent in the oldest group.

The difference in survival between patients with diabetic nephropathy and those with all other primary renal diseases taken together is also shown in Figure 4 for the age group 45–54 after starting hospital haemodialysis (or

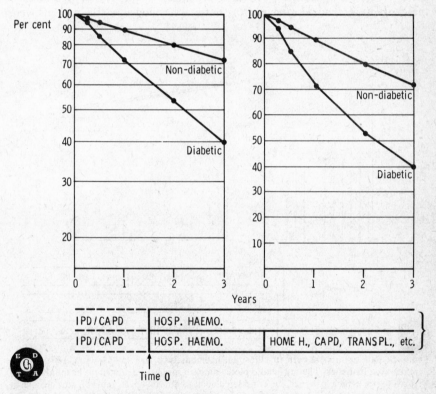

Figure 4. Patient survival *after starting* first hospital haemodialysis, age 45–54 years, 1979–1982, non-diabetics and diabetics. Semilogarithmic plot is shown on the left and arithmetic on the right. The inclusion of patients' histories irrespective of any change in therapy is illustrated at the foot of the figure. Sample size: non-diabetic = more than 10,000, diabetic=2,518

19

haemofiltration) for the first time. The lower part of the figure illustrates how first hospital haemodialysis may have been preceded by a period of peritoneal dialysis, but this is not included in the survival calculation. The righthand panel shows that a large proportion of the initial diabetic population died during the first year. The semilogarithmic lefthand graph demonstrates impressively how the two survival curves continue to diverge. The virtually straight lines indicate that interval mortality was almost constant through the three year course and continued to be much higher in the diabetic group. Three year survival reached 40 per cent versus 72 per cent in the non-diabetic population. These survival rates as well as those after starting first hospital haemodialysis in all the other age groups were all but equal to those on renal replacement therapy given in Table VII.

Survival *on* hospital haemodialysis (or haemofiltration) is compared to that *after starting* hospital haemodialysis for the identical patient group aged 45–54 at commencement of therapy (Figure 5). The lower part of the figure illustrates how the treatment sequence is handled by the two conventions. In the convention denoted *after starting* hospital haemodialysis the patients were

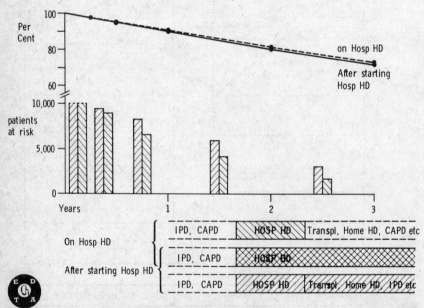

Figure 5. Patient survival with first hospital haemodialysis, age 45–54 years, 1979–1982, excluding diabetics. The arithmetic plots compare survival calculated *on* hospital haemodialysis (in which patients are considered lost to follow-up at time of any change in therapy) with that calculated *after starting* hospital haemodialysis (in which patients are included irrespective of any change in therapy). These two conventions are illustrated at the foot of the figure and their different effects on the numbers of patients at risk at each time interval are shown by the vertical blocks

kept in the analysis whatever happened to them after this first period of hospital haemodialysis. They could be surviving with a functioning transplant or could have died on CAPD after a failed second graft and would still be considered in the calculation of mortality or survival. In contrast, *on* hospital haemodialysis is survival restricted to that treatment modality with patients considered as lost to observation at the moment of changing to other forms of therapy. Therefore, the number at risk at successive intervals declines more rapidly *on* haemodialysis than it does for survival *after starting* haemodialysis. However, the difference in survival at three years — 73 per cent *on* versus 72 per cent *after starting* hospital haemodialysis — was negligible. This can be explained, among other reasons, by the fact that the majority of patients who commenced hospital haemodialysis were not changed to other modes of therapy.

CAPD and patient survival

Patient survival *after starting* CAPD in 1981 or 1982 is depicted in Figure 6 for 15–34 and 55–64 year old patients with all primary renal diseases except diabetes up to 24 months and separately for the small number of diabetics up to 12 months. The differences in survival between patients starting their first CAPD and patients on any form of renal replacement therapy were marginal

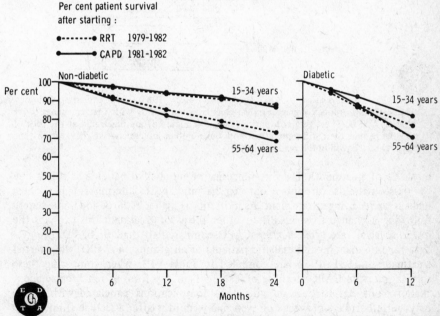

Figure 6. Patient survival *after starting* CAPD 1981–1982 compared to patient survival after starting renal replacement therapy (RRT) 1979–1982 in non-diabetics (lefthand panel) and diabetics (righthand panel) aged 15–34 and 55–64 years

in non-diabetic patients. In patients with diabetic nephropathy, survival at one year after starting CAPD was equal or better, particularly in the young diabetics aged 15–34 with 82 per cent versus 77 per cent for the entire diabetic population of that age group after starting renal replacement therapy.

Figure 7 compares results of the two conventions for survival calculation in patients aged 45–54. Survival *on* CAPD was 80 per cent at two years compared to 75 per cent *after starting* CAPD (which includes subsequent periods on other

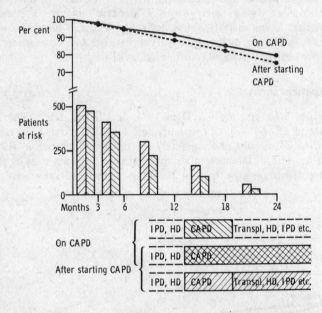

Figure 7. Patient survival with CAPD, aged 45–54 years, 1981–1982, excluding diabetics. The arithmetic plots compare survival calculated *on* CAPD with that calculated *after starting* CAPD. These two conventions (see also Figure 5) are illustrated at the foot of the figure and their different effects on the numbers of patients at risk at each time interval are shown by the vertical blocks

methods of treatment). The difference in the number of patients at risk is due to those patients 'dropping out' to haemodialysis, intermittent peritoneal dialysis or receiving a transplant. As mortality is higher in the period immediately following a change from CAPD to other forms of treatment this explains the lower survival rate *after starting* CAPD compared to that *on* CAPD. Survival data for non-diabetic and diabetic patients of all groups *on* CAPD, who started treatment in 1981–1982, are compiled in Table VIII. When comparing these survival rates *on* CAPD to those of Table VI on any form of renal replacement therapy, one has to bear in mind that complications associated with CAPD may be lethal days or weeks or even many months after a change from CAPD to haemodialysis. This mortality fails to be considered when calculating survival *on* CAPD.

TABLE VIII. Patient survival on continuous ambulatory peritoneal dialysis, 1981–1982, according to age group; non-diabetics and diabetics

MONTHS ON CONTINUOUS AMBULATORY PERITONEAL DIALYSIS
Per cent survival and number (N) at risk

Age group years	Sample size	3		6		12		18		24	
		%	(N)	%	(N)	%	(N)	%	(N)	%	(N)
NON-DIABETICS											
15 - 34	351	99	(301.5)	99	(211.0)	97	(128.0)	97	(56.5)	+	(16.0)
35 - 44	353	99	(311.0)	98	(234.0)	96	(144.0)	91	(62.0)	+	(17.0)
45 - 54	553	98	(481.5)	95	(356.5)	92	(223.0)	85	(101.5)	80	(30.5)
55 - 64	775	96	(685.0)	91	(510.5)	84	(326.0)	79	(140.0)	71	(37.5)
65+	698	95	(618.0)	89	(461.0)	75	(303.5)	64	(127.0)	52	(33.5)
DIABETICS											
15 - 34	104	97	(87.5)	92	(60.0)	92	(33.0)	+	(10.5)	+	(1.5)
35 - 44	107	98	(92.5)	89	(65.5)	77	(38.5)	+	(15.0)	+	(2.0)
45 - 54	104	93	(90.0)	89	(66.5)	80	(48.5)	+	(22.5)	+	(5.5)
55 - 64	140	97	(119.5)	91	(88.5)	71	(64.0)	+	(28.0)	+	(7.5)
65+	53	95	(43.0)	+	(29.0)	+	(21.0)	+	(9.0)	+	(1.0)

+ Number at risk less than 30

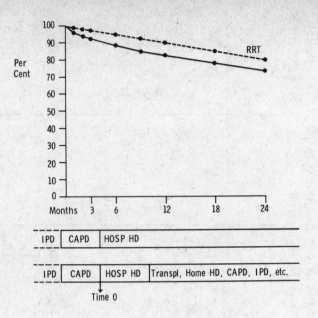

Figure 8. Patient survival *after starting* hospital haemodialysis following CAPD, aged 45–54 years, 1979–1982, excluding diabetics, compared to survival after starting renal replacement therapy. The convention used is illustrated at the foot of the figure. Sample size (N) = 164

What happened when CAPD failed as a technique is illustrated in Figure 8. The majority of CAPD failures, unless they ended with the patient's death, were probably changed to hospital haemodialysis. The increased mortality during the early days, weeks and months after this change caused the initial drop in the survival curve of these unfortunate patients compared to standard survival on renal replacement therapy. However, after six months, interval survival was again similar to that on renal replacement therapy. Failure of CAPD thus seemed to have little, if any, long-term adverse sequelae at least as far as mortality six to 24 months after quitting CAPD was concerned.

Despite these limitations and in contrast to previous years, it would appear that Europe has learnt how to apply CAPD and make adequate use of its potential to achieve better treatment, particularly in young diabetics.

Survival after transplantation

Many aspects of graft survival have been covered in previous years. This time we present data on patient survival after transplantation in 1979–1982, again separately for diabetic nephropathy and for all other primary renal diseases (Table IX). Patient mortality after first cadaveric grafting has long been known to be higher in the early post-transplant months compared to standard survival on renal replacement therapy (Figure 9). In young adults aged 15–34, however,

24

TABLE IX. Patient survival after first cadaver transplantation, 1979–1982, according to age group; non-diabetics and diabetics

Age group years	Sample size	MONTHS AFTER CADAVER TRANSPLANTATION Per cent survival and number (N) at risk									
		3 %	(N)	6 %	(N)	12 %	(N)	24 %	(N)	36 %	(N)
NON-DIABETICS											
15 - 34	3,816	96	(3,690.5)	95	(3,351.0)	93	(3,010.0)	91	(2,241.0)	89	(1,187.0)
35 - 44	2,686	95	(2,595.0)	93	(2,295.5)	90	(2,044.0)	86	(1,517.5)	82	(789.0)
45 - 54	2,159	91	(2,090.0)	88	(1,790.5)	84	(1,565.5)	79	(1,111.0)	74	(551.0)
55 - 64	728	89	(698.5)	82	(569.5)	77	(469.5)	66	(329.5)	61	(150.0)
65+	125	84	(118.5)	80	(89.0)	77	(74.0)	76	(56.0)	71	(30.5)
DIABETICS											
15 - 34	173	87	(168.0)	79	(135.5)	72	(110.0)	59	(75.0)	55	(31.0)
35 - 44	171	87	(166.0)	81	(135.5)	77	(113.5)	72	(84.0)	65	(41.0)
45 - 54	94	80	(92.0)	73	(69.0)	63	(56.5)	51	(37.0)	+	(17.0)
55 - 64	16	+	(15.5)	+	(10.0)	+	(6.5)	+	(5.0)	+	(2.0)
65+	2	+	(2.0)	+	(2.0)	+	(2.0)	+	(1.0)	+	(0.0)

+ Number at risk less than 30

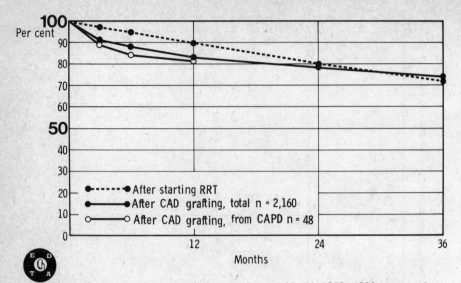

Figure 9. Patient survival after first cadaver graft, aged 45–54, 1979–1982, compared to survival of the same age group after starting renal replacement therapy and showing survival in a small group (N=48) grafted from CAPD

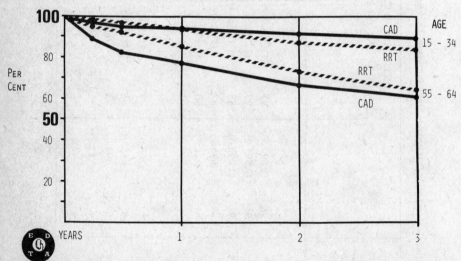

Figure 10. Patient survival after first cadaver graft, aged 15–34 and 55–64, excluding diabetics and compared with survival of the same age groups after starting renal replacement therapy

early post-transplant mortality was barely greater than that of standard RRT, whilst relatively old recipients aged 55–64 ran a definitely increased risk of dying early on (Figure 10). After the first few months, whatever the age of the recipients, interval mortality decreased below that of all forms of renal replace-

26

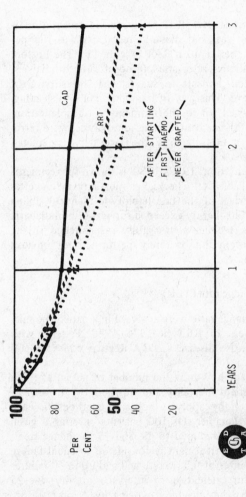

Figure 11. Patient survival after first cadaver graft, 1979–1982, aged 35–44 in diabetics compared to survival after starting renal replacement therapy in diabetics of the same age range. The lower line gives the survival *after starting* first haemodialysis in diabetics of the same age group from which transplanted patients have been excluded. Note: this lower curve should not be compared to the others – see text for explanation

TABLE X. Patient survival after first living donor transplantation, 1979–1982, aged 15–44, including diabetics

MONTHS AFTER LIVING DONOR TRANSPLANTATION
Per cent survival and number (N) at risk

Age	Source of graft	Sample size	3 %	(N)	6 %	(N)	12 %	(N)	18 %	(N)	24 %	(N)	36 %	(N)
15	Parent	564	98	(542.5)	96	(497.5)	95	(442.0)	92	(369.5)	90	(276.5)	88	(122.0)
to	Sibling – 2 haplo.	331	99	(320.0)	98	(297.5)	97	(271.5)	97	(230.5)	96	(187.5)	95	(98.0)
44	Sibling – 1 haplo.	90	97	(86.5)	95	(76.0)	95	(65.0)	95	(54.0)	95	(44.5)	+	(26.0)

+ Number at risk less than 30

ment therapy combined (see also Figure 16). Thus the survival curve after transplantation crossed that on renal replacement therapy at one year in the age group 15—34 (Figure 10) and in the course of the third year in recipients aged 45—54 (Figure 9), whilst the survival curve of the 55—64 year old group was about to reach that on renal replacement therapy at three years (Figure 10). Post-transplant survival of the small number of patients transplanted from CAPD, although slightly inferior, probably does not really differ from the total group (Figure 9).

The difference of patient survival after first cadaveric transplantation is particularly striking in the 35—44 year old diabetic recipients with 65 per cent at three years compared to 47 per cent on RRT (Figure 11). The bottom curve, which shows survival in diabetics after starting hospital haemodialysis, but excluding all those ever grafted, appears to suggest that the survival of these diabetics is worse than standard. This way of handling data is misleading, because all the patients who survived up to the moment of transplantation, that is a patient group that had 100 per cent survival on dialysis, were retrospectively removed from the analysis. Consequently, the lower curve is depicted only to stress that it should be ignored [3].

Survival after live donor transplantation, 1979—1982, is shown for recipients aged 15—44 including diabetics (Table X). The higher mortality in diabetics probably explains why patient survival of the one haplotype identical sibling or parent donor graft recipients all but slightly exceeded survival of non-diabetic cadaveric graft recipients. The six recipients of a fully mis-matched sibling donor graft, a type of transplantation that is rarely performed for obvious reasons, have nevertheless, so far survived.

Interval mortality and treatment change rate (TCR)

Interval mortality and treatment change rates were analysed in a patient population aged 15—54 at commencement of RRT in 1976—1982. Patients with multi-system, malignant or hypertensive diseases (EDTA Registry codes 52—99) were excluded (Figure 12).

Figure 13 is a simple example to show how the number of patients at risk are derived in order to calculate patient mortality and, furthermore, how treatment change rate can be calculated by applying actuarial methods to each mode in a sequence of integrated therapies. Of 100 patients entering a given interval on a particular therapy, 15 are assumed to die and 25 to change treatment during the interval. If change of treatment is considered to equal failure of that mode of therapy, then the interval failure rate will add up to 40 failures in 100 patients or 40 per cent. For calculation of interval mortality, the 25 patients who changed treatment have to be considered as being 'lost to observation' during the interval. The actuarial method (which assumes an even distribution of drop-outs throughout the interval) considers half of those 'lost to observation' as being 'at risk of dying' during the interval. Interval mortality is thus 17 per cent. Similarly, for calculation of treatment change rate (TCR) the 15 patients who died must be considered 'lost to observation' because of the theoretical possibility of their changing to other methods of treatment had they not died.

28

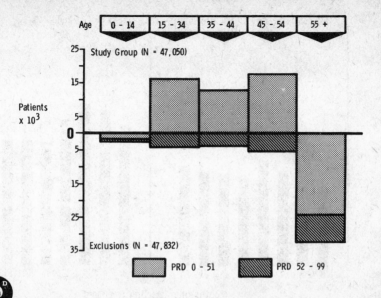

Figure 12. Distribution of new patients who commenced treatment 1976–1982 according to age and primary renal disease (PRD) to show how a study group was derived in which to compare results of different therapies. PRD 0–51 and 52–99 refer to codings used by the EDTA Registry to record diagnosis of PRD on the patient questionnaire

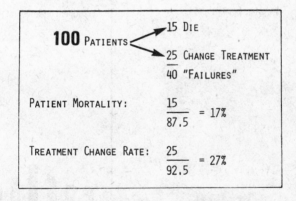

Figure 13. Example to illustrate the calculation of patient mortality and treatment change rate

Therefore, half of the patients who died are considered 'at risk of changing treatment', resulting in an interval treatment change rate of 27 per cent.

Figure 14 shows that interval mortality on hospital haemodialysis was between two per cent and three per cent per three month interval, and because it was fairly constant, it would produce an exponential survival curve which becomes

29

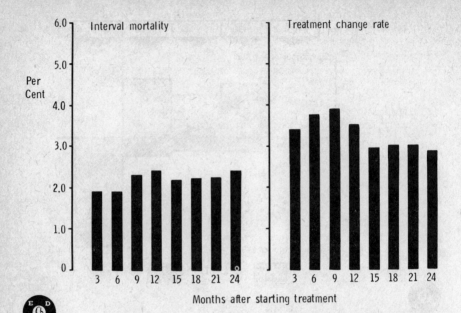

Figure 14. Interval mortality and treatment change rate in study group patients on first hospital haemodialysis (sample size = 41,721)

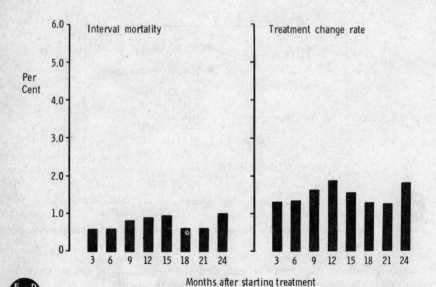

Figure 15. Interval mortality and treatment change rate in study group patients on first home haemodialysis (sample size = 6,393)

30

a straight line when depicted semilogarithmically. The TCR was just under four per cent and, again, constant. Home haemodialysis (Figure 15) had the lowest interval mortality and TCRs.

First cadaveric transplantation (Figure 16) gave a high initial mortality – this is patients who died before returning to dialysis – which after one year diminished to less than one per cent per three months, similar to home haemodialysis. TCR was over 10 per cent in the first three months falling to around one per cent per three months after the first year.

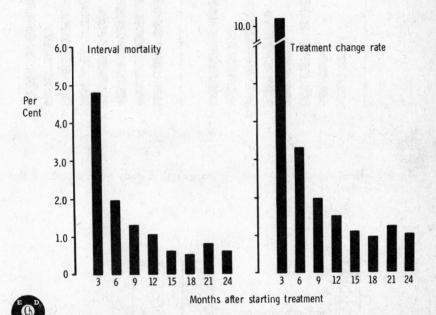

Figure 16. Interval mortality and treatment change rate in study group patients with first cadaver graft (sample size = 9,290)

CAPD (Figure 17) resulted in three monthly interval mortalities which did not compare unfavourably with hospital haemodialysis but the TCR was higher in most intervals emphasising the use of other methods of treatment to back-up CAPD. It should be borne in mind that patients commencing treatment during the early years of CAPD are included in this analysis and that some of the patients who changed from CAPD to other treatments returned to CAPD after a short interruption.

Causes of first cadaver graft failure

Traditionally the individual patient questionnaire has asked for a single cause of graft failure and the options listed in Figure 18 have been offered. Almost

31

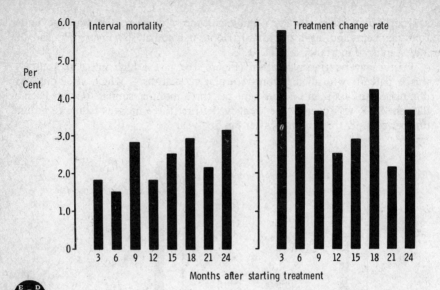

Figure 17. Interval mortality and treatment change rate in study group patients on first CAPD (sample size = 2,059)

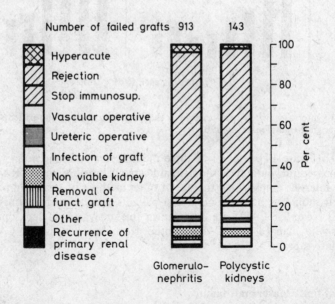

Figure 18. Cause of first cadaver graft failure, 1980–1982, in patients whose PRD was glomerulonephritis and polycystic kidney disease

32

80 per cent of the failures were accounted for by rejection including one to two per cent by rejection after stopping all immunosuppressive drugs and only 1.5 per cent by recurrent primary renal disease in the glomerulonephritic patients. The differences between the major categories of primary renal diseases were small.

Per cent distribution of causes of graft failure differed slightly according to time after transplantation (Figure 19). Ten per cent of early failures resulted

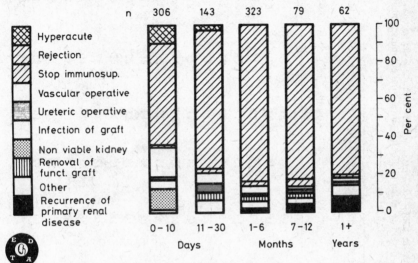

Figure 19. Cause of first cadaver graft failure, 1980–1982, in patients whose PRD was glomerulonephritis, according to time after transplantation

from hyperacute rejection and another 55 per cent from rejection. After the first month, rejection was thought to cause 85 per cent of graft failures. Despite the fact that hyperacute rejection was defined as 'leading to failure within 48 hours of transplantation' some centres still erroneously reported cases of hyperacute rejection causing graft failure 10 days or more after transplantation.

Vascular operative problems caused 16 per cent of early failures and decreased in frequency with time. Ureteric operative failures peaked with five per cent of failures between days 11 and 30. Over 10 per cent of early failures were attributed to non-viability of the cadaveric organs. The percentage due to recurrence of glomerulonephritis increased with time, beginning between the second and sixth months and causing eight per cent of failures in the second and subsequent years. However, the total number of graft failures due to recurrence of glomerulonephritis was small. The Registry will collect additional information on the types of glomerulonephritis that recur and cause failure of grafts.

Primary renal diseases

Age distribution and geographical variation of primary renal diseases at commencement of renal replacement therapy were analysed for the years 1980–1982.

TABLE XI. Age distribution of patients who commenced treatment in 1980–1982 in 32 countries. Crude acceptance rates per year per million of population and the total patients accepted in the three year period are given in the first and second columns; remaining columns show the percentages of patients in each 10 year age group

Country	Acceptance per year per million pop.	Total patients 1980–82	PER CENT PATIENTS ACCORDING TO AGE AT START OF TREATMENT								
			0–9	10–19	20–29	30–39	40–49	50–59	60–69	70–79	80+
Algeria	1.6	90	1	13	19	7	31	19	9	1	0
Austria	37.4	841	0	4	10	13	21	31	18	3	0
Belgium	44.1	1,296	2	2	7	11	18	27	21	11	1
Bulgaria	13.9	374	1	6	17	15	27	28	3	0	3
Cyprus	54.4	98	0	5	5	10	30	24	23	4	0
Czechoslovakia	16.2	740	1	6	17	27	28	17	3	0	0
Denmark	32.6	498	1	5	7	14	21	27	22	3	1
Egypt	4.9	574	0	4	15	27	29	15	5	1	5
Fed Rep Germany	47.4	8,696	1	3	7	11	22	26	20	10	1
Finland	34.8	501	0	3	12	23	17	25	17	2	0
France	38.6	6,185	2	4	10	13	15	23	20	13	1
German Dem Rep	22.9	1,156	1	6	18	17	30	22	6	1	0
Greece	28.0	782	0	3	8	13	25	27	18	5	1
Hungary	7.0	225	0	4	28	31	24	10	2	0	0
Iceland	23.3	14	0	14	14	7	7	50	7	0	0
Ireland	20.7	205	1	10	22	19	22	18	8	0	1
Israel	57.6	657	2	5	10	12	16	21	21	12	1
Italy	38.1	6,490	1	3	7	10	17	28	24	10	1

TABLE XI. *Continued*

Country	Acceptance per year per million pop.	Total patients 1980–82	PER CENT PATIENTS ACCORDING TO AGE AT START OF TREATMENT								
			0–9	10–19	20–29	30–39	40–49	50–59	60–69	70–79	80+
Lebanon	7.0	57	0	11	16	16	25	23	4	7	0
Libya	10.6	92	0	14	24	21	19	12	7	2	2
Luxembourg	40.0	48	4	2	8	13	8	17	27	21	0
Netherlands	32.8	1,377	2	4	10	13	16	24	24	7	0
Norway	44.5	547	1	6	11	13	12	22	30	5	0
Poland	4.4	472	3	8	32	26	22	8	1	0	1
Portugal	25.5	749	0	6	14	18	23	21	12	2	4
Spain	37.2	4,127	1	6	12	15	20	27	16	3	1
Sweden	43.3	1,079	1	2	7	18	14	23	26	8	0
Switzerland	44.9	877	1	4	8	10	19	28	24	6	0
Tunisia	5.2	96	0	3	23	27	27	15	5	0	0
Turkey	2.3	308	0	6	34	20	24	13	2	0	0
United Kingdom	23.1	3,873	2	8	14	17	22	24	10	1	1
Yugoslavia	19.7	1,307	1	4	14	16	28	29	7	1	0
TOTAL REGISTRY	25.8	44,431	1	5	11	14	20	25	18	7	1

Age distribution of all patients accepted for renal replacement therapy is listed countrywise in Table XI. Figure 20 depicts age distribution for the total Registry and two selected countries. Countries with limited facilities, like Poland, preferentially accepted younger patients with a median age below 40, whilst France, a country with adequate facilities, treated more patients who were in their sixties or seventies when commencing renal replacement therapy. In the total Registry the highest acceptance was in the decade 50–59 with 24 per cent of all patients. Half of the patients were 50 or younger, the other half older than 50.

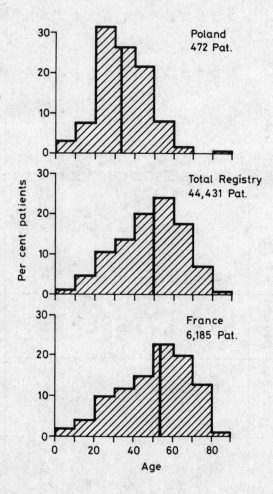

Figure 20. Age distribution of new patients, all diseases, at start of renal replacement therapy 1980–1982, total Registry (centre panel) compared with Poland (upper panel) and France (lower panel)

Age distribution of glomerulonephritis (Figure 21) shows a higher proportion of younger patients with a median age between 42 and 43 for the total Registry as well as for France where glomerulonephritis has been diagnosed particularly

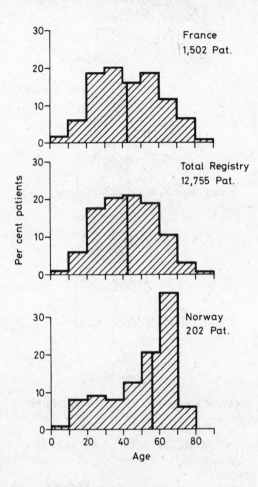

Figure 21. Age distribution of new patients with glomerulonephritis 1980–1982, total Registry (centre panel) compared with the United Kingdom (upper panel) and Italy (lower panel)

frequently in 20–40 year old patients. Norway (lower panel) shows a peculiar age distribution for glomerulonephritis with a tremendous peak in the seventh decade and a median age of 56. All forms of pyelonephritis/interstitial nephritis (Figure 22) show an age distribution which differs little from that for all patients irrespective of primary renal disease. United Kingdom, a country with limited facilities, has treated a larger proportion of young pyelonephritics who often

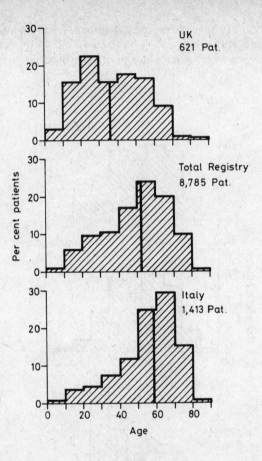

Figure 22. Age distribution of new patients with pyelonephritis 1980–1982, total Registry (centre panel) compared with the United Kingdom (upper panel) and Italy (lower panel)

owe their disease to malformations of the urinary tract. This is in sharp contrast to Italy, where the median age was almost 60 in patients diagnosed as pyelonephritic.

Figure 23 shows three diseases. Two-thirds of the 1,324 patients reported to have *analgesic nephropathy* were accepted in the Federal Republic of Germany (436 patients), Switzerland (228 patients) and Belgium (213 patients). Analgesic nephropathy, rarely, if ever, occurred before age 30 and had a mean age of almost 60. *Adult polycystic kidney disease* usually causes end-stage renal failure between the ages of 40 and 70 with a few patients below as well as above these ages being accepted for renal replacement therapy. There was no particular geographical variation in the frequency of adult polycystic kidney disease. *Hereditary nephritis with nerve deafness (Alport's Syndrome)* often leads to end-stage renal failure around age 20–30. The younger groups were

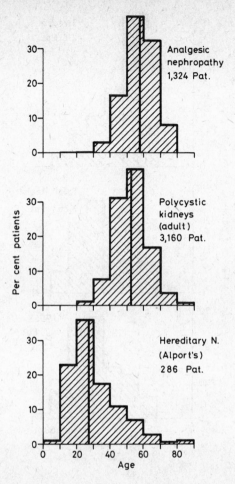

Figure 23. Age distribution of new patients 1980–1982, analgesic nephropathy (upper panel), adult polycystic kidneys (centre panel) and hereditary nephropathy (lower panel)

mostly male, whilst females prevailed among the older patients with this disease.

Age at start of RRT for diabetic nephropathy (Figure 24) was never below 20. Sweden like other Scandinavian countries had a markedly high incidence of young diabetics aged 30–40 and a median age of just below 40. France, by contrast, had taken on a much higher percentage of older diabetics, the median age being 55.

There has been a continuous increase in the proportion of new patients who were diabetic accepted for RRT during the last 10 years. It rose from just below two per cent of all new patients in 1973 to over seven per cent in 1981 [4].

Figure 25 shows how the crude acceptance rate, that is, the number of new diabetics per million of total population, increased strikingly in Sweden,

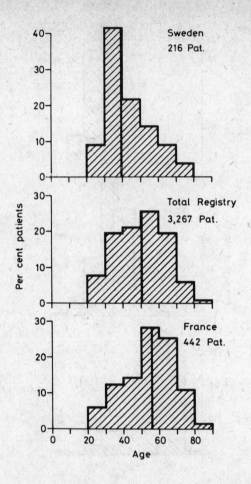

Figure 24. Age distribution of new patients with diabetes, 1980–1982, total Registry (centre panel), compared with Sweden (upper panel) and France (lower panel)

Finland and Norway and to a lesser extent in central European, southern and eastern countries. Age specific acceptance, that is the number of patients with diabetic nephropathy per million of population of the same age accepted for RRT is listed in Table XII for 17 countries reporting to the EDTA Registry. Countries with adequate facilities treated more old diabetics above 60 years of age per million population as opposed to countries with limited facilities. With an age specific acceptance of 13.6 diabetics per million population in 1982, Israel reported the highest acceptance of old diabetics. The high frequency of young and probably insulin dependent diabetics developing end-stage renal failure in Scandinavia and Finland has yet to find an adequate explanation.

Renal stone disease and hypertension were chosen as nephrological topics

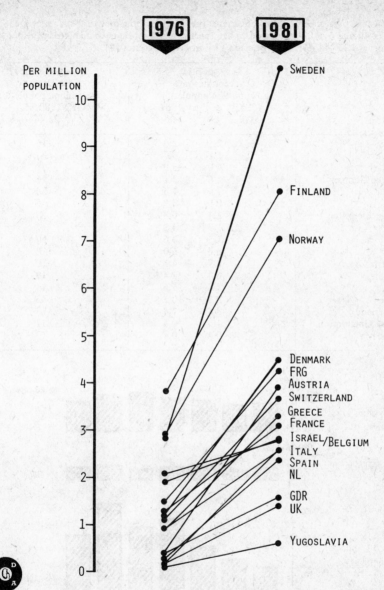

PER MILLION
POPULATION

SWEDEN
FINLAND
NORWAY

DENMARK
FRG
AUSTRIA
SWITZERLAND
GREECE
FRANCE
ISRAEL/BELGIUM
ITALY
SPAIN
NL

GDR
UK

YUGOSLAVIA

Figure 25. Crude acceptance rate of new diabetics (all ages) in 17 selected countries in 1976 and 1981 [4]

for this Congress. Renal stone disease accounted for 3.5 per cent and hypertensive disease for 7.2 per cent of the 93,037 new patients who commenced treatment in 1976–1982.

Renal stone disease included the following diagnoses: gout, nephrocalcinosis (or hypercalcaemic nephropathy) and pyelonephritis due to urolithiasis. Figure

TABLE XII. Age specific acceptance rates (per million population) for diabetics aged less than 40 and over 60 compared to age specific death rate due to diabetes in the population aged 25–44 (WHO statistics) in 17 European countries [4]

DIABETES Country	Age specific Acceptance rate Per million population EDTA Registry 1981 AGE	<40	>60	Age specific Death rate Per million population WHO 1980/81 25–44
Austria		2.1	2.0	16
Belgium		1.1	3.7	N/A
Denmark		4.0	3.0	28
Fed Rep Germany		1.6	7.1	16
Finland		7.9	1.3	38
France		0.9	6.7	8
German Dem Rep		1.1	0.3	N/A
Greece		1.9	4.3	12
Israel		1.5	13.6	N/A
Italy		0.6	6.0	10
Netherlands		0.9	4.5	10
Norway		6.7	2.4	19
Spain		1.0	5.6	11
Sweden		8.1	10.5	33
Switzerland		3.6	2.6	13
United Kingdom		1.3	0.4	12
Yugoslavia		0.4	0.4	13

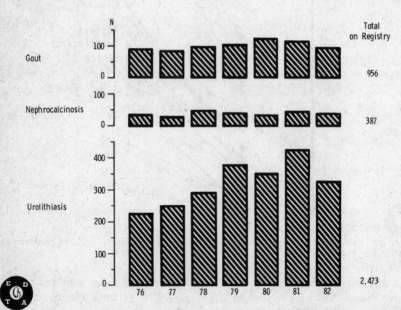

Figure 26. Renal stone diseases: yearly incidence of new patients 1976–1982 with a diagnosis of gout (upper panel), nephrocalcinosis or hypercalcaemic nephropathy (centre panel) and pyelonephritis due to urolithiasis (lower panel)

26 shows that the yearly incidence of ESRF due to gout was about 100 patients; it was less than 50 due to nephrocalcinosis and urolithiasis has increased to about 400 ESRF patients per year with nearly 2,500 in all during the last seven years.

Figure 27 gives the age and sex distribution of renal stone diseases. Gouty nephropathy affected more males than females (M:F = 10.2) and 50 per cent were males in the age range 15—54. Mean age at presentation with ESRF was similar for gout and urolithiasis but younger for nephrocalcinosis with a few children and a fair proportion of women aged more than 55. Male to female ratio was close to unity for both nephrocalcinosis and urolithiasis.

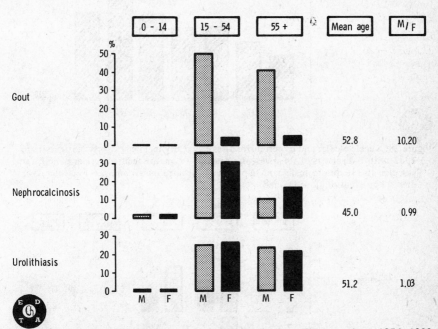

Figure 27. Renal stone diseases: age and sex distribution of new patients 1976–1982 with a diagnosis of gout (upper panel), nephrocalcinosis or hypercalcaemic nephropathy (centre panel) and pyelonephritis due to urolithiasis (lower panel)

Hypertensive disease included the following diagnoses: renal vascular disease — type unspecified, due to malignant hypertension or due to hypertension (Figure 28). The yearly incidence of renal vascular diseases has increased year by year, particularly that due to hypertension, and 1,000 patients with these diagnoses were added in each of the last few years. During the seven years reviewed in this figure, almost 10,000 patients with renal vascular and hypertensive diseases were added to treatment programmes.

Figure 29 gives the age and sex distribution for renal vascular and hypertensive diseases. For each of these diseases M:F ratio exceeded 2.0. The mean age of patients with malignant hypertension (43.7 years) was 10 years younger

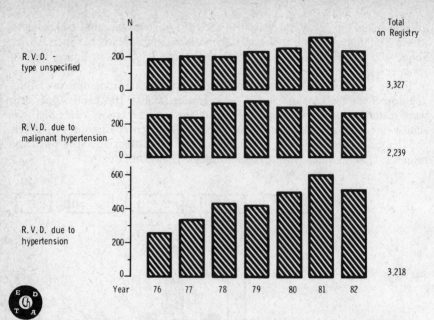

Figure 28. Renal vascular and hypertensive diseases: yearly incidence of new patients 1976–1982 with a diagnosis of renal vascular disease – type unspecified (upper panel), renal vascular disease due to malignant hypertension (centre panel) and renal vascular disease due to hypertension (lower panel)

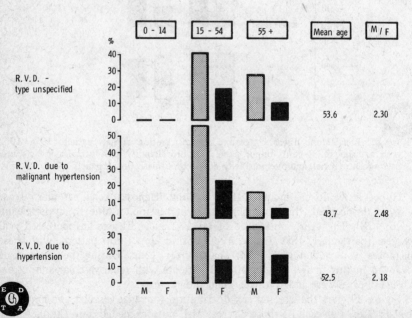

Figure 29. Renal vascular and hypertensive diseases: age and sex distribution of new patients 1976–1982 with a diagnosis of renal vascular disease – type unspecified (upper panel), renal vascular disease due to malignant hypertension (centre panel) and renal vascular disease due to hypertension (lower panel)

than the other types and 50 per cent of patients with ESRF due to malignant hypertension were males aged 15–54.

Comparison of interval mortality on RRT shows that hypertensive diseases had a higher risk than urolithiasis and nephrocalcinosis (Figure 30). The risk

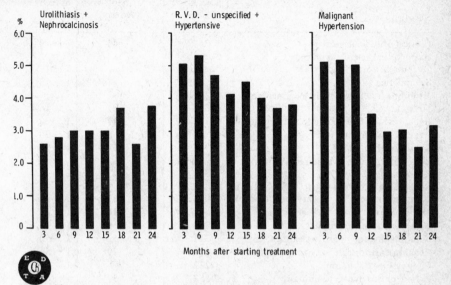

Figure 30. Interval mortality on renal replacement therapy in patients with a diagnosis of urolithiasis combined with nephrocalcinosis (lefthand panel), renal vascular disease – type unspecified combined with renal vascular disease due to hypertension (centre panel), and renal vascular disease due to malignant hypertension (righthand panel)

was particularly high in the early intervals in hypertensives with five per cent three month interval mortality. Risk declined in patients with malignant hypertension who were treated successfully for the first nine months.

Recovery of function

We last reported in 1979 on those rare patients in whom recovery of function of their own kidneys had been sufficient to make further dialysis unnecessary. We included only patients who received at least six weeks RRT before recovery and in whom recovery had been documented to last for a minimum of three months. Patients who commenced treatment in the years 1976–1982 numbered 93,037 and 1,174 recoveries occurred amongst them – one in 79.2 patients. This represents twice the frequency we have previously recorded which was one in 168 patients. The possibility of recovery was higher in certain PRDs. Thus patients with urolithiasis had a one in 61 chance of recovery; in malignant hypertension it was one in 29 and in polyarteritis and Wegener's granulomatosis it was one in 20 (Table XIII).

In 1980 we followed up these interesting patients with a mini-questionnaire.

45

TABLE XIII. Recovery of function of patients' own kidneys after at least six weeks renal replacement therapy and lasting for at least three months according to primary renal disease

Diagnosis	Total patients	Number of patients with recovery	Incidence of recovery
Cortical or tubular necrosis	357	41	1 : 9
Haemolytic Uraemic Syndrome (Moschcowitz Syndrome)	302	30	1 : 10
Scleroderma	88	7	1 : 13
Nephropathy caused by drugs or nephro-toxic agents – cause not specified	341	21	1 : 16
Renal vascular disease due to polyarteritis	334	17	1 : 20
Wegener's Granulomatosis	40	2	1 : 20
Lupus Erythematosus	770	33	1 : 23
Pyelonephritis due to acquired obstructive uropathy	1,300	47	1 : 28
Renal vascular disease due to MALIGNANT hypertension (NO primary renal disease)	2,023	69	1 : 29
Myelomatosis	525	18	1 : 29
Henoch-Schoenlein purpura	265	6	1 : 44
Nephropathy due to analgesic drugs	341	53	1 : 50
Renal vascular disease – type unspecified	1,624	29	1 : 56
Goodpasture's Syndrome	232	4	1 : 58
Pyelonephritis due to urolithiasis	2,257	37	1 : 61
Glomerulonephritis, histologically examined	9,914	150	1 : 66
Nephrocalcinosis and hypercalcaemic nephropathy	269	4	1 : 67
Medullary cystic disease, including nephronophthisis	349	5	1 : 70
Tuberculosis	1,071	14	1 : 77
ALL PRDS	93,037	1,174	1 : 79
Pyelonephritis/Interstitial nephritis – cause not specified	11,245	132	1 : 85
Gout	719	8	1 : 90
Chronic renal failure, aetiology uncertain	10,738	109	1 : 99
Renal vascular disease due to hypertension (NO primary renal disease)	3,053	30	1 : 102
Congenital renal hypoplasia – type unspecified	777	6	1 : 130
Pyelonephritis due to vesico-ureteric reflux (excluding dysplasia)	1,770	13	1 : 136
Glomerulonephritis, histologically NOT examined	18,906	118	1 : 160
Amyloid	1,272	6	1 : 212
Polycystic kidneys, adult type	6,647	28	1 : 237
Hereditary nephritis with nerve deafness (Alport's syndrome)	600	2	1 : 300

TABLE XIV. Recovery of function; reason that diagnosis of recovery was first suggested and method by which it was proved. Data from mini-questionnaire

DIAGNOSIS FIRST SUGGESTED BY: (N=386 patients)		
Patient		5.9%
Biochemical results		89.9%
Clinical course of transplant		0.3%
'Other'		3.9%

PROVED BY: (N=403 patients)		
Stopping dialysis		92.6%
Removal of transplant		1.5%
Special test — X-ray	0.7%	
Radio-nucleide	3.2%	
Catheter	0	5.9%
Other	2.0%	

One question asked was how the diagnosis of recovery was first suggested, and another, how it was proved (Table XIV). In nearly 90 per cent of 386 patients the diagnosis was first suggested by biochemical results and in nearly six per cent by the patient himself. Recovery of function was proved in the vast majority (92.6%) of 403 patients by stopping dialysis; in a small proportion (1.5%) by removal of a transplant.

Dialyser reuse in 1981

The pattern of reuse of dialysers was analysed for the years 1975 to 1981 according to type of dialyser, type of dialysis and country.

Figure 31 shows the use of the different types of dialyser for all countries between 1975 and 1981. Whereas the popularity of both Kiil and coil dialysers has declined over the seven year period, there has been a continuous increase in the use of the capillary (hollow fibre) type. The per cent of patients using parallel flow dialysers has remained constant at about 40 per cent. Capillary (hollow fibre) dialysers were used by almost 50 per cent of patients in 1981.

Figure 32, showing reuse of dialysers according to type, between 1975 and 1981 should be considered in conjunction with Figure 31 which shows the trends in use. The per cent of patients reusing Kiil dialysers increased despite their waning use; more than 50 per cent of patients on Kiil dialysers reused them in 1981, compared with 10 per cent or less for other types, in the same year. The reuse of capillary dialysers has declined in the face of their increasing popularity. Reuse practice for both parallel flow and coil dialysers has changed little between 1975 and 1981.

Figure 33 compares reuse of dialysers for selected countries in the years 1975, 1978 and 1981. Practice varied considerably between nations, and in 1981 reuse ranged between one per cent in Sweden to almost 90 per cent in

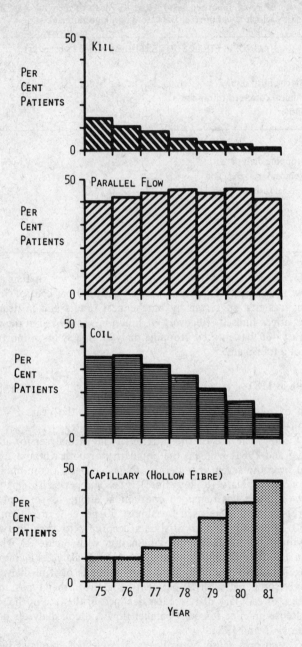

Figure 31. Proportions of patients for whom the four groups of dialysers were reported as the ones most frequently used in each of the years 1975–1981

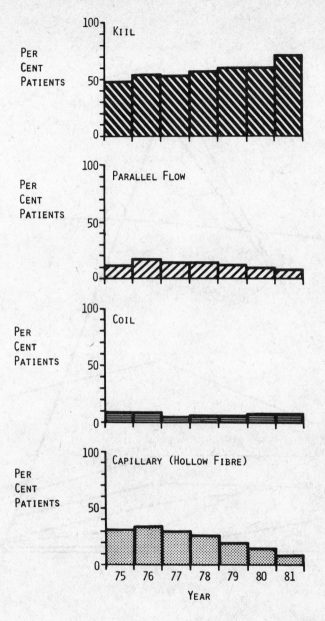

Figure 32. Proportions of patients who reused their dialysers, according to dialyser type in each of the years 1975–1981

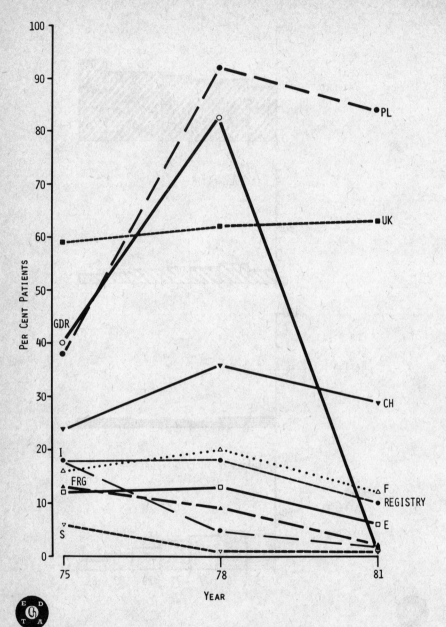

Figure 33. Per cent of patients who reused their dialysers in selected countries 1975, 1978 and 1981

50

Poland. The figure shows that reuse declined in most countries between 1975 and 1981, despite an upsurge in 1978. The one exception was the United Kingdom where there was a small but consistent rise in reuse of dialysers between 1975 and 1978, and 1978 and 1981.

Figure 34 shows the per cent of patients reusing dialysers between 1975 and 1979 according to whether haemodialysis was performed at home or in hospital. Reuse was practised more often by home haemodialysis patients, but declined between 1975 and 1979.

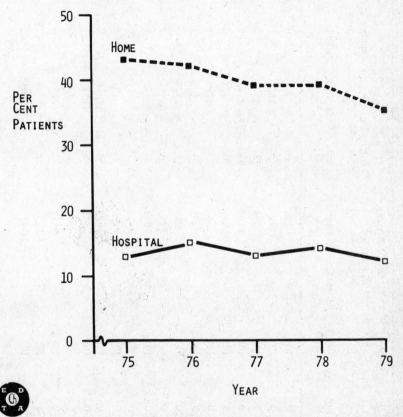

Figure 34. Per cent of patients who reused their dialyser in home and hospital haemodialysis 1975–1979

Table XV gives in detail the reuse practice of each country according to type of dialyser in 1981. The figure in brackets shows the numbers of patients using each dialyser. The final column is the per cent of patients reusing dialysers irrespective of type.

51

TABLE XV. Reuse of dialysers: per cent of patients who reused dialysers in 1981 according to country and type of dialyser

| Country | TYPE OF DIALYSER | | | | | | | | | Per cent patients reusing dialysers of any kind in 1981 |
| | Kiil | | Disposable parallel flow | | Disposable coil | | Capillary hollow fibre | | |
	Patients %	Patients (N)	Patients %	Patients (N)	Patients %	Patients (N)	Patients %	Patients (N)	
Algeria	0	(0)	0	(10)	0	(0)	0	(17)	0
Austria	0	(0)	0	(170)	0	(128)	<1	(777)	<1
Belgium	0	(0)	13	(789)	38	(52)	3	(973)	8
Bulgaria	0	(0)	97	(116)	93	(14)	98	(248)	97
Cyprus	0	(0)	0	(0)	0	(92)	0	(8)	0
Czechoslovakia	0	(0)	3	(36)	<1	(679)	86	(7)	1
Denmark	0	(0)	8	(373)	0	(0)	2	(173)	6
Egypt	20	(51)	59	(96)	7	(202)	0	(24)	22
Fed Rep Germany	50	(44)	2	(3,525)	0	(44)	2	(9,075)	2
Finland	0	(0)	1	(206)	0	(8)	1	(115)	1
France	40	(309)	12	(4,845)	2	(341)	10	(5,544)	12
German Dem Rep	0	(0)	33	(3)	0	(0)	1	(1,254)	1
Greece	0	(0)	0	(369)	0	(401)	0	(256)	0
Hungary	0	(0)	0	(7)	0	(153)	87	(40)	17
Iceland	0	(0)	0	(11)	0	(0)	0	(0)	0
Ireland	0	(0)	0	(41)	3	(219)	0	(0)	3
Israel	95	(22)	7	(129)	1	(479)	40	(144)	12
Italy	0	(0)	1	(7,343)	1	(500)	<1	(2,230)	<1

TABLE XV. *Continued*

Country	Patients %	Patients (N)	Disposable parallel flow Patients %	Disposable parallel flow Patients (N)	Disposable coil Patients %	Disposable coil Patients (N)	Capillary hollow fibre Patients %	Capillary hollow fibre Patients (N)	Per cent patients reusing dialysers of any kind in 1981
Lebanon	0	(0)	0	(0)	0	(17)	0	(18)	0
Libya	0	(0)	0	(58)	0	(0)	0	(0)	0
Luxembourg	0	(0)	32	(50)	0	(3)	0	(20)	22
Netherlands	0	(0)	<1	(1,064)	0	(4)	0	(897)	<1
Norway	0	(0)	29	(58)	0	(0)	1	(248)	6
Poland	100	(1)	80	(185)	86	(356)	100	(3)	84
Portugal	0	(0)	0	(235)	0	(188)	0	(277)	0
Spain	0	(0)	2	(2,095)	1	(1,718)	11	(2,266)	5
Sweden	0	(0)	1	(470)	0	(0)	1	(475)	1
Switzerland	0	(0)	19	(623)	18	(118)	47	(419)	29
Tunisia	0	(0)	0	(0)	0	(203)	0	(24)	0
Turkey	0	(0)	10	(20)	1	(203)	0	(13)	2
United Kingdom	83	(921)	56	(1,642)	51	(352)	60	(1,572)	63
Yugoslavia	0	(0)	<1	(1,109)	2	(573)	<1	(258)	1

Continuous ambulatory peritoneal dialysis (CAPD)

Nineteen hundred and eighty-two was the first year in which we asked the number of catheter insertions during the year. Over 80 per cent of patients who began CAPD in 1982 required no more than the initial insertion, and three-quarters of patients who commenced CAPD before 1982 did not require a single re-insertion in 1982 (Figure 35).

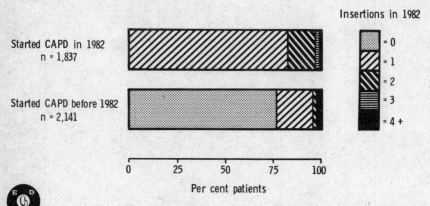

Figure 35. CAPD: proportions of patients who had 0, 1, 2, 3 or 4 plus catheter insertions in 1982 according to whether they started CAPD in 1982 (n=1,837) or before 1982 (n=2,141)

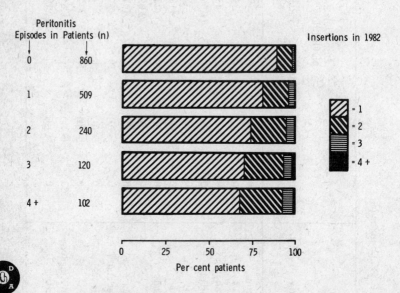

Figure 36. CAPD: proportions of patients who had 1, 2, 3 or 4 plus catheter insertions in 1982 related to the number of episodes of peritonitis during 1982

Figure 36 relates the number of catheter insertions to episodes of peritonitis. The more numerous the episodes of peritonitis, the greater the likelihood of multi-catheter replacements. In patients with no episodes of peritonitis, 89 per cent required only the initial catheter placement, but in patients with four or more episodes of peritonitis, 32 per cent required catheter replacements.

Peritonitis was given as the main reason for abandonment of CAPD in 304 patients in 1982 (Figure 37). Other abdominal complications and inadequate

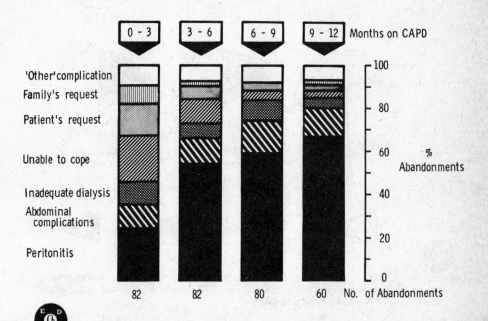

Figure 37. CAPD: main reason for abandonment of CAPD in 1982 according to time on CAPD

dialysis were reasons which accounted for a regular proportion of abandonments at all intervals from commencement of the treatment. The proportion of patients who abandoned because they were unable to cope with CAPD or because of their own or of their family's request was larger in the earlier than in the later months.

Figure 38 is an analysis of hospitalisation for peritonitis according to time on CAPD, whether this was less or more than three months during 1982, and the patient's age. Eighty per cent of patients avoided hospitalisation for peritonitis during the first three months, but only half of those treated for longer did so. There was little difference in the pattern of hospitalisation according to the age of patients. The proportions admitted for up to two weeks, two to six weeks, and more than six weeks do not suggest that older patients are any more costly to treat in this respect than younger ones.

55

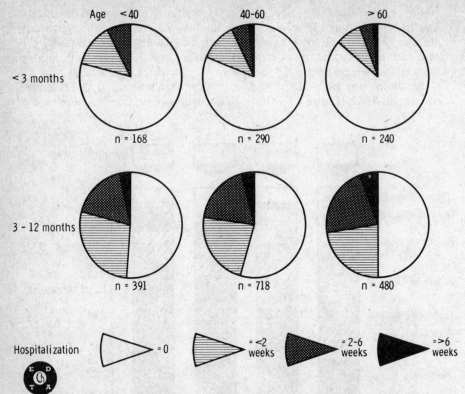

Figure 38. CAPD: hospitalisation for peritonitis according to whether patient was on CAPD for less than three months or for three to 12 months in 1982 and in age groups less than 40, 40–60 and more than 60 years

Malignant diseases

The data we have been collecting on malignant diseases since 1979 are of great importance and interest. Figure 39 is a preliminary analysis of this data carried out as a joint study with the CRC Cancer Epidemiology Group in Oxford. The calculation of the incidence ratio 'observed to expected' cases involves sophisticated programming applying the latest cancer data for different countries to the person-years at risk in each five year age group either on dialysis or following transplantation. A ratio greater than one indicates an excess of cases in the group of patients concerned and is not only of clinical importance for our patients but may also shed light on oncogenic processes. When all cancers were considered together the O/E ratio was little different from unity in the five countries considered. When individual cancers were considered some excess of non-Hodgkin's lymphoma and of skin cancers became apparent (Figure 40). The O/E ratio exceeded eight for non-Hodgkin's lymphoma in transplanted patients in the United Kingdom and four in Sweden and skin cancers also showed an excess incidence in transplanted patients in Sweden, France and

56

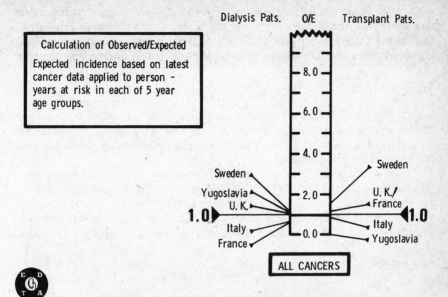

Figure 39. Incidence of malignant diseases in patients treated by dialysis and transplantation – all cancers. Preliminary results of joint study with CRC Cancer Epidemiology Group, Oxford

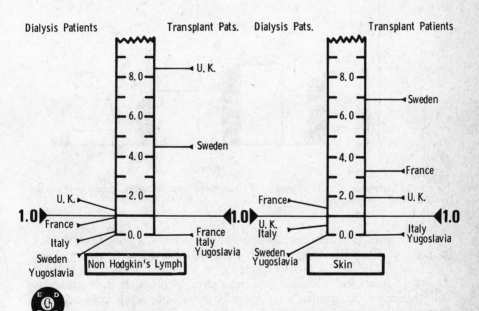

Figure 40. Incidence of malignant diseases in patients treated by dialysis and transplantation – non-Hodgkin's lymphomas and skin cancers. Preliminary results of joint study with CRC Cancer Epidemiology Group, Oxford

the United Kingdom. The data from Italy and Yugoslavia appears incomplete and we would, therefore, ask for particular care in completion of this part of the patient forms. The Registry has a unique opportunity to answer pressing questions on malignant disease in uraemic and immunosuppressed patients.

Transplantation

Several aspects of centre transplantation practice such as use of machine perfusion, longest accepted cold ischaemia time, use of a special transplant co-ordinator, diagnostic facilities and blood transfusion policy were analysed from the centre questionnaire.

Use of machine perfusion to achieve better conservation of cadaveric organs was far from widespread. Eighty-seven per cent of 181 transplant centres did not perfuse a single kidney with a machine in 1982.

Information on the longest cold ischaemia times a centre was normally prepared to accept for cadaver kidneys in 1982 was supplied by 160 centres.

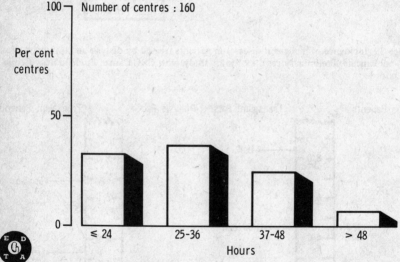

Figure 41. Transplantation practice in 1982: accepted cold ischaemia times reported by 160 active transplant centres

This time varied from less than 24 hours up to 72 hours. Figure 41 shows that 33 per cent of centres accepted cold ischaemia times up to 24 hours, 35 per cent between 25 and 36 hours (mostly 30 to 36 hours), 25 per cent between 37 and 48 hours and seven per cent more than 48 hours. It is of interest to note that many centres that were normally prepared to accept cold ischaemia times of 50 and even longer hours did so without having used machine perfusion in 1982.

Accepted cold ischaemia times varied according to centre size (Figure 42).

Almost half of the small centres performing up to 10 grafts in 1982 would not accept kidneys with cold ischaemia times above 24 hours, whereas 43 per cent of centres doing 11—25 and 46 per cent of those doing 26—50 grafts in 1982 accepted cold ischaemia times between 25 and 36 hours. The 27 big centres performing more than 50 grafts, however, accepted the longest cold ischaemia times: 37—48 hours in 44 per cent and more than 48 hours in 11 per cent of centres.

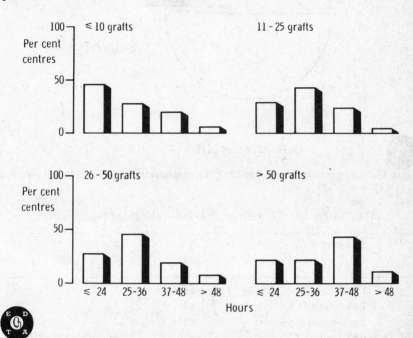

Figure 42. Transplantation practice in 1982: accepted cold ischaemia times reported by 160 active transplant centres according to the number of grafts performed in 1982

Information about a special transplant co-ordinator was supplied by 178 centres (Figure 43). The co-ordinator was said to be a nurse in five per cent of centres, a technician in one per cent, an administrator or secretary in 10 per cent and 'other' in five per cent, but none were students. Half of the centres did without a co-ordinator. A substantial number of centres (28%) claimed to use a doctor as co-ordinator but most of these centres were rather small. Thus, the majority of small centres doing up to 25 grafts had no special transplant co-ordinator. At least 55 per cent of centres with 26—50 grafts had nobody, whilst only one-third of those centres with 51 or more grafts in 1982 managed without a transplant co-ordinator.

A high percentage of the 181 centres doing cadaveric transplantation in 1982 had a wide array of diagnostic facilities available for regular investigation of transplants (Table XVI).

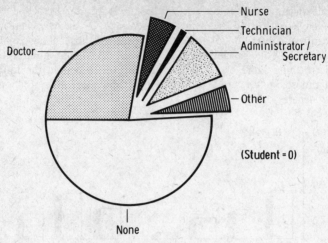

Figure 43. Transplantation practice in 1982: use of special transplant co-ordinator reported by 178 centres

Number of centres : 178

TABLE XVI. Per cent of active transplant centres with stated diagnostic facility

Diagnostic facility	Yes %	No %	? %
Ultrasound (Echography)	91	3	6
Radio-nucleide Renography	86	7	7
Radio-nucleide Scanning	83	10	7
CAT Scan	61	29	10
Angiography	92	3	4
Percutaneous biopsy	87	8	5

Deliberate blood transfusions in preparation for cadaveric transplantation were administered by some 70 per cent of centres in 1978. Four years later, in 1982, there remained a few centres only who abstained from giving deliberate transfusions; 88 per cent of centres performing up to 25 grafts, 89 per cent of those performing 26–75 grafts and 100 per cent of large centres with more than 75 grafts in 1982 deliberately transfused some or all of their prospective recipients of cadaveric transplants.

Opinion about donor specific blood transfusion in living donor transplantation appears to be divided. Forty-four centres which performed a total of 248 living donor grafts in 1982 gave donor specific transfusions compared to 63 centres which performed a total of 241 living donor grafts but did not give pre-transplant blood transfusions from the kidney donor to the recipient.

60

Hepatitis

Table XVII shows the number of new cases of hepatitis in patients and staff reported on the centre questionnaire for 1982. A similar table has been published in each of our Reports for the last three years.

Figure 44 shows an analysis of the new cases of hepatitis in patients during each of these last four years in order to demonstrate the proportion due to B, A, and non-A-non-B. The numbers of new cases progressively declined in each of these years. The proportion due to hepatitis B diminished and there was only a small proportion in each year due to hepatitis A. However, the proportion attributed to non-A-non-B hepatitis increased year by year to reach 28 per cent of all new cases in patients in 1982.

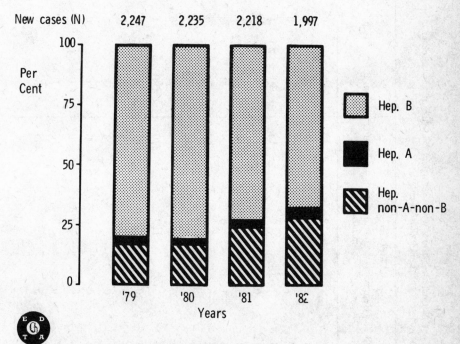

Figure 44. New cases of hepatitis in patients (including those with serological evidence of new disease) in each of the years 1979–1982 showing proportion attributed to hepatitis B, A and non-A-non-B. Data from centre questionnaire

Figure 45 reviews the data collected during the past 18 years concerning numbers of cases of hepatitis in staff. This has been expressed as a ratio showing the number of patients on hospital haemodialysis for each member of staff infected. Following the appalling experience of 1965–1975 with only 20 patients on treatment for every case in staff, experience has consistently improved and in the last four years the ratio increased from 58 to 134 [5].

61

TABLE XVII. New cases of hepatitis (including those with serological evidence of new disease) in patients and staff in 1982: data from centre questionnaires. †Staff deaths not yet confirmed by direct enquiry

Country	PATIENTS				STAFF				Deaths (staff)
	Hep. B	Hep. A	Hep. non-A -non-B	Total	Hep. B	Hep. A	Hep. non-A -non-B	Total	
Algeria	17	1	2	20	10	0	3	13	0
Austria	57	1	8	66	8	0	0	8	0
Belgium	53	2	16	71	4	0	0	4	0
Bulgaria	14	1	0	15	10	1	2	13	0
Cyprus	3	0	0	3	0	0	0	0	0
Czechoslovakia	64	14	0	78	12	0	1	13	0
Denmark	3	1	0	4	0	0	0	0	0
Egypt	38	10	0	48	0	2	1	3	0
Fed Rep Germany	117	3	98	218	47	2	5	54	0
Finland	2	0	0	2	0	0	0	0	0
France	230	13	127	370	38	1	18	57	0
German Dem Rep	138	0	23	161	31	0	4	35	4
Greece	23	0	4	27	5	0	0	5	0
Hungary	21	0	3	24	8	0	0	8	0
Iceland	0	0	0	0	0	0	0	0	0
Ireland	0	0	0	0	0	0	0	0	0
Israel	7	0	9	16	0	2	1	3	0
Italy	161	3	72	236	46	0	7	53	0

TABLE XVII. *Continued*

Country	PATIENTS				STAFF				Deaths (staff)
	Hep. B	Hep. A	Hep. non-A -non-B	Total	Hep. B	Hep. A	Hep. non-A -non-B	Total	
Lebanon	1	0	0	1	0	0	0	0	0
Libya	0	0	0	0	0	0	0	0	0
Luxembourg	4	0	0	4	1	0	0	1	0
Netherlands	4	2	11	17	0	0	0	0	0
Norway	3	0	1	4	0	0	0	0	0
Poland	53	1	3	57	22	0	2	24	0
Portugal	34	0	4	38	6	1	0	7	0
Spain	154	9	102	265	30	2	2	34	0
Sweden	0	0	10	10	0	0	0	0	0
Switzerland	4	1	19	24	4	0	1	5	0
Tunisia	11	0	0	11	5	0	0	5	0
Turkey	13	5	23	41	3	1	5	9	0
United Kingdom	2	1	26	29	1	0	0	1	0
Yugoslavia	129	3	5	137	24	0	0	24	1
TOTAL REGISTRY	1,360	71	566	1,997	315	12	52	379	5†

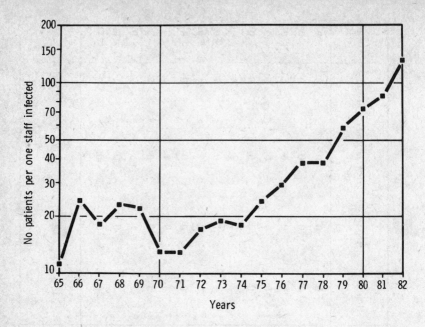

Figure 45. Ratio of patients on hospital haemodialysis to staff infected with hepatitis in years, 1965–1982

Acute (reversible) renal failure

Table XVIII shows the number of patients with acute (reversible) renal failure (ARF) in whose care reporting centres were involved during 1982. These exclude post-transplantation acute renal failure. The methods used for the treatment of ARF in centres reporting to the EDTA Registry are shown with the numbers of patients for whom these methods were employed either alone or in combination in Table XIX. The dominance of haemodialysis and relatively low representation of peritoneal dialysis (Table XIX) reflects practice in units treating ESRF. Each method of treatment required back-up by some other method as is shown by that proportion of patients for whom combined treatments were necessary.

In Figure 46 we show the correlation between new ESRF patients per million population and ARF patients per million population in those countries which had at least 1,000 ESRF patients on therapy. Clearly, the more dialysis skills available the greater the number of patients with ARF who were treated. Obviously, these cases of ARF are likely to be an underestimate of the numbers actually treated in each country since some treatments will be carried out by units which do not treat ESRF.

TABLE XVIII. Acute (reversible) renal failure: numbers of patients in whose care centres were involved in 1982 (excluding post-transplantation acute renal failure). Data from centre questionnaire

Country	Number of Centres treating patients	Per million population	Number of Patients treated	Per million population
Algeria	1	0.1	7	0.4
Austria	17	2.3	317	42.2
Belgium	42	4.3	589	59.9
Bulgaria	15	1.7	120	13.6
Cyprus	1	1.7	3	4.8
Czechoslovakia	14	0.9	187	12.3
Denmark	5	1.0	179	35.0
Egypt	5	0.1	125	3.2
Fed Rep Germany	146	2.4	4,378	71.4
Finland	17	3.5	193	40.5
France	92	1.7	1,625	30.4
German Dem Rep	35	2.1	376	22.4
Greece	9	1.0	101	10.8
Hungary	4	0.4	21	2.0
Iceland	1	5.0	5	22.7
Ireland	2	0.6	62	19.3
Israel	20	5.3	261	70.7
Italy	151	2.7	2,231	39.3
Lebanon	2	0.7	533	177.1
Libya	2	0.7	10	3.6
Luxembourg	4	10.0	28	77.8
Netherlands	27	1.9	535	38.4
Norway	9	2.2	74	18.2
Poland	20	0.6	300	8.6
Portugal	4	0.4	62	6.3
Spain	66	1.8	2,221	59.8
Sweden	16	1.9	152	18.4
Switzerland	20	3.1	278	43.8
Tunisia	2	0.3	13	2.1
Turkey	8	0.2	185	4.3
United Kingdom	37	0.7	1,237	22.2
Yugoslavia	21	1.0	169	7.7
TOTAL REGISTRY	815	1.4	16,577	28.9

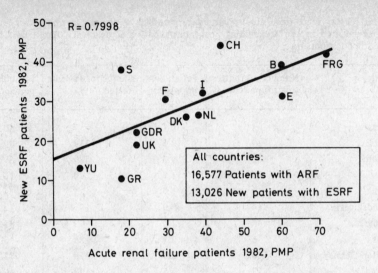

Figure 46. Relation between numbers of cases of acute (reversible) renal failure (ARF) treated in 1982 per million population and number of new cases of end-stage renal failure (ESRF) accepted for treatment in 1982 per million population in countries which treated more than 1,000 ESRF patients. Data on ARF from centre questionnaire which were sent only to centres with a programme of treatment for ESRF

Conclusions

1　The Registry now has nearly 150,000 patient records with individual case histories extending over more than 20 years.

2　Patient survival on CAPD was comparable with overall survival on renal replacement therapy in patients starting treatment in 1981–82. Patient survival from one year after first cadaveric grafting onwards was higher than average on renal replacement therapy in young recipients.

3　Interval mortality and treatment change rates have been suggested for assessing and comparing results.

4　Graft failure resulted from rejection in some 80 per cent and that due to recurrence of glomerulonephritis rose to eight per cent of failures which occurred after the first year post-transplantation.

5　Age distribution of primary renal diseases showed striking geographical variation. Diabetic nephropathy was particularly frequent in young Scandinavians.

6　Demographic data on renal stone disease (3.5% of patients with ESRF) and hypertension (7.2% of patients with ESRF) have been presented because these diseases were themes for this year's Congress.

7   Recovery of function of the patients' own kidneys was recognised in one in 79 patients, and occurred more commonly in certain renal diseases.

8   The use of capillary (hollow fibre) dialysers has increased over the past five years but has not been accompanied by an increase in the proportion of patients reusing dialysers.

9   Interesting early results are emerging from the data on malignant diseases with excess of non-Hodgkin's lymphomas and skin cancers in transplanted patients.

10 Centre transplantation practice: machine perfusion was used rarely; large centres accepted longer cold ischaemia times (40–72 hours) than small centres; deliberate blood transfusions in preparation for transplantation were administered by some 90 per cent of centres.

11 More than one case with acute renal failure was treated for each new ESRF patient.

References

1   Drukker W, Haagsma-Schouten WAG, Alberts Chr, Spoek MG. *Proc EDTA 1969; 6:* 99
2   Gurland HJ, Brunner FP, Chantler C et al. *Proc EDTA 1976; 13:* 3
3   Wing AJ, Brunner FP, Brynger H et al. *Proc EDTA 1978; 15:* 3
4   Jacobs C, Brunner FP, Brynger H et al. *Diabetic Nephropathy 1983; 2, No.2:* 12
5   Wing AJ, Broyer M, Brunner FP et al. *Proc EDTNA 12 1983:* in press

Appendix

1. Late returns

Most of the analyses and tabulations presented in this Report are based on the data of centres whose returns were received in time for processing before the London Congress, June, 1983. However, those Tables marked with an asterisk (*) against the title of the Table and the numbers given in the sections on demographic data from patient questionnaires include data on patients whose entry to the file was delayed through late reporting and problems associated with processing transferred patients.

2. Survival rates and sample size

The mathematical formulae used for the calculation of survival rates have been stated in our appendices to our previous Reports (see Appendix, Report V, 1974).

3. Computer programs

The programs for analysing the questionnaires have been written in the FORTRAN programming language and are used on a PDP11/44 under the RSX-11M operating system.

TABLE XIX. Treatment of acute (reversible) renal failure in 1982, showing the number of patients treated by each method either alone or in combination with other methods. Data from centre questionnaire

Country	Intermittent Haemodialysis			Intermittent Haemofiltration			Continuous Haemofiltration		
	Alone	Combined	Total	Alone	Combined	Total	Alone	Combined	Total
Algeria	0	0	0	0	0	0	0	0	0
Austria	277	71	348	9	56	65	8	2	10
Belgium	508	16	524	5	2	7	0	1	1
Bulgaria	174	44	218	0	21	21	0	0	0
Cyprus	5	0	5	0	0	0	0	0	0
Czechoslovakia	139	15	154	0	0	0	0	0	0
Denmark	202	3	205	0	0	0	1	0	1
Egypt	140	10	150	0	0	0	0	0	0
Fed Rep Germany	3,753	549	4,302	1,011	197	1,208	466	208	674
Finland	135	1	136	1	1	2	0	0	0
France	1,562	103	1,665	58	6	64	17	2	19
German Dem Rep	369	33	402	3	0	3	2	0	2
Greece	141	6	147	0	0	0	0	0	0
Hungary	63	7	70	0	0	0	0	0	0
Iceland	4	0	4	0	0	0	0	0	0
Ireland	44	1	45	0	0	0	0	0	0
Israel	108	28	136	0	0	0	0	5	5
Italy	1,740	99	1,839	39	2	41	11	3	14

TABLE XIX. *Continued*

Country	Intermittent Haemodialysis			Intermittent Haemofiltration			Continuous Haemofiltration		
	Alone	Combined	Total	Alone	Combined	Total	Alone	Combined	Total
Lebanon	530	0	530	0	0	0	0	0	0
Libya	4	3	7	0	0	0	0	0	0
Luxembourg	22	0	22	2	0	2	0	0	0
Netherlands	449	76	525	10	5	15	0	5	5
Norway	75	7	82	0	0	0	0	0	0
Poland	295	58	353	0	0	0	0	0	0
Portugal	19	12	31	0	0	0	0	0	0
Spain	1,234	110	1,344	18	38	56	0	0	0
Sweden	102	11	113	0	0	0	13	2	15
Switzerland	245	35	280	6	0	6	3	6	9
Tunisia	16	0	16	5	0	5	5	0	5
Turkey	58	5	63	0	0	0	0	0	0
United Kingdom	506	137	643	10	14	24	10	5	15
Yugoslavia	316	3	319	1	2	3	22	1	23
TOTAL REGISTRY	13,235	1,443	14,678	1,178	344	1,522	558	240	798

69

TABLE XIX. *Continued*

Country	Intermittent Peritoneal Dialysis			Continuous Peritoneal Dialysis			Plasmapheresis		
	Alone	Combined	Total	Alone	Combined	Total	Alone	Combined	Total
Algeria	0	0	0	6	0	6	0	0	0
Austria	3	2	5	4	7	11	18	3	21
Belgium	5	0	5	13	10	23	11	7	18
Bulgaria	0	0	0	0	0	0	10	0	10
Cyprus	0	0	0	0	0	0	0	0	0
Czechoslovakia	17	1	18	5	0	5	2	3	5
Denmark	41	1	42	0	0	0	18	1	19
Egypt	2	0	2	16	0	16	0	0	0
Fed Rep Germany	108	7	115	61	19	80	157	128	285
Finland	28	1	29	32	0	32	7	0	7
France	63	10	73	76	31	107	65	31	96
German Dem Rep	23	1	24	36	0	36	27	2	29
Greece	41	0	41	2	0	2	2	1	3
Hungary	14	1	15	0	0	0	2	0	2
Iceland	0	0	0	0	0	0	0	0	0
Ireland	14	1	15	0	0	0	0	0	0
Israel	116	17	133	1	0	1	0	7	7
Italy	385	14	399	89	1	90	67	50	117

TABLE XIX. *Continued*

Country	Intermittent Peritoneal Dialysis			Continuous Peritoneal Dialysis			Plasmapheresis		
	Alone	Combined	Total	Alone	Combined	Total	Alone	Combined	Total
Lebanon	0	0	0	0	0	0	0	0	0
Libya	1	0	1	0	0	0	0	0	0
Luxembourg	0	0	0	0	0	0	0	0	0
Netherlands	19	7	26	19	1	20	22	7	29
Norway	1	0	1	0	0	0	4	7	11
Poland	62	20	82	0	6	6	0	0	0
Portugal	20	0	20	8	1	9	0	1	1
Spain	544	62	606	12	4	16	24	27	51
Sweden	24	2	26	7	0	7	48	4	52
Switzerland	0	0	0	23	24	47	53	32	85
Tunisia	29	0	29	12	0	12	0	0	0
Turkey	120	0	120	29	0	29	0	0	0
United Kingdom	356	97	453	116	10	126	8	23	31
Yugoslavia	14	0	14	1	0	1	42	103	145
TOTAL REGISTRY	2,050	244	2,294	568	114	682	587	437	1,024

Open Discussion

ANDREUCCI (Chairman) Thank you Dr Wing for your excellent presentation. I think it is very interesting to look at this data. The life of patients on dialysis is apparently approaching the life of patients without dialysis: let us hope we reach that goal. I am happy that you have mentioned also some important data on the nephrological topics of this Congress, hypertension and renal stone disease. You have also mentioned what we will discuss later on the controversies of short and long dialysis, and finally you have mentioned your heroes. I have now my own hero, who is an 85-year old lady who has been on dialysis for five years. I first saw her five years ago when she was in uraemic coma: she is alright now, is 85 years old and as far as I know there has been no recovery of function as yet.

CAMBI (Parma) I have a question to raise about the grouping of the dialysis duration: you put together people that are treated eight to 12 hours. I think that the difference of 50 per cent between eight and 12 may be misleading, because within this group surely there is adequate and inadequate dialysis treatment? In the past you used to separate groups of dialysis time with a smaller interval and I would be happy to see these smaller intervals again.

WING Thank you very much for your suggestion, Professor Cambi. I think we should certainly follow up your idea, and you know that we would like to do that with you.

CAMERON (London) In view of the very big difference in the severity and the incidence of chronic renal failure from hypertension in different races reported from the United States, have any differences between the countries in Europe emerged from your study of renal failure from hypertension?

WING We have only done a demographic analysis concerning the numbers of patients with the different forms of hypertensive disease in the different countries, so I do not have any qualitative data about whether they are doing better in one country as compared to another. It could be done.

GABRIEL (London) Is the increased incidence of non-Hodgkin's lymphoma and skin neoplasia post grafting geographically determined with the increase in skin tumours being in the more southern part of Europe?

WING I showed the skin tumours and the tumour data separately for the individual countries because when you do this calculation it is important to look for the expected numbers of tumours in any particular geographical area. That would be taken care of for the southern countries. When you express the results as observed over expected, that takes into account the different cancer data for the different geographical areas. The data that we use for the present analysis was collected subsequently to that published in an earlier paper: there may have been an overlap for one year. This collaborative study

72

which we have done with Dr Kinlen* in Oxford is EDTA collected data up to 1979. Obviously the numbers of cases involved are extremely small. I showed you that Sweden had a rather higher observed to expected ratio for non-Hodgkin's lymphoma, but that is based on only one case, because the expected incidence of those cases is so very, very small.

MARSH (London) I am not quite clear whether the interval mortality expressed for CAPD refers only to those patients continuing on CAPD or whether it is the mortality for all patients accepted for CAPD, many of whom would be transferred to other treatments. If the latter, then perhaps it is not too surprising that the interval mortality approaches that of hospital haemodialysis.

WING As you know, we do not have any information on what is the intent of the physician when he puts the patient onto treatment. We have only a date on which the patient began CAPD. We start counting from that point, and as I showed you on our example slide our method is such that if they change treatment they are treated then as lost to follow-up for the subsequent interval mortality calculation. It is very important that anybody presenting survival or mortality data does tell you very clearly the assumptions that they have used, particularly when we are dealing with these patients who change from one treatment to another. We do not know what is in the physician's mind when they do so and what his primary intention with a given patient.

MION (Montpellier) I want to ask you something which relates to the previous question. I agree completely in the important analysis you have given at looking at interval mortalities and transfer rates from one technique to the other, but then you get a difficult problem. How long after transfer do you consider a transferred patient's death as a consequence of the previous technique or from the new technique? This is particularly important with CAPD when a patient might be transferred and die from peritonitis for instance.

WING You are absolutely right. As far as we are concerned we have to treat them as moving to the next treatment at the date at which they are reported to us as doing so. We could, of course, do the analysis in a different way and given an arbitary inclusion at any time interval that you wish to prescribe after such a change. This is as Dr Nolph is doing with the American study where a CAPD patient is considered at risk, in respect of his CAPD treatment, for two weeks after he switches from CAPD to haemodialysis. We just have the dates at which they commence and change their different treatments and I use them as I have shown you. There are other ways of doing this and you can bias the answer a little by how you work it out.

MION My question was not a criticism: I think it is a difficulty with the technique. For instance with peritoneal dialysis we have seen that related to peritoneal dialysis for as long a time as 18 months the patient develops a disease such as

* Kinlen LJ, Eastwood JB, Kerr DNS. *Br Med J 1980; 1:* 1,401

73

sclerosing peritonitis. I mean when we look at our data for intermittent or continuous ambulatory peritoneal dialysis for two years it seems that we have the same survival as with haemodialysis. But if we include these late deaths then we have a drop and I think that this is one thing we should be aware of.

WING Yes, we are aware of it. It is very difficult. You can look at the patients after they return when they have given up CAPD and see how they do from that point of time. They are casualties of CAPD in the same way as those patients who have a failed renal transplant and return to haemodialysis or any other form of dialysis are casualties of transplantation. They are patients at a very high risk with very high mortality rates.

McGEOWN (Belfast) Do you have data on the longevity of cadaver transplants: you mentioned only live donors in your presentation?

WING I am sure we have got the data but we did not analyse it: we will have to do that.

EL-MATRI (Tunisia) I would like to put a question about acute renal failure. Do you mean by ARF acute renal failure on previously normal kidneys or ARF superimposed on chronic renal failure, and what is the rate of each one of them?

WING Yes, we have simply used the phrase 'acute (reversible) renal failure'. We did not actually define that the patient was ill enough to require supportive dialysis. Perhaps we should have done that as well.

ANDREUCCI Thank you Dr Wing for this excellent presentation and this excellent discussion.

*****

ANDREUCCI Thank you Dr Brunner for your presentation. Can I ask if in your analysis of chronic pyelonephritis you excluded cases of obstruction?

BRUNNER We reported what was given on the patient questionnaire as diagnosis and pyelonephritis which includes all the obstructive causes, malformations and part of it might be infection. In any case we have to report what is reported to us.

ANDREUCCI I understand, but I think it is difficult, especially with a retrospective diagnosis, to say this is a primary pyelonephritis unless you have excluded obstruction and other causes.

ROSENFELD (Tel-Aviv) You showed a three year survival in the younger group of 89 per cent and you showed in the same category survival from parental living donors will be similar, almost identical, to the results from cadavers.

74

BRUNNER There is one minor difference in that the cadaveric group excluded diabetics aged 15–34 years. Living donors included diabetics and were 15–44 years of age, so they are not quite comparable, but I think there is no doubt that the young group of the cadaveric transplant recipients survive well and that the living donor recipients may survive just marginally better.

VAN YPERSELE (Brussels) I have to congratulate you once again on giving us an excellent presentation. I am a little bit puzzled by the number of patients whose graft failure is attributed beyond one year to recurrence of glomerulonephritis. Although recurrence of glomerulonephritis is a significant phenomenon it does not usually lead to terminal renal failure and my question is: have you any idea of the histological type of glomerulonephritis whose recurrence lead to terminal graft failure after one year?

BRUNNER I have some ideas from the literature which is known to you, but we would like to follow this up and find out which histological diagnosis is most important in recurrences causing graft failure. It was eight per cent of the total number of failures and so it is still a small number.

VAN YPERSELE You mean eight per cent of the failures after one year?

BRUNNER Yes.

VAN YPERSELE Yes. Well that is still a significant number.

ANDREUCCI Do you have any idea how long the patients with recurrent glomerulonephritis had been on dialysis prior to transplantation?

BRUNNER I do not have the data on this.

KURUVILA (Denver, Colorado) Do you have any data on transplantation using Cyclosporin A?

BRUNNER We do not yet have any data on transplantation using Cyclosporin. We plan to include a question on Cyclosporin for next year.

KERR (Chairman) I find it hard to believe that latitude is the main determinant of whether people die from diabetes at a young or an old age. Are you planning any questions to find out whether there are differences in the management of diabetes or whether it is genetic factors in Scandinavia and Italy?

BRUNNER This would be a nice thing to do, but I think that goes beyond the scope of our possibilities.

COMBINED REPORT ON REGULAR DIALYSIS AND TRANSPLANTATION OF CHILDREN IN EUROPE, XII, 1982

Members

M BROYER	Hôpital Necker Enfants Malades, Paris, France
F P BRUNNER	Departement für Innere Medizin, Universität Basel, Switzerland
H BRYNGER	Department of Surgery I, Sahlgrenska Sjukhuset, Göteborg, Sweden
R A DONCKERWOLCKE	Het Wilhelmina Kinderziekenhuis, University of Utrecht, Utrecht, Netherlands
C JACOBS	Centre Pasteur-Vallery-Radot, Paris, France
P KRAMER	Medizinische Universitätsklinik, Göttingen, Federal Republic of Germany
N H SELWOOD	UK Transplant, Bristol, United Kingdom
A J WING*	St Thomas' Hospital, London, United Kingdom

* Chairman

Research Fellows

S CHALLAH	Department of Community Medicine, St Thomas' Hospital, London, United Kingdom
N GRETZ	EDTA Registry, St Thomas' Hospital, London, United Kingdom and Klinikum Mannheim, University of Heidelberg, Federal Republic of Germany

CONTENTS

For Appendix please see page 67 of the Adult Report

Acknowledgments

This work was supported by grants from the Governments or National Societies of Nephrology of Austria, Belgium, Bulgaria, Cyprus, Czechoslovakia, Denmark, Egypt, the Federal Republic of Germany, France, the German Democratic Republic, Greece, Iceland, Ireland, Israel, Italy, Luxembourg, the Netherlands, Norway, Sweden, Switzerland and the United Kingdom.

Generous grants were made by Asahi Medical GmbH, Bellco S.p.A., B Braun Melsungen AG, Cordis Dow B.V., Cobe Laboratories Inc, Enka AG, Extracorporeal Inc, Dr E Fresenius KG, Gambro AB, Hospal Ltd, Sorin Biomedica S.p.A., Travenol Laboratories Ltd.

The post of Research Fellow to the EDTA Registry, currently held by Dr Norbert Gretz, was funded by the National Kidney Research Fund, United Kingdom.

We acknowledge the support of UK Transplant, Bristol, United Kingdom.

We particularly thank those doctors and their staff who have completed questionnaires. Without their collaboration, this Report could not have been prepared.

COMBINED REPORT ON REGULAR DIALYSIS AND TRANSPLANTATION OF CHILDREN IN EUROPE, XII, 1982

M Broyer, **R A Donckerwolcke**, F P Brunner, H Brynger, S Challah, N Gretz, C Jacobs, P Kramer, N H Selwood, A J Wing

Introduction

The twelfth combined report concerning children on dialysis and after kidney transplantation is based on information available from the patient questionnaire, centre questionnaire and the special paediatric mini-questionnaire. The special paediatric enquiry was concerned mainly with growth on dialysis and after transplantation and with the characteristics of aseptic necrosis of bone in transplanted patients. Differences in sample size of data on patients with aseptic necrosis of bone are due to incomplete recording of data reported on the paediatric questionnaire.

Numbers of patients and methods of treatment

The number of paediatric patients on the register was 3,649 of whom 2,312 were alive on treatment on 31 December, 1982 (Tables I and II). A further 24 had recovered function of their own kidneys and 71 had been reported lost to observation. There were 343 records of patients alive on 31 December, 1981 which had not been updated with 1982 data at time of going to press. These numbers include all patients under the age of 15 years at the time of first treatment. However, 1,270 of the children on treatment were older than 15 on 31 December, 1982. Table II shows the number of children alive on treatment in December, 1982, together with the proportion on different modes of treatment; it includes children over 15 in December, 1982, but under 15 years at start of treatment. Calculation of numbers of patients per million child population (pMCP) in Table II are restricted to population and patients aged less than 15 years at the end of 1982.

Figure 1 compares treatment modalities in selected countries in 1981 and 1982. In the Federal Republic of Germany, France and the United Kingdom, the proportion of patients surviving with a transplanted kidney continued to increase. The percentage of patients on peritoneal dialysis grew particularly

TABLE I. Numbers of paediatric patients registered alive on treatment on 31 December, in each of the years 1973–1982 according to country. (pMCP=per million child population). Data from individual patient questionnaires (including some late returns)*

Country	PATIENTS ALIVE ON TREATMENT									
	1973		1974		1975		1976		1977	
	N	pMCP†	N	pMCP	N	pMCP	N	pMCP	N	pMCP
Austria	7	4.0	12	6.8	13	7.4	16	9.1	22	12.6
Belgium	20	9.0	26	11.8	25	11.3	34	15.4	39	17.6
Bulgaria	3	1.6	5	2.6	3	1.6	5	2.6	6	3.1
Cyprus	0	–	2	11.3	2	11.3	2	11.3	4	22.6
Czechoslovakia	0	–	0	–	1	0.3	3	0.9	5	1.5
Denmark	14	12.2	20	17.4	19	16.5	22	19.1	28	24.4
Fed Rep Germany	71	5.3	101	7.6	138	10.4	187	14.1	220	16.6
Finland	7	6.7	6	5.7	8	7.6	8	7.6	11	10.5
France	117	9.5	149	12.1	194	15.8	236	19.2	277	22.6
German Dem Rep	9	2.5	10	2.8	13	3.7	13	3.7	18	5.1
Greece	1	0.5	6	2.8	7	3.2	8	3.7	10	4.6
Hungary	0	–	1	0.5	1	0.5	1	0.5	2	0.9
Ireland	1	1.0	2	2.1	3	3.1	4	4.1	5	5.1
Israel	8	7.0	10	8.8	11	9.7	17	15.0	21	18.5
Italy	57	4.2	81	6.0	107	8.0	122	9.1	142	10.6
Luxembourg	0	–	0	–	0	–	0	–	0	–
Netherlands	28	8.1	38	11.0	45	13.0	58	16.7	77	22.2
Norway	8	8.4	8	8.4	9	9.4	11	11.5	14	14.7
Poland	2	0.2	2	0.2	4	0.5	7	0.9	7	0.9
Portugal	0	–	0	–	0	–	0	–	1	0.4
Spain	16	1.7	26	2.7	35	3.6	52	5.4	78	8.1
Sweden	17	10.0	20	11.8	24	14.2	25	14.7	27	15.9
Switzerland	12	8.6	16	11.4	23	16.0	25	17.8	30	21.4
Turkey	1	–	1	–	2	–	5	–	7	–
United Kingdom	107	8.2	132	10.1	160	12.2	178	13.6	203	15.5
Yugoslavia	4	0.7	7	1.3	12	2.2	19	3.5	18	3.3
TOTAL	510		681		859		1058		1272	

† pMCP=per Million Child Population

TABLE I. *Continued*

Country	PATIENTS ALIVE ON TREATMENT									
	1978		1979		1980		1981		1982	
	N	pMCP†	N	pMCP	N	pMCP	N	pMCP	N	pMCP
Austria	29	16.6	32	18.3	34	19.4	29	16.6	30	17.4
Belgium	51	23.1	69	31.2	73	33.0	93	42.0	86	40.2
Bulgaria	6	3.1	8	4.1	9	4.7	13	6.7	10	5.1
Cyprus	4	22.6	4	22.6	4	22.6	4	22.6	3	20.0
Czechoslovakia	3	0.9	6	1.8	9	2.7	16	4.8	17	4.9
Denmark	30	26.1	32	27.9	34	29.6	41	35.6	29	25.4
Fed Rep Germany	250	18.8	294	22.1	329	24.8	413	33.6	336	27.0
Finland	16	15.2	18	17.1	20	19.0	23	21.9	15	14.7
France	321	26.2	364	29.7	423	34.5	524	41.7	495	40.3
German Dem Rep	24	6.8	26	7.3	34	9.6	39	11.0	43	12.4
Greece	14	6.5	19	8.8	22	10.2	30	13.8	15	6.9
Hungary	5	2.3	4	1.9	4	1.9	3	1.4	1	0.4
Ireland	10	10.3	16	16.4	19	19.5	21	21.6	21	21.0
Israel	23	20.3	30	26.4	32	28.2	41	36.1	49	40.8
Italy	177	13.2	213	15.9	231	17.2	301	22.4	267	20.0
Luxembourg	0	–	3	41.7	6	83.3	4	57.1	3	42.9
Netherlands	91	26.3	102	29.5	117	33.8	148	42.7	135	40.3
Norway	15	15.7	17	17.8	21	22.0	29	30.4	34	36.2
Poland	11	1.3	17	2.0	18	2.2	30	3.6	19	2.4
Portugal	1	0.4	1	0.4	2	0.8	7	2.6	9	3.3
Spain	117	12.2	139	14.5	179	18.6	218	22.7	212	22.0
Sweden	33	19.5	32	18.9	34	20.0	42	24.8	42	24.7
Switzerland	39	27.8	42	30.0	44	31.4	52	37.1	51	38.6
Turkey	5	–	6	–	4	–	6	–	5	4.7
United Kingdom	242	18.5	275	21.0	325	24.9	399	30.5	333	26.0
Yugoslavia	18	3.3	17	3.1	28	5.1	43	7.8	40	7.3
TOTAL	1535		1786		2055		2569		2300	

† pMCP=per Million Child Population

TABLE II. Numbers of patients on the paediatric register who were aged less and more than 15 years on 31 December, 1982 and proportions on different modes of treatment according to country. This table includes data from countries recently reporting children to the Registry (Algeria, Egypt, Lebanon and Libya). Data from individual patient questionnaires (including some late returns)*

| Country | AGE <15 YEARS | | | | | | | AGE ≥15 YEARS | | | | | |
| | MODES OF TREATMENT | | | | | Alive total | pMCP† | MODES OF TREATMENT | | | | | Alive total |
	Hosp. HD %	Home HD %	IPD %	CAPD %	Transplant %	N	N	Hosp. HD %	Home HD %	IPD %	CAPD %	Transplant %	N
Algeria	0	0	0	100.0	0	1	0.2	0	0	0	0	0	0
Austria	54.5	0	27.3	0	18.2	11	6.4	36.8	5.3	0	0	57.9	19
Belgium	23.9	0	0	0	76.1	46	21.5	35.0	2.5	0	5.0	57.5	40
Bulgaria	83.3	0	0	0	16.7	6	3.1	100.0	0	0	0	0	4
Cyprus	0	0	0	0	0	0	–	0	0	0	0	100.0	3
Czechoslovakia	80.0	0	0	10.0	10.0	10	2.9	57.1	0	0	0	42.9	7
Denmark	64.3	0	0	14.3	21.4	14	12.3	33.3	0	0	0	66.7	15
Egypt	100.0	0	0	0	0	4	0.4	0	0	0	0	0	0
Fed Rep Germany	39.1	6.3	0	7.0	47.7	128	10.3	36.1	8.2	0	0.5	55.3	208
Finland	33.3	0	0	0	66.7	3	2.9	41.7	0	8.3	0	50.0	12
France	52.2	2.8	2.0	5.5	37.5	253	20.6	41.3	9.5	0	0.8	48.3	242
German Dem Rep	72.2	0	0	0	27.8	18	5.2	52.0	0	0	0	48.0	25
Greece	40.0	0	0	0	60.0	5	2.3	50.0	0	0	0	50.0	10
Hungary	0	0	0	0	0	0	–	100.0	0	0	0	0	1
Ireland	36.4	0	9.1	0	54.5	11	11.0	20.0	0	0	10.0	70.0	10
Israel	26.1	0	4.4	26.1	43.5	23	19.2	65.4	0	0	0	34.6	26

TABLE II. Continued

	AGE <15 YEARS							AGE ≥15 YEARS					
	MODES OF TREATMENT					Alive total	pMCP†	MODES OF TREATMENT					Alive total
	Hosp. HD %	Home HD %	IPD %	CAPD %	Transplant %	N	N	Hosp. HD %	Home HD %	IPD %	CAPD %	Transplant %	N
Italy	62.9	3.2	0	13.7	20.2	124	9.3	56.6	8.4	0	2.8	32.2	143
Lebanon	100.0	0	0	0	0	1	1.1	0	0	0	0	0	0
Libya	100.0	0	0	0	0	2	1.9	100.0	0	0	0	0	4
Luxembourg	100.0	0	0	0	0	2	28.6	0	0	0	0	100.0	1
Netherlands	36.8	1.8	0	10.5	50.9	57	17.0	15.4	1.3	0	0	83.3	78
Norway	11.8	0	0	0	88.2	17	18.1	17.6	0	0	0	82.4	17
Poland	88.9	0	0	0	11.1	9	1.1	60.0	0	0	0	40.0	10
Portugal	85.7	0	0	0	14.3	7	2.6	50.0	0	50.0	0	0	2
Spain	60.4	6.3	4.5	8.1	20.7	111	11.5	60.4	1.0	1.0	2.0	35.6	101
Sweden	16.7	0	0	16.7	66.7	12	7.1	16.7	10.0	0	3.3	70.0	30
Switzerland	27.8	0	0	16.7	55.6	18	13.6	15.2	3.0	0	9.1	72.7	33
Turkey	100.0	0	0	0	0	2	1.9	100.0	0	0	0	0	3
United Kingdom	10.2	6.3	3.2	19.7	60.6	127	9.9	9.2	19.9	0	3.4	67.5	206
Yugoslavia	95.0	0	0	0	5.0	20	3.7	85.0	0	0	0	15.0	20
TOTAL	46.0	3.4	1.8	9.1	39.7	1042	7.9	36.9	8.0	0.2	1.8	53.1	1270

† per Million Child Population

in the under 15 year olds but the increase was not as great as that observed in previous years in France and the United Kingdom. Peritoneal dialysis did not become the substitute for home haemodialysis as might have been expected from trends in earlier years, and home haemodialysis remained popular for the over 15 year olds. The proportion of children on hospital haemodialysis in the United Kingdom is remarkably small in comparison with other countries.

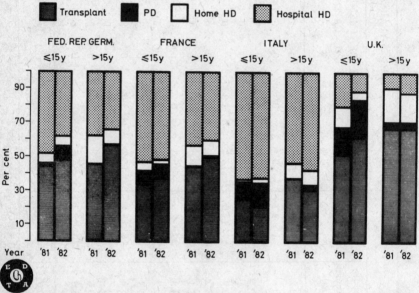

Figure 1. Proportions of patients on the paediatric register, according to age, on different modes of treatment in 1982 in four selected countries

In 1982, 288 children started treatment. In several European countries patients from abroad have been accepted for treatment. In France and the Federal Republic of Germany respectively 18 and 11 new patients from abroad were accepted for dialysis treatment in 1982. Table III shows the acceptance rates of new patients over the last 10 years in most countries reporting to the Registry. For some countries the acceptance of foreign patients may have been an important influence on the number of new patients.

Patient survival

Tables IV, V and VI give information on patient survival. Results in children who commenced treatment before 1 January, 1978 are compared with those who commenced treatment after 1 January, 1978.

Patient survival on renal replacement therapy was considerably better among the latter group of patients (Table IV). Overall five year patient survival was 68 per cent for 1,760 patients treated before 1978 and 76 per cent for 1,874 patients treated since 1978. The results have also been analysed according to patient's age at the start of treatment. Results in the 5–10 and 10–15 year old groups showed improvement since 1978. The improvement noticed at six months and one year in the 0–5 year old group encourages us to hope that a similar increase in long-term patient survival in these small children will be attained in subsequent years.

Table V shows survival after starting haemodialysis in hospital and in home and according to age at the start of treatment. Patient survival has been computed after starting haemodialysis, that is, irrespective of changes in therapy. Survival after starting home haemodialysis was better than survival after starting hospital haemodialysis and this holds when the results were analysed for the 5–10 and 10–15 year age groups separately. It is interesting to note the small number of children under five years undergoing home haemodialysis.

Patient survival following transplantation (Table VI) has been analysed according to the alternative convention which excludes patients as lost to follow-up from the date of any change of treatment (and, therefore, considered at risk of dying with their grafts, only until a change of treatment). Using this method, patient survival was analysed according to source of donor kidney and period of treatment. When all patients on the register were considered, survival at five years showed little difference between recipients of living donor or cadaver donor transplants. Patient survival showed only a slight improvement in recent years in recipients of both living and cadaver donors.

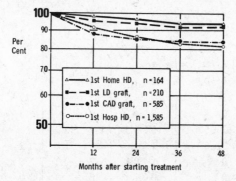

Figure 2. Patient survival after starting treatment according to mode of treatment in patients whose first treatment was after 1 January, 1978

Patient survival after starting different modes of treatment during the last five years is illustrated in Figure 2. Survival at four years was better in the home haemodialysis group (95%) and live donor transplant group (94%) than in those on hospital haemodialysis (82%) or after first cadaver donor transplantation (84%). Notice that when all the patient's history after grafting is included, survival following living donor kidney transplantation is superior to survival in recipients of cadaver donor kidneys.

85

TABLE III. Numbers of new patients who were registered as having commenced treatment in each of the years 1973–1982, according to country. (pMCP=per million child population). This table excludes data from Algeria, Egypt and Libya. Data from individual patient questionnaires (including some late returns)*

| Country | NEW PATIENTS (1973–1977) | | | | | | | | | |
| | 1973 | | 1974 | | 1975 | | 1976 | | 1977 | |
	N	pMCP†	N	pMCP	N	pMCP	N	pMCP	N	pMCP
Austria	4	2.3	5	2.9	7	4.0	4	2.3	6	3.4
Belgium	5	2.7	5	2.7	2	0.9	14	6.3	5	2.7
Bulgaria	3	1.6	5	2.6	3	1.6	5	2.6	3	1.6
Cyprus	0	–	2	11.3	0	–	0	–	2	11.3
Czechoslovakia	0	–	0	–	1	0.3	2	0.6	2	0.6
Denmark	1	0.8	6	5.2	3	2.6	4	3.5	6	5.2
Fed Rep Germany	35	2.8	38	3.0	46	3.7	66	5.3	51	4.1
Finland	0	–	0	–	2	1.9	0	–	3	2.9
France	39	3.2	45	3.6	62	5.0	57	4.6	52	4.2
German Dem Rep	6	1.7	3	0.8	7	2.0	5	1.4	15	4.2
Greece	0	–	5	2.3	2	0.9	2	0.9	4	1.9
Hungary	0	–	2	0.9	1	0.5	0	–	1	0.5
Ireland	0	–	1	1.0	1	1.0	1	1.0	1	1.0
Israel	1	0.9	2	1.8	3	2.5	8	7.0	8	7.0
Italy	23	1.7	28	2.1	38	2.8	29	2.2	31	2.3
Luxembourg	0	–	0	–	0	–	0	–	0	–
Netherlands	13	3.8	12	3.5	9	2.7	14	4.0	21	6.0
Norway	3	3.1	1	1.0	1	1.0	2	2.1	4	4.2
Poland	0	–	1	0.1	2	0.2	6	0.7	2	0.2
Portugal	0	–	0	–	0	–	0	–	1	0.4
Spain	7	0.7	14	1.4	16	1.6	25	2.6	29	3.0
Sweden	5	3.0	3	1.8	5	3.0	6	3.5	4	2.4
Switzerland	8	5.8	4	2.9	8	5.8	4	2.9	8	5.8
Turkey	1	–	0	–	2	–	5	–	3	–
United Kingdom	30	2.4	41	3.2	41	3.2	35	2.6	41	3.2
Yugoslavia	1	0.2	3	0.5	7	1.3	12	2.1	4	0.7
TOTAL	185		226		269		306		307	

†pMCP=per Million Child Population

86

TABLE III. *Continued*

Country	NEW PATIENTS (1978–1982)									
	1978		1979		1980		1981		1982	
	N	pMCP†	N	pMCP	N	pMCP	N	pMCP	N	pMCP
Austria	7	4.0	8	4.6	2	1.1	1	0.6	5	2.9
Belgium	14	6.3	24	11.2	15	7.0	12	5.6	5	2.3
Bulgaria	4	2.1	6	3.1	4	2.1	4	2.1	5	2.6
Cyprus	0	–	0	–	0	–	0	–	0	–
Czechoslovakia	1	0.3	3	0.9	4	1.2	9	2.6	4	1.2
Denmark	3	2.6	5	4.4	4	3.5	7	6.1	4	3.5
Fed Rep Germany	44	3.5	66	5.3	58	4.7	56	4.5	34	2.7
Finland	6	5.8	5	4.8	0	–	4	3.9	0	–
France	61	4.9	65	5.3	72	5.9	85	6.9	49	4.0
German Dem Rep	8	2.6	6	1.7	12	3.4	8	2.6	4	1.2
Greece	5	2.3	11	5.1	7	3.2	6	2.8	1	0.5
Hungary	3	1.4	1	0.5	0	–	0	–	0	–
Ireland	6	6.2	6	6.2	5	5.0	2	2.0	2	2.0
Israel	9	7.5	13	10.8	5	4.2	7	5.8	12	10.0
Italy	52	3.9	49	3.7	41	3.1	50	3.8	38	2.9
Luxembourg	0	–	3	42.9	3	42.9	0	–	0	–
Netherlands	14	4.0	17	5.2	21	6.0	26	7.8	7	2.1
Norway	3	3.1	3	3.1	6	6.4	5	5.3	6	6.4
Poland	9	1.1	10	1.2	6	0.7	12	1.4	2	0.3
Portugal	0	–	0	–	1	0.4	6	2.2	5	1.8
Spain	50	5.2	30	3.1	51	5.3	33	3.4	29	3.0
Sweden	9	5.3	1	0.6	5	2.9	3	1.8	4	2.4
Switzerland	9	6.4	6	4.5	6	4.5	5	3.8	4	3.0
Turkey	0	–	2	–	0	–	3	–	2	1.9
United Kingdom	57	4.5	54	4.2	66	5.1	65	5.1	48	3.8
Yugoslavia	3	0.5	2	0.4	17	3.1	11	2.0	12	2.2
TOTAL	377		396		411		420		282	

†pMCP=per Million Child Population

TABLE IV. Patient survival after starting renal replacement therapy, according to age at start of treatment and year of first therapy

Treatment period	Age group years	Sample size	MONTHS AFTER STARTING RENAL REPLACEMENT THERAPY											
			6		12		24		36		48		60	
			N at risk	%	N at risk	%	N at risk	%	N at risk	%	N at risk	%	N at risk	%
Before 1 January 1978	0 – 5	88	83.0	85	75.0	81	70.5	72	62.0	69	60.0	66	53.0	66
	5 – 10	443	416.0	89	392.0	81	359.0	73	321.5	67	292.0	62	262.5	59
	10 – 15	1229	1189.5	94	1157.0	88	1073.5	82	988.0	77	923.0	74	856.5	71
	All	1760	1688.5	93	1624.0	86	1503.0	79	1371.5	74	1275.5	71	1172.0	68
After 1 January 1978	0 – 5	232	188.5	92	163.5	87	118.5	74	58.5	69	28.0	+	8.5	+
	5 – 10	551	489.5	97	446.5	93	346.5	88	221.5	81	114.5	81	39.5	73
	10 – 15	1091	974.0	96	873.5	94	693.5	90	452.0	87	232.0	85	67.5	81
	All	1874	1652.0	96	1483.5	93	1158.5	88	732.0	83	374.5	82	115.5	76

+ Number at risk less than 30

TABLE V. Patient survival after starting hospital or home haemodialysis, according to age at start of treatment and year of first therapy

Modes of treatment	Age group years	Sample size	MONTHS AFTER STARTING HOSPITAL OR HOME HAEMODIALYSIS											
			6		12		24		36		48		60	
			N at risk	%	N at risk	%	N at risk	%	N at risk	%	N at risk	%	N at risk	%
1st Hospital haemodialysis	0 – 5	231	202.0	90	177.5	85	146.5	74	103.5	71	80.0	68	57.0	67
	5 – 10	866	782.5	93	731.5	88	629.5	81	491.0	74	369.5	71	276.5	67
All years	10 – 15	2131	1938.5	95	1864.0	90	1627.0	85	1331.0	81	1078.5	77	865.0	74
	All	3228	2968.0	94	2773.0	89	2403.0	83	1925.5	78	1528.0	75	1198.0	72
1st Home haemodialysis	0 – 5	7	6.0	+	6.0	+	4.5	+	4.0	+	3.5	+	2.5	+
	5 – 10	88	86.0	99	85.5	97	79.5	93	67.0	89	53.0	85	40.5	83
All years	10 – 15	290	278.0	97	264.5	96	246.0	94	214.0	90	178.0	87	146.5	84
	All	385	370.0	98	356.0	96	330.0	93	285.0	90	234.5	86	189.5	84

+ Number at risk less than 30

89

TABLE VI. Patient survival with a renal transplant in patients aged less than 15 years at transplantation, according to source of donor kidney and whether grafted before or after 1 January, 1978. Note: patients excluded at time of change to any other therapy

Period of treatment	Source of kidney	Sample size	MONTHS WITH GRAFT											
			6		12		24		36		48		60	
			N at risk	%	N at risk	%	N at risk	%	N at risk	%	N at risk	%	N at risk	%
Before 1 January 1978	Living donor	187	156.5	96	151.5	94	141.5	92	126.0	89	110.0	89	94.5	86
	1st Cadaver	428	298.0	92	280.5	89	251.0	88	227.5	86	207.5	84	192.5	83
	2nd Cadaver	59	38.0	92	35.0	86	28.5	+	23.0	+	20.5	+	19.5	+
After 1 January 1978	Living donor	210	184.5	98	169.5	97	134.5	96	83.5	94	39.5	94	11.5	+
	1st Cadaver	585	439.0	95	386.5	93	286.0	92	172.5	92	93.5	92	31.5	89
	2nd Cadaver	56	35.0	91	26.5	+	16.5	+	9.0	+	5.0	+	1.0	+
All	Living donor	397	341.0	97	321.0	96	276.0	94	209.5	92	149.5	91	106.0	89
	1st Cadaver	1013	737.0	94	667.0	92	537.0	90	400.0	89	301.0	87	224.0	87
	2nd Cadaver	115	73.0	91	61.5	87	45.0	83	32.0	81	25.5	+	20.5	+

+ Number at risk less than 30

Causes of death

Tables VII and VIII analyse causes of death. When all years were considered, cardiovascular causes (that is, the first seven causes given in Tables VII and VIII) comprised a larger proportion (55.6%) of 545 deaths in the 5–15 year olds than of the 59 (42.5%) in the less than five year olds. Problems related to dialysis treatment — hyperkalaemia, fluid overload and haemorrhage — were not more common in the younger age group. Both infections and malignant disease were more common in the less than five year olds. The cause of death on home haemodialysis was often unknown (cardiac arrest, cause unknown). Infection accounted for a large proportion of deaths in transplanted children, 12.8 per cent died because of graft failure, and 4.4 per cent because of malignant disease, probably nephroblastoma.

Figure 3 compares the deaths before and after 1 January, 1978 and shows that the proportion of dialysis deaths attributed to cardiac failure diminished, but that attributed to hyperkalaemia remained high, drawing attention to the

TABLE VII. Causes of deaths in children on renal replacement therapy according to last mode of treatment

Causes of death	Hospital haemodialysis %	Home haemodialysis %	CAPD %	Transplant %
Hyperkalaemia	9.3	4.3	0	2.5
Haemorrhagic pericarditis	3.7	0	0	0.5
Other causes of cardiac failure	9.1	8.7	0	3.0
Cardiac arrest, cause unknown	13.7	34.7	0	8.4
Hypertensive cardiac failure	14.2	4.3	22.2	2.5
Fluid overload	1.4	0	11.1	0
Cerebrovascular accident	12.1	4.3	11.1	10.3
Haemorrhage from graft site	1.6	8.7	0	3.4
Other haemorrhage	3.3	8.7	0	4.0
Infection	11.4	21.7	22.2	28.6
Liver disease	1.4	0	0	1.0
Social (therapy ceased)	1.9	0	0	1.9
Uraemia caused by graft failure	0	0	0	12.8
Cachexia	2.3	0	11.1	0
Malignant disease	1.1	0	0	0
Accident related to treatment	0	0	0	4.4
Others	13.5	4.6	22.2	16.7
TOTAL DEATHS† (N)	569	23	9	203

† Includes patients on Paediatric Register who were older than 15 years at time of death

91

TABLE VIII. Causes of death in children on dialysis according to age at time of death

Causes of death	0–5 years %	5–15 years %
Hyperkalaemia	5.1	7.7
Haemorrhagic pericarditis	0	3.5
Other causes of cardiac failure	3.4	7.9
Cardiac arrest, cause unknown	11.9	11.7
Hypertensive cardiac failure	6.8	13.6
Fluid overload	1.7	1.3
Cerebrovascular accident	13.6	9.9
Haemorrhage from graft site	1.7	2.2
Other haemorrhage	1.7	3.7
Infection	20.3	14.7
Liver disease	0	0.9
Social (therapy ceased)	3.4	3.3
Uraemia caused by graft failure	6.8	3.3
Cachexia	3.4	1.6
Malignant disease	5.1	1.5
Accident related to treatment	0	0
Others	15.1	13.2
TOTAL DEATHS (N)	59	545

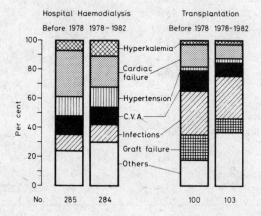

Figure 3. Causes of death before and after 1 January, 1978 in patients whose last mode of treatment was hospital haemodialysis or transplantation

importance of dietary care in children. Proportions of causes of death following cadaver transplant show a reduction in cardiac failure, cerebrovascular accident and graft failure.

CAPD

The percentage of paediatric patients treated with CAPD continued to grow in 1982 as is shown in Table II and Figure 1.

Peritonitis remained the principal complication with one episode per 6.8 patient-months (excluding three patients with more than four episodes) versus one episode per 5.4 patient-months in 1981 (excluding one patient with more than four episodes). However, the proportion of patients who remained peritonitis-free in 1982 was 30 per cent after three to six months on CAPD (Figure 4), lower than in 1981 [1].

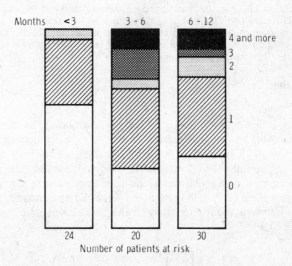

Figure 4. CAPD in children: proportion of paediatric patients with stated number of episodes of peritonitis in 1982 according to time on CAPD

In spite of this persisting problem the survival of 170 children who started CAPD during the last two years was better than the 56 who started in 1979–80 (Figure 5). Furthermore, technique survival also improved. The lower lines of the right part of Figure 5 give technique survival when all deaths and changes in treatment are considered as failures. The upper lines show a recalculation in which grafted patients were excluded and any patient who died was considered 'lost to observation' from the date of death. The improvement amongst patients treated in 1981–82 indicates much more successful use of the technique.

93

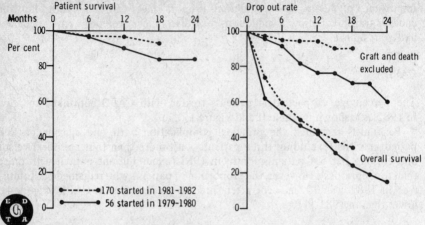

Figure 5. CAPD in children: (lefthand panel) patient survival and (righthand panel) drop out rate. There are two calculations of drop out rate: 'Overall survival' is the technique survival considering all deaths and changes in treatment as failures, 'Graft and death excluded' considers any patients who died as lost to observation from the date of death and excludes all grafted patients from the calculation

Transplantation

Organisation

We used the centre questionnaire to collect information on the organisation of kidney transplantation in children. Out of the 233 transplants claimed to have been performed in 1982 in patients less than 15 years of age, 103 were carried out in combined adult-paediatric programmes and 130 in specialised paediatric programmes. Special paediatric centres predominated in France and Spain, and combined centres in the Federal Republic of Germany, while the two types of centre were reported equally in the United Kingdom and the Netherlands (Figure 6).

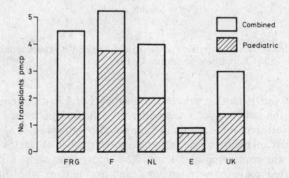

Figure 6. Numbers of transplants (pMCP) performed in paediatric and combined transplant programmes in 1982 in five selected countries

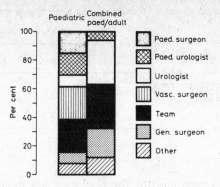

Figure 7. Organisation of paediatric transplantation: (i) surgeon performing transplantation

In the combined programmes more than 75 per cent of the operations were performed either by a urologist, by a team of specialised surgeons or by a general surgeon (Figure 7). In the paediatric programmes, paediatric surgeons, paediatric urologists, vascular surgeons or teams of specialised surgeons performed 75 per cent of the transplants.

The responsibility for the care of these patients following the operation was invariably assumed by a paediatric nephrologist in the paediatric programmes, but nephrologists, surgeons or paediatricians were in charge of patients transplanted in combined centres. In these centres the early post-operative care was carried out mainly by surgeons and long-term follow-up by paediatric nephrologists (Figure 8).

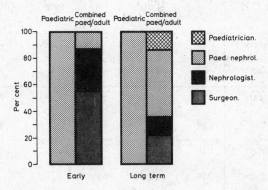

Figure 8. Organisation of paediatric transplantation: (ii) doctor responsible for early and long-term follow-up

Only three centres, all paediatric ones, performed more than 10 transplant operations in children in 1982 (Table IX). A large majority of the combined programmes performed less than six transplantations during the year.

TABLE IX. Paediatric transplant activity in 1982 according to type of programme

Number of transplants in 1982	1–5	6–10	11–20	>20
Centres with paediatric programme	9	3	2	1
Centres with combined paediatric/adult programme	25	4	–	–

Source of donors

Sources of kidney transplants for the first graft are given in Table X. This information is given according to age and date of grafting before and after 1 January, 1978. Twenty-four per cent of all the first paediatric transplants in Europe were performed using living donors, the majority of them being father or mother. Siblings were rarely used and there was only one identical twin donor. The percentage of living donors decreased slightly in the last five years in comparison with the years before, except for the youngest recipients aged less than five years for whom almost one-third of transplants were performed using a kidney from the father or mother.

TABLE X. Source of donor kidney (first grafts) in patients on the paediatric register according to age and year of grafting (before and after 1 January, 1978)

Age group years	Before/After 1 Jan 1978	Cadaver	Father/ Mother	Siblings	Identical twin	Other living donor	%LD Transplant
<5	Before	12	4	–	–	–	25
	After	33	15	–	–	–	31
5 – 15	Before	422	175	5	–	5	30
	After	558	183	8	1	4	26
15+	Before	128	25	–	–	1	17
	After	234	16	6	–	–	9
Subtotal	Before	562	204	5	–	6	28
	After	825	214	14	1	4	22
TOTAL		1387	418	19	1	10	24

The source of second transplants was also studied. Out of 257 second grafts, 232 were cadaver transplants, and 25 living related donor transplants (22 parents and three siblings), that is to say, living donors represented only 10 per cent of second transplants and this percentage has not changed over the years.

Graft survival

Graft survival in children aged less than 15 years at the time of transplantation is reported in Tables XI, XII and XIII respectively for first cadaver, second cadaver and living donor grafts. The results are presented separately for transplants performed before and after 1 January, 1978. The improvement varies from five to 10 per cent in the last five years, where the best survival was observed with living donors.

TABLE XI. Graft survival after first cadaver transplant in patients aged less than 15 years at time of grafting (before and after 1 January, 1978)

	Sample size	MONTHS AFTER 1st CADAVER TRANSPLANT						
		3	6	12	24	36	48	60
Before 1 Jan 1978	430							
N at risk		411.0	300.0	289.0	262.0	236.0	211.0	195.5
% survival		70	67	61	55	49	46	45
After 1 Jan 1978	586							
N at risk		553.5	442.0	391.0	292.5	176.0	95.5	32.5
% survival		80	75	69	62	58	55	50

TABLE XII. Graft survival after second cadaver transplant in patients aged less than 15 years at time of grafting (before and after 1 January, 1978)

	Sample size	MONTHS AFTER 2nd CADAVER TRANSPLANT						
		3	6	12	24	36	48	60
Before 1 Jan 1978	86							
N at risk		79.0	53.0	51.0	46.0	36.0	33.0	32.0
% survival		62	59	53	42	38	37	35
After 1 Jan 1978	106							
N at risk		99.5	73.5	56.5	38.0	21.0	12.5	3.0
% survival		73	64	58	50	+	+	+

+ Number at risk less than 30

TABLE XIII. Graft survival after first living donor transplant in patients aged less than 15 years at time of grafting (before and after 1 January, 1978)

	Sample size	MONTHS AFTER 1st LIVING DONOR TRANSPLANT						
		3	6	12	24	36	48	60
Before 1 Jan 1978	188							
N at risk		185.0	159.0	153.0	147.0	130.0	116.0	99.0
% survival		85	81	79	71	64	55	49
After 1 Jan 1978	210							
N at risk		206.5	186.0	171.5	139.5	85.0	40.0	11.5
% survival		92	89	85	77	71	67	+

+ Number at risk less than 30

Causes of graft failure

Causes of graft failure in paediatric patients (aged less than 15 years at time of grafting) are reported in Table XIV for first and second cadaver as well as living donor transplants.

TABLE XIV. Causes of graft failure in paediatric patients

1 January 1978 ⟶	1st Cadaver				2nd Cadaver		1st living donor		TOTAL	
	Before		After		Before	After	Before	After		
	N	(%)	N	(%)	N	N	N	N	N	(%)
Hyperacute rejection	13	(4)	5	(2)	3	5	3	2	31	(4)
Rejection while taking Immunosuppressive drugs	214	(73)	159	(68)	45	43	82	31	574	(73)
Rejection after stopping all Immunosuppressive drugs	14	(5)	3	(1)	1	–	4	1	23	(3)
Recurrent PRD	23	(8)	13	(6)	1	1	4	2	44	(6)
Vascular operative problem	4	(1)	20	(9)	–	–	2	4	30	(4)
Ureteric operative problem	10	(3)	5	(2)	3	–	1	–	19	(2)
Infection of graft	7	(2)	9	(4)	3	2	–	–	21	(3)
Removal of functioning graft	8	(3)	6	(3)	2	–	2	2	20	(3)
'Non-viable' kidney	–	(0)	11	(5)	–	–	–	–	11	(1)
Other	1	(<1)	3	(1)	–	5	1	–	10	(1)
TOTAL	294		234		58	56	99	42	783	(100)

When the causes of graft failure before and after 1978 were compared, rejection remained the most important cause of graft loss. The decrease of graft failure related to hyperacute rejection and to rejection after stopping all immunosuppressive drugs in recipients of first cadaver grafts should be noted. This decrease is balanced by an increase in the proportion of grafts lost due to 'other causes' which merit detailed consideration. Recurrence of primary renal disease represents a significant cause of graft failure following both cadaver and living donor grafts; vascular operative complications increased during the last five years and this is probably related to an increase in the number of small children undergoing transplantation. Non-viable kidneys also emerged as a significant cause of graft failure. No living donor grafts were lost due to infection, but this cause of graft failure still occurred in recipients of cadaver grafts during the last five years.

Aseptic necrosis of bone

Data on aseptic necrosis of bone were requested on the paediatric mini-questionnaire and were recorded in 596 paediatric patients. In 148 only clinical symptoms were reported and in 448 an X-ray examination was performed. Of these, 372 had no abnormalities but 76 (17%) had radiological evidence of aseptic necrosis. Thirty-eight (50%) of these also had clinical symptoms and in 22 pain was persistent, despite surgery which was carried out in six. In 10 cases, the symptoms were transient.

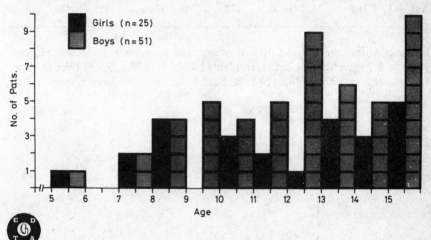

Figure 9. Aseptic necrosis of bone (ANB) in transplanted patients: 76 patients according to age and sex

Of the 76 patients with aseptic necrosis, 25 were girls and 51 were boys (Figure 9). Aseptic necrosis was diagnosed in all age groups, except in the under fives. Before puberty, the disease affected girls and boys equally, but the majority of affected patients older than 11 years at the time of transplantation were boys (Table XV). The incidence of aseptic necrosis was slightly higher in pubertal (20.8%) than in prepubertal children (18.3%).

Although aseptic necrosis is often diagnosed several years after transplantation, the data we have collected do not suggest that the risk of this complication

TABLE XV. Aseptic necrosis of bone (ANB) in transplanted patients according to sex and age at time of transplantation

Age group years	GIRLS			BOYS			ALL		
	Transplant N	ANB N	% N	Transplant N	ANB N	% N	Transplant N	ANB N	% N
<5	2	0	–	7	0	–	9	0	–
5–6	6	1	(16.7)	5	1	(20.0)	11	2	(18.2)
6–7	4	0	–	10	0	–	14	0	–
7–8	10	2	(20.0)	14	2	(14.3)	24	4	(16.7)
8–9	10	4	(40.0)	15	4	(26.7)	25	8	(32.0)
9–10	16	0	–	23	5	(21.7)	39	5	(12.8)
10–11	12	3	(25.0)	17	4	(23.5)	29	7	(24.1)
11–12	18	2	(11.1)	22	5	(22.7)	40	7	(17.5)
12–13	14	1	(7.1)	20	9	(45.0)	34	10	(29.4)
13–14	20	4	(20.0)	28	6	(21.4)	48	10	(20.8)
14–15	20	3	(15.0)	27	5	(18.5)	47	8	(17.0)
>15	37	5	(13.5)	34	10	(29.4)	71	15	(21.1)
ALL	169	25	(14.8)	222	51	(23.0)	391	76	(19.4)

increases with time (Figure 10). However, the prevalence of aseptic necrosis was much higher for patients transplanted before 1978 (25.9%) than in those transplanted in 1978–1982 (14.6%). Several factors may have contributed to

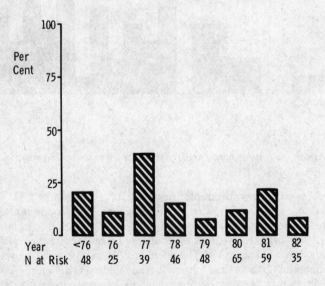

Figure 10. Aseptic necrosis of bone (ANB): per cent affected, according to year of transplant

100

this decrease in aseptic necrosis in recent years such as a better outcome of transplantation, smaller doses of steroids and changes in treatment of renal osteodystrophy.

We were not able to demonstrate a relationship between the dose of steroids administered during the first month after transplantation and the development of aseptic necrosis of bone. The amount of intravenous methylprednisolone and the mean oral dose of prednisone administered during the first month after grafting was not significantly different in patients with symptomatic aseptic necrosis of bone, in patients with only radiological evidence of aseptic necrosis of bone and in patients without aseptic necrosis of bone (Figure 11 and Table XVI).

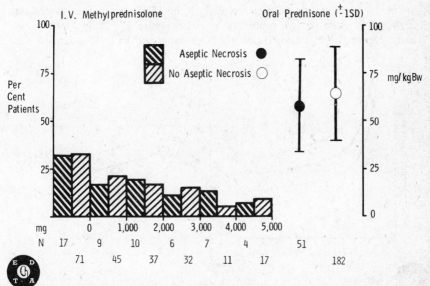

Figure 11. Aseptic necrosis of bone (ANB) and total steroid dose during the first month after grafting

TABLE XVI. Aseptic necrosis of bone (ANB) and mean oral dose of prednisone administered during first month after transplantation

Aseptic necrosis of bone	No abnormalities	Only X-ray abnormalities	X-ray abnormalities and clinical symptoms
Mean dose oral prednisone (mg/kg/BW/month)	64.1	58.0	60.2
Patients (N)	182	32	19

Growth in prepubertal children

Data for this year's study on growth were collected from patient questionnaires and from a special paediatric mini-questionnaire. Growth was studied in prepubertal children, assuming that boys were prepubertal if they were less than 11 years old and girls if they were less than 10 years on 31 December, 1982. Children with a bone age of more than 10 years were excluded. For inclusion in these studies patients must not have undergone any change in mode of treatment during 1982, and only linear growth between December, 1981 and December, 1982 was considered. Patients with cystinosis and oxalosis were excluded. Linear growth in each patient in 1982 was compared to the mean normal for age [2]. Thus we calculated the ratio, observed to expected growth.

On dialysis

Growth of prepubertal children on dialysis in 1982 was better in children less than five years of age, especially in boys (Figure 12, Table XVII) as previously reported [1]. Growth on CAPD remains difficult to compare with

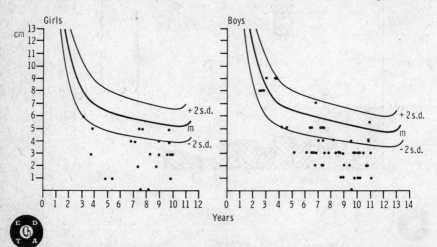

Figure 12. Linear growth of prepubertal girls and boys on dialysis throughout the year 1982

TABLE XVII. Linear growth of prepubertal children on dialysis in 1982 (ratio of observed to expected growth)

| | AGE (years) | | | | | | | | | |
	2–3	3–4	4–5	5–6	6–7	7–8	8–9	9–10	10–11	2–11
Haemodialysis										
n patients	1	5	1	–	7	10	12	14	11	61
Mean	0.93	0.94	0		0.61	0.62	0.45	0.49	0.57	0.57
± SD		±0.34			±0.26	±0.26	±0.21	±0.24	±0.32	±0.30
CAPD										
n patients	1	2	2	2	2	4	–	–	2	15
mean	0.84	0.87	0.75	0.30	0.76	0.56			0.60	0.63
± SD						±0.22				±0.24

102

growth on haemodialysis since the number of patients treated for a full year by CAPD remains small. The mean (± 1SD) observed to expected growth ratio in the 15 children on CAPD was 0.63 (±0.24), higher than the figure of 0.57 (±0.3) observed in the 61 children on haemodialysis. But the age distributions are not similar in the two groups and children on CAPD were younger. In the under fives, growth was greater on haemodialysis, 0.80 (±0.43) (n=7) versus 0.67 (±0.26) (n=7). It is certainly important to emphasise that in any comparative study of growth on dialysis the age of patients must be taken into account.

Growth on dialysis was compared to residual creatinine clearance. Growth was slightly better in patients with residual function, 0.61 (±0.31) (n=29) versus 0.54 (±0.26) (n=30) in patients without residual clearance (NS). No relationship was found between growth and the residual clearance in spite of a relatively wide range in clearances (0.5 to 8ml/min/1.73m^2).

Weight for height in prepubertal children dialysed for more than one year is shown in Figures 13 and 14. There was a difference between patients aged less than six years and the older ones. The younger children tended to have a low weight for height, but this was no longer the case after six years, and after eight years weight for height was equally distributed around the mean. Patients on CAPD did not behave differently from those on haemodialysis. Considering growth according to weight for height (Table XVIII) a generally

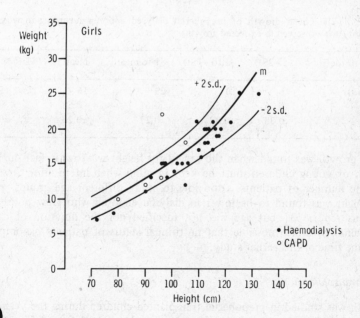

Figure 13. Prepubertal girls at least one year on dialysis: weight for height in December 1982

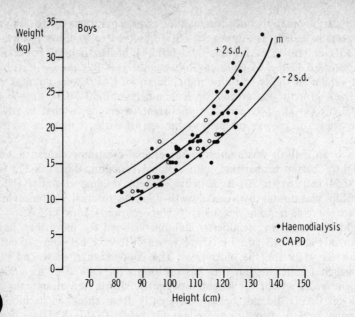

Figure 14. Prepubertal boys at least one year on dialysis: weight for height in December 1982

TABLE XVIII. Linear growth of prepubertal dialysed children according to weight for height (ratio observed to expected growth)

Weight for height	< −2SD	−2 to −1SD	−1 to mean	mean to +1SD	> +1SD
n patients	6	21	29	16	5
mean	0.75	0.55	0.61	0.58	0.47
± SD	±0.33	±0.32	±0.27	±0.28	±0.19

better growth was found when the weight for height was low; in fact the better growth of young children must be kept in mind when interpreting these data and the number of patients is too low to study different age groups. Weight for height was found to be lower in dialysed children who grew poorly in a previous report [3] but age was not specified nor the duration of dialytic treatment. It is also possible that nutritional status of patients has improved since the time of this earlier study.

After transplantation

Growth was studied in prepubertal transplanted children during the year 1982. For this study we selected the 50 patients who were 1.5 to 3.5 years post grafting on 31 December, 1982, and who retained a functioning first graft at this time.

104

Growth was very variable in these patients: the ratio, observed to expected growth in 1982 ranged from 0.19 to 1.80. Looking for the factors which could be involved in the differences of growth velocity we found that the level of renal function probably played a role (Figure 15). In patients with a mean

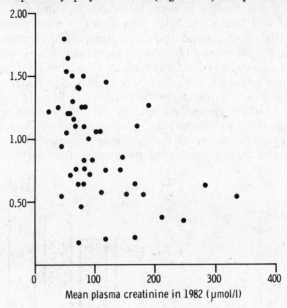

Figure 15. Ratio observed/expected growth in 1982 in transplanted prepubertal children according to mean plasma creatinine concentration

plasma creatinine above 120μmol/L the mean growth (±SD) was: 0.51 (±0.19) (range 0.20–0.85, n=11) compared to 1.01 (±0.38) (range 0.17–1.81, n=36) in patients with a mean plasma creatinine less than 120μmol/L (p<0.001). Consequently it seems that moderate chronic renal insufficiency can slow down growth velocity, especially in transplanted children, since the same level of renal function is generally compatible with normal growth in children during the period of conservative management prior to ESRF.

TABLE XIX. Growth in prepubertal transplanted children with a mean plasma creatinine less than 120μmol/L in 1982, according to daily prednisone dose

Mean daily prednisone dose in 1982 (mg/kg/BW)	0.10–0.20	0.20–0.30	0.30–0.40	0.40–0.50	>0.50
n patients	2	12	11	9	4
Mean growth (observed/expected)	0.94	1.05	1.19	0.81	0.91
± SD		±0.31	±0.40	±0.36	±0.34

Growth was also studied according to the mean daily dose of prednisone received in 1982 (Table XIX). For this study, transplanted children with a mean plasma creatinine above 120μmol/L were excluded. No influence of the daily dose of prednisone could be found on the ratio, observed to expected growth. Growth was finally compared in children receiving alternate day and daily corticosteroid treatment. Again patients with a mean plasma creatinine above 120μmol/L were excluded. In 14 transplanted children receiving alternate day treatment the mean ratio observed to expected growth (±1SD) was 1.09 (±0.33) versus a mean ratio of 0.98 (±0.40) in 23 children receiving daily treatment (NS). Previous reports from the EDTA Registry did not allow firm conclusions since one showed a better growth on alternate day [4] and another no difference on alternate versus daily therapy [5]. Many transplanted children are nevertheless receiving alternate day prednisone and this is apparent in an analysis performed in relation to the time after transplantation in December, 1982 (Figure 16). During the second six months, four per cent were given

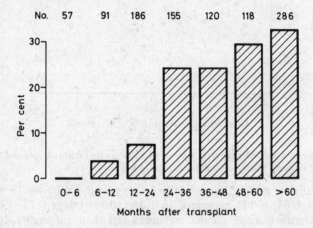

Figure 16. Per cent of transplanted children on alternate day prednisone in 1982 according to time after grafting

alternate day steroids, and between the first and second year this proportion was 7.5 per cent. The switch to alternate day therapy was made more frequently following the second year after transplantation. In patients two to four years after transplantation, the proportion rose to 25 per cent and five years after to 33 per cent.

Conclusions

1 The contribution of transplantation to the treatment of children varied between countries and was still increasing in many.

2 A significant increase in patient survival for all modes of treatment

106

was found when survival for patients treated before and after 1 January, 1978 was compared.

3   A better integration of different modes of treatment may have contributed to the better survival.

4   Although the use of CAPD increased, it did not become a substitute for home haemodialysis and peritonitis remained its major complication with one episode per 6.8 patient-months in 1982.

5   Transplantation was performed both in specialised paediatric and in combined adult-paediatric programmes. Paediatricians were much more involved in patient care in specialised paediatric programmes.

6   Graft survival has clearly improved during recent years.

7   Aseptic necrosis of bone was diagnosed in 17 per cent of the transplanted children, and was more common in boys than girls. No relationship between aseptic necrosis of bone and the amount of steroids administered during the first month post-transplant could be demonstrated.

8   Growth on haemodialysis was better in boys less than five years in spite of a rather low weight for height in this age group.

9   Growth rate in transplanted prepubertal children was better if plasma creatinine was less than 120μmol/L.

10 Of the transplanted children, 33 per cent were on alternate day steroid treatment five years after transplantation.

References

1   Donckerwolcke RA, Broyer M, Brunner FP et al. *Proc EDTA 1982; 19:* 61
2   Sempe M, Roy MP, Filliuzat AM. *Rapport terminal de l'enquête sur la croissance.* Paris: CIE. 1976: 63
3   Donckerwolcke RA, Chantler C, Brunner FP et al. *Proc EDTA 1978; 15:* 77
4   Chantler C, Donckerwolcke RA, Brunner FP et al. *Proc EDTA 1979; 16:* 74
5   Donckerwolcke RA, Chantler C, Broyer M et al. *Proc EDTA 1980; 17:* 87

Open Discussion

ANDREUCCI (Chairman)   Thank you Dr Donckerwolcke for the important data you have given concerning the behaviour of children on dialysis and transplantation. The paper is now open for discussion.

I have observed many improvements, but in haemodialysis patients there is an increasing incidence of death due to hyperkalaemia and this is said because we should by now have better means of avoiding this. Do you have any explanation for this observation?

DONCKERWOLCKE   No, none at all. I think you are right: it should be better and not worse.

GABRIEL (London) Amongst the causes of death in children on dialysis I presume some die of malignant disease. Do you, as yet, have data to suggest whether there is an increased incidence of malignancy in these children?

DONCKERWOLCKE I cannot give the data at present but we will try to add this to later reports.

AHMED (Liverpool) This is not a question but a suggestion to Dr Wing as Chairman of the EDTA Registration Committee. This is the first time in about 12 or 14 years that we have not been presented with any data on hepatitis. Because of the pre-transplant blood transfusion policy, vital data on the incidence and effect of hepatitis will be lost, and so can you continue to ask questions about the incidence of hepatitis on a yearly basis on our registration forms?

WING Thank you for that question. I shall be presenting data on hepatitis to the EDTNA meeting tomorrow. I agree it is very important and we will continue to collect this information. Our nursing colleagues are most concerned about hepatitis.

MacLEOD (Aberdeen) Have you looked at the patient survival of children who are looked after in specialised paediatric units and compared that to the survival of those who are looked after in combined units?

DONCKERWOLCKE We have not looked at that this year as we did it several years ago. I think that we will have to review this again in the future.

KURUVILA (Denver, Colorado) With reference to the aseptic necrosis of bone, do you have any data on the duration of renal failure and the use of steroids prior to transplantation, and also on the use of Vitamin D in these children?

DONCKERWOLCKE The EDTA Registry is not collecting data on patients with chronic renal failure, so we have no data relating to events prior to starting renal replacement therapy. We did not look at the duration of dialysis before transplantation to see if there was any difference and also unfortunately we do not have any data on Vitamin D administration in these patients.

ANDREUCCI Thank you Dr Donckerwolcke for your presentation and thanks to the Registration Committee and the excellent work they have done.

PART II

GUEST LECTURES – DIALYSIS

Chairmen: C Mion
             R A Baillod

SHORT DIALYSIS

V Cambi, G Garini, G Savazzi, L Arisi, S David,
P Zanelli, F Bono, F Gardini

University of Parma, Parma, Italy

Introduction

The frequency and duration of dialysis treatment has become a subject of interest to the EDTA Registry since the report of 1974 [1]. At that time, in most European Centres, the duration of a dialysis session was generally adjusted to the availability of dialysis facilities. Among the European population, hospital patients dialysed for longer than 23 hours weekly were 21.3 per cent, whereas at home the same treatment duration was performed in 61.9 per cent of the population.

In the early sixties, thanks to the known association between dialysis time and peripheral neuropathy, long and frequent dialysis sessions seemed the only way of preventing the catastrophic consequences of nerve damage. In the late sixties, the middle molecule (MM) hypothesis [2] stimulated research in two directions: first the search in patient's serum for those solutes in the range of 300–1500 daltons and subsequently the search for biological assays capable of demonstrating their potential toxicity; secondly numerous clinical trials devised to confirm or exclude the consequences of MM related uraemic toxicity. Low flow dialysis [3] and short dialysis [4] represented the first clinical attempts respectively for and against the MM hypothesis. The purpose of low flow dialysis conducted with a Q_D of 100ml/min and a Q_B of 150–200ml/min was to demonstrate that uraemic toxicity could be prevented, despite an increase in small molecules (SM) retention, providing there was an adequate clearance of MM as in standard Kiil dialysis. At present, looking retrospectively at that trial we now realise that MM clearance was, by definition, identical to that obtained with standard Kiil dialysis; SM in the same patients were higher. However, the absolute predialysis values of serum urea ranged between 60 and 80mg% [3]. A few years later a long-term American study [5] reached the conclusion that within a time duration of up to five hours the clinical condition is good if the predialysis urea is below 80mg% and bad with serum concentrations between 110 and 130mg%. In addition the patient remains in a relatively good condition provided there is a predialysis urea below 80mg% even if the dialysis time is shortened to 2.5 hours.

111

With the technology available in the early seventies it was not difficult to alter the removal rate of SM relative to MM. In fact in 1971 by switching from Kiil to coil dialysers and from the external shunt to the A-V fistula (Q_B 250–300) we created conditions in which we could obtain predialysis BUN values similar to standard Kiil dialysis despite a time reduction from 10 to four hours.

However, according to the square metre hour hypothesis, this treatment was unquestionably inefficient in removing MM: in patients treated with coil dialysis and very reduced dialysis time, such as we performed, there should have been a high incidence of severe peripheral neuropathy.

The purpose of this paper is to summarise the early studies devoted to the evaluation of peripheral nerve function, to estimate the actual nutritional status of a homogenous short dialysis population and finally to analyse the cardiovascular complications observed in the long-term.

Population and methods

Peripheral nerve studies

Motor nerve conduction velocity (MNCV) was measured with a dual channel Hewlett Packard 1510 A electromyograph, with a variable persistence storage scope. Motor action potentials (MAP) recorded from ulnar and peroneal nerves were obtained with a sensitivity of 2mV/cm, a sweep time of 2ms/cm and orthodrome single stimulation with a pulse width of 200μsec and variable voltage from 0–325 volts to obtain a supramaximal response. Routine use was made of bipolar needle electrodes. A longitudinal study was performed (Figure 1) in 13 consecutive patients treated for over 12 months with standard Kiil dialysis (10 hours thrice weekly) and successively with short dialysis (four hours thrice weekly). Ulnar and peroneal MNCV were recorded.

Nutritional aspects

One hundred and thirty-seven patients willing to co-operate were selected from the dialysis population during the year 1982. Mean age was 50 ± 13 years. Time on dialysis 6 ± 3 years. The following anthropometric data were collected: mid arm muscle circumference, fat relative to body weight, mean body weight, and in addition total serum proteins and albumin were measured.

Survival and cardiovascular complications

Two hundred and fifty-six patients (165 men and 91 women) treated by chronic haemodialysis since 1974 were studied. The follow-up period extended from January 1974 to December 1982. Six patients with malignancy prior to haemodialysis were excluded from the study. The mean time on dialysis was 34.4 ± 30 (SD) months. Mean age at the start of haemodialysis was 52.3 ± 15 (SD) years (51.8 ± 15 for men and 52.9 ± 16 for women). Main causes of the initial nephropathy were chronic glomerulonephritis (24.6% of patients), chronic pyelonephritis (21.9%), nephroangiosclerosis (12.9%), polycystic kidney disease (8.6%) and diabetic nephropathy (3.5%).

112

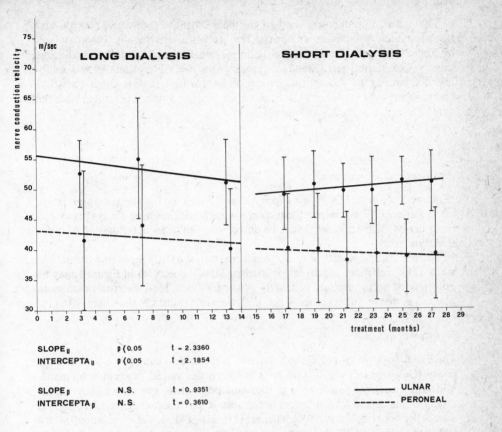

Figure 1. Ulnar and peroneal nerve conduction velocity in 13 patients dialysed with standard Kiil dialysis (10 hours thrice weekly) and later with one square metre coil dialyser four hours thrice weekly

Dialysis technique

All patients dialysed four hours thrice weekly with one square metre coils or parallel flow dialysers; for a limited period of time coils of 1.5 square metres and capillary kidneys of 1.3 square metres have been used. Blood flow was 250ml/min or more, and dialysate flow 500ml/min. Dialysate composition (in mEq/L) was Na 140, K 0–3, Mg 1.5, Ca 4, Cl 104, acetate 40, glucose 1g/L.

Statistical analysis

Seventy-one deaths were registered during the follow-up period. They comprised 27 non-cardiovascular (NCDV) deaths and 44 cardiovascular (CDV) deaths, including 17 patients with myocardial infarction and 11 with cerebrovascular accidents. Autopsies were performed on 22 of 71 patients who died during the study period.

113

Life table methods were used to calculate both the cumulative survival and the cumulative probability of death. The statistical analysis of these data was by the Cutler and Ederer method. Comparison between survival distributions was by Cox-Mantel test. Standard error for all life table estimates was established according to the approximation of Greenwood [6—8]. Other statistical comparisons were made with the Student unpaired and paired t-test and with the contingency table 2 x 2.

Results

Peripheral nerve studies

Ulnar and peroneal MNCV were longitudinally followed in the same population of 13 patients. The treatment duration for each trial has been always prolonged for a period of months sufficient to detect any potential deterioration of nerve function.

Neither clinical neuropathy nor deterioration of MNCV appeared during the study. The statistical improvement in ulnar MNCV described in Figure 1 may be only related to the normal variability of the methods. More extensive studies on peripheral nerve function in short dialysis are published elsewhere [9—11].

Nutritional aspects

The mean body weight of dialysis patients compared to controls of the same age group (Geigy tables) was 100 per cent in 55 females and 95 per cent in 82 males. Mid arm muscle circumference in the same population was respectively 23.6 ± 2.0cm in males and 21.9 ± 2.1cm in females. Relative muscle circumference was 94 ± 8 per cent (males) and 95 ± 9 per cent (females) [12]. Fat represented 15 ± 4 per cent (males) and 26 ± 6 per cent (females) relative to dry body weight. Total serum proteins were 7.0 ± 0.5g/dl and albumin 4.0 ± 0.3g/dl.

Survival and cardiovascular mortality

Mean age of patients at start of treatment was 52.3 ± 15 years, (46.7 years in 1974, and 62.1 years in 1982). More than a half of the population was over 55 years at start of treatment (Table I). Figure 2 shows the age distribution: 15 per cent of the patients were over 70 years. The present population on haemodialysis per million population is 450. Figure 3 and Table II show respectively five year patient survival according to the age groups and life table analysis [6].

In all age groups the survival of patients on short dialysis was superior to the European population treated with variable dialysis schedules. Nine years prospective survival is 75 per cent below 34 years, 57 per cent between 35—54 years. Survival has been also referred to a selected group of renal disease; nine years survival of patients with chronic glomerulonephritis (63 cases, mean age 44 ± 16) was significantly better than control (p<0.005) whereas the survival of nephro-angiosclerosis for a similar period (33 cases, mean age 55.9 ± 10) was significantly worse (p<0.05). Seventy-one of the 256 patients died: 62 per cent from cardio-

114

TABLE I. Characteristics of the nine years (January 1974 to December 1982) unselected population coming from an area of 400,000 inhabitants

	Males		Females		Total	
	Number	(%)	Number	(%)	Number	(%)
Number of patients	165	(64.4)	91	(35.6)	256	
Mean age (years ± SD) at start of treatment	51.8 ± 15*		52.9 ± 16*		52.3 ± 15	
Mean time (months ± SD) on dialysis	34.8 ± 30*		33.7 ± 28*		34.4 ± 30	
Age distribution:						
≤34 years	33	(20.0)	11	(12.1)	44	(17.2)
35–54 years	47	(28.5)	34	(37.4)	81	(31.6)
≥55 years	85	(51.5)	46	(50.5)	131	(52.2)

* p = not significant

AGE AND SEX DISTRIBUTION OF DIALYSIS PATIENTS (n. 256)

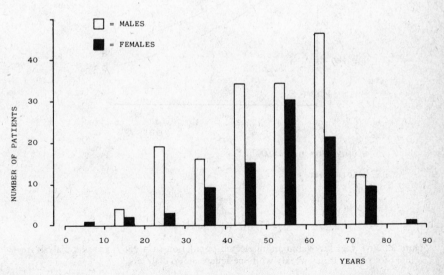

Figure 2. Age and sex distribution in the population described in Table I

115

PER CENT PATIENT SURVIVAL ACCORDING TO AGE GROUPS ON HAEMODIALYSIS (HOSPITAL OR HOME) IN PATIENTS IN TREATMENT SINCE 1974

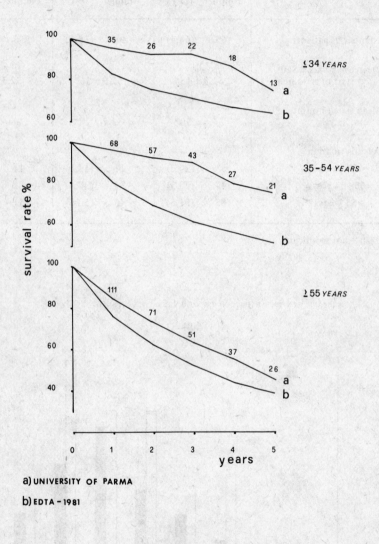

Figure 3. Five year survival in an unselected population (n = 256) in regular dialysis treatment four hours thrice weekly with one square metre dialysers

116

TABLE II. Life table analysis of mortality data of 256 dialysis patients

Months	Number alive	Living withdrawals	Number of deaths	Cardiovascular deaths	Myocardial infarction deaths	Probability of death			Cumulative probability of death*	Cumulative probability of death of cardiovascular cause*	Cumulative probability of death of myocardial infarction*
						From all causes	From cardiovascular causes	From myocardial infarction			
0–6	256	33	9	4	2	3.8	1.7	0.8	3.8 ± 1.2	1.7 ± 0.8	0.8 ± 0.6
7–12	214	17	14	9	5	6.8	4.4	2.5	10.3 ± 2.0	6.0 ± 1.6	3.3 ± 1.2
13–18	183	23	6	3	0	3.5	1.7	0	13.5 ± 2.3	7.6 ± 1.8	3.3 ± 1.2
19–24	154	15	7	6	3	4.8	4.1	2.1	17.6 ± 2.7	11.4 ± 2.3	5.3 ± 1.7
25–30	132	11	6	4	2	4.7	3.2	1.6	21.5 ± 3.0	14.2 ± 2.6	6.8 ± 2.0
31–36	115	8	3	3	1	2.7	2.7	0.9	23.6 ± 3.2	16.6 ± 2.9	7.7 ± 2.1
37–42	104	14	7	5	2	7.2	5.2	2.1	29.1 ± 3.6	20.9 ± 3.3	9.6 ± 2.5
43–48	83	10	3	1	0	3.8	1.3	0	31.9 ± 3.8	21.9 ± 3.4	9.6 ± 2.5
49–54	70	8	2	1	0	3.0	1.5	0	33.9 ± 3.9	23.1 ± 3.6	9.6 ± 2.5
55–60	60	7	6	3	1	10.6	5.5	1.9	40.9 ± 4.4	27.3 ± 4.1	13.0 ± 2.9
TOTALS			63	39	16						

* Probability (mean ± SE) of dying by the end of the period

vascular complications (23.9% of them from myocardial infarction), 15.5 per cent from infectious disease, 7.0 per cent from malignant disease and 15.5 per cent for other reasons (Table III).

TABLE III. Total deaths registered in nine years (January 1974 to December 1982) among 256 patients dialysed four hours thrice weekly with disposable square metre dialysers

	Males		Females		Total	
	Number	(%)	Number	(%)	Number	(%)
Number of deaths	44	(62.0)	27	(38.0)	71	
Mean age (years ± SD)	61.9 ± 11*		61.6 ± 15*		61.8 ± 12	
Mean time on dialysis (months ± SD)	30.3 ± 25*		29.7 ± 21*		30.1 ± 23	
Age distribution:						
≤34 years	1	(2.3)	3	(11.1)	4	(5.6)
35–54 years	10	(22.3)	3	(11.1)	13	(18.3)
≥55 years	33	(75.0)	21	(77.8)	54	(76.1)

* p = not significant

Death from myocardial infarction occurred in 17 patients; mean age 62.6 (range 34–77 years); mean blood pressure at start of HD was 121 ± 6, whereas on HD was 102 ± 12. Five of 17 patients recorded at least one previous episode of myocardial infarction. The interdialysis weight gain of this group was 3.1 per cent. Table IV presents the individual analysis of the clinical findings of this group.

Conclusion

In the most recent report of EDTA [13] short dialysis was indicated as responsible for a significant increase in mortality especially from myocardial infarction. To us, at present, the term short dialysis appears obsolete and ambiguous. In fact the duration of a dialysis session is just one step in a sophisticated approach to the therapy of uraemia. However, in the eighties we do not have any reason to go back to unmotivated modalities of treatment.

On the contrary it must be emphasised that an awareness that short dialysis was the right direction for treatment stimulated a continuous flow of studies to optimise both removal of small and larger molecular weight solutes. Until recently the goal of removing uraemic toxins had to face the dilemma of the choice between highly efficient dialysis and cardiovascular instability or a more

TABLE IV. Clinical findings of 17 dialysis patients who died from myocardial infarction

Patient	Age (years)	Sex	Duration of dialysis (months)	Cause of renal failure	Mean blood pressure at start of HD (mmHg)	Mean blood pressure on HD (mmHg)	Angina pectoris	Previous myocardial infarction	Interdialysis weight gain kg	%BW
1) RE	60	F	73	Pyelonephritis	119	90	Yes	No	2.0	2.9
2) RL	48	M	8	Pyelonephritis	115	93	No	No	2.1	2.0
3) SM	66	F	41	Pyelonephritis	121	92	Yes	No	1.6	3.4
4) CP	69	M	3	Pyelonephritis	118	112	Yes	Yes	1.4	1.9
5) CG	71	F	11	Pyelonephritis	119	106	No	No	2.4	4.5
6) GE	59	M	18	Nephroangiosclerosis	110	95	Yes	Yes	2.9	3.9
7) GO	67	M	32	Nephroangiosclerosis	123	110	Yes	No	2.7	3.5
8) MG	54	M	40	Nephroangiosclerosis	127	119	No	No	1.5	2.5
9) LE	53	M	23	Nephroangiosclerosis	125	118	Yes	Yes	2.9	3.5
10) GG	34	F	5	LES glomerulonephritis	129	109	No	No	1.4	2.9
11) BV	77	M	24	Glomerulonephritis	117	98	No	No	1.9	2.6
12) II	65	F	11	Glomerulonephritis	120	106	No	No	1.7	4.7
13) MM	67	M	25	Glomerulonephritis	119	97	Yes	Yes	3.4	5.5
14) FC	73	F	11	Diabetic nephropathy	127	102	No	No	1.9	2.3
15) PN	59	M	10	Diabetic nephropathy	125	121	Yes	No	1.5	2.5
16) SE	68	M	59	Cystic kidney disease	118	91	Yes	Yes	1.9	2.7
17) DL	74	M	27	Chronic renal failure, aetiology uncertain	123	105	Yes	No	1.0	2.0
M	62.6		24.8		122*	104*			2.0	3.1
SD	11		19		6	10			0.6	1

* p > 0.001

prolonged dialysis schedule. Today everybody agrees that attention must be paid to the removal of both small and middle molecules.

The optimal goal should be the greatest removal of uraemic toxins compatible with cardiovascular stability and performed in a limited period of time. These goals cannot be obtained either with traditional short dialysis (low SM removal) or with efficient short dialysis (cardiovascular instability). The presently much older dialysis population cannot be adequately treated with presently available highly efficient dialysers which greatly increases the problem of cardiovascular instability (Table V).

TABLE V. Logic steps in dialysis treatment

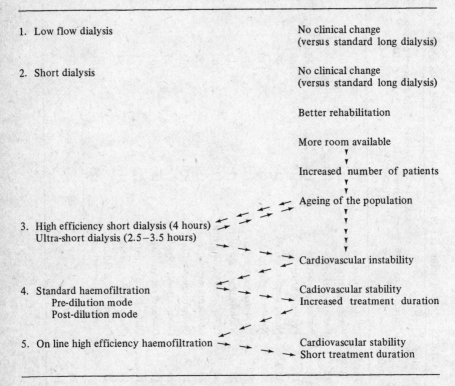

1. Low flow dialysis — No clinical change (versus standard long dialysis)

2. Short dialysis — No clinical change (versus standard long dialysis)

Better rehabilitation

More room available

Increased number of patients

Ageing of the population

3. High efficiency short dialysis (4 hours) / Ultra-short dialysis (2.5–3.5 hours)

Cardiovascular instability

4. Standard haemofiltration / Pre-dilution mode / Post-dilution mode — Cadiovascular stability / Increased treatment duration

5. On line high efficiency haemofiltration — Cardiovascular stability / Short treatment duration

In recent years a new equilibrium has been obtained with standard haemofiltration; unfortunately, once more, inefficient in removing SM unless the dialysis time and the amount of infusate are increased. Today technology seems capable of facing the new needs we have just analysed. Present studies conducted in our centre with high efficiency haemofiltration seem to confirm the possibility of obtaining within three to four hours of treatment adequate removal of both small and larger molecular weight solutes together with a cardiovascular stability superior to any of present modalities of similar efficiency.

References

1   Parsons FM, Brunner FP, Bruck HC et al. *Proc EDTA 1975; 11:* 3
2   Babb AL, Popovich RP, Christopher TG. *Trans ASAIO 1971; 17:* 81
3   Christopher TG, Cambi V, Harker LA. *Trans ASAIO 1971; 17:* 92
4   Cambi V, Dall'Aglio P, Savazzi G et al. *Proc EDTA 1972; 9:* 67
5   National Cooperative Dialysis Study. Lowrie EC, Laird NM, eds. *Kidney Int 1983; Suppl 13:* S1
6   Cutler SJ, Ederer F. *J Chronic Dis 1958; 8:* 699
7   Cox DR. *J R Stat Soc 1972; B34:* 187
8   Mantel N. *Cancer Chemother Rep 1966; 50:* 163
9   Cambi V, Arisi L, Buzio C et al. *Proc EDTA 1973; 10:* 342
10 Cambi V, Savazzi G, Arisi L et al. *Proc EDTA 1974; 11:* 112
11 Cambi V, Savazzi G, Arisi L et al. *Proc EDTA 1973; 10:* 271
12 Blackburn GL, Thornton PA. *Med Clin North Am 1979; 63:* 1103
13 Broyer M, Brunner FP, Brynger H et al. *Proc EDTA 1982; 19:* 2

LONG DIALYSIS: A REVIEW OF FIFTEEN YEARS EXPERIENCE IN ONE CENTRE 1968–1983

G Laurent, E Calemard, B Charra

Centre de Rein Artificiel, Tassin, France

Since 1961 it has been our policy to increase the dialysis time when a haemo-dialysis patient is not doing well. Technical progress has been made in dialyser design and in dialysis methods; however, it remains our conviction that longer dialysis is still the answer for the patients with problems. In the EDTA Registry annual report presented last year, long dialysis was defined as more than 13 hours dialysis weekly [1]. For the year 1977 the same Registry reported that only 6.2 per cent of centre patients and 11.7 per cent of home patients in Europe received more than 20 hours a week of treatment [2].

In Tassin, in 1983, all patients are still treated for more than 20 hours every week. In reviewing here our 15 years' experience with long dialysis our aim is to remind those who have forgotten it or to teach those who ignore it, the quality, the simplicity and the value of this good first method to which we remain faithful. We await valid reasons and strong evidence demonstrating the better quality of other treatment modalities.

Our cumulative experience with long dialysis consists of 3250 patient-treatment years with an unchanged technique. The total population was 373 patients with 233 presently on dialysis, 208 of them have been treated for more than one year. The residual renal function is less than 1ml per minute in all patients.

TABLE I. Long dialysis population. Age of patients at start of haemodialysis

Age groups	Number of patients	%
< 35	91	24.4
35–44	78	21.0
45–54	114	30.6
55+	90	24.0
Total*	373	100.0

* All patients admitted since 1968

Patients were equally distributed among four age groups (Table I) at the start of treatment. They are an unselected population. The important development of transplantation in our area has increased the mean age of the group: half of the present population is more than 55 years old. The distribution of primary renal disease shows no difference from that generally described (Table II).

TABLE II. Distribution of primary renal diseases – 1983

	N	% total
Chronic glomerulonephritis	81	34.8
Pyelonephritis/interstitial nephritis	28	12.0
Cystic kidney disease	30	12.9
Heredo-familial	28	12.0
Renal vascular	10	4.3
Multi-system	13	5.6
Other/unknown	43	18.4
Total	233	100.0

There are almost twice as many males as females. Fifty patients have dialysed for more than 10 years, 10 of them more than 15 years. Fifty-five per cent of the patients dialyse in the centre while 45 per cent do so at home or in a self-care unit. Thirty patients dialyse twice a week (for 10 or 12 hours) and have done so for more than 10 years. Nearly two-thirds of the sessions are performed overnight.

Diet is free with a liberal amount of protein but a low sodium intake is advocated. The only drugs widely used in our unit are for calcium and phosphorus control. We never transfuse and only three patients are on hypotensive drugs.

The main features of our experience is that our technique has remained unchanged since the beginning. We continue to use standard or multipoint Kiil Kidneys, reused only at home six times.

A central dialysate delivery system is used in the centre and our standard sodium is 140mmol/L. The individual equipment at home includes a programmable automatic cleansing and rinsing system, reducing the technical burden for the patients. They can set the day and hour when they propose starting their next dialysis session. We use continuous heparin infusion.

Ninety per cent of the patients use a fistula and when they are unable to have a fistula we prefer the Thomas shunt. Two patients have needled their own brachial artery for two and five years respectively. We have almost no need for vascular prostheses.

Dialysis duration is prolonged: 24hr weekly for the twice and 22hr for the thrice weekly group. We would like to explain the reasons for such a long time spent on dialysis every week.

An important point is the low intradialytic morbidity. We compared the

TABLE III. Intradialytic morbidity – Tassin vs Diaphane

| | Number of incidents per 1000 haemodialyses | | | |
| | Males | | Females | |
	Tassin	Diaphane	Tassin	Diaphane
Hypotension	34	174	79	277
Cramps	56	106	76	95
Vomiting	1	33	2	65
Headache	2	29	2	30
Mean dialyses duration/week	24.1	14.0	23.4	12.9
(hours ± haemodialysis)	(±1.0)	(±3.1)	(±1.9)	(±2.6)

frequency of major incidents arising during dialysis with data of a French dialysis registry (Diaphane) (Table III). Hypotension, headache and vomiting are much less frequent during our long dialysis schedule.

Our study was performed on hospital dialysis patients but we know that during home dialysis incidents are exceptional. We think that this is due to smoothness of slow long dialysis and in these conditions time has not the same value.

Post-dialysis tiredness is mild, most patients after treatment have a quick breakfast and then drive their own car to their work. Sleep can be a problem with long dialysis but our visitors are often surprised to see that everybody is sleeping in the dialysis ward, sometimes even the two nurses taking care of the 18 patients are also asleep! A survey on quality of sleep has been performed to which 236 patients responded. Mean duration of sleep was estimated at eight hours nightly for daytime dialysis patients and a mean of 6.5 hours for the dialysis night of overnight dialysis patients. Eighty-six per cent of overnight patients are satisfied with their dialysis schedule.

Comfortable sessions help the patients to come to the treatment without anxiety; this is what we call *non-emotional* dialysis. This also allows *them* to take charge of their own treatment which is very important in our philosophy. More than half of centre patients and all home patients insert their own needles, most of them prepare their equipment, perform their tests, set their heparin pump and connect themselves to the artificial kidney machine. Many disconnect themselves at the end of the session.

We established a six point scale to estimate the degree of independence of our centre patients. Criteria for assessing patient's independence in conducting their treatment were:

    Self needling
    Self care for starting haemodialysis
    Self care for discontinuing haemodialysis
    Self estimation of adequate transmembrane pressure
    Trouble shooting ability
    Knowledge of own biological data

More than half of them score positive for four or more of these criteria. The natural choice for independence is of course home dialysis wherever possible.

Another interesting feature in our experience is that in spite of long-term treatment very few blood access problems arise in our population. After 12 years 50 per cent of the fistulas are still in use. We think there are several reasons for that:

1. The high incidence of self-needling

2. Our particular technique of always using the same puncture site for each needle (some patients have used the same site for 14 or 15 years)

3. The length of dialysis allows for correct solute removal even with a modest fistula blood flow.

The long-term acceptance of the programme is good, dialysis patients are generally lively and active. Morbidity is low; in 1982, 40 per cent of the patients did not need hospitalisation, 27 per cent were hospitalised for less than eight days. The mean hospitalisation time for the population as a whole was 9.7 days/ year including all medical and surgical problems. Altogether this allowed for a better rehabilitation which we evaluated according to the classes defined by our association. Eighty-three per cent of the home patients and 47 per cent of the hospital patients are back to work.

Until recently, very few patients asked for transplantation as they were satisfied that dialysis provided them with a good physical and psychological condition, and no damage appeared with time. Unfortunately, a new event changed our and their attitude and that is the appearance of the carpal tunnel syndrome after 10 or 15 years of treatment. It was observed in 73 patients, 42 of them were operated on, the mean time between the start of haemodialysis and surgery was 12.6 years. In 75 per cent of these cases a very disabling scapular periarthritis of the shoulder has been observed. Among the patients operated on we found amyloid deposition in 83 per cent. This new pathology is probably not linked to long dialysis *per se* but reduces presently our optimism about dialysis for more than 10 or 15 years. Today, we tend to recommend transplantation to our younger patients. Transplant team psychologists are generally quite surprised to record the demand for transplantation of these patients dialysing for more than 10 years, satisfied with the method with good rehabilitation but distressed by the shoulder pain they experience or fear for. This change of policy is due exclusively to the appearance of this painful complication and not to dialysis intolerance.

We cannot skip the classical complications of dialysis and we will say a few words about it. No clinical motor neuropathy has ever appeared in our 3250 patient-years experience. We have had to care for eight patients coming from other units with severe neuropathy: five were paraplegic, three tetraplegic. They have all improved with an increased protein intake combined to long dialysis treatment.

We have observed three episodes of pericarditis which all recovered after serious fluid removal. No pulmonary oedema has been seen.

The control of anaemia has been obtained without blood transfusion. Patients treated for more than one year have a mean haematocrit of about 30. Twenty-six patients constitute a low haematocrit group with a female predominance (19/26) and four of the nine anephric patients. Twenty-seven patients have a high haematocrit including 10 with polycystic kidney disease and only four females.

The mean interdialytic weight gain is less than 2kg. Patients do not complain of thirst. Thirty patients have a weight gain of less than 1kg, their blood pressure is slightly lower than the general mean. Thirty patients (almost all males) gain more than 3kg; their blood pressure is not significantly different from the mean. Generally speaking weight gain is not a problem with long dialysis and we do not need to give dietary restriction. Long dialysis allows for a very complete and easy fluid removal, enabling control of the extracellular volume and the avoidance of hypertension. The mean blood pressure of our patients is 134/80; a hypotensive group includes 17 patients, mostly women, with a mean blood pressure of 86/50. The hypertensive group includes four patients, three of them being the only patients taking blood pressure medication. This good blood pressure control seems to be a most important point for the long-term patient survival.

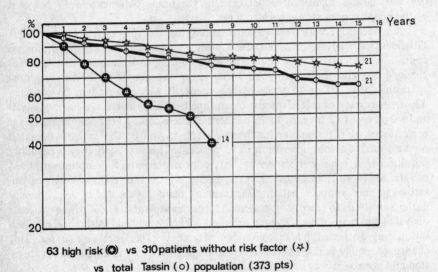

63 high risk (◉) vs 310 patients without risk factor (✰)

vs total Tassin (o) population (373 pts)

Figure 1. Cumulative patient survival

The overall survival of 373 patients treated since the beginning is 75 per cent at 10 years and 65 per cent at 15 years (Figure 1). If we exclude the 63 high-risk patients because of their initial disease (15 diabetes mellitus, 15 systemic disease 7 malignant disease) or their preceding vascular history (angina and/or myocardial infarction 17, cerebrovascular accident 11, arthritis 4), the survival of these patients is only 50 per cent after seven years of treatment, whereas

126

the other 310 patients without high risk factors have a 75 per cent survival rate at 15 years.

Curiously, the different age groups do not show important differences in terms of survival except for patients starting dialysis treatment before 35 years of age. This group of 91 patients has an actuarial survival rate of 93 per cent at 15 years.

The annual death rate of 2.3 per cent was compared with EDTA data for the year 1978 for 1000 patients at risk (Table IV) [3]. The difference is in

TABLE IV. Annual death rate per 1000 patients at risk according to cause – patients on haemodialysis, all ages

Causes of death*	EDTA 1978	Tassin† 1968–1983
Cardiovascular deaths	70.5	8.7
Infection	14.5	4.0
Malignant diseases	6.6	1.9
Therapy ceased/suicide	3.3	1.9
Other/unknown	14.1	6.8

* According to EDTA classification
† Based on 3213 patient-treatment years

the cardiovascular mortality about 10-fold *less* in our experience. Infection and malignant disease also appear less frequently as a cause of death in our group. Can we believe that these differences are primarily due to long dialysis which allows for good blood pressure control, a free diet and a physical condition not far from normal?

The overall number of deaths was 75: nine were due to myocardial infarction, seven of them occurred in diabetic patients.

Let us compare the mortality in the year 1981 for patients alive at January 1 (Figure 2) using the same presentation as at the last meeting in Madrid [1]. The difference in mortality rate between short and long dialysis becomes obvious with the extra long dialysis. We had no myocardial infarction this year and the general mortality was the same rate as in our overall experience.

One question arises from our experience: is long dialysis an efficient prevention of cardiovascular complications observed in long-term haemodialysed patients? If it is so, why should we switch to short dialysis?

Anyway, no medical advantage seems to derive from such a change; of course, most patients have heard about shorter dialysis schedules and ask questions about it, but when they are able to perform dialysis during the night they prefer a method free of intradialytic complications which provides them with good physical status. We rather often receive demands from patients to be accepted in our centre for longer sessions or asking us how they could get longer schedules in their own units. We have frequently had the opportunity to treat patients coming from a short dialysis programme and to observe that within a few weeks

127

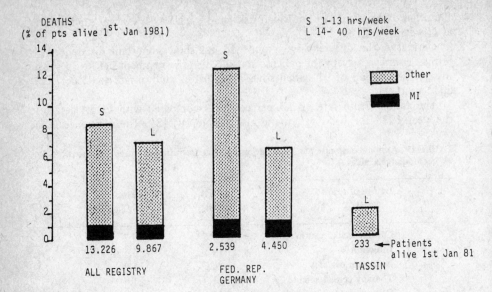

Figure 2. Deaths due to myocardial infarction (MI) and other causes in patients on haemodialysis during 1981 in relation to time on dialysis

the haematocrit rises and the blood pressure comes to normal so that blood
pressure medication can be discontinued.

The administrative regulations limiting the number of available stations
dictated the trend towards shorter dialysis. We think it is important to draw
attention to long dialysis from a purely medical standpoint and to reflect on
the real choice.

Dialysis costs are clearly important. For those who fear that long dialysis
could be more expensive, suffice it to say that our running cost is the lowest in
our country. Rehabilitation means economy, home dialysis is less expensive,
and non-emotional dialysis is a strong argument towards home dialysis (50 per
cent in our case when the national mean is 18 per cent). Low morbidity and
hospitalisation rate save money as well as the lower requirements for medications and routine biochemical tests.

In addition the 13 per cent of patients dialysing only twice a week cost less
to society.

The long soft dialysis has remained the only dialysis technique used at our
centre. The main reasons for this consistent policy have been:

A low intradialytic morbidity resulting in non-emotional comfortable
haemodialysis

Easy control of extracellular volume and blood pressure without hypotensive drugs

Excellent long-term survival

Our overall experience was characterised by a low mortality (75 deaths in

128

373 patients). Cardiovascular accidents accounted for only 33.3 per cent of all deaths compared to 70.6 per cent of all deaths among home haemodialysis patients [1].

References

1 Broyer M, Brunner FP, Brynger H et al. *Proc EDTA 1982; 19:* 2
2 Wing AJ, Brunner FP, Brynger H et al. *Proc EDTA 1978; 15:* 4
3 Brunner FP, Brynger H, Chantler C et al. *Proc EDTA 1979; 16:* 2

Open Discussion

MION (Chairman) Thank you very much Dr Laurent for your very nice presentation of this unique experience: you are a true exponent of long dialysis and I think that nobody can challenge you in this field. Now both our presenters have stimulated your minds and I hope there are many questions for discussion.

BAILLOD (Chairman) I would like to put one question to both the speakers because I really thought that in working out the quality of dialysis they might mention the problem of parathyroid hormone and whether they needed to perform more parathyroidectomies and whether they could control calcium and phosphate adequately? I would like each speaker to comment on this.

CAMBI Parathyroidectomy was undertaken in 14 per cent of all patients treated in the last nine years. We have checked the dietary intake of phosphate in our cases and we try not to exceed 600—800mg daily. Following the suggestion of the Fournier group, who presented a paper last year at EDTA* we have been substituting calcium carbonate and we are actually eliminating the use of aluminium hydroxide.

LAURENT We have undertaken about 70 parathyroidectomies in our group of patients. We have some patients starting their treatment before 1963 and at that time we did not know how to manage phosphate and calcium. Many patients use phosphate-binders; we have no problems with the long-term intake of aluminium.

NUBÉ (Alkmaar) We have heard this morning about short dialysis and long dialysis, but everyone knows we are using many artificial kidneys with many different clearances. Would it not be better to talk about clearance of solutes per week, instead of the dialysis time?

CAMBI That is an important question, and I do not know the answer. Actually we underline that short dialysis is a word that at present is without meaning and there are other qays of quantifying the dialysis treatment. The title of this session was "Short or Long Dialysis" because the EDTA statistics show an

* Moriniere Ph, Roussel A, Tahiri Y et al. *Proc EDTA 1982; 19:* 784

increased myocardial mortality with short dialysis. I would like to add that my presentation on short dialysis would have been totally different without the failure of the computer facility of the EDTA Registry. I think that it is almost useless to present some statistics about our own population when there are enormous differences in the ages of our patients. How can you evaluate a group of patients over 70 years old dying of myocardial infarction? That is the reason we are considering the possibility of starting again this study by comparing groups of patients selected from the EDTA Registry.

AHMED (Liverpool) I have reduced the hours of dialysis, just out of mercy, in two of our long-term overnight home dialysis patients who had undergone long hours of dialysis. They came back to say that they felt so awful that they wanted to go back to long hours of dialysis. We have also seen the carpal tunnel syndrome in the non-fistula arm. Can I ask Dr Laurent whether he has seen the carpal tunnel syndrome in the contralateral arm to the fistula?

LAURENT We have not seen any relation to the fistula. Some patients had their first carpal tunnel symptoms in the other arm to the fistula and they have never had vascular surgery on that side.

DRUEKE (Paris) I doubt that the assessment of motor nerve conduction velocity alone is a good means of evaluating clinically important uraemic poly-neuritis. I would like to ask Dr Cambi in how many patients did he consider increasing dialysis time, dialyser surface area or both in order to correct or to improve clinically important polyneuritis?

CAMBI In the last 12 years we have never seen a single case of polyneuritis. We have seen a group of patients, independent of dialysis treatment, deteriorating without developing the clinical signs of polyneuritis and then stabilising over four years. At the beginning, in the early 70s, we did change between long and short dialysis but we did not find any difference.

DRUEKE This is very different from our personal experience, and we do not dialyse for shorter times or with smaller surfaces than you. We continue to see cases every year of clinically important, but minor, forms of polyneuritis.

WALLS (Leicester) I think we would all congratulate Dr Laurent on his very low incidence of cardiovascular mortality. He must have a unique experience in exposing his patients to greater amounts of acetate in the dialysate than anybody else in the world. I wonder if he would like to make any comment about the longitudinal lipid studies that he might have done in his patients to see whether we are chasing an epiphenomenon or not or whether this is concerned in the cardiovascular mortality?

LAURENT We did not find any change in the lipids in our patients. We had mean values after five, 10 and 15 years and the values were the same. We always use acetate in all our patients.

KERR (Newcastle upon Tyne) Both authors have presented such wonderful results that I wish we could achieve the same. It suggests to me that perhaps the physician has more influence than the duration of dialysis, but I would like to ask one question of Professor Laurent and one of Professor Cambi. Your results, Professor Laurent, with fistula survival are extraordinarily good in spite of needling in the same place, which in our patients often seems to produce aneurysm; we also have a substantial incidence of excessive fistula flow. Are you using an end-to-side, a side-to-side fistula or some modification that allows your fistulas to survive so long? My question to Professor Cambi: you said that your schedule was so designed that middle molecular clearance must be poor, but I wonder whether that takes account of the recent recognition that middle molecules are largely confined to extracellular space which should make quite short dialysis adequate in removing them?

LAURENT We do assess the fistula and they are side-to-side. I think that one point is that our patients are not hypertensive and this is important for the survival of fistula. We have not seen any aneurysm and the technique of the same site puncture is chosen for the comfort of the patients and to make home dialysis more easy. It is very easy to put the needles always in the same place as there is a channel for insertion and we have not seen aneurysm formation.

CAMBI I cannot answer Professor Kerr's questions because I think that we have now to follow a different philosophy because now we know that all retained solutes may be toxic. We have to remove them in a way different to that of 12 to 15 years ago. I am not sure that we can state that middle molecules are confined to the extracellular space. We do not know the target of these toxins. I think that the only thing we can say is that we have to remove as many as possible without cardiovascular instability.

ELIAHOU (Tel-Aviv) I think that Professor Laurent has a very unique experience which should not be ignored, but it lacks intra-institutional controlled comparison. May I suggest that Professor Laurent switches his patients to six to 10 hours weekly, i.e. half their present time, for the next two years and then reports the outcome to us?

LAURENT I apologise, but I think that my patients would never accept that.

BARTOVA (Prague) You have mentioned the carpal tunnel syndrome from amyloid deposition. Have you come across any other complication from amyloid deposition in the patients treated by long hours dialysis?

LAURENT Yes, as I mentioned we have seen shoulder pains and we have two cases of bone disease due to amyloid deposition.

RONCO (Vicenza) I would like some information about the diet of Professor Cambi's patients. We have to deal with a system in which, in association with a rapid removal of solutes, we have a 24-hour production. Do you not think that the first condition in planning a short dialysis schedule should be a metabolic control to obtain a constant positive nitrogen balance?

CAMBI Of course short dialysis is totally unphysiological while CAPD is very physiological: there is no question that normal urinary function is even better. What we conclude from the metabolic studies we performed, but did not present, is that these patients have a normal nitrogen balance and they are not wasting. Why should we increase the dialysis time, especially when we have the chance of avoiding cardiovascular instability during the course of treatments. I am wondering if it is really correct only to concentrate our attention about dialysis and cardiovascular instability, because in order to do that we should have clean statistics. We should clean the statistics of EDTA that last year presented patients treated for 1—13hr/week and for 14—40hr/week and also this year they are considering patients between 8—12hr/week. This can be done, but the other point is that if dialysis is adequate in social terms and in terms of cost I would like to ask the long dialysis people how many patients per million are being treated: if you are able to treat 500 patients per million I am happy.

LAURENT I think that one point with long dialysis is that it is the most easy way to establish patients on home dialysis. If you want to treat many patients per million I think it is very important to have a very easy method of converting them to home treatment.

ZAZGORNIK (Vienna) What was the frequency of uraemic pericarditis in your patients on short and long dialysis treatment?

CAMBI Unfortunately I do not have any figures, but what we notice is that sometimes there are epidemics of pericarditis, maybe once every two or three years. I think this is probably virus dependent and not dialysis dependent, but this does not worry us as much as clinical neuropathy.

LAURENT I reported in my paper that for the 3,000 patient-years experienced we have had three episodes of pericarditis.

PAPADIMITRIOU (Thessalonika) If I understand Dr Laurent correctly, 10 per cent of your deaths are due to car accidents. If this is right, do you have autopsies from these patients as some of your patients who died during the car accident may have had a myocardial infarction immediately before.

LAURENT No, in many cases they were not themselves driving and they were involved in very big accidents. I think it is because patients are travelling for many kilometres to go to the Unit. The statistics of Insurance Companies show that there is one death every million kilometres. We calculated the number of kilometres for the patients to come to the Unit was eight million kilometres. We are, therefore, in the statistics of kilometres.

CAMBI You are saying that they are travelling many kilometres. Isn't this an indication of inadequate facilities because of long dialysis hours? Once again, how many patients per million are you treating in your area?

LAURENT In our area there are many patients treated, because we started with Professor Traeger in 1960 the treatment by dialysis for chronic patients. At the beginning there were no dialysis facilities in a very large area and some patients came from 200 or 300 kilometres away. Some for personal reasons could not have home dialysis.

NAGA (Alexandria) Could I ask about the incidence of pruritus during short term dialysis and the best way of management?

CAMBI Pruritis is a problem associated with hyperparathyroidism, and we noticed that only some of the patients with secondary hyperparathyroidism presented with pruritus. Of course pruritus may also be iatrogenic if we make mistakes with Vitamin D therapy, but I cannot give you numbers.

LAURENT Pruritus was a reason for increasing dialysis in some patients. I think pruritus due to hyperparathyroidism is very different to the pruritus of insufficient dialysis. When symptoms occur in the warmth and during the night in bed we increase dialysis and the symptoms improve.

WAUTERS (Lausanne) I would like to ask Dr Cambi on which data is based his statement that three times four hourly is adequate and three times three hourly inadequate treatment?

CAMBI We noticed, only on a clinical basis, that the majority, I will say 100 per cent, were in a safe condition considering the result in terms of survival with four hours. I stress once again that talking about timing in 1983 is totally meaningless because we have to talk about several other problems related to the removal and to the treatment. I totally agree that we may reach different dialysis duration but also with different modalities of treatment.

FUNCK-BRENTANO (Paris) I wonder if the actual challenge is between short dialysis or long dialysis. I believe that the real challenge is between good dialysis and bad dialysis. It might be easier to promote a good dialysis with a long procedure because all the changes are going slowly. This does not mean that short dialysis cannot be good. General comparisons between the two methods are in fact inadequate. Each method must be adjusted according to the patient's will and benefit. Each method has to be tested in terms of medical adequacy and economical adequacy. So the results might be different in different countries.

SODENSTROM (Stockholm) I wonder how many of your patients used single needle versus double needle monitors?

CAMBI No, we do not regularly use single needles. We are very perplexed con-

133

sidering what type of renal substitution treatment we are going to follow. We anticipated that we would need a high blood flow, much higher than 300ml/min and the problems of recirculation with single needles may be very dangerous associated with short dialysis.

LAURENT We never use single needle systems.

BAILLOD I would like to make a comment about the fact that Dr Laurent has introduced a problem that I think people who have had patients on dialysis for 15 years plus must be getting very worried about. It is the problem of the carpal tunnel syndrome followed by the shoulder joint pains followed by the stiffening hands and patients with low blood pressures, all of which may be due to amyloid. Although when I have asked our histologist to prove amyloid they have not always been able to do so. I think that this is an area that unfortunately Professor Cambi did not talk about: patients in the 15 year group with this problem. Perhaps later on we will know whether short dialysis avoids this problem. It is not so much the mortality and the death of patients but the morbidity that these patients have to live with when they are untransplantable. This is painful for them and for us to observe.

MION I think that this is a very important comment.

BRYNGER (Göteborg) Patients are very different in protein intake and body-weight. Do you consider this in using different dialyser clearances or blood flows?

CAMBI This is another difficult question to answer, because we can just say that they are in a steady state and that means that the balance between what they need and their intake is correct. The protein intake of my patients is around 1 gram per kilogram body weight.

FIRBANK (Belgium) When comparing short and long dialysis schedules I think it could be important to know the patient's residual renal clearance. Professor Laurent mentioned it was less than 1ml per minute. Perhaps I missed it, but could I ask Professor Cambi for his data on that point?

CAMBI Yes. I did not mention this because I thought it was clear that after 12 years 90 to 95 per cent of the patients are almost anuric.

WIZEMANN (Giessen) We have identified overhydration as a major risk for coronary perfusion. I would like to ask both speakers what are the weight gains of your patients in the interval between dialyses?

LAURENT I would say that weight gain between dialyses was a mean of 2kg with 30 patients having less than 1kg and 30 patients with more than 3kg.

CAMBI We just evaluated and presented this morning the interval weight gain in the patients dying from myocardial infarction and this was 3.1 per cent.

ANDREUCCI (Naples) Our patients are always asking for shorter dialysis, so I think that it is not only the problem with the patients whether they want a long dialysis, as Guy Laurent is saying, or a short dialysis: it depends on the doctor. If the doctor suggests a short dialysis they will do even shorter and shorter as they are always asking for shorter dialysis. I am sure that even if most of the participants listening to this discussion seem to be close to what Dr Laurent is saying, I think that most of the people here are using schedules similar to those of Dr Cambi.

LAURENT We must always believe in what we do.

SHORT HAEMODIALYSIS LONG-TERM RESULTS

J P Wauters, S Pansiot, J D Horisberger

University Hospital, Lausanne, Switzerland

Introduction

During the past few years haemodialysis treatment schedules of end-stage renal failure have been progressively shortened: 3 x 5 hours per week is at present the most widely used schedule [1]. Last year however Kramer et al questioned the long-term safety of short haemodialysis (SHD) since an increased cardio-vascular mortality was reported in females and in males aged more than 55 when dialysed for 3 x 4 hours per week or less [2]. Since 1976 all patients in our unit underwent a 3 x 3 hours per week haemodialysis treatment which was adapted individually according to clinical and biochemical criteria. The present report analyses the results obtained six years after the introduction of this programme.

Patients and methods

Fifty-eight patients aged 22 to 71 years at start of treatment (mean 52 years) were treated for more than three years with SHD. Residual renal function estimated by creatinine clearance was less than 5ml/min, at the start of treatment. A diet containing 1g/kg/day of protein was prescribed. Dialysis schedules were adapted in order to maintain a stable clinical status and pre-dialysis blood values below 30mmol/L for urea and 1200μmol/L for creatinine. High efficiency dialysers, exclusively capillary filters, were used. Blood flow in the extra-corporeal circuit was between 250 and 300ml per minute, dialysate flow was at 500ml per minute. Dialyser re-use was practised following standard re-use methods [3].

Results

The clinical and biochemical results observed in the 58 patients are summarised in Table I. It appears that when compared to 0.5 yr of SHD the results at three, five and six years do not show any significant change in the parameters usually used to assess clinically the adequacy of dialysis therapy i.e. blood pressure,

TABLE I. Long-term results observed in 58 patients treated by short haemodialysis

Yr	n	Blood pressure mmHg	Urea mmol/L	Creatinine μmol/L	Ht vol %	MNCV m/sec	Treatment time hrs/week
0.5	58	148±4/84±2	28±1	1015±32	24±0.8	50±2	9.15±2.41
3	58	155±3/86±2	29±1	1082±24	25±0.8	47±1	8.63±1.25
5	34	149±4/87±2	30±1	1116±32	29±1.4	45±1	9.15±1.22
6	11	138±5/77±4	28±2	1177±67	30±2.7	48±2	9.25±1.47

(Mean ± SE); n = number

blood urea, creatinine and haematocrit values, motor nerve conduction velocity, as well as serum Ca, P and alkaline phosphatase.

Two subgroups of patients were analysed depending on the time they had started dialysis therapy.

1. A subgroup of 44 patients had been exclusively treated with SHD for at least three years. As shown in Table II, no significant differences were observed between six months after the start of haemodialysis and five or six years after the start of haemodialysis, in weight, blood pressure, blood urea and creatinine values both pre- and post-dialysis. After five years of SHD, serum creatinine was 1112 ± 178μmol/L pre- and 577 ± 98μmol/L post-dialysis. Calcium, phosphate and alkaline phosphatase could be maintained at near normal values by the long-term prescription of aluminium hydroxide to every patient and by vitamin D substitution in most of them. During this period no parathyroidectomy had to be performed. The haematocrit values tended to increase while motor nerve conduction velocity measured on the sciatic popliteal nerve remained within the normal limits.

TABLE II. Long-term results in 44 patients treated exclusively by short haemodialysis

Yr	Blood pressure mmHg	Urea mmol/L	Creatinine μmol/L	Calcium mmol/L	P mmol/L	Alk. Phosph. IU/L	Ht vol %	MNCV m/sec
0.5	148±21/84±11	27.8±5.7	1014±201	2.26±0.19	1.63±0.53	42±22	24±5	50±8
3	152±24/83±12	28.6±7.2	1056±174	2.27±0.29	1.85±0.61	50±29	25±6	47±7
5	153±24/86±13	30.9±7.4	1112±178	2.32±0.30	1.84±0.40	42±21	27±8	45±6
6	137±16/82±12	30.0±8.8	1181±251	2.28±0.42	1.50±0.40	44±27	26±9	46±8

(Mean ± SE)

2. Fourteen patients had been treated first with long haemodialysis for periods ranging from one to six years (mean 3.2 yrs) and subsequently with SHD. When the results obtained at the end of the long dialysis schedule were compared with the results obtained after five to six years of SHD it appears that blood urea and

creatinine levels pre- and post-dialysis remained within the usual limits (Table III). A diminution of patient weight, an increase in motor nerve conduction velocity and an increase in haematocrit values were observed. The potassium fluctuations were decreased by the use of a dialysate containing 2mmol/L potassium and the liberal use of potassium exchanging resins. Fluctuations of phosphate increased while those of calcium decreased with the use of less calcium in the dialysate.

TABLE III. Comparison of values obtained in 14 patients at the end of 3 x 5 hrs/week haemodialysis and after five or six years short haemodialysis

	Long haemodialysis			Short haemodialysis		
BP (mmHg)	147 ±	22/88	± 13	142 ±	25/86 ±	12
Urea (mmol/L)	28 ±	6		28 ±	5	
Creatinine (μmol/L)	1302 ±	292		1142 ±	201	
Calcium (mmol/L)	2.39 ±	0.23		2.50 ±	0.38	
P (mmol/L)	1.51 ±	0.58		1.65 ±	0.46	
Alk. Phosph. (IU/L)	38 ±	34		54 ±	25	
Ht (vol %)	25.5 ±	6		32.6 ±	7	
MNCV (m/sec)	44 ±	4		47 ±	5	

(Mean ± SE)

The mortality among the 58 patients treated for at least three years with SHD was also analysed. Seven patients died during the six years observation period, which represents 12 per cent: two patients died of cardiovascular events. Four hospitalisations were needed for problems directly related to the dialysis sessions: disequilibrium syndrome in two cases and haemolytic episodes in two cases. Nine patients were transferred to other treatment modalities, renal transplantation or CAPD.

Discussion

The increased individual, social and professional rehabilitation which can be obtained with shorter dialysis schedules prompted us six years ago to adapt the patients treated by haemodialysis in our unit to a 3 x 3 hrs/week treatment programme. Mid-week pre-dialysis values of 30mmol/L for blood urea and 1200μmol/L for plasma creatinine were taken as the upper acceptable limits. In a multicentre study, Lowry et al showed however that when short haemodialysis

141

is applied, blood urea values of 40mmol/L were associated with increased morbidity [4]. Therefore short dialysis should be performed with very efficient dialysers and high blood flow.

Using this approach at six years no prejudicial effect can be detected clinically or biochemically. The mortality in particular of cardiovascular origin remained comparable to that described with longer schedules.

Conclusion

In 58 haemodialysed patients treated 3 x 3 hours per week for more than three years, it appears that SHD:

1. May be safely applied for at least six years;

2. Maintain biological values within the expected limits, provided efficient dialysers and high blood flows are used;

3. Has a mortality and morbidity comparable to those of longer treatment schedules;

4. Is preferred by the patients.

References

1   Brynger H, Brunner FP, Chantler C et al. *Proc EDTA 1980; 17:* 63
2   Kramer P, Broyer M, Brunner FP et al. *Proc EDTA 1982; 19:* 2
3   Wauters JP, Brunner HR, Boudry JF. *Artif Organs 1978; 2:* 373
4   Parker TF, Laird NM, Lowrie EG. *Kidney Int 1983; 23:* S42

Open Discussion

KLINKMANN (Chairman)   How often did you re-use your dialysers and did you see any adverse effect of re-use during short haemodialysis?

WAUTERS   The re-use methods we used were classical. We re-use hollow fibre kidneys, as published previously, by passing decalcified water through the blood compartment and storing the filters with formalin. There is nothing very difficult about this. The creatinine clearances measured after three uses of the filter did not show a significant change. At the present time the only check for good re-use is visual checking; we don't routinely perform blood clearance determinations.

PARSONS (London)   Have you not changed your dialysers at all over this long period of time? What matters is the physics of the clearance either of low molecular or middle weight molecular substances. We all know that time is not what matters, it's the efficacy of the dialyser that matters. I would be surprised to find that you have not changed your dialyser over six years. The other interesting point is the residual function of your patients. You said the mean or the mode was 5ml per minute and that gives you 7 litres of GFR daily

142

and you are adding, by your dialysis, something in the order of 10 litres a day. You are not really adding a great deal to your dialysis efficiency and I would suspect that some of your patients have clearances in excess of 5ml per minute and this may be why these patients are doing extremely well.

WAUTERS Concerning the dialyser we have chosen, we have, during the six year period, systematically opted for high efficiency capillary dialysers. First we used the CF 15.00 (Travenol) or C-DAK® 2.5 (Cordis-Dow) and now we treat mostly with the CF 15.11 (Travenol), and we measured the clearances in vivo for urea and creatinine, and as I mentioned we have, at a blood flow of 300ml/min a clearance of 182ml/min for urea and a clearance for creatinine at 157ml/min.

PARSONS You had dialysers that cleared at 182ml/min at the beginning and 182ml/min at the end of your six-year study?

WAUTERS Yes, and this is reflected by the fact that our mean dialysis treatment time per week in fact decreased during the six years. Among our sub group of 32 patients, they were treated 10 hours per week at the beginning, now they are treated nine hours per week.

WIZEMANN (Giessen) When we performed ultrashort haemodiafiltration for two hours three times a week for a period of over 15 months we had no problems with uraemic control compared with conventional haemodialysis. Would you agree that the pitfalls of ultrashort treatment lie in cardiovascular stability? What do you do with patients who suffer from symptomatic hypotension and what proportion of your patients suffer from symptomatic hypotension?

WAUTERS Symptomatic hypotension is certainly a problem during short haemodialysis. I think that by choosing different blood lines and filters this can be prevented in many cases; in the few cases where it appears frequently we change to bicarbonate dialysis.

COMTY (Minneapolis) Have you made an assessment of nutrition in these patients? Serum urea and creatinine values can be notoriously misleading in the long term patient as evidence of adequate dialysis. If he is not eating because of anorexia or too strict a diet he may have low serum creatinine values because of loss of muscle mass and a low urea value because of a low urea generation rate. You did not mention serum values of your patients.

WAUTERS We have the assistance of a dietitian. Patients are instructed to eat 1g per kg per day of protein and we calculated for our centre patients a protein catabolic rate which was about 1g per kg per day, which is the usual measured value in dialysis patients.

CLINICAL EVALUATION OF A NEW THROMBIN INHIBITOR AVAILABLE FOR HAEMODIALYSIS

K Ota, H Kawaguchi, S Nakagawa*, S Koshikawa†, K Maeda‡, N Matsui§, Y Hirasawa¶, T Sasaoka★

Tokyo Women's Medical College, *Tokyo Medical and Dental University, †Showa University Fujigaoka Hospital, ‡Nagoya University Branch Hospital, § Tsuchiura Kyodo Hospital, ¶ Shinrakuen Hospital, and ★Yokosuka Kyosai Hospital, Japan

Summary

A new thrombin inhibitor MD-805 was synthesised and used for clinical haemodialysis instead of heparin. It effectively prevented clotting even in the absence of antithrombin III (AT III). The serum triglyceride concentration decreased with concomitant elevation of free fatty acid concentration during heparin dialysis, while these remained almost unchanged during dialysis using MD-805. The predialysis concentration of AT III four weeks after changing from heparin to MD-805 was significantly increased. No serious systemic and local complications were encountered. MD-805 appears to be a promising anticoagulant applicable to haemodialysis.

Introduction

Heparin has been widely used as the anticoagulant for haemodialysis. It is well known, however, that the drug has inherent side effects on lipid and bone metabolism. A completely new anticoagulant, tentatively called MD-805 has been synthesised [1] and evaluated clinically. This report is a summary of a study carried out in six dialysis centres.

Materials and methods

The drug, MD-805, is a thrombin inhibitor which has arginine in its molecular structure (Figure 1). The mechanism of anticoagulation lies in the fact that the drug has a higher affinity to thrombin than does fibrinogen, formation of fibrin is inhibited even in the absence of antithrombin III. The drug is metabolised by the liver and excreted mainly through the biliary tract. The half life is calculated to be less than 30 mintues.

144

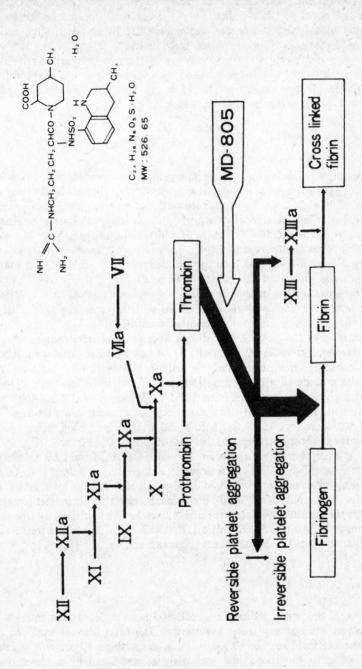

Figure 1. Molecular structure and sites of action of MD-805

145

The drug was infused to the arterial line at 25mg/hour during dialysis and was discontinued either at the termination of dialysis or 30 minutes prior to the termination of dialysis. The dosage was modified to fit each individual patient depending on the residual blood volume in the dialyser.

Fifty-one patients were studied, 21 males and 30 females (average weight 50kg). For these patients the anticoagulant used for haemodialysis was changed from heparin to MD-805 and maintained for 12 weeks. Data obtained were compared with those of previous regular heparin dialysis.

Results

Haemodialysis was carried out successfully in all cases using MD-805. No serious side effects were observed in any of these cases, although the use of the drug was discontinued in eight cases for various reasons, such as: prolongation of bleeding at puncture sites, aggravation of haemorrhoidal bleeding, palpitation, headache, and elevation of transaminase. Changes of white blood cell, and platelet counts were similar to those observed in dialysis using heparin. However, pO_2 showed a significant elevation compared with heparin dialysis. The residual blood volume in dialysers was greater in the inductive phase of this study. It was, however, reduced by adjusting the dosage of infusion. Reduction rates of urea, creatinine and uric acid were similar to those obtained with heparin dialysis. Predialysis values of these nitrogen compounds remained unchanged.

Examination of the clotting time during dialysis using various methods such as KCT, Hepaquick, ACT, PT, and APTT revealed a similar prolongation compared to those obtained during heparin dialysis. However, using the Lee-White method the prolongation of clotting time was found to be less with MD-805.

Serum triglycerides decreased from 167.7 ± 73.9mg/dl to 104.8 ± 46.9mg/dl ($p < 0.01$), with a concomitant rise in free fatty acids from 0.656 ± 0.682mEq/L to 1.077 ± 0.646mEq/L ($p < 0.01$) before and after dialysis using heparin, while these remained almost unchanged in dialysis using MD-805 (Figure 2).

With the exception of antithrombin III which elevated from 22.9 ± 4.8mg/dl to 24.5 ± 5.6mg/dl ($p < 0.01$) at four weeks and to 25.4 ± 3.8mg/dl ($p < 0.01$) at 12 weeks predialysis serum values of other parameters such as total cholesterol triglyceride, HDL cholesterol, α-, β-, pre-β-lipoproteins and fibrinogen remained unchanged throughout the course of the 12 weeks. The predialysis free fatty acids changed from 0.656 ± 0.682mEq/L to 0.452 ± 0.335mEq/L at four weeks, but this was not statistically significant (Figures 3 and 4).

Discussion

The results of this study indicate that MD-805 is an anticoagulant suitable for haemodialysis without any other medication. The total amount used for one dialysis was 125 to 150mg, or 12.5 to 15ml in cases using a 10 per cent solution. Administration to the blood line was easily accomplished by a conventional infusion pump.

146

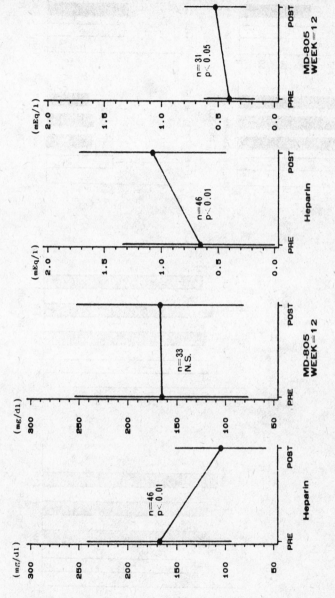

Figure 2. Changes of triglyceride and free fatty acid concentrations before and after dialysis

147

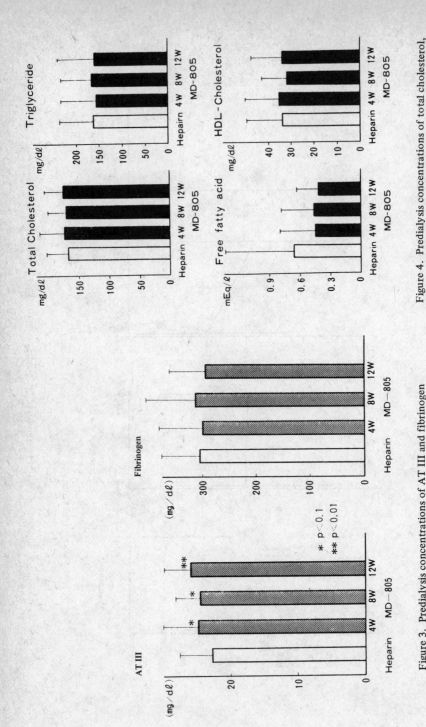

Figure 4. Predialysis concentrations of total cholesterol, triglyceride free fatty acid and HDL cholesterol

Figure 3. Predialysis concentrations of AT III and fibrinogen

148

The advantages of this drug over heparin are:

1. Pure, chemically synthesised drug;

2. No side effects on lipid metabolism;

3. Applicable to patients with antithrombin III deficiency.

One disadvantage of the drug is that it has no specific antagonist, such as protamine sulphate for heparin.

The beneficial effects on lipid metabolism and antithrombin III observed in the short-term study should be evaluated on a long-term basis. In addition it would be advisable to conduct a long-term study to determine whether MD-805 has any effect on bone metabolism.

Conclusions

1. Haemodialysis can be successfully carried out using MD-805 as the sole anticoagulant.

2. Significant prolongation of clotting time is obtained by MD-805.

3. Significant elevation of AT III is observed.

4. No influence is observed on lipid metabolism.

5. No serious systemic or local complications were detected.

Reference

1 Okamoto S, Hijikata A, Kikumoto R et al. *Biochem Biophys Res Commun 1981; 101:* 440

Open Discussion

CATTELL (Chairman) If you have some untoward event, such as a major haemorrhage, is it possible to inactivate this new thrombin quickly? Secondly, what is the half life of the action of the drug. In other words, if you cease its administration, how long is it before you have inactivation of its effects?

OTA One of the disadvantages of this drug is that it has no antagonist, like protamine sulphate for heparin, but the half life of the drug is short, about 20 minutes. Therefore this drug can be used in such a situation, but another drug, a proteinase inhibitor, is now being used experimentally in our country and it also has a very short half life, so it is available in such cases.

RITZ (Heidelberg) If I understand your introduction correctly, the principle of it is interaction with fibrinogen by virtue of the amino acid analogue. In the presence of fibrinogen or fibrin degradation products one would anticipate that the efficacy of the drug would be diminished. Do you have any experience of this?

OTA No I have not, since the drug is infused continuously thrombin is absorbed by the drug and anticoagulation continues.

Proc EDTA (1983) Vol 20

TRANSFUSED AND PHARMACOLOGICAL IRON: RELATIONSHIP OF OVERLOAD TO HLA ANTIGENS

M Taccone-Gallucci, G D Di Nucci, C Meloni, M Valeria, D Adorno, M Elli, G Mariani, F Mandelli, C U Casciani

University of Rome, Italy

Summary

Forty-eight haemodialysis patients were divided in two groups according to presence or absence of haemochromatosis alleles (HA). Serum ferritin concentrations were determined and analysed according to blood transfusion history. Furthermore 20 patients were given iron saccarate and post treatment ferritin concentrations were determined at 15 and 30 days.

Following blood transfusion, only HA+ patients increased ferritin concentrations, while intravenous iron administration produced increased ferritin both in HA+ and HA- patients. Therefore it is advisable to minimise transfusions in HA+ patients, while intravenous iron administration should be avoided regardless of HA status.

Introduction

Blood transfusion and the administration of parenteral iron are used frequently to correct chronic anaemia in haemodialysis patients (HD). However, this often causes iron overload [1]. It has also been shown that 'haemochromatosis alleles' HLA A_3, B_7, B_{14} predispose to iron overload [2].

To evaluate the importance of blood transfusion and parenteral iron administration in causing iron overload, we have studied patients undergoing chronic haemodialysis, dividing them according to the presence or absence of 'haemochromatosis alleles' (HA). As ferritin is considered a reliable marker of total body iron [3,4], we have used this to determine iron overload.

Material and methods

Forty-eight patients (27 males and 21 females, mean age 45 yr, range 7–74) on chronic haemodialysis four hours thrice weekly, for a mean of 44 months duration (range 6–139) for end-stage renal disease of various aetiology, have

150

been studied. None of the patients had evidence of active liver disease or ongoing infection and there were no apparent differences in dietary iron intake. None of the patients had received iron supplements during the three months preceding the study. None had received any blood transfusion in the same period; furthermore a group of patients (n = 28) had received no transfusions for at least 15 months prior to the study (non-transfused), the others (n = 20) had received at least one unit of blood between three and 15 months prior to the study (transfused).

HLA typing was determined by a standard microlymphocytotoxicity technique [5]. Haematological parameters and serum iron were determined using standard techniques. Serum ferritin was assayed by a RIA method [6] using a commercial kit (Becton-Dickinson, Milano, Italy); the 95 per cent confidence limit for both sexes in our laboratory was: 18–185ng/ml. A patient was said to have 'iron overload' when the serum ferritin concentration exceeded 400ng/ml.

For the purpose of the study, the patients were divided into two groups according to the presence (HA+, n = 15) or absence (HA–, n = 33) of at least one of A_3, B_7, and B_{14} antigens. Age, sex, red blood cell count, haemoglobin concentration, serum iron, duration and frequency of dialysis and transfusion regimen did not differ significantly in the two groups (Table I).

TABLE I. Baseline data

Parameters	HLA+ (15 patients)	HLA– (33 patients)	
Age (years)	49.0 ± 4.60	42.0 ± 2.93	NS
Time on dialysis (months)	51.0 ± 9.55	38.0 ± 6.09	NS
Red blood cell count (x 10^9/L)	2874.17 ± 188.23	2800.69 ± 91.33	NS
Haemoglobin (g/dl)	8.71 ± 0.57	8.77 ± 0.29	NS
Serum iron (g/dl)	87.0 ± 9.80	71.06 ± 4.22	NS
Patients transfused	8/15	12/33	
Units of blood/patient*	3.5 ± 1.23	2.08 ± 0.35	NS

Entries: $\overline{X}$ ± SEM
NS: not significant
*: in the last 15 months

Furthermore, from the total number of patients, 20 patients (7 HA+ and 13 HA–) with normal baseline ferritin values were selected and treated with 200mg x 5 i.v. iron saccarate.

Statistical analysis was carried out using Fisher's exact test, p>0.05 was considered non significant. In the text and tables the data are expressed by the average values and the Standard Error of the Mean (SEM).

All the patients gave informed consent to the study.

Results

Mean serum ferritin concentrations were significantly higher in HA+ patients compared to HA– patients: 439.21 ± 178.47ng/ml vs 166.22 ± 33.79ng/ml (p<0.05). The difference between serum ferritin values was statistically significant in HA+ patients who had received blood transfusions within 15 months prior to the study in comparison to those who had not (760.37 ± 296.16ng/ml vs 70.31 ± 24.66ng/ml, p<0.05). Previous transfusions did not influence serum ferritin concentrations in HA− patients (190.16 ± 52.52ng/ml, transfused vs 152.54 ± 44.48ng/ml, non transfused). In addition, serum ferritin concentrations were significantly higher in transfused HA+ patients in comparison to transfused HA− ones (760.37 ± 296.19ng/ml vs 190.16 ± 52.52ng/ml, p<0.05). The difference between serum ferritin concentration related to HA status is not statistically significant in non-transfused patients (70.31 ± 24.16ng/ml, HA+ vs 152.54 ± 44.48ng/ml, HA−, NS) (Table II).

TABLE II. Ferritin concentrations in transfused and non-transfused dialysis patients in relation to haemochromatosis alleles

	All patients	Transfused	Non-transfused
		↓ * ↓	
HA+	439.21 ± 178.47 (15)	760.37 ± 296.19 (8)	70.31 ± 24.66 (7)
	↕*	↕*	NS ↕
HA−	166.22 ± 33.79 (33)	190.16 ± 52.52 (12)	152.54 ± 44.48 (21)
		↑ NS ↑	

Entries: ng/ml of serum ferritin ($\overline{X}$ ± SEM)
* p<0.05 ** p<0.005
NS: not significant
In brackets: number of patients

TABLE III. Effect of parenteral iron on serum ferritin concentrations in relation to the haemochromatosis allele status

	Time 0	After 15 days	After 30 days
HA+ (7)	109.7 ± 29.28	367.14 ± 82.09	247.57 ± 57.60
	↑ ↑ **	↑	
		**	
HA− (13)	86.0 ± 21.94	320.38 ± 42.72	261.92 ± 38.88
	↑ ↑ **	↑	↑
		**	

For legends see Table II

The intravenous administration of iron saccarate caused a significant increase of ferritin as assayed both 15 and 30 days after iron administration in all 20 treated patients, regardless of the HA status (Table III).

Discussion

Ferritin represents the most important detectable form of iron storage in the body. Interest in ferritin is due to recent studies demonstrating that serum ferritin reflects the quantity of iron in the tissues [4]. Hence serum ferritin has a clinical value in assessing both iron deficiency and iron overload [4]. In haemodialysis patients iron stores depend on a balance between blood loss during dialysis and iron uptake [7]. The latter depends on the absorption of dietary iron and both therapeutic and transfusion iron. Iron overload is a common problem in haemodialysis patients; its prevalence is as high as 70 per cent among patients receiving parenteral iron [2]. It has been suggested that the tendency to iron overload is related to genetic factors, i.e. the presence of at least one of the HA antigens [2]. Our results confirm these observations; in fact in our patients, iron overload was demonstrated only in the HA+ transfused patients. It is of interest that recently [8] a correlation has been demonstrated between serum ferritin concentrations and the number of blood transfusions. In addition our study shows that the increase of serum ferritin following intravenous iron saccarate is independent of the HA status of the patient.

In conclusion, our results suggest that a strict blood transfusion policy should be applied, particularly to the HA+ patients as these patients are at particular risk of transfusional iron overload. The increase in serum ferritin concentrations, regardless of the HA status, following intravenous iron supports the theory that transfused and oral iron follow two different metabolic pathways. The impressive findings of Ali et al [9] that intravenous iron supplements, although increasing serum ferritin concentrations, may not increase iron stores in the bone marrow should lead to a ban of intravenous supplement therapy in the treatment of anaemia in haemodialysis patients regardless of the HA status of the patients.

Acknowledgments

The authors acknowledge the help given by Mrs Gina Del Gallo and the expert secretarial assistance of Mrs Gabriella Valente.

References

1   Eschbach JW. In Drukker W, Parson FM, Maher JF, eds. *Replacement of Renal Function in Dialysis*. The Hague: Nijhoff. 1978: 557
2   Bregman H, Gelfand MC, Winchester J et al. *Trans ASAIO 1980; 26:* 366
3   Eschbach JW, Cook JD. *Trans ASAIO 1977; 23:* 54
4   Lypschitz DA, Cook JD, Finch CA. *N Engl J Med 1974; 290:* 1213
5   Terasaki P, McClelland JD. *Nature 1964; 204:* 998
6   Barnett MD, Gordon YB, Aness JAL et al. *J Clin Path 1978; 31:* 742
7   Linn KL, Mitchell TR, Shepperd J. *Clin Nephrol 1980; 14:* 124
8   Müller-Wiefel DE, Lenhard V, Scharer K. *Proc EDTA 1981; 18:* 524
9   Ali M, Fayemi AO, Frascino J et al. *Lancet 1982; i:* 652

Open Discussion

CATTELL (Chairman) Given the iron kinetics and the fact that you measured the serum ferritin immediately on concluding the five week course of intravenous iron is this sufficient time to reach a steady state?

ELLI We performed the determination at 15 and 30 days after completing the administration. The administration was given on a weekly basis, 200mg i.v. once a week, and 15 and 30 days after the last infusion we determined the serum ferritin.

CATTELL But you may not at that stage have reached a steady state in respect to serum ferritin values. Does it then reflect the true iron status of the body?

ELLI The haematologists tend to agree that the steady state for iron balance is reached almost immediately. The totally insignificant difference between the values found at day 15 and day 30 seems to support this view.

COMTY (Minneapolis) We presented similar but less elegant studies in 1978 to the American Society of Nephrology. One of the problems is that the gastro-enterologists tell us that serum ferritin is not a good method of measuring iron stores in patients with acute liver disease. I agree with you because we have seen acute iron overload develop in patients as they evolved acute hepatitis and we have seen a very high incidence of what might be considered to be haemochromatosis in our patients with chronic aggressive hepatitis. On the other hand we have seen another phenomenon in the dialysis patients over the years. Certain patients do seem to hyper-absorb dietary iron in the absence of hepatitis, and absence of abnormal liver function tests, and with a normal liver biopsy. I agree with you that there is something different about patients with HBsAg+ but I'm not sure what it is. The question of whether ferritin is a valid measure of iron stores in the hepatitis patient needs evaluation, meanwhile we use serum ferritin as an indicator of iron stores.

ELLI All of our patients had negative hepatitis antigens, and we made sure that our patients had no on-going liver diseases before entering them into the study. In the follow-up it turned out that they actually were not having any liver disease or any infection, that is another cause of possible mistake in ferritin determinations. As far as the intestinal iron absorption is concerned our patients were on a diet which could be considered homogenous. They were not supplemented with oral therapeutic iron; they were just on a free diet.

PECCHINI (Cremona) We have made a similar study but we have given iron only once (you have given the dose four times). Maybe the differences in overload between transfusion and therapeutic iron is related to HLA.

ELLI Theoretically this could be the cause, but we have to take into account the free interval from the last preceding therapeutic iron administration, and possibly the total amount of iron the patients had received during their life. Our patients had received no therapeutic iron for at least three months prior to the study. Furthermore it is our policy to limit as much as possible iron supplementation to our patients.

Proc EDTA (1983) Vol 20

DOPAMINERGIC CONTROL OF SYMPATHETIC ACTIVITY AND BLOOD PRESSURE IN HAEMODIALYSIS PATIENTS

A Sturani, E Degli Esposti, A De March*, A Santoro, G Fuschini*, A Zuccalà, C Chiarini, C Flamigni*, P Zucchelli

Malpighi Hospital, and *S. Orsola Hospital, Bologna, Italy

Summary

Bromocriptine was used to test the hypothesis that the abnormality of the dopaminergic system described in haemodialysis patients may cause enhanced sympathetic activity and high blood pressure. Bromocriptine significantly reduced supine mean blood pressure and plasma noradrenaline. Moreover, although the increments in plasma noradrenaline during tilt tests were reduced by bromocriptine there was a significant improvement in the response of blood pressure. These results suggest that dopaminergic control of sympathetic activity may be impaired in haemodialysis patients and may be a cause of high blood pressure. Moreover, a restoration of a normal relationship between noradrenaline and adrenergic receptors would be consistent with the present results.

Introduction

It has been suggested that the central dopaminergic system contributes to the regulation of blood pressure. The administration of the dopamine agonist, bromocriptine, causes orthostatic hypotension in some normotensive subjects [1] as well as inducing a significant reduction in blood pressure in essential hypertension [2, 3]. The hypotensive effect of bromocriptine seems to be more marked when prolactin [2] and noradrenaline [3] plasma concentrations are high. Therefore, it has been postulated that bromocriptine may exert its anti-hypertensive action by stimulating central dopaminergic activity, thereby reducing sympathetic outflow [3].

The aim of the present study was to test the hypothesis that the abnormality of the dopaminergic system, which has been described in haemodialysis patients [4], causes enhanced sympathetic activity and high blood pressure.

Material and methods

Six haemodialysis patients aged between 27 and 50 years were studied. In all cases informed consent was obtained. Underlying renal diseases were glomerulonephritis (four patients), polycystic disease (one patient) and hypertensive nephroangiosclerosis (one patient). The patients had been established on maintenance haemodialysis for at least 12 months at the time of the study. Their clinical status was stable, and there were no known intercurrent diseases. The patients were not nephrectomised. They were all males and presented both high blood pressure (supine mean blood pressure ≥100 mmHg) and high plasma prolactin (mean value 22 ± 3ng/L, range 15.2–33ng/L). The patients were treated with disposable multilayer dialysers for four to five hours, thrice weekly. The dialysate composition was as follows: Na 140mEq/L, K 1.8mEq/L, Ca 3.6mEq/L, Mg 0.5mEq/L, acetate 37mEq/L and glucose 1g/L. The patients were advised to maintain their usual diet. All drugs were stopped two weeks prior to the study except for calcium supplements, aluminium hydroxide preparations and vitamin D derivatives.

The study was performed in the interdialytic day, 20 hours after the last dialysis. In the morning of the study, an 18 gauge butterfly needle was inserted into a forearm vein in all patients. At 9 a.m., after one hour of resting supine, blood pressure and heart rate (Critikon DI-NAMAP 845) were recorded and blood was taken for the determination of prolactin and noradrenaline. Subsequently, a seven minute tilt test and a two minute cold pressor test with determination of blood pressure, heart rate and plasma noradrenaline were performed. Thereafter, blood pressure and heart rate were recorded after 15 minutes of walking. This protocol was performed twice, after a week of treatment with a placebo and after a week of treatment with bromocriptine 2.5mg/day orally.

Mean arterial pressure was calculated as diastolic blood pressure plus one-third of pulse pressure. Noradrenaline was determined according to the fluorimetric method of Renzini et al [5]. Prolactin was determined by a radioimmunoassay method [6]. Tilt and cold pressor tests were performed as previously described [7].

Statistical methods

The results are presented as mean values ± SE mean. Statistical analysis of the results were performed by the paired Student t-test. Simple linear regression analysis was used for testing the relation between two variables.

Results

No significant differences were found between the two periods of treatment in haematocrit, total plasma proteins, blood calcium, plasma electrolytes and body weight. Mean supine blood pressure was significantly reduced by bromocriptine therapy in all patients (Table I). In particular, four patients became normotensive (mean blood pressure <110mmHg). In addition, mean walking blood pressure was significantly reduced by bromocriptine (from 122 ± 5.4 to 112 ± 5.3mmHg, p<0.01) without the appearance of orthostatic hypotension in any patient. No significant changes were observed in supine and walking heart rate. Both plasma prolactin and plasma noradrenaline, however, were

157

TABLE I

	Placebo	Bromocriptine	p
Mean blood pressure (mmHg)	119 ± 4.7	106 ± 4.9	<0.01
Heart rate (beats/min)	77 ± 3.1	74 ± 2.2	NS
Plasma noradrenaline (ng/L)	278 ± 58	173 ± 45	<0.05
Plasma prolactin (ng/ml)	22 ± 3.1	3 ± 0.6	<0.01

significantly reduced by bromocriptine (Table I). A significant relationship was observed between the pretreatment plasma noradrenaline and the changes in mean supine blood pressure induced by bromocriptine (r = 0.758, p<0.05). In other words, patients with higher pretreatment plasma noradrenaline showed a greater reduction in blood pressure after bromocriptine therapy. The response of blood pressure and plasma noradrenaline to the tilt and cold pressor tests is reported in Figure 1. Although the increments in plasma noradrenaline during

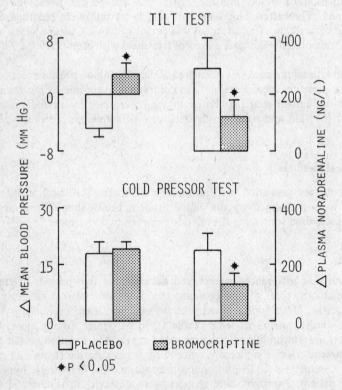

Figure 1

the tilt test were reduced by bromocriptine (from 288 ± 110 to 124 ± 57ng/L, $p<0.05$), there was a significant improvement in the response of mean blood pressure (from -4.8 ± 1.1 to 2.8 ± 1.7mmHg, $p<0.05$). The same behaviour was observed during the cold pressor test: the increment of mean blood pressure was not changed (from 18 ± 3.2 to 19 ± 3.5mmHg, $p =$ NS), in spite of a significant reduction in the noradrenaline increment (from 252 ± 56 to 137 ± 43ng/L, $p<0.05$).

Discussion

In the present study we have demonstrated that in male haemodialysis patients with high plasma prolactin concentrations and hypertension the administration of bromocriptine causes parallel decreases in blood pressure, plasma prolactin and sympathetic tone, as shown by the decrease of plasma noradrenaline concentration. Moreover, a significant relationship between the pretreatment sympathetic tone and the blood pressure-lowering effect of bromocriptine was observed. Basal high plasma prolactin concentration and lack of prolactin responsiveness to suppressive and stimulatory agents has been documented in haemodialysis patients [8]. These disturbances, due to a decreased central tuberoinfundibular-dopaminergic system activity, seem to be reversible, as they are corrected both by renal transplantation [8] and chronic administration of bromocriptine [4]. Furthermore, increases in plasma noradrenaline concentration have been also demonstrated in haemodialysis patients [9]. Our data support the hypothesis that a defective dopaminergic control is the common cause of a high plasma prolactin and increased sympathetic tone in some haemodialysis patients, and may be a factor in the maintenance of elevated blood pressure. A return to normal of central dopaminergic activity by bromocriptine therapy leads to the restoration of plasma prolactin, sympathetic tone and normal blood pressure.

Our study also demonstrated that while there was a significant reduction in plasma noradrenaline increments, the blood pressure response to the cold pressor and tilt tests was unchanged or improved. This phenomenon, which has also been observed in essential hypertensive patients [3], suggests that central suppression of sympathetic activity may enhance the response to endogenous noradrenaline. It is known that chronic exposure of adrenergic receptors to increased noradrenaline in the circulation and possibly at the receptor sites, leads to a down-regulation of the receptors with a consequent diminished responsiveness [10]. A restoration of a normal relationship between noradrenaline and adrenergic receptors would be consistent with the present results.

References

1   Whitfield L, Sowers JR, Tuck ML, Golub MS. *J Clin Endocrinol Metab 1980; 51:* 724
2   Stumpe KO, Kolloch R, Higuchi M et al. *Lancet 1977; ii:* 211
3   Kolloch R, Kobayashi K, DeQuattro V. *Hypertension 1980; 2:* 390

4   Verzetti G, De Leo M, De Leo V, Genazzani AR. *Minerva Nefrol 1981; 28:* 321
5   Renzini V, Brunori CA, Valori C. *Clin Chim Acta 1970; 39:* 587
6   Ehara Y, Silver T, Vandenberg G et al. *Am J Obstet Gynecol 1973; 117:* 962
7   Sturani A, Chiarini C, Degli Esposti E et al. *Br J Clin Pharmacol 1982; 14:* 849
8   Lim VS, Kathapalia SC, Frohman LA. *J Clin Endocrinol Metab 1979; 48:* 101
9   Zuccalà A, Degli Esposti E, Sturani A et al. *Int J Artif Organs 1978; 1:* 76
10   Davies AO, Lefkowitz RJ. In Turner P, Shand DG, eds. *Recent Advances in Clinical Pharmacology.* Edinburgh: Churchill Livingstone. 1980: 35

Open Discussion

MANN (Heidelberg) Bromocriptine has significant adrenergic blocking properties, did you test in your patients whether at the doses used there was some alpha-blockade?

STURANI   No. I know that many studies in essential hypertension have demonstrated that the blocking action of bromocriptine is only on the central dopaminergic system, not at the peripheral site. We think that in our patients we have probably the same result as in some haemodialysis patients. The dosage we administered was 2.5mg, relatively small in comparison to the high dosage used in essential hypertensive patients.

CATTELL (Chairman)   In using bromocriptine, as we and many others have done, for the treatment of impotence, patients do in fact develop tolerance to the dose given. Did you notice that you lost your effect in any of your patients with prolonged use?

STURANI   Yes I agree with you, but our study did not examine this. We wanted only to test the hypothesis that alteration in the central dopaminergic activity may be a cause in the genesis of hypertension in some haemodialysis patients. In some cases we observed a return to high blood pressure after long term administration of bromocriptine.

Proc EDTA (1983) Vol 20

EFFECT OF VACCINATION SCHEDULE AND DIALYSIS ON HEPATITIS B VACCINATION RESPONSE IN URAEMIC PATIENTS

J Bommer, E Ritz, K Andrassy, G Bommer, F Deinhardt*, W Jilg*, G Darai

University of Heidelberg and *University of München, FRG

Summary

Antibody response to vaccination with hepatitis B vaccine (HB-Vax®) was evaluated in 43 staff, 81 dialysis patients and 12 non-dialysed uraemic patients. We confirmed less frequent seroconversion and lower concentration of antibody to hepatitis B surface antigen (anti-HBs) in dialysis patients despite a higher dose (40μg vaccine). However, more frequent vaccination (5 times vs 3) increased anti-HBs concentration to almost normal. Concomitant administration of hepatitis B immunoglobulin (HBIG) and hepatitis B vaccine (passive/active) did not interfere with vaccination success. Antibody response was equally poor in dialysed and non-dialysed uraemic patients.

Introduction

Hepatitis B continues to be an important unsolved problem of haemodialysis as demonstrated by the figures of the EDTA report [1]. The availability of a vaccine containing hepatitis B surface antigen (HBsAg) for active immunisation [2–5] is promising, but studies have shown impaired anti-HBs response in dialysed patients [5].

The present investigation examines (a) whether with hepatitis B vaccine (HB-Vax®, Merck, Sharp and Dohme) the anti-HBs response is impaired in dialysis patients; (b) whether anti-HBs responses can be improved by changes in the vaccination schedule; (c) whether simultaneous administration of hepatitis B immunoglobulin interferes with vaccination success and (d) whether impaired anti-HBs response is present even in non-dialysed uraemic patients.

Patients and methods

Hepatitis B vaccine (HB-Vax®, Merck, Sharp and Dohme) was given to 43 staff (19 male; 24 female; age 39.6 ± 8.6 years), 81 dialysis patients (51 male; 30 female; age 46.4 ± 10.1 years) and 12 non-dialysed patients with preterminal

TABLE I

	No.	male/female	age (y)	duration of dialysis (m) median (range)	6 months a) seroconversion b) anti-HbS-titre (mIU/ml) median (range)	7 months	9 months
Staff	43	19/34	31.6 ± 8.6		a) 36/43 (84%) b) 62.5 (2.7–4006)	39/43 (91%) 462 (4–8681)	39/43 (91%) 285 (4–9316)
group I	29	14/15	47.7 ± 12.1	41 (9–85)	a) 10/29 (34%) b) 7.9 (2.4–58)	13/29 (45%) 125 (2.6–637)	16/29 (55%) 71 (2.6–501)
group II	26	20/6	47.0 ± 9.2	31 (3–122)	a) 15/26 (58%) b) 355 (3.5–5284)	15/25 (64%) 404 (2.9–11900)	15/24 (63%) 232 (2–4851)
group III	26	19/7	44.4 ± 9.9	38 (2–112)	a) 13/26 (50%) b) 353 (6.7–18316)	14/26 (54%) 377 (11–18874)	15/26 (58%) 107 (7.8–1279)
predialysis	12	10/2	41.7 ± 11.2		a) 4/12 (33%) b) 25 (3.4–68)	5/12 (41%) 153 (2–3517)	7/12 (58%) 46 (2.1–2563)

uraemia (serum creatinine > 500μmol/L) (10 male; 2 female; age 41.7 ± 11 years). Staff members received a dose of 20μg HB-Vax® per vaccination; uraemic patients 40μg per vaccination. The following time intervals were chosen for vaccination:

Staff:		months 0, 1, 6
Dialysed patients:	group I	months 0, 1, 6
	group II	months 0, 1, 2, 4, 6
	group III	months 0, 1, 2, 4, 6
	with 3ml	
	HBIG i.m.	months 0, 1, 6
Non-dialysed patients:	group IV	months 0, 1, 6

Hepatitis B immunoglobulin of Merck, Sharp and Dohme (Hep B Gamma GE®) was used for passive immunisation in group III. Anti-HBs was measured monthly with RIA (Ausab®, Abbott Labs, North Chicago/Ill); anti-HBs values are given as mIU/ml according to Hollinger et al [6].

Results

As shown in Table I and in Figure 1, 91 per cent of staff seroconverted after three vaccinations. In contrast, using the same schedule with double dose, only 45 per cent of the dialysed patients (group I) seroconverted after seven months and 55 per cent after nine months. In parallel, median anti-HBs concentrations were significantly lower as compared to healthy staff. However, in dialysis patients more frequent vaccinations (group II) caused some increase of the rate of seroconversion and particularly a notable increase in anti-HBs concentrations which almost reached the concentrations observed in staff. Simultaneous administration of hepatitis B immunoglobulin (group III) did not markedly interfere with either the rate or seroconversion of the anti-HBs concentrations achieved.

The anti-HBs response after three vaccinations was comparable in dialysed (group I) and non-dialysed (group IV) uraemic patients. Within the population of dialysed patients, no relation of vaccination response to age, sex or number of blood transfusions was observed (data not given). Of interest are anecdotal observations of vigorous anti-HBs response in patients with Goodpasture's syndrome despite several months of cyclophosphamide treatment.

Short lasting pain at the site of injection was reported by 17 per cent of staff and patients after first and repeated vaccinations. In November and December 1981, vaccination was followed by fever and arthralgia in 20–30 per cent of cases. However, similar symptoms compatible with viral illness were present in non-vaccinated persons and no such symptoms occurred after vaccination at other times.

163

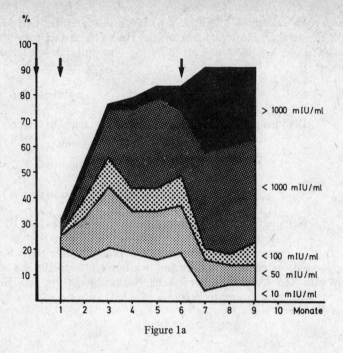

Figure 1a

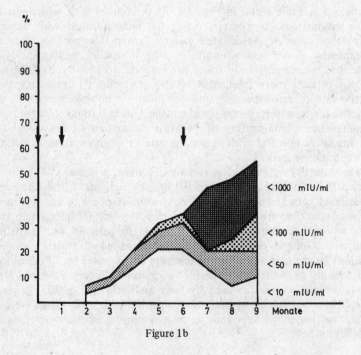

Figure 1b

164

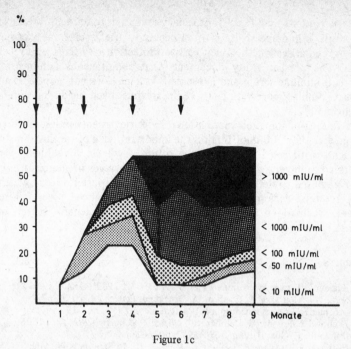

Figure 1c

Figure 1a,b and c. This demonstrates the anti-HBs response and the distribution of anti-HBs concentrations (mIU/ml) in staff (1a), dialysis patients with three vaccinations (1b, group I) or five vaccinations (1c, group III)

Discussion

The present study confirms previous reports and demonstrates that after hepatitis B vaccination the anti-HBs response is diminished in dialysis patients when compared to non-uraemic controls [4,5,7]. A similarly diminished response was also noted in non-dialysed patients with preterminal uraemia; this observation illustrates that uraemia, and not the dialysis procedure, interferes with vaccination success. Impaired anti-HBs response was not explained by age, malnutrition, polytransfusion or antecedent immunosuppressive therapy of our dialysis patients. The impairment of anti-HBs response was not only reflected by a lower rate of seroconversion, but also by lower anti-HBs concentrations in those patients who seroconverted.

The major finding of the present study is the demonstration that higher anti-HBs concentrations can be achieved if dialysis patients are vaccinated more frequently. Indeed, anti-HBs concentrations in dialysis patients who seroconverted were then comparable with anti-HBs concentrations in healthy individuals. This finding is of obvious practical importance.

This study does not answer the question at what intervals further revaccinations will be necessary. But it is of note that during the limited period of observation median anti-HBs concentrations did not decrease more rapidly

165

in dialysis patients than in staff. Especially in dialysis units, acute administration of hepatitis B immune serum is often necessary after accidental exposure. The question then arises whether such passive protection interferes with vaccination success. The present study documents that simultaneous administration of hepatitis B immune serum and hepatitis B vaccine does not jeopardise anti-HBs response. Similar observations have meanwhile been made in non-uraemic individuals [4].

The finding of impaired vaccination response in patients with serum creatinine levels greater than $500\mu mol/L$ raises the important issue of vaccination strategies in patients with renal disease. In the future it will be advisable to vaccinate patients who may progress to uraemia at earlier stages of the disease. Further work is required to define the level of glomerular filtration rate at which vaccination response is impaired. For patients with advanced renal failure more frequent vaccinations provide a practicable way to achieve better anti-HBs response.

References

1   Kramer P, Broyer M, Brunner FP et al. *Proc EDTA 1982; 19:* 4
2   Maupas P, Coursaget P, Goudeau A, Drucker J. *Lancet 1976; i:* 1367
3   Crosnier E, Jungers P, Couroucé A-M et al. *Lancet 1981; i:* 455
4   Zachoval Z, Frösner G, Deinhardt F. *Münch Med Wschr 1981; 123:* 1506
5   Deinhardt F, Gust ID. *Bull WHO 1982; 60:* 661
6   Hollinger FB, Adam E, Heiberg D, Melnick JL. In Szmuness W, Alter HJ, Maynard JE, eds. *Viral Hepatitis.* Philadelphia: Franklin Inst Press. 1982: S451–466
7   Crosnier E, Jungers P, Couroucé A-M et al. *Lancet 1981; i:* 797

Open Discussion

ROTTEMBOURG (Paris) You investigated 12 patients in pre-terminal uraemia. We studied about 56 pre-terminal uraemic patients with a creatinine clearance between 5 and 20ml/min who received the vaccine of Institute Pasteur three times at one-monthly intervals with a booster one year after. Seroconversion was about 80 per cent one month after the third injection, and about 85 per cent after the booster injection. Why do you say that pre-terminal status is too late? Is it a problem of the vaccine and what is the titre you consider an effective serum conversion?

BOMMER The mean serum creatinine in our patients was on average 8mg/100ml. The data in the literature relating to patients with a serum creatinine of 5mg/100ml who were vaccinated have a higher rate than our patients. We cannot decide at the moment what's the best time to vaccinate patients with renal insufficiency. It may be that we have to vaccinate at creatinine values of 2–4mg/100ml.

HAMILTON (Glasgow) Dialysis patients vary in their immune response from almost normal immune reactivity down to anergic status. It may well be that the anergic patients are the very ones who do not respond to your vaccine and they are also the patients who are liable to get persistent hepatitis. Have you any data on the degree of immune reactivity in the patients you vaccinated?

BOMMER No, I am sorry we have no data of immune reactivity of these patients.

COMTY (Minneapolis) Do you have any idea whether an antibody titre of say 40 leaves the patient more susceptible to hepatitis B than say an antibody titre of 200. We have looked at antibody titres in our staff and patients over the years after clinical hepatitis B, and they vary considerably and I really don't know the answer. We have patients and staff vaccination figures exactly the same as yours but having followed them a little bit longer we are seeing staff losing measurable antibody. The questions arise: Do we revaccinate our staff too? Do we change the sequence of injections? Do we give them more frequent injections and try and maintain antibody titres? This is going to be a very costly exercise in the long-term planning of the use of hepatitis vaccine in most centres.

BOMMER We have similar experience. Please remember the slides of the graphical data. After the third vaccination patients of group II have the same antibody titres as patients of group I, at the seventh month. I agree with you that the time intervals between the vaccination are not as important as the number of vaccinations.

FUNCK BRENTANO (Paris) We have observed the same resistance to vaccination in about 40 per cent of our patients in end-stage renal failure. I would like to know if you have any data about the aetiology of the kidney disease of these patients and whether they have so-called immunological kidney disease such as glomerulo-nephritis or a non-immunological cause such as hereditary diseases? Do you have any data on the resistance to vaccination between these two categories of patients?

BOMMER No, we have not differentiated our patients with different diseases. We can tell you that two patients with Goodpasture's syndrome treated with cyclophosphamide and prednisone had a good response and good antibody production.

SCHICHT (Leiden) We have also actively and passively vaccinated patients. I think we used a similar schedule to you and we had a conversion rate which is higher than yours. I wonder if it is because we have a rather large number of higher immunised patients who are capable of giving some immune response? We achieve 68 per cent success when regularly vaccinating actively and passively together.

BOMMER I think it's perhaps a question of definition. What is a positive response? We defined as a positive response if we detect positive anti-HBs antibodies three times at monthly intervals. Sometimes we found an antibody against hepatitis B surface antigen, but one month later no antibody titre was detectable. I agree with you, the antibody response in our patients was not very high. In addition we have performed further vaccination, e.g. in the patients in group II. Then we found again some seroconversion in these patients. In three of the 12 patients who had no antibodies after five vaccinations we found HBs antibodies after the sixth injection.

SCHICHT When you give passive vaccination to patients they passively acquire HBs antibodies and if you give enough of the very strong immunoglobulin, it is not enough to state that they need to have twice the normal amount. You have to prove that you have an increase in HBs antibodies.

BOMMER In the passive/active group antibody response was positive if there was an increase of the antibody titre three months after the last injection of immunoglobulin.

CAPPELLI (Genoa) In your follow-up do you have any patients who seroconvert from HBs negative to HBs positive due to exposure to antigens?

BOMMER After the second month after the last vaccination, we have not observed an increase of seroconversion in our patients.

KLINKMANN (Chairman) Would it be too early to ask you to give us certain suggestions about the strategy you would prefer at this time?

BOMMER I think it's a little bit too early as it is necessary to collect more data to confirm our results. For example, the Paris group have also performed a lot of vaccinations. I do not know the exact results, but for the moment we can say it is better to revaccinate many times. Every vaccination gives you a chance that some patients seroconvert.

OPEN HEART SURGERY IN PATIENTS WITH END-STAGE RENAL DISEASE

J Rottembourg, T Mussat, I Gandjbakhch, A Barthelemy,
D Toledano, G M Gahl, C Cabrol

Groupe Hospitalier Pitié-Salpétrière, Paris, France

Summary

Seventeen patients on maintenance dialysis therapy or with severe impaired kidney function required correction of cardiovascular diseases by open heart surgery. Ten aortic, two mitral valvular replacements and five coronary artery bypass grafts were performed. Special attention was taken for these patients, including pre-operative dialysis, cardiopulmonary bypass with complete haemodilution, composition of extracorporeal circuit volumes, arterial and venous access and myocardial protection.

Prosthetic valves were preferred to porcine heterografts for valve replacements and autogenous saphenous veins were utilised for coronary artery bypass grafts. Follow-up of 14 patients was available from one to 84 months. Carefully planned open heart surgery can be successfully carried out in uraemic patients without an increased operative risk.

Introduction

The number of patients on dialysis and transplantation programmes is steadily increasing [1]. The prolongation of life in these patients has gradually improved with an overall expected yearly mortality rate of 10 per cent [1,2]. Cardiovascular diseases are recognised as accounting for approximately one-half of all mortalities reported in haemodialysis patients [1–3]. Myocardial infarction and other cardiac diseases are the immediate causes of death in about one-third of the fatalities in the haemodialysis population of the Diaphane Registry in France [2].

Co-existence of coronary artery disease or valvular heart disease and chronic renal failure presents a challenge when patients require major surgical procedures which have acceptable morbidity and mortality [4]. Careful consideration must be given to the special management problems associated with chronic renal failure and open heart surgery and close co-operation must be maintained between the surgeon, cardiologist, nephrologist and anaesthetist.

Clinical data and management

Patients

From October 1974 to December 1982, 17 major cardiac operations requiring cardiopulmonary bypass were performed on 17 patients with end-stage renal failure. These 17 surgical procedures were as follows: eight aortic valve replacements (three for endocarditis, one aortic valve replacement for bacterial septal aneurysm), two mitral valve replacements, one Pezzi Laubry syndrome (interventricular communication associated with aortic insufficiency) and five coronary artery bypass grafts (CABG).

The 17 patients (14 males and three females) ranged in age from 27 to 58 years (mean age 38.2 years). Of this group, 11 patients were treated by intermittent haemodialysis for one to 84 months (average 18 months), two patients by continuous ambulatory peritoneal dialysis (CAPD) for seven and 40 months respectively, one patient was operated on after five years on haemodialysis followed by two years with a poorly functioning kidney transplant (creatinine clearance 12ml/min), three patients had severe renal failure (creatinine clearance less than 10ml/min) at time of surgery and began dialysis therapy two to four months after the surgical procedure.

The aetiology of renal failure was chronic glomerulonephritis in 11 patients, pyelonephritis: two, diabetic nephropathy: one, nephroangiosclerosis: one, polycystic kidney disease: one and unknown nephropathy in one. Most patients were suffering from multiple associated diseases: hypertension in five patients, hyperlipidaemia: six, secondary hyperparathyroidism: eight and peripheral vascular disease: five. Four patients with previous arteriovenous fistula infections (staphylococcus epidermidis in two, staphylococcus albus in one, and an unknown organism in the last) had a bacterial endocarditis.

Clinical cardiac functional status was defined pre-operatively. The four patients with bacterial endocarditis were in class IV in the New York Heart Association (NYHA) functional classification. In the seven patients suffering from rheumatic valvulopathy (two mitral, five aortic) two were in class IV and five in class III. The Pezzi Laubry syndrome was in class III with severe pulmonary hypertension. The five patients who received coronary grafts were in class IV. Four patients had a previous history of myocardial infarction and four were suffering from angina pectoris.

Management

Pre-operative preparation, centred around adjustment in fluid and electrolyte balance by dialysis. Immediately pre-operatively patients required normal dialysis treatment in order to lower serum potassium and to reach an ideal dry weight. When necessary patients were transfused with packed red cells to increase their haematocrit to 30 per cent. For patients on CAPD treatment was stopped immediately pre-operatively and patients were operated with an empty peritoneal cavity. Induction and maintenance of anaesthesia was routine using sodium pentothal, curare, morphine and nitrous oxide.

Cardiopulmonary bypass was instituted with complete haemodilution. Arterial cannulation was performed in the aorta in 14 cases and in the external iliac artery in three cases. For the venous cannulation two large venous cannulae were inserted through the appendage of the right atrium into the superior and inferior venae cavae. The arterial blood pressure, usually monitored by an indwelling catheter inserted in the radial artery, was controlled in these patients by cannulation of pedal artery in six cases, femoral artery in eight cases, and contralateral radial artery in three cases. Only internal and external jugular veins were used as venous access. The composition of the extracorporeal circuit is given in Table I. Heparinisation of the pump was normal.

TABLE I. Volume loading from the bypass (ml) lines: 700ml − pump oxygenator:800ml

	Normal patients	Dialysis patients
Ringer's lactate	500ml	200ml
Bicarbonate 14‰	500ml	500ml
Mannitol 10%	500ml	−
Fresh frozen plasma	−	800ml
Potassium	26mmol	−

Myocardial protection was achieved by hypothermia. General moderate hypothermia (26°C) was induced through the extracorporeal circulation by the heat exchanger. Ringer lactate solution (two to four litres) was used to maintain the hypothermic cardiac arrest. This solution, which is normally infused in the extracorporeal circulation, was for these dialysed patients drained off to avoid fluid overload. Surface cooling completed the hypothermic management using isotonic saline solution (four to eight litres) cooled to 4°C.

Dialysis access must be protected; if an arteriovenous fistula is present, the extremity must be well guarded to prevent pressure and occlusion on the operating table, and no blood pressure cuffs or intravenous needles are used in that arm. If a shunt is present the two limbs are perfused with heparinised saline solution. Routine antibiotics were administered with adaptation to renal failure when necessary. Bladder catheterisation was not routinely performed during surgery. Post-operative dialysis was generally not necessary until the second or third post-operative day. Most patients without bleeding problems were heparinised immediately post-operatively in relation to the presence of a prosthetic valve or coronary artery bypass grafts. Therefore dialysis sessions were performed without heparin as we have described previously [5].

Results

Prosthetic valves used in the 11 cases were Starr-Edwards and Bjork-Shiley valves. No porcine heterografts were used. Saphenous vein grafts were utilised for coronary artery bypass surgery. Woven Dacron tube graft with coronary

171

artery implantation to the graft was performed in the Pezzi-Laubry syndrome. Weight gain was moderate during the cardiopulmonary bypass (1.100 ± 0.400kg). Mean post-operative bleeding was 1200ml (360—2400ml) which was replaced by packed red cells. Only one patient was re-explored for bleeding. Mean daily infusion was about 300ml of hypertonic glucose. Vasoactive drugs were needed in five patients for a period of one to five days.

There was no operative mortality in this series. Three early post-operative deaths occurred: two patients with bacterial endocarditis died with poor cardiac output and intractable ventricular arrhythmias. Another death was due to an extension of a myocardial infarction after coronary bypass. Follow-up of the 14 survivors from one month to seven years has been obtained: one patient died after six months from hypoglycaemia, another after nine months from recurrent endocarditis; a third died five years after surgery from a cerebrovascular accident. To date 11 patients are surviving from one to 84 months with a mean period of 36 months. Three patients who received coronary artery bypass improved their functional status; two are treated by CAPD, one by haemodialysis. Only one patient with previous endocarditis is surviving five years after open heart surgery with functional class I. This patient received a kidney transplant three years ago. Six patients who had aortic or mitral valve replacement improved one functional class respectively. The patient with Pezzi Laubry syndrome returned to functional class II.

Discussion

Experience with open heart surgery in uraemic patients can be accomplished with acceptable results [4,6,7]. Uncontrolled heart failure, low cardiac output, bacterial endocarditis and coronary artery diseases were recognised as major cardiac complications of long-term dialysis therapy [2]. In this group of patients the incidence of subacute bacterial endocarditis is between 2.7 and 6.6 per cent [9] due to: 1) depression of immunity; 2) presence of an arteriovenous fistula whether infected or not; and 3) transient episodes of bacteriaemia, during dialysis. The surgical mortality rate was 30 per cent in a recent review of the literature [10] in 26 cases with subacute bacterial endocarditis compared to a 60 per cent mortality rate with medical treatment.

It has been claimed that accelerated atherogenesis is present in the dialysis population [3]. Exact reasons have not been completely identified: however, hypertension, glucose intolerance, hypertriglyceridaemia, vascular calcifications and hyperparathyroidism obviously contribute to the increased incidence of coronary artery disease. Sudden changes in intravascular volumes and electrolyte composition, effects of anaemia, acidosis, arteriovenous fistula and stressful life situations add to the haemodynamic demands required of an ischaemic myocardium. These factors may make medical control of angina more difficult. Many reports suggest that coronary angiography and coronary artery bypass graft surgery are suitable, with a mortality rate of about 10 per cent in both dialysed and transplanted patients.

A co-ordinated approach to the peri-operative period should ensure good results. To prevent acidosis, hyperkalaemia and hypervolaemia during surgery, dialysis treatment should be performed just before surgery. Induction and maintenance of anaesthesia can be undertaken routinely. Haemodilution technique seems to decrease the chance of coagulation difficulties in these uraemic patients. Our haemodilution technique using a minimal fluid infusion allows us to decrease weight gain during cardiopulmonary bypass to 1.100kg in dialysis patients compared to 2.6kg in patients with normal kidney function. Vascular access protection has been emphasised by many authors and occasional heparin infusion has been recommended.

Valve replacement can be undertaken using either porcine heterografts or prosthetic valves. The risk of prosthetic infection and the risk of anticoagulation has led some to prefer porcine heterografts. Secondary hyperparathyroidism with high serum calcium and vascular calcification is common in dialysed patients and suggests the use of prosthetic rather than biological grafts despite the fact they need more anticoagulation therapy. For CABG grafts most workers prefer autogenous saphenous grafts for the bypass conduit. When the saphenous vein cannot be utilised the internal mammary artery has been successfully employed.

Post-surgery dialysis therapy is controversial. Some prefer systematically to initiate peritoneal dialysis after surgery to avoid anticoagulation, while others recommend regional heparinisation. In our department CAPD was reintroduced immediately post-operatively, and haemodialysis sessions were performed without heparin 36 to 48 hours after surgery with no bleeding problems.

Reports of the literature summarised together 122 surgical procedures in uraemic patients: 63 (52%) valve replacements, 56 (45%) CABG and three other procedures. The operative mortality rate was 12 per cent (15 patients) and late operative mortality 14 per cent (18 patients). Subacute bacterial endocarditis accounted for most of the early deaths (10 of 15 patients).

In summary, our experience with major cardiac surgical procedures in patients with end-stage renal failure demonstrates their ability to tolerate such operations with acceptable morbidity and mortality. The proper selection of these patients combined with intensive and co-ordinated peri-operative care should ensure similar results in patients undergoing open cardiac procedures. Early surgical intervention in uraemic patients with subacute bacterial endocarditis should be considered, and bypass surgery has been shown to be safe in this population.

References

1   Kramer P, Broyer M, Brunner FP et al. *Proc EDTA 1982; 19:* 3
2   Degoulet P, Legrain M, Reach I et al. *Nephron 1982; 31:* 103
3   Lowrie EG, Lazarus JM, Hampers CL et al. *N Engl J Med 1974; 290:* 737
4   Love JD. *Cardiac Surgery in Patients with Chronic Renal Disease.* New York: Futura Publishing Co. 1982
5   Rottembourg J, Bouayed F, Durande JP et al. *Proc Europ Soc Artif Organs 1979; 6:* 121
6   Monson BK, Wickstrom PH, Haglin JJ et al. *Ann Thorac Surg 1980; 30:* 267
7   Kuehnel E, Lunch H, Benneth W et al. *Trans ASAIO 1976; 22:* 14
8   Chawla R, Gaiuunas P, Lazarus JM et al. *Trans ASAIO 1977; 23:* 694
9   Cross AS, Steigbigel RT. *Medicine 1976; 55:* 453
10   Dupon H, Michaud JL, Duveau D et al. *Arch Mal Coeur 1980; 73:* 1087

Open Discussion

KLINKMANN (Chairman) Thank you Dr Rottembourg for this really very impressive result. It shows us quite clearly how far we have come from the early days of Professor Alwall.

COMTY (Minneapolis) What do you do with your patient post-operatively in terms of anticoagulation and in the coronary artery bypass grafts in terms of using beta-blockers?

ROTTEMBOURG For anticoagulation post-operatively, patients are for one to three weeks on heparin with subcutaneous injections three times per day and after that with oral anticoagulation for long periods.

COMTY Are you continuing with beta blockers in your patients after coronary artery bypass grafts in the absence of angina?

ROTTEMBOURG If hypertension persists then we use beta-blockers.

COMTY I was thinking of their use as an anti-arrhythmic in patients who have good left ventricular function.

ROTTEMBOURG When there is an improvement of the left ventricular function and no other requirement, we stop them.

SCHIEFT (Leiden) Why don't you dialyse patients while they are on the heart machine? It is easy, you don't use anything extra.

ROTTEMBOURG I know that is possible, but we prefer to do it immediately pre-operatively.

SCHIEFT It's easy: they are already heparinised and you can easily do without dialysis after the operation. The anaesthetist can give whatever he wants because you dialyse it out.

ROTTEMBOURG I did not know you worked in a cardiac operating theatre!

SCHIEFT We do. We dialyse our patients during surgery.

ROTTEMBOURG There are many people, many machines and one more I think is not necessary when dialysis can be performed immediately before surgery. We perform dialysis in the morning from seven to 11am and the patient is operated on at 11.30am. Surgeons are unhappy at having too many people in their operating room and I think that it is better to leave them quiet with a normal patient without any additional machine.

KLINKMANN Dr Schieft, do you dialyse during cardiac surgery?

SCHIEFT Routinely.

KLINKMANN And no surgeon chases you out?

SCHIEFT They are quite happy to have us there.

KLINKMANN Alright, you are lucky, you're a lady.

KRAMER (Linz) In many centres haemofiltration is done during the operation to remove excess water and it is very easily done by the pump. Do you think that angioplasty is a good technique in a single vessel stenosis on dialysis patients? I see from your results there are a few patients undergoing cardiac surgery for one vessel disease.

ROTTEMBOURG Of the five patients who received coronary artery bypass two of them received only one saphenous, two of them two, and one of them three grafts. These operations were performed I think in 1976 or 1977. At that time angioplasty was not available in France. I think from now angioplasty could at least be tried on these patients, but you know that those performing angioplasty do not like to have patients with long-standing hypertension because they know perfectly well that the angioplasty is not performed with great success if the patient has been hypertensive for 10 or 15 years. Most of our uraemic patients have long-term hypertension, so I am not sure that angioplasty will be the right treatment, but it could be tried.

HAEMODIALYSIS IN A SINGLE AND A TWO NEEDLE VASCULAR ACCESS SYSTEM: A COMPARATIVE STUDY

R Vanholder, N Hoenich*, M Piron, J M Billiouw, S Ringoir

Renal Division, University Hospital, Gent, Belgium, and
*University of Newcastle-upon-Tyne, Royal Victoria Infirmary,
Newcastle-upon-Tyne, United Kingdom

Introduction

On theoretical grounds, single needle dialysis has often been claimed to be characterised by a lower dialyser blood flow and a certain degree of recirculation, if compared to the two needle access method. This should result in a lower dialysis performance for the single needle technique, especially as far as small and middle molecular clearances are concerned. However, studies directly investigating the importance of this theoretical disadvantage are relatively scarce.

In our renal division, pressure-pressure monitored single needle haemodialysis was introduced as a routine vascular approach since 1973 [1, 2] and has been performed since then in more than 100,000 dialysis sessions, with good results in patient survival and clinical status. Recent attempts by our group to define dialyser blood flow, small molecular clearances and recirculation rate in several applications of this pressure-pressure single needle technique [3–5], revealed performance data comparable to those obtained with the two needle technique. The present article reviews corresponding in vivo and in vitro performance data of the single and two needle vascular access methods.

Methods

Figure 1 is a flow diagram of the pressure-pressure monitored double headed pump system, as first described by Ringoir and co-workers [1, 2]. A single electric motor (BL 760, Bellco Mirandola, Italy) is coupled to an arterial and a venous pump head by a clutch mechanism. Both pump heads work occlusively and alternately. In the arterial phase, blood is withdrawn from the patient, and a positive pressure is built up in the dialyser blood compartment. When a pre-selected maximum pressure has been reached, the arterial pump head stops rotating, and the venous pump head starts working, until a preset pressure minimum is reached.

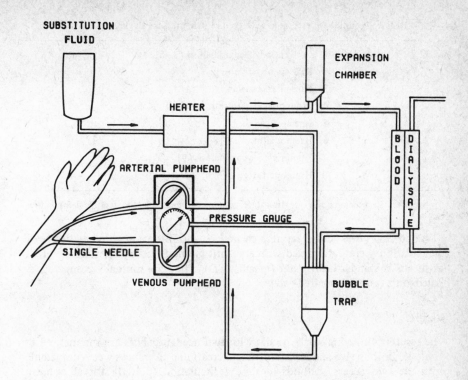

Figure 1. Flow diagram of haemodialysis unit, using conventional unipuncture dialysis equipment

The equipment is completed by an arterial expansion chamber, a venous bubble trap chamber, a heparin pump and a bed scale weight monitor with digital display. In those dialysis strategies where a substitution fluid is infused (haemofiltration, haemodiafiltration, plasmapheresis), a fluid substitution pump and a fluid heater are added.

Single needle dialysis with this pressure-pressure device has been adapted in our unit to all new haemodialysis strategies, introduced since 1976 (Table I).

The present study can be subdivided into two different parts. First, in vivo and in vitro clearances were determined with both single and two needle access method, making use of the same types of haemodialysers. Second, dialyser performances obtained during conventional fistula single needle haemodialysis and during subclavian catheter haemodialysis are compared in the same patients, making use of the same dialysers and working under the same conditions for both access methods. Intravenous catheters introduced into the subclavian vein are regularly used as a vascular access method in our unit [10].

For subclavian catheter haemodialysis a 30cm long modified Shaldon dialysis catheter (Extracorporeal Medical Specialties, King of Prussia, Pennsylvania, USA) was used. Single needle dialysis was performed with the 14-gauge x 25mm Deseret haemodialysis angiocath (Deseret Co, Sandy, Utah, USA).

TABLE I. Techniques performed with the pressure-pressure single needle system*

1. Conventional haemodialysis [3–5]
2. RP6 open system [6]
3. Pure ultrafiltration
4. Sequential ultrafiltration and diffusion
5. Haemofiltration [7]
6. Haemodiafiltration [8]
7. Membrane plasmapheresis [9]
8. Haemoperfusion

* Numbers in brackets refer to literature references describing the technical modalities

Blood flow, urea and creatinine clearances, ultrafiltration rates and degree of recirculation were determined with standard methods [3–5]. Results are given as means ± standard deviation (mean ± SD). They are mutually compared by Wilcoxon's test for unpaired values.

Results

The results comparing single needle with two needle dialysis are summarised in Table II. Both in vivo and in vitro urea and creatinine clearances were comparable with the two access methods, despite recirculation ($p > 0.05$ for all values). Average calculated recirculation was 6 ± 1 per cent in unipuncture.

TABLE II. Small molecular clearance characteristics at a blood flow of 200ml/min

	In vitro		In vivo	
	Urea	Creatinine	Urea	Creatinine
Two needle	155 ± 5	127 ± 5	143 ± 7	119 ± 8
Single needle	157 ± 6	130 ± 7	144 ± 5	116 ± 4
Corrected for recirculation			140 ± 7	112 ± 5

The results comparing single needle fistula dialysis with subclavian catheter dialysis are summarised in Table III. With identical blood flows, both urea and creatinine clearance appeared to be lower in subclavian catheter haemodialysis. This can mainly be attributed to a higher recirculation rate. Dialyser clearances, uncorrected for recirculation, appeared to be similar for both access methods over a wide range of blood flows.

Figure 2 illustrates the ultrafiltration capacity obtained with filters with different ultrafiltration characteristics. It is illustrated that, according to the

TABLE III. In vivo haemodialysis performance in single needle haemodialysis

	Blood flow	Urea clearances	Creatinine clearances	Percentage recirculation
Fistula needle	271 ± 5	157 ± 6	124 ± 5	12 ± 1
Subclavian vein catheter	277 ± 5	144 ± 5*	111 ± 5*	19 ± 1*

* p < 0.05 versus fistula needle

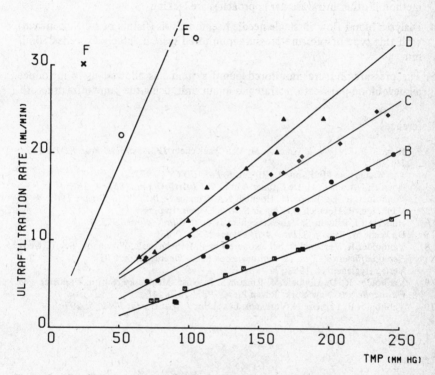

Figure 2. Ultrafiltration characteristics of different filters used with the pressure-pressure monitored single needle technique. Filters A (▫), B (●), C (◆) and D (▲) are regularly used in conventional haemodialysis. Filter E (○) is a high flux haemodialyser used for haemodiafiltration. Filter F (✕) is used in plasmapheresis

individual transmembrane pressures and the properties of the membrane, the ultrafiltration volume can be adapted to the individual needs of each patient and each situation. The pressure-pressure monitored single needle system thus allows an excellent ultrafiltration control, which is especially useful in haemofiltration, haemodiafiltration and plasmapheresis.

179

Conclusions

1. Although recirculation reduces small molecular clearances in single needle haemodialysis, overall dialyser performance is not significantly different from that obtained in two needle dialysis.

2. The pressure-pressure monitored single needle system allows an excellent ultrafiltration control.

3. Haemodialysis performance with a subclavian catheter as an access method is inferior to the results obtained with conventional single and two needle fistula haemodialysis. However, dialysis performance remains sufficient for patient treatment, so that the subclavian catheter remains a valuable access method if other intravascular approaches are lacking.

4. Dialyser blood flow in single needle haemodialysis (fistula or subclavian vein) with this type of pressure-pressure monitored system, largely exceeds 250ml/min.

5. The pressure-pressure monitored pump system has allowed us to introduce all new blood purification strategies in our unit, using the same infrastructure.

References

1 Ringoir S, De Broe M, Cardon M, Van Waeleghem JP. *Abstracts. Proc EDTA 1973; 10:* 200
2 Van Waeleghem JP, Boone L, Ringoir S. *Proc EDTNA 1973; 1:* 10
3 Hoenich NA, Piron M, De Cubber A et al. *Int J Artif Organs 1981; 4:* 168
4 Vanholder R, De Paepe M, Hoenich NA, Ringoir S. *Int J Artif Organs 1981; 4:* 72
5 Vanholder R, Hoenich N, Ringoir S. *Artif Organs.* In press
6 Hilderson J, Ringoir S, Van Waeleghem JP et al. *Clin Nephrol 1975; 4:* 18
7 De Paepe M, Ringoir S. *Int J Artif Organs 1982; 5:* 87
8 Vanholder R, Verbanck J, Schelstraete J et al. In Schütterle, Wizemann, Seyffart, eds. *Hemodiafiltration. Proc 1st Symp Giessen 1981.* Oberursel/Ts, FRG: Verlag Hygieneplan. 1981: 76–80
9 Vanholder R, De Clippele M, Ringoir S. In Nosé, Malchesky, Smith, Krakauer, eds. *Plasmapheresis.* New York: Raven Press. 1983: 145–148
10 Vanholder R, Lameire N, Verbanck J et al. *Int J Artif Organs 1982; 5:* 297

MYOCARDIAL PERFUSION AND LEFT VENTRICULAR PERFORMANCE DURING LONG AND SHORT HAEMODIALYSIS IN PATIENTS WITH CORONARY HEART DISEASE

V Wizemann, W Kramer, J Thormann*, M Kindler*, G Schütterle, M Schlepper*

*Zentrum für Innere Medizin Gissen, and
Kerckhoff-Klinik Bad Nauheim, FRG

Summary

In seven patients with confirmed coronary heart disease and stable blood pressure control acetate haemodialysis improved left ventricular performance and exercise tolerance. Similar positive effects were obtained by a four hour dialysis (one litre fluid removal/hour) and a two hour dialysis (two litre fluid removal/hour). In this group of patients weight gain and overhydration between dialyses appears to be the major risk for myocardial perfusion and rapid weight reduction by acetate dialysis appears adequate therapy. One practical consequence from our study is to minimise fluid overload in coronary heart disease and we try to avoid iatrogenic induction of thirst by decreasing dialysate sodium from 140mmol/litre to 125–135mmol/litre. As far as myocardial risk factors are concerned it appears that it is more important to focus on interdialysis weight gains than on acute dialysis therapy.

Introduction

Epidemiological studies suggest that during regular dialysis therapy coronary heart disease (CHD) does not represent a major mortality risk in patients who have not had symptoms of CHD prior to haemodialysis [1] and that the incidence of death due to myocardial infarction is surprisingly low in large dialysis populations [2, 3]. However, in patients undergoing maintainance dialysis therapy with evidence of pre-established CHD mortality risk is increased [1]. A high incidence of asymptomatic ischaemic causing electrocardiographic changes during dialysis indicates the uncertain significance in the clinical evaluation of myocardial ischaemia [4]. The majority of patients registered by the EDTA in 1981 were treated by short dialysis (<13 hours/week). The necessity of rapid volume removal in short and ultrashort dialysis methods can result in a rapid decrease of cardiac stroke volume [5] and thereby might result in myocardial hypoperfusion. The aim of the present study was to evaluate the cardiac responses to varying fluid volume removal rates in patients with confirmed CHD

181

and stable blood pressure during acetate haemodialysis. Each patient was dialysed for four hours (fluid removal one litre/hour) and for two hours (fluid removal two litres/hour). Before and after each dialysis an ECG, radionuclide angiography (technetium-99) and thallium-201 imaging were performed during rest and exercise conditions.

Patients and methods

Seven male patients (mean age 47 years, range 36—56 years) with a history of arterial hypertension and confirmed CHD were studied. All had a history of stable exertional angina (NYHA II-III) for at least three months with at least three attacks weekly. Two had previous transmural myocardial infarctions and in three coronary angiography was performed. Mean duration of dialysis therapy was 3.6 years (range 0.5—9.5 years), mean haematocrit was 30 per cent (range 28—37%). Drug therapy (e.g. beta-blockers, clonidine, etc.) was withdrawn 72 hours before the measurements were undertaken.

Study protocol: All measurements were performed immediately before and after haemodialysis (Fresenius 2008 C with volume balanced controlled ultra-filtration, hemoflow D6, Q_B 300ml/min, Q_D 500ml/min, dialysate sodium 140mmol/litre, potassium 2.0mmol/litre) and dialysis was carried out in the gamma-camera room. A standardised weight gain between dialyses of 4kg ± 0.3kg for all patients was achieved. Haemodialysis lasted 120 and 240 minutes for each patient. Exercise was performed in a supine position with a bicycle ergometer. During rest and exercise a 12 lead ECG, technetium-99 angiography (Pho/Gamma, L.E.M., Searle, on line computer Osborne-1), and thallium-201 imaging was performed. Statistical analysis was performed by the paired t-test. All data are expressed as mean ± SEM.

TABLE I. Predialysis and postdialysis data during rest and exercise testing (mean ± SEM)

| | | Four hour dialysis | | Two hour dialysis | |
		Pre	Post	Pre	Post
Heart rate (beats/min)	Rest	67 ± 5	70 ± 5	66 ± 4	66 ± 4
	Exercise	123 ± 5	121 ± 4	122 ± 4	122 ± 4
Systolic blood pressure (mmHg)	Rest	153 ± 5	146 ± 4	149 ± 6	149 ± 6
	Exercise	187 ± 9	187 ± 9	178 ± 7	184 ± 8
Wall motion abnormalities	Rest	4.6 ± 1.5	2.6 ± 1.0**	4.3 ± 1.5	2.6 ± 1.0*
	Exercise	6.0 ± 1.4	5.4 ± 1.8**	6.1 ± 1.4	5.1 ± 1.4**

* $p < 0.05$, ** $p < 0.01$ when compared to predialysis values

Results

Comparison of predialysis and postdialysis data

Predialysis heart rate and systolic blood pressure during rest and exercise did not differ from those postdialysis (Table I).

Exercise duration increased from 178 ± 32 seconds predialysis to 415 ± 49 seconds after four hour dialysis (p<0.01) and from 190 ± 33 to 394 ± 37 seconds after two hour dialysis (p<0.01).

Maximal ST-shift in the ECG decreased after both four hour and two hour dialysis when the respective data for rest and exercise conditions were compared (Figure 1) and the same observation was made for exercise pain score (Figure 1).

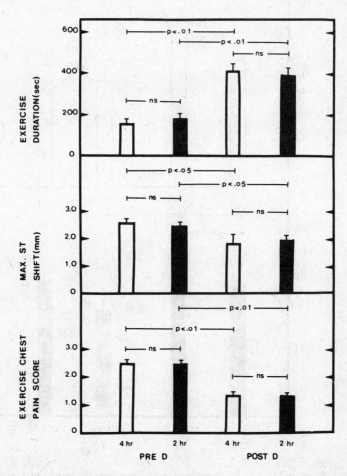

Figure 1. Exercise duration, ST-shift and exercise chest pain score before and after a four hour and a two hour acetate haemodialysis

183

Resting and exercise wall motion abnormalities improved significantly after a four hour and two hour dialysis (Table I).

As shown in Figure 2 ejection fraction decreased during exercise stress predialysis and postdialysis as expected in CHD. Ejection fraction increased from $56 \pm 9\%$ to $65 \pm 9\%$ (resting conditions, $p<0.05$) and from $48 \pm 7\%$ to $54 \pm 8\%$ (exercise conditions, $p<0.05$) after a four hour dialysis. A two hour dialysis led to an increase of ejection fraction from $58 \pm 9\%$ to $68 \pm 10\%$ (resting conditions, $p<0.05$) and from $54 \pm 9\%$ to $61 \pm 10\%$ (exercise conditions, $p>0.05$).

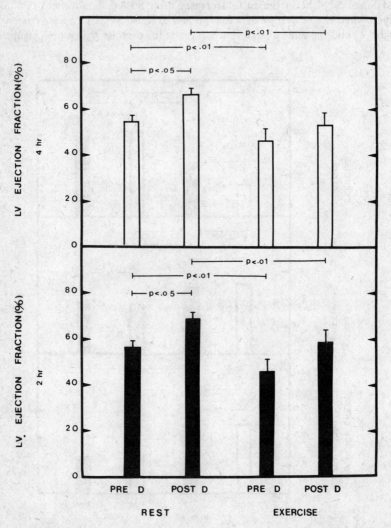

Figure 2. Left ventricular ejection fraction during rest and exercise stress before and after acetate haemodialysis, four hour dialysis (upper panel), two hour dialysis (lower panel)

There was no significant difference in heart rate and systolic blood pressure during rest and exercise conditions when four hour dialysis was compared to two hour dialysis (Table I). The same result was obtained concerning exercise duration, maximal ST-shift, pain score (Figure 1), wall motion abnormalities (Table I) and percentage of ejection fraction during rest and exercise (Figure 2).

Discussion

Most published studies dealing with cardiovascular problems during haemodialysis focus on cardiac output, peripheral vascular resistance and the incidence of symptomatic hypotension. Short dialysis therapy is contraindicated when unstable blood pressure control occurs. On the other hand the majority of haemodialysis patients show a stable blood pressure regulation during volume removal by dialysis [6] but as indicated in a study of 382 dialysis patients the presence of coronary heart disease cannot be ignored [1].

Our study clearly demonstrates that haemodialysis improves left ventricular function and exercise tolerance in patients with CHD and stable blood pressure control and that fluid removal rates of even two litres/hour are beneficial in these patients. It remains to be clarified if the positive cardiac responses are caused by fluid withdrawal and a consequent reduction in preload, removal of a hypothetical cardiodepressant agent by dialysis, a potential positive inotropic action of acetate [7] or by changes in serum electrolytes. Although limited by methodological validity M-mode echocardiography studies support our observations concerning stable haemodialysis patients without confirmed CHD [8, 9] and comparable results were obtained in a study with technetium radionuclide ventriculography [10]. However, in these studies only resting data were analysed. The addition of exercise testing and simultaneous thallium perfusion imaging and technetium radionuclide ventriculography confirm the validity of measurements.

References

1   Rostand SG, Grets JC, Kirk KA et al. *Kidney Int 1979; 16:* 600
2   Roguska J, Simon NM, del Greco F, Krumlovsky FA. *Trans ASAIO 1974; 20:* 579
3   Degoulet P, Legrain M, Réach I et al. *Nephron 1982; 31:* 103
4   Diskin CJ, Salzsieder KH, Solomon RJ et al. *Nephron 1981; 27:* 94
5   Wizemann V, Kramer W, Knopp G et al. *Clin Nephrol 1983; 19:* 24
6   Degoulet P, Réach I, di Giulio S et al. *Proc EDTA 1981; 18:* 133
7   Idelson BA, Redline RC, Schick EC et al. *Abstr ASAIO 1983; 12:* 51
8   Macdonald L, Uldall R, Buda RJ. *Clin Nephrol 1981; 15:* 321
9   Ireland MA, Mehta BR, Shin MF. *Nephron 1981; 29:* 73
10   Hung J, Harris PJ, Uren RF et al. *N Engl J Med 1980; 302:* 347

Proc EDTA (1983) Vol 20

A DEMONSTRATION OF NEUTROPHIL ACCUMULATION IN THE PULMONARY VASCULATURE DURING HAEMODIALYSIS

N J Dodd, M P Gordge, J Tarrant, V Parsons, M J Weston

King's College Hospital Renal Unit, Dulwich Hospital, London, United Kingdom

Summary

[111] Indium oxine labelled autologous neutrophils were used to investigate neutropenia occurring during haemodialysis. Continuous surface counts demonstrated accumulation of labelled neutrophils in the lung, reaching a peak at 15 minutes after commencing dialysis, coincident with a fall in arterial blood and dialyser radioactivity, and a fall in arterial blood neutrophil count. Lung radioactivity returned to baseline after one hour implying reflux of labelled neutrophils into the circulation, whilst dialyser activity rose progressively and remained high even after washback of blood from the dialyser reflecting accumulation of neutrophils on the membrane.

Introduction

Up to 98 per cent of circulating neutrophils may be lost from the peripheral blood 15 minutes after commencing haemodialysis with cuprophane membrane dialysers. Thus $25-30 \times 10^9$ cells (for a patient with a five litre blood volume) disappear from the circulation at a time when only three litres of blood has passed through the dialyser (blood flow 200ml/minute). This dramatic phenomenon has been ascribed to generation of leuco aggregating complement fragments by alternative pathway activation, following blood passage across the polysaccharide cuprophane membrane [1]. Animal experiments have shown that complement mediated leuco aggregation leads to pulmonary leucostasis and consequent disturbance of gas transfer [2]. Similarly, during human haemodialysis the profound neutropenia has been linked with arterial hypoxia and a related increase in the alveolar-arterial oxygen gradient [1].

Brubaker and Nolph [3] used in vitro labelling of neutrophils with ^{32}P diisopropylfluorophosphate, to show that the majority of labelled cells which disappear from the circulation after 15 minutes, have returned by one hour of dialysis. They also found that a rebound neutrophilia occurred and concluded that this reflected bone marrow release of neutrophils in response to neutropenia.

We have used [111]Indium labelled autologous neutrophils with continuous surface counting to plot the time course and sites of neutrophil accumulation or loss during cuprophane haemodialysis.

Methods

Two patients on long-term haemodialysis gave informed consent to participate in this study. Each patient was studied twice, once using labelled neutrophils, and a week later, using labelled platelets prior to the neutrophil experiments; 40ml of venous blood was taken from the patient, heparinised, and leucocyte rich plasma prepared by spontaneous sedimentation of erythrocytes. Neutrophils were then separated from the lymphocytes and platelets by 'Ficoll-Hypaque' density gradient centrifugation, and any residual red cells were removed by hypotonic lysis. After washing in Hank's balanced salt solution the neutrophils were labelled with 250μCi [111]Indium oxine, washed again and finally resuspended in 0.9% saline prior to re-injection. A 5ml suspension containing approximately 1×10^8 labelled cells was injected intravenously one hour prior to haemodialysis.

Platelets, prepared by centrifugation of heparinised whole blood to produce platelet rich plasma, were labelled with 200μCi [111]Indium oxine and similarly re-injected to the patient one hour prior to commencing haemodialysis.

All four study dialyses were performed with a Lucas machine and Gambro Lundia major flat plate dialysers. Continuous surface counting was carried out over the right lung upper zone and spleen, using two inch shielded sodium iodide crystal scintillation detectors, whilst dialyser radioactivity was measured with a three inch shielded crystal. A print-out record was taken every 20 seconds for the first two hours from the lung and spleen detectors, and throughout the entire four hour dialysis from the dialyser detector. Blood samples were taken before, and at intervals during dialysis, for measurement of neutrophil and platelet count, and peripheral blood radioactivity.

Results

All results (Figure 1) are expressed as percentages of the values at the start of dialysis. Graphs A and B show the results of the two labelled neutrophil dialyses. There was a rise in radioactivity over the lung reaching a maximum 15 minutes after starting dialysis, subsequently falling to baseline or below by one hour. This pulmonary accumulation of labelled neutrophils was reflected by a fall in activity over the dialyser and in arterial blood, and by a fall in the neutrophil count. Blood radioactivity and neutrophil count then rose but had not returned to baseline values after two hours. In contrast, there was a progressive rise in dialyser radioactivity above baseline value reaching a maximum at the end of dialysis. This activity fell only slightly after a 500ml washback of the dialyser and a one litre flush with saline.

Mean results of the two labelled platelet dialyses are shown in Graph C. There was a fall in blood radioactivity closely reflecting the platelet count.

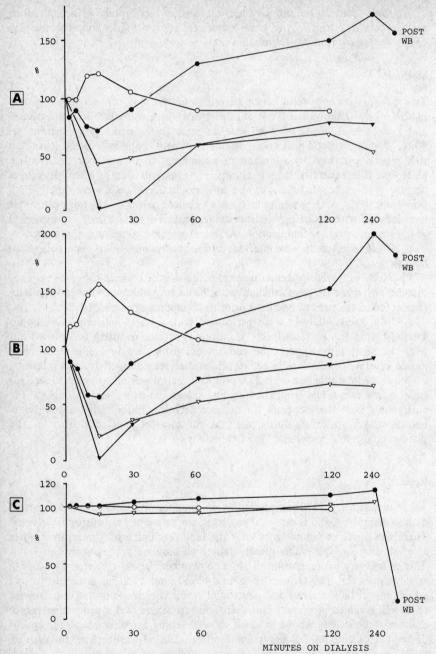

Figure 1. Graphs A and B: Labelled neutrophil dialyses. Graph C: Mean results of labelled platelet dialyses. ○—○ Lung activity; ●—● Dialyser activity; △—△ Blood activity; ▲—▲ Neutrophil count

188

Lung radioactivity remained at baseline initially, showing a small fall later in dialysis. Dialyser activity rose slowly to 14 per cent above baseline but was substantially reduced after washback and a one litre flush with saline.

Surface counts over the spleen during platelet and neutrophil dialyses were high and did not change significantly reflecting pre-dialysis sequestration of cells.

Discussion

We have demonstrated directly accumulation of neutrophils in the lungs during haemodialysis. This accumulation is transient, with activity returning to baseline after one hour indicating a reversible process. However, superoxide production by granulocytes in response to activated complement [4] is potentially damaging to the pulmonary vascular endothelium, and it may be that such a process, repeated twice a week for prolonged periods is related to pulmonary calcification seen in some chronic haemodialysis patients [5].

The subsequent accumulation of neutrophils in the dialyser may have some bearing on dialyser efficiency, particularly towards the end of dialysis. We have previously reported a case in which neutrophil accumulation on the cuprophane membrane was so marked as to substantially reduce dialyser efficiency and necessitate change to a cellulose acetate dialyser [6]. In this study we found that the accumulated neutrophil activity was only slightly reduced after saline flush of the dialyser suggesting that the cells are adherent to the membrane. In contrast, dialyser platelet activity which rose only slightly during four hours' dialysis, was substantially removed after saline flush.

Acknowledgment

We would like to thank Martin Clarke, of the Department of Medical Physics for his assistance.

References

1 Craddock PR et al. *N Engl J Med 1977; 296;* 769
2 Toren M, Goffinet JA, Kaplow LS. *Blood 1970; 36:* 337
3 Brubaker LH, Nolph KD. *Blood 1971; 38:* 623
4 Goldstein IM et al. *J Clin Invest 1975; 56:* 1155
5 Conger JD et al. *Ann Intern Med 1978; 83:* 330
6 Dodd NJ, Parsons V, Weston MJ. *Int J Artif Organs 1982; 5:* 275

HAEMODIALYSIS, CONTINUOUS AMBULATORY PERITONEAL DIALYSIS AND CELLULAR IMMUNITY

F Collart, C Tielemans, M Dratwa, L Schandene*,
J Wybran*, E Dupont*

*Brugmann University Hospital, and *Erasme University
Hospital, Brussels, Belgium*

Summary

The cellular immunity of haemodialysis and continuous ambulatory peritoneal dialysis (CAPD) patients was studied with regards to T-lymphocyte subsets and to suppressor T-cell function. The two groups of patients showed similar alterations: low proportions of suppressor-cytotoxic T-cells and low suppressive activity. In both groups there is a deterioration of this suppressive activity with time on dialysis.

Introduction

The accumulation of middle molecules is one of the many factors implicated in the alterations of cellular immunity in uraemic patients [1]. As these middle molecules are better cleared by continuous ambulatory peritoneal dialysis (CAPD) than by haemodialysis it has been suggested that CAPD should be able to restore normal cellular immunity in those patients [2, 3]. To assess this hypothesis we evaluated the cellular immunity of haemodialysis and CAPD patients with regards to their T-lymphocyte subsets and to their suppressor T-cell activity.

Patients

Thirty-six haemodialysis and 12 CAPD patients were studied. All patients suffering any disease or nephropathy known to be associated with alterations of the T-cell subsets have been excluded from the study [4]. Mean age and mean time on dialysis are reported in Table I.

190

TABLE I. Comparison of T-cell subsets and suppressor T-cell function of 12 CAPD patients and 36 haemodialysis patients

	Normal values	CAPD (n = 12)	p*	HD (n = 36)	p*	p**
Time on dialysis (months)		35.6 ± 3.8		40.4 ± 6.0		NS
Age (years)		65.7 ± 2.8		50.3 ± 2.5		<0.02
OKT3$^+$ cells, %	68.0 ± 2.0	64.6 ± 2.6	NS	60.0 ± 2.0	NS	NS
OKT4$^+$ cells, %	47.0 ± 2.0	43.8 ± 2.5	NS	42.0 ± 2.0	NS	NS
OKT8$^+$ cells, %	27.0 ± 8.0	21.1 ± 1.0	<0.001	19.0 ± 1.0	<0.001	NS
T4/T8	1.6 ± 0.1	2.2 ± 0.2	<0.02	2.5 ± 0.2	<0.001	NS
Con-A test, %	45.1 ± 10.3	32.1 ± 6.3	<0.02	27.2 ± 4.3	<0.005	NS
MLC test, %	50.2 ± 12.7	31.2 ± 11.4	NS	20.0 ± 5.3	<0.001	NS

p*   versus normal controls

p** CAPD versus haemodialysis (HD) patients

Results are given as means ± SEM

Methods

T-lymphocyte subsets were enumerated by an indirect immunofluorescence assay with monoclonal antibodies produced by mouse hybridomas [5]. Three monoclonal antibodies were used: OKT3, reacting with all peripheral T-cells, OKT4 identifying only T-cells with helper or inducer function and OKT8 directed against a T-cell subset with suppressor-cytotoxic function.

The suppressive activity was generated by incubation of the patients' lymphocytes with concanavalin-A (Con-A) for 24 hours and then assayed by measuring their inhibitory potency on the proliferative response of autologous monocytes to Con-A or in mixed lymphocytes culture (Con-A test and MLC test). We measured the proliferative response by the amount of ^{3}H-thymidine incorporated into cellular DNA in the presence and absence of the suppressor cells. The inhibition of the proliferative response was expressed as a percentage of suppression following the formula:

$$\% \text{ suppression} = \left(1 - \frac{\text{CPM in the presence of suppressor cells}}{\text{CPM in the absence of suppressor cells}}\right) \times 100$$

Results

Haemodialysis and CAPD patients presented similar profiles of their T-lymphocyte subsets (Table I): normal proportions of total T-cells, of helper T-cells, low proportions of suppressor-cytotoxic T-cells and increased ratio of helper to suppressor cells. In both haemodialysis and CAPD patients there was a profound decrease in the suppressive function. No differences with regards to those parameters were observed between haemodialysis and CAPD patients. It should be

191

noted that our CAPD patients were older than our haemodialysis patients. As it is known that age alters cellular immunity [6], we also compared smaller groups of CAPD and haemodialysis patients matched for age, sex and time on dialysis (Table II). In those two groups we found no difference in T-lymphocyte subsets

TABLE II. Comparison of nine CAPD and nine haemodialysis (HD) patients matched for age, sex and time on dialysis

	CAPD	HD	p
OKT8$^+$ cells, %	21.2 ± 1.3	22.1 ± 2.2	NS
T4/T8	2.2 ± 0.2	2.0 ± 0.3	NS
Con-A test, %	26.3 ± 8.0	23.9 ± 7.9	NS
MLC test, %	35.2 ± 11.4	17.1 ± 9.6	NS

Results are given as means ± SEM

nor in suppressive activity, ruling out a possible age effect. To evaluate the possible influence of the dialysis method on cellular immunity we then searched for a correlation between suppressive activity and time on dialysis (Figure 1). In both groups a negative correlation was found between those two parameters. This correlation was statistically significant in haemodialysis patients but not in CAPD patients. However, statistical comparison of the two regression lines show that they are not different. Thus it may be concluded that the evolution of suppressor T-cell activity is not different in CAPD and haemodialysis patients.

Discussion

The present study confirms that haemodialysis is not able to improve the cellular immunity of uraemic patients; furthermore it shows a real deterioration of T-cell suppressive function. The low suppressive activity did not correlate with other parameters commonly implicated in the alterations of the cellular immunity of uraemic patients (plasma albumin, plasma zinc, vitamin deficiency) so that we can only conclude that the progressive alteration of this parameter is due to the accumulation of one or more poorly or non-dialysable substances. The evolution of CAPD patients seems not to be different.

Our results are in agreement with those of Singh et al [7] who studied the changes of T-lymphocyte subsets of patients transferred from haemodialysis to CAPD in whom they found similar alterations and no improvement with CAPD treatment. Recent work by two Italian groups have shown that the results of the E-rosette test in vitro and of the tuberculin hypersensitivity skin test improve with time on CAPD [2, 3]. In apparent opposition to the latter, the present study does not show any improvement with time in the suppressive activity of CAPD patients. It should be pointed out that in those reports other parameters of the cellular immunity were studied: the E-rosette test evaluates the number of T-cells possessing sheep red-blood cell receptors and the tuberculin hyper-

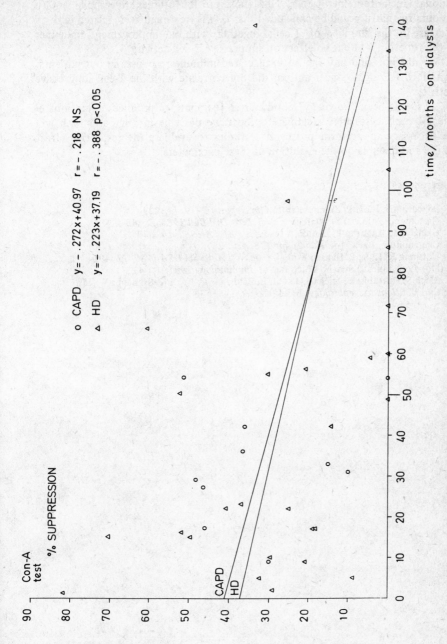

Figure 1. Correlation between time on dialysis and suppressive activity in haemodialysis and CAPD patients

sensitivity skin test reflects the activity of different immunocompetent cells among which are helper T-cells. Thus those previous studies are complementary to ours so that it could be concluded that CAPD treatment is associated with an increase in the number of T-cells together with an improvement in helper T-cell function, but has no effect on suppressive T-cell activity.

We did not find any sign of exaggerated immune responses in our patients: IgA, IgE, IgG, IgM concentrations did not correlate with the T-cell suppressive activity.

As it has been shown by Moody et al [6] that age produces alterations in the T-lymphocyte subsets similar to those we describe in our patients, it will be necessary to perform prospective studies to evaluate the respective effect of age and uraemia on the evolution of these parameters.

References

1   Bergström J, Fürst P, Zimmerman L. *Clin Nephrol 1979; 11:* 229
2   Giacchino F, Alloatti S, Quarello F et al. *Perit Dial Bull 1982; 2:* 165
3   Giangrande A, Cantu P, Limido A et al. *Proc EDTA 1982; 19:* 372
4   Chatenoud L, Bach M-A. *Kidney Int 1981; 20:* 267
5   Hoffman R, Kung P, Hansen W et al. *Proc Natl Acad Sci USA 1980; 77:* 4914
6   Moody C, Innes J, Staiano-Coico L et al. *Immunology 1981; 44:* 431
7   Singh S, Hurtubise P, Michael G et al. In Baldamus C, Koch K, Schoeppe W, eds. *Contributions to Nephrology.* Basel: Karger. 1983: 36

GLUCOSE, INSULIN AND C-PEPTIDE KINETICS DURING CONTINUOUS AMBULATORY PERITONEAL DIALYSIS

T-E Wideröe, L C Smeby, O L Myking*, T Wessel-Aas

*University of Trondheim, and *University of Bergen, Norway*

Summary

The insulin and C-peptide kinetics due to glucose (50g), given intraperitoneally or enterally has been compared in five non-diabetic patients on continuous ambulatory peritoneal dialysis (CAPD). The fasting C-peptide concentrations were three to ten times the normal values whereas the fasting plasma insulin concentrations were within normal limits. After intraperitoneal glucose administration a more marked hyperglycaemia ($p < 0.05$) and a more long lasting hyperinsulinaemia ($p < 0.05$) was found than after the enteral glucose load. The relative change in plasma C-peptide was slower and less pronounced in both experiments. C-peptide concentration in plasma did not differ significantly between the two experiments. Estimated total body clearance (K_t) for insulin was higher than for C-peptide ($p < 0.01$), but dialysis clearance (K_d) for C-peptide was higher than for insulin in both experiments ($p < 0.01$).

Introduction

Insulin and C-peptide, which has no recognised metabolic activity [1, 2], are produced in the pancreatic β-cells by cleavage of pro-insulin and subsequently secreted into portal circulation in equimolar concentrations [3]. The liver removes about 60–70 per cent of the insulin [1, 2], but only minor fractions of the C-peptide [1, 2]. It has been suggested that C-peptide is metabolised mainly by the kidney [1]. Normally, 5–20 per cent of pancreatic secretion of C-peptide and 0.1 per cent of endogenous insulin is excreted in urine [1, 3]. Half time disappearance rates are about 11–33 minutes for C-peptide and about five minutes for insulin [1, 3, 4]. In the fasting state, the molar concentration of C-peptide in blood is five to seven times higher than that of insulin because of the slower turnover of C-peptide. After stimulation, the relative increase in insulin concentration is higher than for C-peptide, because of its lower basal concentration [1].

Transperitoneal glucose administration would be expected to give a response similar to intravenous glucose loading. C-peptide measurements in plasma and in dialysate during CAPD could be of value as an indicator of the β-cell function in patients on CAPD treatment.

This study investigates insulin and C-peptide responses to equimolar glucose loads given either by the peritoneal or the oral route, and the transperitoneal transport of these compounds in patients on CAPD treatment.

Methods

Five patients, mean age 44 years (range 21—57), were selected for the investigation after informed consent was given. All patients had been well controlled on CAPD treatment for 3—16 months. The exchange procedure for all patients was four two litre bags daily.

Each patient was examined twice with a one week interval between studies.

Experiment 1: A peritoneal glucose infusion of 429mmol (77g) was given using two litre dialysate (Dianeal®, Travenol Industries, Halden, Norway). Simultaneous blood and dialysate samples for measurements of insulin, C-peptide and glucose concentrations were taken before instillation, and at the subsequent dwell-times (T_d): seven (during infusion), 15 (end of infusion, 20, 25, 30, 40, 45, 75, 135, 195 and 255 (end of drainage) minutes after the start of dialysate infusion.

Experiment 2: 278mmol (50g) anhydrous glucose dissolved in 75ml water (corresponding to the mean three hours transperitoneal absorption of glucose during the first investigation) were given by mouth while one litre Ringer lactate (Knut Spærens Laboratories A/S, Tønsberg, Norway) was instilled into the peritoneal cavity. Samples from blood and the instilled Ringer solution were obtained at the start and then at the following dwell-times: 30, 40, 60, 80, 210 and 180 (during drainage) minutes. Drained dialysate volumes were measured in both experiments.

The patients were fasting during each investigation period. During the night before the test, two litre dialysate containing 1.5g glucose/100ml were instilled for nine hours and the peritoneal cavity was drained just before starting the investigation the next morning.

Insulin and C-peptide concentrations were determined by commercial RIA-kits: 'C-peptide II kit', Aiichi, Tokyo, Japan, and 'Phadebase Insulin Test', Pharmacia, Uppsala, Sweden.

The calculation of total body clearance (K_t) for insulin and C-peptide was based on a single compartment model with first order disappearance kinetics. Distribution of volume was chosen as 16 per cent of body weight [5].

The calculation of dialysis clearance (K_d) for insulin and C-peptide must be referred to the plasma concentration of these compounds, and we chose to use estimated mean plasma values ($\overline{C}_p$) during each of the two experiments, which gives a dialytic clearance as:

$$K_d = \frac{(V_d \cdot C_d) - (V_{d0} \cdot C_{d0})}{\overline{C}_p \cdot T}$$

For calculation of K_t and K_d, four hours were used in experiment one and three hours in experiment 2.

196

TABLE I. Individual kinetic changes in plasma concentrations of glucose, insulin and C-peptide during peritoneal and enteral glucose load. The changes are expressed as ΔC_{max}: maximal change in absolute concentration relative to initial value; ΔC_{3h}: change in absolute concentration at three hours relative to initial value; and $\Delta C\%$: mean change in relative plasma concentration (in per cent of initial value) during three hours

$$\left(=\frac{1}{T}\int_{o}^{T}\Delta C\% \times dt\right).$$

The significances of the differences between peritoneal and enteral glucose load are given for the mean values of such substance.

PATIENTS	GLUCOSE (mmol/L or %) Peritoneal			Enteral			INSULIN (mU/L or %) Peritoneal			Enteral			C-PEPTIDE (µg/L or %) Peritoneal			Enteral		
	ΔC_{max}	ΔC_{3h}	$\overline{\Delta C}\%$	ΔC_{max}	ΔC_{3h}	$\overline{\Delta C}\%$	ΔC_{max}	ΔC_{3h}	$\overline{\Delta C}\%$	ΔC_{max}	ΔC_{3h}	$\overline{\Delta C}\%$	ΔC_{max}	ΔC_{3h}	$\overline{\Delta C}\%$	ΔC_{max}	ΔC_{3h}	$\overline{\Delta C}\%$
A. S. A.	4.4	1.6	59.1	2.5	-0.5	14.5	14	7.3	283.7	63	-2.6	159.9	5.4	4.6	46.1	5.1	1.7	66.1
L. G.	4.3	0.6	58.3	2.6	0.5	37.0	59	6.3	343.0	56	-2.3	147.5	7.8	3.3	80.9	7.2	4.6	81.1
E. W.	3.3	0.6	36.7	3.9	-1.0	32.5	137	43.5	212.5	111	11.2	76.7	6.0	5.2	17.7	18.2	13.3	26.7
B. B.	6.1	2.3	184.2	1.9	-0.7	26.8	44	6.4	267.3	64	0.9	228.0	6.1	4.1	56.6	3.4	0.5	24.3
P. S.	4.2	0.4	45.5	3.1	0.1	24.9	57	2.5	206.2	97	2.4	250.4	7.4	6.5	54.8	5.2	1.3	30.1
Mean ± SEM	4.5 ±0.5	1.1 ±0.4	76.8 ±27.2	2.5 ±0.2	-0.3 ±0.3	27.1 ±3.8	62.2 ±20.4	13.3 ±7.6	262.5 ±25.1	78.2 ±10.9	1.9 ±2.5	172.7 ±31	6.6 ±0.5	4.7 ±0.5	51.2 ±10.2	7.8 ±2.7	4.3 ±2.4	45.7 ±11.7
Significance	p<0.05	p<0.05	p<0.1	-	-	-	n.s.	p<0.01	p<0.05	-	-	-	n.s.	n.s.	n.s.	-	-	-
Norm. values	3.6 - 5.8						0 - 70						1.13 - 2.73					

197

Statistical methods

Statistical calculations were based on Student's t-test for paired data and all values are given as mean ± SEM.

Results

The mean (± SEM) drained volume for all patients from the peritoneal cavity was 2810 ± 49ml after four hours dwell-time during experiment 1, and 776 ± 47ml after three hours dwell-time during experiment 2.

The individual differences of the time dependent changes in blood concentrations of glucose, insulin and C-peptide between enteral and peritoneal glucose absorption are given in Table I. One patient (EW) was an obese, hyperinsulinaemic female with a completely different glucose/insulin relationship than the other patients, and results from patient EW had a great influence on the statistical significance of the differences between the two experiments. The following differences relative to the initial plasma concentration were found: maximal increase (ΔC_{max}) and the change after three hours (ΔC_{3h}) in blood glucose were highest (p<0.05) during peritoneal glucose administration. A similar difference was found when the mean increase during three hours in the relative blood glucose concentration ($\Delta C\% = (C - C_0/C_0) \times 100\%$) was compared (p<0.05). $\Delta C\%$ and ΔC_{3h} for insulin was higher (p<0.05 and p<0.01, respectively) during the peritoneal glucose absorption as compared to the enteral absorption. No differences between the two experiments could be detected for C-peptide measurements.

The increase in plasma values was slower and reached a plateau only about 70 per cent higher than initial concentration for C-peptide as compared to 400 per cent for insulin. The fasting concentrations of C-peptide were elevated as compared to normal values (Table I), i.e. 11.3 ± 3.4 to 19.1 ± 5.9μg/L in experiment 1 and 11.9 ± 4.2 to 18.5 ± 4.1μg/L in experiment 2. Fasting insulin values were within the normal range, i.e. 26.3 ± 15.9 to 105. 2 ± 25.2mU/L in experiment 1 and 14.2 ± 6.0 to 76.2 ± 26.2mU/L in experiment 2.

After three hours instillation time the insulin concentration in the instilled fluids was 25.5 ± 8.6 and 26.5 ± 2.3% of mean plasma concentration ($\bar{C}_p$) during the first and second experiment respectively. The corresponding C-peptide concentrations were 35.4 ± 3.6 per cent and 50.8 ± 6.8 per cent. Calculated mean total body clearance (K_t) and dialysis clearance (K_d) for insulin and C-peptide for the two experiments are shown in Table II, and the following

TABLE II. Calculated mean total body clearance (K_t) and dialysis clearance (K_d) for insulin and C-peptide during enteral and transperitoneal glucose load

| Glucose load | K_t (ml/min) | | K_d (ml/min) | |
	Insulin	C-peptide	Insulin	C-peptide
Enteral	208.0 ± 39.8	28.6 ± 6.0	1.13 ± 0.10	2.22 ± 0.40
Transperitoneal	117.2 ± 13.2	28.1 ± 2.7	2.75 ± 0.64	4.35 ± 0.40

differences should be noted: estimated K_t for insulin was higher than for C-peptide ($p<0.01$), while K_d for C-peptide was higher than for insulin ($p<0.01$) in both experiments. When changing from one litre Ringer solution to two litre 4.25 per cent dialysate in the peritoneal cavity, K_d increased for insulin ($p<0.05$) and for C-peptide ($p<0.01$). K_t for insulin was lower during enteral as compared to peritoneal glucose load ($p<0.025$), while K_t for C-peptides was unchanged in the two experiments.

Discussion

Peritoneal absorption takes a longer time than intestinal absorption. To absorb a dose of 50g glucose from an intraperitoneal pool of about 70g (measured value) in two litres, three hours dwell-time was needed. The individual variability in absorption following this route of administration was about 30 per cent. A more pronounced initial and longer lasting hyperglycaemia was found when glucose was given through the peritoneal membrane, and after one hour all patients remained more hyperinsulinaemic during the peritoneal glucose load.

The lasting hyperglycaemia and hyperinsulinaemia after peritoneal glucose administration can be explained by the slow and continuous absorption of glucose together with peripheral carbohydrate intolerance in uraemic patients [6,7]. The different initial (0—45 minutes) hyperglycaemia in the two experiments can be due to differences in both glucose absorption and transport to peripheral blood. However, it is difficult to depict differences in these mechanisms. More than 60 per cent of orally ingested, highly concentrated glucose solutions is absorbed within the first minutes [8, 9]. After intraperitoneal glucose administration the glucose concentration decreased from about 190 to 110mmol/L after 45 minutes. If the ultrafiltration volume at 45 minutes dwell-time is estimated to be about 500ml, calculated glucose absorption is 19g. These findings, which are in agreement with earlier measurements are, however, in contrast with the higher blood glucose values found during peritoneal load in this study.

An explanation to the different degree of initial hyperglycaemia in these experiments could be that a larger part of peritoneally absorbed glucose bypasses the portal circulation than glucose absorbed from the intestine. It is uncertain from this study if the insulinotropic properties of gastric hormones are of any importance in this matter.

Increased fasting plasma C-peptide concentration and increased molar ratio between fasting plasma C-peptide and insulin in uraemic patients is reported [10]. Our study confirms these findings, however, both the fasting concentrations in plasma of C-peptide and the ratio between C-peptide and insulin were much higher than found by others in uraemic patients treated with haemodialysis [10]. This could indicate that CAPD treatment results in a continuous increased production of pro-insulin. This assumption could not be reflected by measurement of fasting insulin concentrations which were within the normal range.

The significant higher K_d for C-peptide than for insulin is probably due to the different molecular weights of insulin (~ 6000 daltons) and C-peptide (~ 3000 daltons). As expected from simple diffusion and convection, increased dialysate volume and osmolality resulted in increased K_d for both hormones. We found a significantly higher K_t for insulin than for C-peptide, reflecting the higher metabolic clearance [1, 2]. The lower K_t for insulin during the peritoneal glucose load compared to enteral glucose load can be explained by the model used for calculation of K_t. Continuous glucose absorption through the peritoneum gives a sustained insulin secretion which cause the calculated clearance for insulin during peritoneal glucose administration to be underestimated as the formula used assumes no insulin production.

In conclusion the three to ten times increased fasting C-peptide values in plasma assumes a continuous increased production of pro-insulin during CAPD treatment. C-peptide concentrations in samples from instilled dialysate gives a better estimate of plasma values than corresponding insulin values. Measurements of C-peptide in both plasma and in the instilled peritoneal dialysate could be of value for an evaluation of β-cell function in patients on CAPD treatment needing exogenous insulin and producing antibodies to this exogeneous compound.

Our experiments also show that the peritoneal route results in more prolonged hyperglycaemia and hyperinsulinaemia than the enteral. As insulin augments the hepatic production of triglycerides and very low density lipoproteins, this may contribute to a higher risk of progressive atherosclerosis in patients treated with CAPD. Long-term observations on changes in insulin response during CAPD treatment are still lacking.

Acknowledgments

This work was supported by a grant from Travenol Laboratories A/S, Norway.

References

1   Faber OK, Kehlet H, Madsbad S et al. *Diabetes 1978; 27 (Suppl 1):* 207
2   Kühl C, Gaber OK, Hornes P et al. *Diabetes 1978; 27 (Suppl 1):* 197
3   Gerbitz KD. *J Clin Chem Clin Biochem 1980; 18:* 313
4   Faber OK, Hagen C, Binder C et al. *J Clin Invest 1978; 62:* 197
5   Turner RC, Grayburn JA, Newman GB et al. *J Clin Endocrinol 1979; 33:* 279
6   Mondon CE, Dolkas CB, Reaven GM et al. *Diabetes 1978; 27:* 571
7   Rabkin R, Unterhalter SA, Duckworth WC. *Kidney Int 1979; 16:* 433
8   Wiseman G, ed. *Absorption from the Intestine.* New York and London: Academic Press. 1964: 17
9   Davenport HW, ed. *Physiology of the Digestive Tract.* Chicago: Year Book Medical Publishers Inc. 1973: 183
10 Kajinuma H, Tanabashi S, Ishiwata K et al. In *Symposium on Proinsulin, Insulin and C-peptide, Tokushima, Japan, 1978. International Congress Series 486.* Amsterdam: Excerpta Medica. 1978: 183

USE OF UREA KINETIC MODEL AND HAEMOFILTRATION TO IMPROVE NITROGEN BALANCE IN HAEMODIALYSED CHILDREN

M Giani, M Picca, A Saccaggi, L Capitanio, R Galato, A Bettinelli, N Teotino, L Ghio, A Edefonti

Pediatric Dialysis Unit, University of Milan, Italy

Summary

To improve nitrogen balance and nutritional status, 10 paediatric patients (11.2 ± 2.7 years; 28.5 ± 5.1kg) on regular haemodialysis (HD) for 25.3 ± 1.2 months were treated with haemofiltration (HF) for 12.2 ± 3.4 months. HF was prescribed using a urea kinetic model to ensure a pre-treatment blood urea nitrogen (BUN) of 130mg/100ml. Urea generation rate (Gu) and protein catabolic rate (PCR) were computed by urea kinetics. Protein and calorie intake was assessed in the children on an unrestricted diet by analysis of 10 days' dietary records obtained every two months. During HF treatment a significant decrease of Gu and PCR was obtained and nitrogen balance increased in all the children.

Introduction

Nitrogen (N) balance is often negative in patients on haemodialysis (HD) and this could greatly affect growth in children [1]. N balance constitutes an important critical factor in the treatment of dialysed children for two opposite reasons. On the one hand, these children often have anorexia that results in decreased protein and calorie intake with catabolism of endogenous protein stores [2]; on the other hand, excessive protein intake increases nitrogenous products [3]. As a result an evaluation of the patient's nutritional state is necessary to tailor dialysis treatment to the patient's needs. Urea kinetic analysis provides important information about urea generation rate (Gu) and the amount of catabolised proteins [4] and using this model, we have studied N balance in 10 children during HD and haemofiltration (HF).

Materials and methods

Ten children, on regular HD for 25.3 ± 1.2 months and subsequently treated with HF for 12.2 ± 3.4 months, were studied. The clinical data are shown in

TABLE I. Clinical data of patients

Patient Number	Age (years)	Sex	Pubertal status	Weight (kg)	Diagnosis*	GFR ml/min/1.73m²
1	13.5	M	pre	25	a	–
2	7.2	F	pre	10.8	b	–
3	7.4	F	pre	15.5	b	–
4	12.7	M	pre	22	c	1.9
5	11.3	F	pre	20	d	–
6	15.2	M	pre	25.7	b	–
7	12.8	F	pre	25	a	0.9
8	9.7	M	pre	16	d	1.1
9	10.2	M	pre	25	d	1.3
10	11.4	M	pre	23	b	1.2
Mean	11.2			20.8		
SD	±2.7			±5.1		

* a=Haemolytic uraemic syndrome; b=Heredo-familial diseases; c=Focal glomerulosclerosis; d=Chronic pyelonephritis

Table I. HD treatment was established following the standard requirements for children [5]. Urea kinetic modelling according to Gotch [4] was utilised for Gu and protein catabolic rate (PCR) determination during HD and HF and to determine in HF the amount of ultrafiltrate necessary to maintain the mean pre-treatment BUN less than 130mg/100ml. These assessments were performed over a period of 10 days every two months. At the same time the dietary protein and calorie intake was assessed. All the children were on an unrestricted diet. N balance was expressed as the difference between dietary protein intake (DPI) and PCR kinetically determined.

Results

Table II shows the mean values of DPI, Calories, BUN, Gu and PCR obtained in our patients during HD and HF respectively. Dietary assessments showed

TABLE II. Mean values obtained in 10 children during haemodialysis and haemofiltration

		DPI g/kg/day	CAL kg/day	BUN mg/100ml	Gu mg/min	PCR g/kg/day
HD	Mean	2.04	58.13	158	4.06	2.09
	SD	±0.72	±8.43	±46	±0.7	±0.56
HF	Mean	2	58.59	110	3.2	1.62
	SD	±0.58	±10.28	±25	±0.75	±0.28
		NS	NS	$p < 0.05$	$p < 0.05$	$p < 0.05$

no significant difference in protein and calorie intake between the HD and HF periods of the study. In particular, in seven of 10 patients the protein intake was greater than 100 per cent of the recommended dietary allowances (RDA) [6] according to statural age; in two other children the values were 100 per cent RDA; only one child had lower values. In five of 10 children calorie intake was higher or equal to 75 per cent of the counselled values.

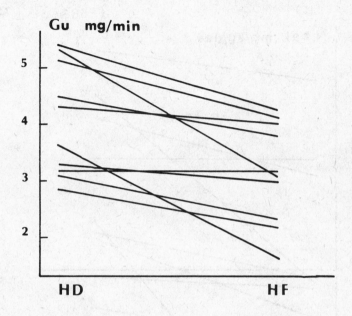

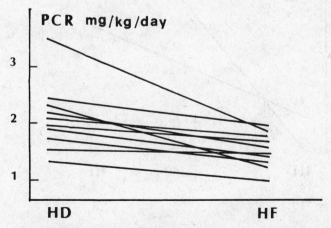

Figure 1 Changes in Gu and PCR for each patient during HD and HF

BUN, Gu and PCR were significantly lower during HF in comparison with HD. The changes in Gu and PCR values for each patient are shown in Figure 1.

N balance had a significant increase changing from a mean value of −14.6mg/kg/day during HD to +53.6mg/kg/day during HF (Figure 2). A significant linear correlation was found between DPI and N balance and between calorie intake and N balance (Figures 3 and 4).

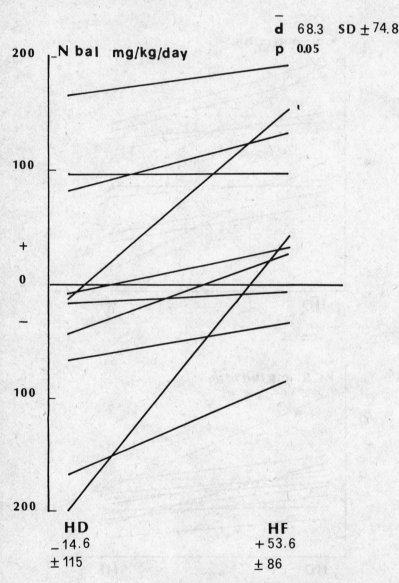

Figure 2. Changes in N balance for each patient during HD and HF

204

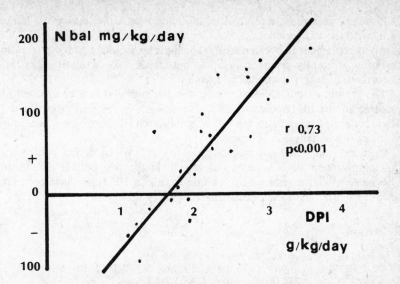

Figure 3. Relationship between DPI and N balance

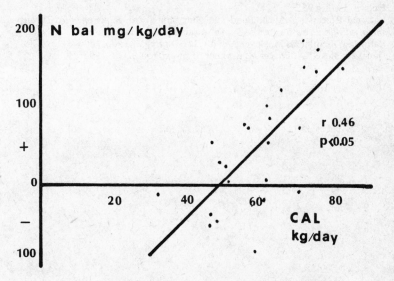

Figure 4. Relationship between calorie intake and N balance

The height of the children improved from a mean value of 2.3 ± 1.4cm/year/patient during HD to 3.28 ± 1.2cm/year/patient during HF.

Conclusions

In our patients, with very similar calorie and protein intake, BUN, Gu and

PCR values were significantly lower and N balance higher during the HF compared with the HD period.

An improvement in N balance after adequate nutritional and dialysis treatment has been previously reported [7]. Our results, in a larger study, confirm the importance of such a combined approach.

The growth in our children during the HD period was very similar to that reported in the EDTA data of 1981 for patients on an unrestricted diet [8]. The accelerated growth in the same patients in HF could be a consequence of the positive changes in N balance.

In conclusion, the different method of dialysis treatment could explain the improvement of N balance and growth in the two periods of our study. The more effective removal of uraemic toxins in HF could have contributed to the amelioration of the protein anabolism.

References

1   Abitbol CL, Holliday MA. *Clin Nephrol 1978; 10:* 9
2   Schoenfeld PY, Henry RR, Laird NM et al. *Kidney Int 1983; 23:* 80
3   Bennett N, Davies RK. *Dial Transplant 1981; 10:* 332
4   Sargent J, Gotch F, Borah M et al. *Am J Clin Nutr 1978; 31:* 1696
5   Linch RE, Mauer SM, Buselmeier TJ et al. In Strauss J, ed. *Pediatric Nephrology, Renal Failure.* 1978; 195
6   National Research Council, Food and Nutrition Board. *Recommended Dietary Allowances, edition 9.* Washington: National Academy of Sciences. 1980
7   Harmon WE, Spinozzi M, Meyer A et al. *Dial Transplant 1981; 10:* 324
8   Donckerwolcke RA, Broyer M, Brunner FP et al. *Proc EDTA 1982; 19:* 84

RISK OF ORALLY ADMINISTERED ALUMINIUM HYDROXIDE AND RESULTS OF WITHDRAWAL

F Bournerias, N Monnier, R J Reveillaud

Centre Hospitalier, Saint-Cloud, France

Summary

In 23 haemodialysis patients, taking regularly aluminium hydroxide ($Al(OH)_3$) of various dosage regimens for more than 18 months, three developed aluminium (Al) related morbidity (fracturing osteopathy 3/3, encephalopathy 2/3, 1/3 died).

In 15 patients followed for 14 months after $Al(OH)_3$ withdrawal the previously elevated serum Al concentrations fell and no worsening of osteodystrophy (especially hyperparathyroidism) could be demonstrated.

Our data and other reports suggest that oral administration of Al containing phosphate binders causes unacceptable morbidity for an unproven benefit, and should be avoided.

Introduction

Despite remaining controversies, there is now increasing evidence that orally administrated aluminium (Al) containing phosphate binders, principally aluminium hydroxide ($Al(OH)_3$), are implicated in dialysis encephalopathy [1] and a particular form of renal osteodystrophy [2].

However, in 1981 90 per cent of European haemodialysis (HD) centres reported using routinely Al containing gels, and only 14 per cent monitored Al serum concentrations regularly [3].

We report here our experience in a haemodialysis centre with a low water Al concentration.

Patients and methods

Patients

Twenty-three haemodialysed patients were studied (11 male, 12 female, mean age 54 years). All were continuously dialysed in our centre and all received

207

various dosage regimens of $Al(OH)_3$ (3–12g/day) for more than 18 months (18–104, mean 55 months) without significant interruption. None presented chronic active hepatitis or other severe intercurrent diseases (prior to October 1981).

Dialysis schedule

All patients were haemodialysed 3 x 4 or 5 hours weekly on a standard dialysate (Ca content 1.75mmol/L).

Water treatment was by conventional softening; it remained unchanged during the study. Water and dialysate Al contents were assayed each six months from 1979 and were constantly $<20\mu g/L$ ($<0.75\mu mol/L$).

Laboratory analyses

Blood samples were obtained immediately before dialysis in each patient and serum calcium (Ca), phosphate (P) and alkaline phosphatase were measured monthly by standard autoanalyser.

Serum Al concentrations were measured by flameless atomic absorption spectrometry, using a graphite furnace, six monthly from 1979 to 1981, and at three and 14 months after $Al(OH)_3$ withdrawal.

Immunoreactive parathormone (iPTH) was measured by radioimmunoassay (CEA antibody detecting C terminal fragment), three months before and 14 months after $Al(OH)_3$ withdrawal.

Radiology and EEG

All patients had an EEG study in 1981, and those with abnormalities again in 1982.

X-ray films of the bones (hands and acromio-clavicular joints) were performed routinely each six months. Films from 1981 and 1982 were closely reviewed, especially for signs of hyperparathyroidism.

Statistical methods

Statistical analysis was performed using the paired Student's t-test.

Results

During $Al(OH)_3$ use, serum Al concentrations were elevated (Figure 1) (five patients had Al$<50\mu g/L$ and high P, suggesting poor compliance).

In 1980–1981, three patients developed Al-related pathology (Table I), two improved markedly after $Al(OH)_3$ was stopped, and one died. EEG studies demonstrated abnormalities in six other patients (grade 1 in four patients, grade 2 in 2) [4].

Complete withdrawal of $Al(OH)_3$ was instituted in October 1981, and patients were given low doses (2–6g/day) of calcium carbonate ($CaCO_3$). The treatment

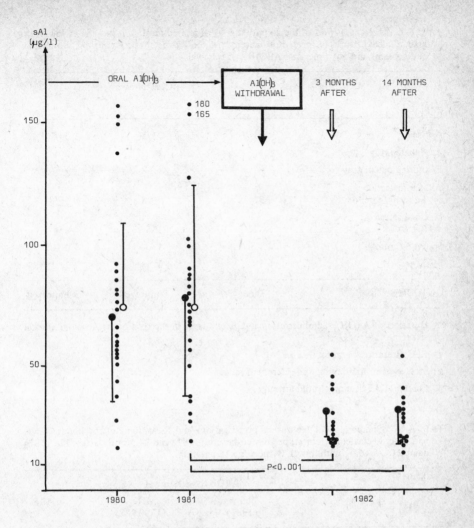

Figure 1. Serum Al before and after Al(OH)₃ withdrawal. Mean serum Al ± SD; n = 23: ○; n = 15: ●; individual patient's values: ●

regimen remained otherwise unchanged.

Of the 22 surviving patients, 15 were followed-up for 14 months after Al(OH)₃ was stopped, and seven were lost for follow-up (two died of unrelated causes, four were transferred and one was transplanted). Laboratory results and X-ray films were compared before and after Al withdrawal in these 15 patients.

Serum Al fell dramatically (Figure 1) and remained low for all patients. No new cases of encephalopathy or fracturing osteopathy were observed. The EEG improved in two out of the four patients with repeat studies.

Serum P increased significantly (Table II) (over 2.5mmol/L in only three patients) and serum Ca remained stable.

TABLE I. Three cases (out of the 23 patients) of Al-related morbidity in 1980–1981, with main clinical features (+: present; 0: absent), Al and P concentrations at time of maximal clinical signs and outcome after $Al(OH)_3$ withdrawal

	Case number		
	1	2	3
Age/sex	61/F	71/M	54/F
Encephalopathy	+	+	0
Fracturing osteopathy	+	+	+
Al administration (months/g per day*)	32/3	70/8	55/8
Maximal serum Al (μg/L)	570	165	154
Serum P (mmol/L)	1.5	1.6	2.10
EEG (grade)†	3	3	1
OUTCOME	Died‡	Improved§	Improved

* Duration of $Al(OH)_3$ administration and daily dosage in the six months preceding clinical signs.

† EEG alterations, grades: 0–3 in [4].

‡ Prescence of microcytic, non-sideropenic anaemia.

§ Cerebral CAT scanning: mild atrophy

TABLE II. Comparison of laboratory investigations and X-ray films of the bones (hands and acrimio-clavicular joints), performed before (1981) and 14 months after (12–1982) complete $Al(OH)_3$ withdrawal, in the same 15 patients

	$Al(OH)_3$ withdrawal		
	Before (1981)	After (12–1982)	n = 15
Serum P (mmol/L)	1.8 ± 0.3	2.1 ± 0.4	$p < 0.05$
Serum Ca (mmol/L)	2.3 ± 0.2	2.4 ± 0.2	NS
Serum alkaline phosphatase (IU/L*)	200 ± 110	203 ± 120	NS
Plasma iPTH (ng/ml†)	4.5 ± 1.9	3.9 ± 1.3	NS
Bone X-ray films‡	No detectable changes		–

* Normal values (not dialysed) < 210 IU/L
† Normal values (not dialysed) < 1.6 ng/ml
‡ Double lecture (one 'blind')

No detectable worsening of hyperparathyroidism was seen during the 14 months following Al(OH)$_3$ withdrawal: serum alkaline phosphatase remained unchanged, plasma iPTH showed a slight but not significant decline, and comparison of X-ray films (1981 versus 1982) showed no detectable changes.

In addition, no patient complained of new bone or muscular pain or of pruritus (vitamin D derivatives were stopped in two cases because of mild hypercalcaemia, and CaCO$_3$ in two others for digestive complaints).

Discussion

Our study, in agreement with that of others [1, 2, 5, 6] demonstrates that the oral administration of Al(OH)$_3$ in haemodialysis patients may lead to Al accumulation, encephalopathy, fracturing osteopathy and occasionally death. In our patients Al-related symptoms and elevated serum Al were partially or fully reversed after Al(OH)$_3$ withdrawal.

Although the toxic role of water Al is clearly predominant in some areas [4], it may have been overemphasised. With the improvement of dialysis water treatment (reverse osmosis and deionisation) in affected centres, this route of intoxication is under control.

The true incidence of morbidity and mortality related to orally administered Al remains unknown. The EDTA 1981 report showed striking discrepancies between countries in reporting encephalopathy and in the use of Al containing gels, and a low rate of regular serum monitoring of aluminium [3]. Such data must be interpreted with caution, but one may infer a great disparity in appreciating the risks of oral Al exposure, probably with an overall underestimation.

Moreover, our data and others [7] suggest that the use of Al(OH)$_3$ for hyperphosphataemia is not as an effective means as generally supposed in the control of secondary hyperparathyroidism in HD patients (who can be treated in severe cases by subtotal parathyroidectomy, a safe and effective procedure).

Many unanswered questions are still pending, which our study did not address, particularly the disparity of serum Al between individual patients (Al hyperabsorption or poor Al compliers) and problems in tissue redistribution [5].

Another important point is the proposal that low Al(OH)$_3$ dosage regimens (i.e. 2g/day) may not be harmful if serum Al is strictly monitored [2–6]; but the literature shows a tendency to reduce the 'safe serum Al concentration' with time and so this assertion remains unproven.

The search for an ideal phosphate binder continues. CaCO$_3$ is not perfect [8]. Magnesium hydroxide has been proposed [1, 9], but well controlled studies are highly desirable before its routine use in dialysis patients.

All the evidence suggests that oral Al(OH)$_3$ administration to HD patients causes an unacceptable morbidity which outweighs a still unproven benefit, and that the warning of Berlyne and others was correct [1, 2, 6, 10]. Al containing phosphate binders should be avoided in dialysis patients.

Acknowledgments

We are highly indebted to Mr J P Clavel (Laboratoire de Biochimie, Hopital La Salpétrière, Paris) for Al measurements. iPTH assays were performed in 'Service d'explorations fonctionnelles' (Pr R Ardaillou), Hopital Tenon, Paris. Thanks to Mr Previer for EEG studies, to Mrs Anglaret for other laboratory analyses and to Mrs Merckel for preparation of the manuscript.

References

1   Alfrey CA, Legendre GR, Kaehny WO. *N Engl J Med 1976; 294:* 184
2   Cournot-Witmer G, Zingraff J, Plachot JJ et al. *Kidney Int 1981; 20:* 375
3   Broyer M, Brunner FP, Brynger H et al. *Proc EDTA 1982; 19:* 45
4   Vecchierini-Blineau MF, Thebaud HE, Brochard D et al. *Néphrologie 1980; 1:* 29
5   Fleming LW, Stewart WK, Fell GS et al. *Clin Nephrol 1982; 17:* 222
6   Rottembourg J, Jaudon MC, Legrain M et al. *Ann Méd Interne (Paris) 1980; 131:* 71
7   Biswas CK, Arze RS, Ramos JM et al. *Br Med J 1982; 284:* 776
8   Moriniere P, Roussel A, Tahiri Y et al. *Proc EDTA 1982; 19:* 784
9   Guillot AP Hood VL, Runge CF et al. *Nephron 1982; 30:* 114
10   Berlyne GM, Ben-Ari J, Pest D et al. *Lancet 1970; ii:* 494

VITAMIN D_3 METABOLITES IN HYPERCALCAEMIC ADULTS AFTER KIDNEY TRANSPLANTATION

P A Lucas, R C Brown, L Bloodworth, J S Woodhead

Welsh National School of Medicine, Cardiff, United Kingdom

Summary

Vitamin D_3 metabolites and iPTH were measured in 26 patients at various times after renal transplantation. Hypercalcaemia (serum $Ca > 2.62mmol/L$, 14 patients) was associated with hyperparathyroidism ($p < 0.02$) and raised $1,25(OH)_2 D_3$ ($p < 0.05$) but raised $1,25(OH)_2 D_3$ was also found in most patients in the normocalcaemic group. Lower $25(OH)D_3$ concentrations were found in the group with normal $1,25(OH)_2 D_3$ compared to the group with elevated $1,25(OH)_2 D_3$ ($p < 0.05$). Low values of $24,25(OH)_2 D_3$ were found in both the normocalcaemic and hypercalcaemic patients ($p < 0.002$). Impaired creatinine clearance ($\leqslant 55$ ml/min, mean: 38ml/min) was not associated with reduced $1,25(OH)_2 D_3$. No difference in D_3 metabolites was found between hypophosphataemic and normophosphataemic patients.

Introduction

Persisting hyperparathyroidism is likely to be an important factor in the development of post-transplant hypercalcaemia [1,2]. By measuring concentrations of D_3 metabolites in hypercalcaemic patients we sought to investigate the effects of hyperparathyroidism on the $25(OH)D_3$ 1α- and 24-hydroxylating system of the functioning allograft. Hypophosphataemia has been reported to stimulate 1α-hydroxylation [3] and hypophosphataemic patients were therefore also studied.

Subjects and methods

We studied 13 normal subjects and 26 selected patients with renal allografts of various durations (Figure 1). Fourteen were hypercalcaemic (corrected total serum calcium $>2.62mmol/L$) of whom five were hypophosphataemic (serum phosphate $<0.8mmol/L$). Twelve were normcalcaemic of whom five were hypophosphataemic. All patients were receiving prednisone 10–20mg daily and

213

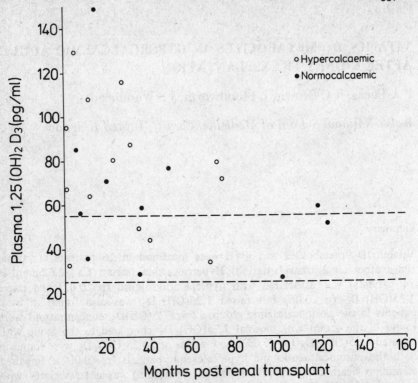

Figure 1. 1,25(OH)$_2$D$_3$ in hypercalcaemic and normocalcaemic post-transplant patients according to the number of months post-transplant. Dotted lines indicate normal range

all but one azathioprine 50–125mg daily. Nine patients were receiving anti-hypertensive medication. Fourteen were receiving diuretic therapy (12 frusemide, two a hydrochlorthiazide and triamterine compound tablet). No patient received cholecalciferol or its metabolites. Parathyroid hormone (iPTH) was measured by immunoradiometric assay which shows poor reactivity with any of the currently available synthetic fragments. It is therefore likely to recognise intact PTH or a large fragment of the molecule. In this assay iPTH is undetectable where hyper-calcaemia has a non-parathyroid cause. Vitamin D$_3$ metabolites were measured by radioimmunoassay following lipid extraction and high performance liquid chromatography [4] (normal values: 25(OH)D$_3$, 3–30ng/ml; 24,25(OH)$_2$D$_3$, 0.1–2ng/ml; 1,25(OH)$_2$D$_3$, 25–55pg/ml). Serum calcium and phosphate were measured by standard autoanalyser techniques.

Statistics

The two-tailed Mann-Whitney U test was utilised throughout.

Results

iPTH was higher in the hypercalcaemic group than in the normocalcaemic group post-transplant (Figure 2). The hypercalcaemic group had spent more time on haemodialysis prior to transplantation (mean: 57.1 v 28.6 months p <0.05).

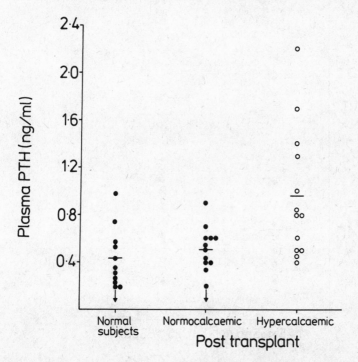

Hypercalcaemic post Tx vs normocalcaemic post Tx (p<0·05)
Hypercalcaemic post Tx vs normal subjects (p<0·02)

Figure 2. iPTH in normal subjects, normocalcaemic and hypercalcaemic transplant patients.
↓ = undetectable concentrations

Up to four years after renal transplantation 63 per cent of $1,25(OH)_2D_3$ values were above 60pg/ml (Figure 1). $25(OH)D_3$ was lower in those patients with $1,25(OH)_2D_3$ concentrations less than 55pg/ml than in those with elevated values (Figure 3). No difference was found in the dosage of prednisone, azathioprine or diuretics nor in transplant duration between those with normal and those with elevated $1,25(OH)_2D_3$. $24,25(OH)_2D_3$ concentrations were strikingly low in 24 of 26 patients (Figure 4). The two patients with normal values had $25(OH)D_3$ greater than 33ng/ml. Decreased creatinine clearance was not associated with reduced $1,25(OH)_2D_3$ (Figure 5). No difference in $1,25(OH)_2D_3$ was found between the hypophosphataemic and normo-phosphataemic groups.

215

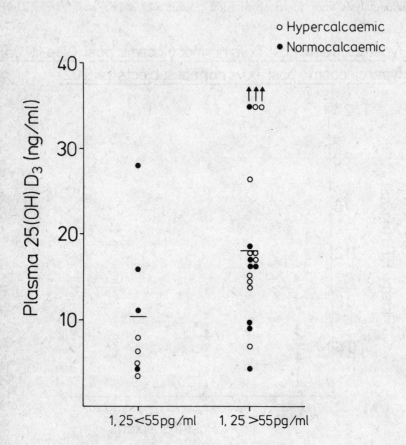

Figure 3. 25(OH)D$_3$ in post-transplant patients divided into those with normal and those with elevated 1,25(OH)$_2$D$_3$. ↑ = concentrations above 33ng/ml

Discussion

Our results support the contention that hypercalcaemia in patients after renal transplantation is related to persisting hyperparathyroidism. The occurrence of raised 1,25(OH)$_2$D$_3$ concentrations (in hypercalcaemic patients) accords with the role of PTH as a major regulator of 1α-hydroxylation [5].

In contrast to our findings in moderate chronic renal failure [6] after transplantation concentrations of 1,25(OH)$_2$D$_3$ are often raised when creatinine clearance is relatively impaired. In this we are in agreement with Garabedian

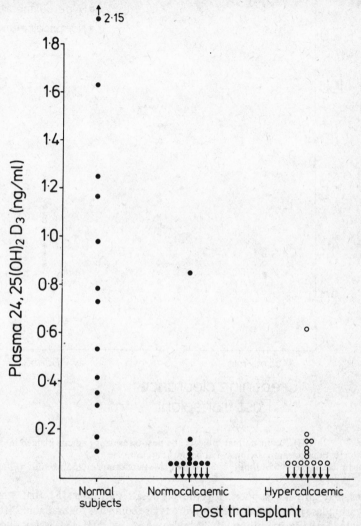

Figure 4.   24,25(OH)$_2$D$_3$ in normal subjects, normocalcaemic and hypercalcaemic post-transplant patients. ↓ = concentrations below 0.07ng/ml

et al [7]. Their subjects differed from ours in being mainly children where ours were all adult and in the fact that all were receiving 25(OH)D$_3$ supplements where none of our patients received either D$_3$ or any D$_3$ metabolite. This may explain why 24,25(OH)$_2$D$_3$ values were strikingly low in all but two of our patients but were elevated in many of theirs [7]. Taken together the two

217

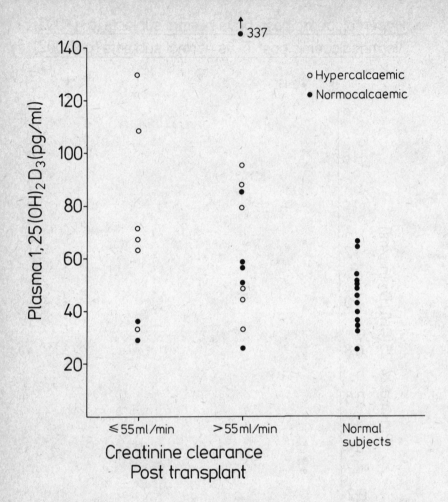

Figure 5. 1,25(OH)$_2$D$_3$ in normal subjects and post-transplant patients divided into groups with creatinine clearances above and below 55ml/min
(Mean clearance ≤55ml/min = 38ml/min. Mean clearance >55ml/min = 70ml/min)

studies may provide support for the proposals of Fraser [5] that while the 1α-hydroxylase is regulated, the 24-hydroxylase competes for available 25(OH)D$_3$ substrate. Specific inhibition of 24-hydroxylase by PTH [8] is not, however, ruled out.

Our findings of low values of 24,25(OH)$_2$D$_3$ and of high values of 1,25(OH)$_2$D$_3$ in many subjects, not only in the hypercalcaemic but also in the less hyperparathyroid, normocalcaemic group, suggests factors other than PTH to be involved. Corticosteroids have been shown to increase PTH secretion [9] and to increase 1,25(OH)$_2$D$_3$ in primary hyperparathyroidism [10]. Their role, and that of other immunosuppressive agents remain to be elucidated.

218

References

1   Conceicao SC, Wilkinson R, Feest TG et al. *Clin Nephrol 1981; 16:* 235
2   Cundy T, Kanis JA, Heynen G et al. *Q J Med 1983; 205:* 67
3   Gray RW, Wilz DR, Caldas AE, Lemann J. *J Clin Endocrinol Metab 1977; 45:* 299
4   Clemens TL, Hendy GN, Papapoulos SE et al. *Clin Endocrinol 1979; 11:* 225
5   Fraser DR. *Physiol Rev 1980; 60:* 551
6   Lucas PA, Brown RC, Woodhead JS, Coles GA. *Kidney Int (Suppl):* In press
7   Garabedian M, Silve C, Levy-Bentolila D et al. *Kidney Int 1981; 20:* 403
8   Boyle IT, Gray RW, DeLuca HF. *Proc Natl Acad Sci USA 1971; 68:* 2131
9   Fucik RF, Kukrega SC, Hargis GK et al. *J Clin Endocrinol Metab 1975; 40:* 152
10   Braun JJ, Juttman JR, Visser TJ et al. *Clin Endocrinol 1982; 17:* 21

219

EFFECTS OF PARATHYROIDECTOMY ON BLOOD PRESSURE DEVELOPMENT IN EUCALCAEMIC, SPONTANEOUSLY HYPERTENSIVE RATS

J F E Mann, E Ritz

Medizinische Klinik, Universität Heidelberg, Heidelberg, FRG

Introduction

The long-term effects of parathyroid hormone on blood pressure remain to be established. Several authors have observed a higher incidence of hypertension in primary hyperparathyroidism than in age-matched controls, irrespective of renal function [1–3]. Hypertension was reversible with parathyroidectomy [3]. It has not been determined whether elevation of arterial blood pressure results from a direct effect of parathyroid hormone or is due to hypercalcaemia. In man, acute experimental hypercalcaemia leads to a rise of blood pressure [4]. On the other hand, acute intravenous (i.v.) injection of parathyroid hormone elicits vasodilatation in several animal species [5].

In the present communication we investigated whether chronic parathyroid hormone deficiency influences blood pressure development in genetic, spontaneously hypertensive (SH) rats. In our study, a group of SH rats were parathyroidectomised and fed a diet with high calcium content to maintain normal serum calcium values.

Material and methods

Two groups of SH rats [6] were investigated at the age of four weeks, 12 rats were parathyroidectomised (PTX), and another 12 were sham-operated (SO). Five days after surgery, hypocalcaemia was present in all PTX-rats. The latter group was then placed on high dietary calcium intake and SO-rats continued on a normal diet. Rats were pairfed. Systolic blood pressure was monitored by tail-plethysmography under light ether anaesthesia.

Three months after surgery, blood volume was determined by the Evans-Blue dilution method. One week later, chronic arterial catheters were placed in the abdominal aorta via the femoral artery. The catheters were placed under the skin to exit at the neck. One day later, direct arterial blood pressure was monitored in the conscious, freely moving rats [7].

Results

Blood pressure development was delayed in SH rats after PTX (Figure 1). This difference became apparent after about four weeks. Upon direct recording after three months, mean arterial blood pressure was 164 ± 6mmHg in PTX-SH rats and 205 ± 6mmHg in SO-SH rats ($p<0.01$). Blood volume was expanded after PTX with 7.4 ± 0.3ml/100g body weight vs 6.9 ± 0.3 ($p<0.05$). Serum calcium values (five days after PTX) were 1.8 ± 0.05mmol/litre in PTX-SH rats as compared

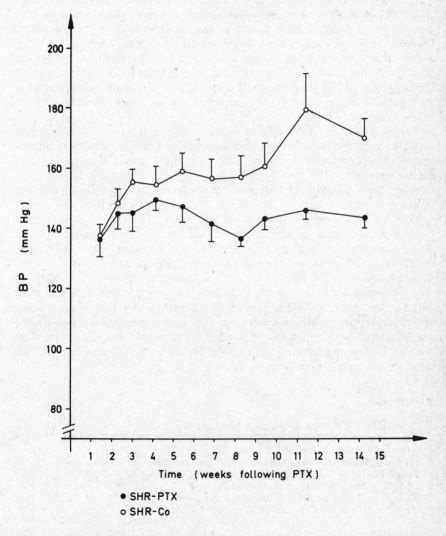

Figure 1. Systolic blood pressure in PTX-SH- and SO-SH-rats. Blood pressure was measured by tail-plethysmography

221

to 2.6 ± 0.05mmol/litre in controls, and increased to 2.7 ± 0.05mmol/litre in PTX-SH rats on high dietary calcium intake.

Discussion

Our data demonstrate that chronic parathyroid hormone deficiency may impede blood pressure development in eucalcaemic SH rats. It is noteworthy that acute i.v. injection of parathyroid hormone induces a remarkable vasodilatation and a fall of arterial blood pressure [5]. It is unknown, however, whether this acute pharmacological effect has any physiological relevance, since extremely high doses of parathyroid hormone have to be given in order to lower blood pressure. One explanation for our findings would be that parathyroid hormone has either a long-term vasoconstrictive action of its own or a permissive effect on the activity of other vasopressor hormones. Preliminary evidence from our laboratory indicates that plasma angiotensin II and norepinephrine are unchanged after PTX (unpublished). However, the responsiveness of arterial resistance vessels has not been tested so far.

The expansion of blood volume following PTX points to increased vascular capacitance in the latter group. This argues against the contention that parathyroid hormone has a permissive effect on blood pressure by sodium and volume retention.

Apart from parathyroid hormone we must consider high dietary calcium intake as a further variable. This point is important, since increased dietary calcium has been shown to lower blood pressure in SH rats [8]. In the present experiment, we chose to supplement oral calcium to PTX-SH rats in order to assure normal serum calcium concentrations. Hypocalcaemia may have its own effects on blood pressure [2]. Although serum calcium concentration was not different between PTX- and SO-SH rats, calcium turnover and urinary excretion were obviously enhanced in the PTX group. Further experiments will show whether this may affect blood pressure independently of parathyroid hormone. We conclude that parathyroid hormone may have a permissive action on the rise of arterial blood pressure independent of calcaemia and volume status in SH rats. Further experiments will consider the combined effects of parathyroid hormone and variations in dietary calcium intake.

References

1 Christenson T, Hellström K, Wengle B. *Eur J Clin Invest 1977; 7:* 109
2 Rambausek M, Ritz E, Rascher W, Kreusser W et al. *Adv Exp Med Biol 1982; 151:* 619
3 Rosenthal FD, Ray S. *Br Med J 1972; 4:* 396
4 Marone C, Beretta-Piccoli C, Weidmann P. *Kidney Int 1980; 20:* 92
5 Pang PKT, Tenner TE, Yee JA, Yang M. *Proc Natl Acad Sci USA 1980; 77:* 675
6 Dietz R, Schömig A, Haebara H, Mann JFE. *Circ Res 1978; 43:* 98
7 Mann JFE, Phillips MI, Dietz R, Haebara H et al. *Am J Physiol 1978; 234:* H629
8 Ayashi S. *Metabolism 1979; 29:* 1234

Proc EDTA (1983) Vol 20

'Y' CONNECTOR SYSTEM FOR PREVENTION OF PERITONITIS IN CAPD: A CONTROLLED STUDY

R Maiorca, A Cantaluppi*, G C Cancarini, A Scalamogna*, A Strada, G Graziani*, S Brasa, C Ponticelli*

*Spedali Civili Brescia, *Ospedale Maggiore Milano, Italy*

Summary

To compare the efficacy of the standard Oreopoulos CAPD system with that of a new method consisting of a Y-shaped set filled with sodium hypochlorite during the dwelling time, a randomised controlled study was performed in 62 new CAPD patients. Life table analysis showed a significantly (p<0.001) less frequent incidence of peritonitis in the group treated with the Y connector system. This study shows that the Y system appears to be effective in reducing the incidence of peritonitis, as compared with the standard technique, in patients on the CAPD programme. The method is simple and economical and the incidence and the severity of side effects appear to be acceptable.

Introduction

Peritonitis is the most frequent complication and the main cause of failure of continuous ambulatory peritoneal dialysis (CAPD) [1]. At present the technique most commonly employed for prevention of peritonitis is that described by Oreopoulos [2]. In order to further reduce risk of dialysate contamination, some modifications of the original system have been suggested [3–5]. Recently, Buoncristiani et al suggested a new device consisting of a Y-shaped set filled with a disinfectant sodium hypochlorite solution during the dwell time [6,7]. With this technique a remarkable reduction of peritonitis incidence has been obtained. However, this study was not performed in a randomised fashion, so that it is difficult to be sure that the same would be true in other treatment centres. In order to compare a technique derived from the Buoncristiani system with the standard Oreopoulos technique, in the last two years all the non-diabetic patients referred to the Spedali Civili of Brescia and Ospedale Maggiore of Milano for CAPD programmes were randomly allocated to the usual spike connector of Oreopoulos [2] or to a modification of the Y system of Buoncristiani [6,7].

Patients and methods

After having prepared peritoneal access, patients were randomly allocated through a closed envelope system to group A or group B techniques.

Group A

Thirty patients, 11 women and 19 men, mean age 55.5 ± 17.5 years (range 14–80), a total experience of 376 patient-months (mean ± SD 12.5 ± 6.4 months, range 3–26). The Travenol spike connector, with the standard bag exchange method [2], was employed for these patients.

Group B

Thirty-two patients, 15 women and 17 men, mean age 55.1 ± 14.3 years (range 12–75), a total experience of 419 patient-months (mean ± SD 12.8 ± 5.9 months, range 3–25). The experimental Y-Solution transfer set (Travenol, Lessines) was employed for this group (Figure 1). Between exchanges the Y-set was filled with sodium hypochlorite solution between the roller clamp (G) and the caps (D and F). After the spike of the inlet tube had been connected to a new plastic bag containing dialysate and before the fresh solution was allowed to flow into the peritoneal cavity, the disinfectant agent and the killed bacteria

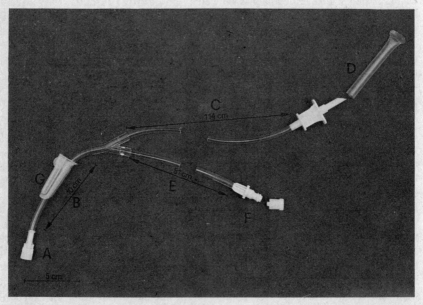

Figure 1. Y-Solution transfer set. The short line (B) connects to the titanium adaptor of the peritoneal catheter by means of a luer-lock (A) and is provided with a roller clamp (G). At the end of the inlet tube (C) there is a spike protected by a cap (D). A screw plug (F) closes the outlet tube (E)

were washed from the Y set through the outlet tube. The disinfectant solution used (Amuchina®, Amuchina SpA, Genova) was a hypochlorite produced by partial electrolysis of a concentrated sodium chloride solution. It was used in a dilution containing 3,000–6,000ppm of available free chlorine. The sterilising effectiveness of this solution has been demonstrated by Buoncristiani et al [8].

The peritoneal access consisted of a double-cuff Tenckhoff catheter with a titanium connector (Baxter Travenol, Deerfield, Illinois). The same type of bag was employed for both groups (Viaflex-Travenol). In group A, 19 patients were treated with four exchanges daily, 10 with three exchanges, and one with five; in group B, 18 patients were treated with four exchanges daily, 13 with three exchanges, and one with five. The dialysis set was changed every six to eight weeks by a skilled nurse. Patients of both groups were trained for 10 to 15 days. The results given are only for patients on CAPD for at least three months. One patient in group A and one in group B were removed from the trial when it became necessary to add drugs (potassium, heparin) to the bags. Peritonitis was diagnosed from the presence of two of the following three findings: 1. Abdominal pain; 2. Dialysate white cell counts over $100/mm^3$; 3. Positive dialysate cultures.

For the two groups, which were comparable for age, dialysis duration and treatment modality, the number and frequency of peritonitis episodes and the percentage of affected patients were evaluated (Yates corrected Chi-square test). Life table analysis, according to the Kaplan-Meier method, was used to calculate the probability that a patient would develop peritonitis within a given time. We took into account all the episodes of peritonitis and used the log-rank test [9] to compare the probability curves for the two groups.

Results

In group A, over a cumulative period of 376 months, 18/30 patients (60%) developed peritonitis, whereas in group B, over a cumulative period of 419 months peritonitis occurred in only 12/32 patients (37%) (χ_c^2 = 2.3, p NS). There were 32 and 13 episodes of peritonitis respectively. Peritonitis incidence during the trial was one episode every 11.7 patient-months in group A and one episode every 32.2 patient-months in group B. Comparing the peritonitis probability curves for the two groups (Figure 2), a statistically significant difference was found (χ^2 = 10.86, p<0.001). Table I gives the results of the dialysate cultures for all the peritonitis cases. From two cases of each group, no bacteria could be grown (6.25% in group A versus 15.4% in group B). There were Gram-positive infections for 43.75 per cent of group A and 61.5 per cent of group B, while Gram-negative peritonitis infections were 50 per cent and 23.1 per cent. Five patients died during the follow-up, two in group A (myocardial infarction) and three in group B (two myocardial infarction and one hepatoma). Two patients (one in each group) were removed from the study, as required by the design of the trial, when it became necessary to add drugs (heparin, potassium) to the bags. Five patients in group A were changed to the Y set after three to four peritonitis episodes. This change was decided upon after the superiority of the Y set over the standard connector had become evident from the statistical

225

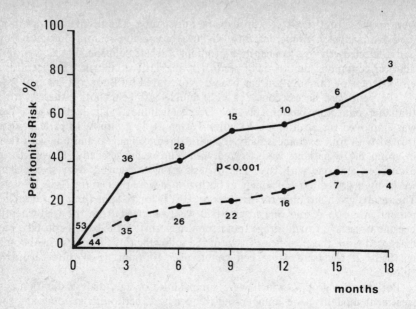

Figure 2. Peritonitis probability curves for the two groups of patients (group A —, group B
- - - -). The numbers indicate patients at risk at each time interval

TABLE I. Organisms causing peritonitis

	Group A	Group B
Staphylococcus epidermidis	8	6
Staphylococcus aureus	4	2
Streptococci	2	–
Acinobacter	1	1
Klebsiella pneumoniae	3	–
Pseudomonas aeruginosa	3	2
Escherichia coli	5	–
Enterobacter cloacae	3	–
Proteus mirabilis	1	–
No growth	2	2

analysis. In these patients, who are not included in group B for calculation, the
peritonitis rate decreased from one episode every 4.5 patient-months to one
episode during 23.2 patient-months. Two other patients of group A had to be
withdrawn because of recurrent tunnel infections. For one patient of group A
and one of B, CAPD was stopped because of ultrafiltration loss. Finally, two
patients (one in each group) were withdrawn at the patients' request, and
another one (group B) became unable to cope with CAPD, because of progressive
atherosclerotic mental deterioration.

226

Technical accidents with the new device

The B line disconnected from the Y-connection in nine patients (13 times) because of defective sticking in one lot of devices. Peritonitis developed in only one patient. There was accidental introduction of the disinfectant solution into the abdomen in eight patients (11 times: three during training and eight at home). The patients experienced sudden abdominal pain that disappeared after two or three rapid bag-exchanges. There were no changes in the biochemical findings nor less of ultrafiltration capacity in these patients.

Discussion

In this prospective controlled trial we compared the incidence of peritonitis in patients treated with the Y connector and patients using the standard Oreopoulos method. The peritonitis rate in patients treated with the Y system (one episode every 32.2 patient-months) was much lower than that in patients using the standard method (one episode every 11.7 patient-months), and life table analysis showed a significantly reduced incidence of peritonitis in the group treated with the Y connector system.

The main characteristic of the system is the sterilisation of the connection site between the administration set and the bag with a disinfectant agent which, after the connection has been made, can be completely discharged to the outside through an outflow branch. In addition to the disinfectant effect, the flushing of the Y connector 'per se' reduces the contamination risk [6]. Additional advantages of the Y-set are to free the patient from the bag during the dwell time and the possibility of adapting the volume of dialysate solution to the anatomical and clinical condition of the patient (e.g. reduced volume requirement in children). The low cost of the device and the disinfectant agent are largely compensated for by not needing sterile gauzes or connector shields. One possible complication of the technique is accidental introduction of the disinfectant agent into the peritoneum. In our patients it occurred only 11 times in more than 40,000 exchanges. In experimental studies the disinfectant agent, Amuchina, was proven to be innocuous [8]. Entrance of the disinfectant agent into the peritoneum was immediately followed by severe abdominal pain but two or three rapid bag exchanges were sufficient to eliminate the pain without any other consequences.

The peritonitis rate of one episode every 32.2 patient-months obtained with the Y system is lower than that of other techniques [2,3–5] and makes peritonitis an almost negligible complication of CAPD in our patients.

On the basis of these results, the Y connector appears to be a simple, safe, and economical system which is very effective in reducing the rate of peritonitis in patients on CAPD.

References

1 Kramer P, Broyer M, Brunner FP et al. *Proc EDTA 1982; 19:* 4
2 Oreopoulos DG, Khanna R, Williams P, Vas SI. *Nephron 1982; 30:* 293

3   Bazzato G, Coli U, Landini S et al. *Proc EDTA 1980; 17:* 266
4   Slingeneyer A, Mion C. *Proc EDTA 1982; 19:* 388
5   Mavichak V, Moriarty MV, Cameron EC et al. *Trans ASAIO 1982; 28:* 253
6   Buoncristiani U, Bianchi P, Cozzari M et al. *Int J Nephrol Urol Androl 1980; 1:* 50
7   Buoncristiani U, Cozzari M, Quintaliani G, Carobi C. *Dial Transplant 1983; 12:* 14
8   Buoncristiani U, Bianchi P, Barzi AM et al. *Int J Nephrol Urol Androl 1980; 1:* 45
9   Peto R, Pike MC, Armitage P et al. *Br J Cancer 1977; 35:* 1

Open Discussion

BAZZATO (Venice) First of all congratulations for this first controlled study of two different techniques in CAPD. We have been using a double bag system in our unit since early 1979 and we have almost abolished exogenous peritonitis. How do you differentiate the incidence of endogenous and exogenous perito-nitis?

CANTALUPPI I have no data on this point. I am not personally convinced endogenous peritonitis really exists.

BINSWANGER (Chairman)   That's an interesting remark. You know in the United States they claim that 30 per cent of all peritonitis is due to endogenous infection. I think it depends very much on the age range of your patients. You have 55 years as the mean age of your patients.

CANTALUPPI   Fifty-five is the mean age of my patients. These data are com-pletely unproven, probably endogenous peritonitis really does exist, but I think that the incidence is negligible.

BAZZATO   Just a comment to your answer: I saw a statistical correlation with bowel constipation in the incidence of peritonitis. There is clinical evid-ence that there is endogenous peritonitis.

CANTALUPPI   I think that peritonitis comes first and bowel constipation second.

BINSWANGER Dr Mion might solve this problem.

MION (Montpellier) Well I can't solve it, I can just give you our data which have shown that about 20 per cent of our peritonitis episodes are clinically related to some kind of bowel disease.
    I wanted first of all to congratulate you again for this very good prospective study. We really need to evaluate new systems in the prevention of peritonitis in CAPD. My question relates to the complexity of the techniques. I was im-pressed by the rather low incidence with disinfectant irrigation but I wanted to know how long a bag exchange takes with this technique.

CANTALUPPI The technique seems complicated: it also appeared complicated to me when I went to Perugia to learn the technique. The technique is a step

228

by step one so the patient cannot make mistakes. The only mistake he can make is to put the disinfectant into his abdomen, so we stress this point very much and thereby avoid this complication. The patient takes about 30 seconds longer than with the usual technique in making an exchange. The 30 seconds are necessary to refill and to flush out the set at the end of the exchange procedure.

GOLDSMITH (Liverpool) Have you seen any eosinophilic peritonitis with your method?

CANTALUPPI No, never.

BINSWANGER May I ask you one question: analysing your data on peritonitis it becomes evident that you have about double the number of peritonitis episodes in your group A. That means some patients have more than one episode of peritonitis. That's different to your group B where you have about the same number of peritonitis episodes and so I would like to ask you whether these two groups are really comparable. I suggest that you have some more dirty patients in your group A.

CANTALUPPI If the theory of randomised control is correct this would be impossible. In practice I think that the simple answer is that the contamination possibilities with the standard system are much more than with the 'Y' system and so we do not have as high a number of patients with recurrent peritonitis with this system.

BINSWANGER We are still all impressed by the very low rate of peritonitis you have reported.

IMPROVED LYMPHOCYTE TRANSFORMATION IN VITRO OF PATIENTS ON CONTINUOUS AMBULATORY PERITONEAL DIALYSIS

E Langhoff, J Ladefoged

Rigshospitalet, Copenhagen, Denmark

Summary

In vitro lymphoblastic transformation and sensitivity to methylprednisolone (MP) was studied in lymphocyte cultures obtained from patients on continuous ambulatory peritoneal dialysis (CAPD), on haemodialysis (HD) and control subjects. The PHA and Con A responses of peripheral blood lymphocytes (PBL) and T cells were identical in CAPD and control cultures, and in both significantly higher than in HD cultures ($p<0.05$). Both PBL and T cells from CAPD and control cultures were more resistant to the suppressive effects of MP than those from HD cultures. There was no relation between the duration of the dialysis period and the lymphocyte mitogen response in HD patients. Enhanced in vitro cell transformation and resistance to steroids during CAPD treatment may reflect an improved form of dialysis of importance for the general immune defence of the uraemic patient.

Introduction

Previous reports have demonstrated a decreased response of lymphocytes to mitogens in chronic uraemia [1, 2]. Recently a beneficial effect of CAPD has been reported [3, 4]. The present investigation examines in patients on CAPD the lymphocyte response to mitogens and the degree of resistance to the suppressive effect of methylprednisolone (MP) on this response in vitro.

Subjects

In vitro lymphocyte functions were investigated in 11 patients on CAPD (five women and six men, aged 23 to 62 years, mean age 44 years, mean dialysis period 1.7 years), 11 patients on HD (seven women and four men, aged 28 to 66 years, mean age 46 years, mean dialysis period 3.7 years), and 11 normal volunteers (five women and six men, aged 30 to 63 years, mean age 40 years). The effect of age and the duration of the dialysis period on in vitro lymphocyte transformation were studied in 32 HD patients, and the effect of age alone was finally studied in 74 control subjects.

Materials and methods

Isolation of PBL and T cells

Twenty millilitres of heparinised blood obtained by venepuncture was added to equal amounts of Hank's balanced salt solution. The PBL were isolated by Lymphoprep® (Nyco, Norway) and washed three times in Hank's solution. The cells were then resuspended to a concentration of 10^6 cells/ml in RPMI-1640 (Gipco, Europe), containing 10 per cent fetal calf serum, 500 IU penicillin/ml (Leo, Denmark), and streptomycin 333μg/ml (Novo, Denmark). The T cells were obtained by the E-rosetting technique. AET- (Sigma 5879, USA) treated sheep red blood cells (SRBC) were added to equal volumes of the above PBL suspension [5]. After centrifugation for five minutes at 160G followed by incubation at 4°C for 60 minutes the sedimented T cell rosettes were resuspended and layered on Lymphoprep® and centrifuged at 500G for 30 minutes. The interface cells were then removed and the sedimented T cell rosettes were isolated and incubated in RPMI-1640 with 15 per cent AB serum for 10–20 minutes at 37°C until lysis of the SRBC. The T cells were washed (Hank's) three times, counted and resuspended to a concentration of 10^6 cells/ml suspension in RPMI-1640 with 10 per cent fetal calf serum and antibiotics.

Lymphocyte cultures

Triplicates of PBL, and T cells from controls, CAPD patients, and HD patients were cultured in microtitre plates (Nunc, Denmark) containing 5×10^4 cells/well. Mitogen stimulated triplicates contained optimal mitogen concentrations, PHA (Difco, Detroit, USA) 20μg/well, or Con A (Pharmacia Fine Chemicals, Sweden) 10μg/well. MP succinate (Urbason®, Hoechst, FRG) was added to the triplicates. The following concentrations were used: 0, 0.05, 0.25, 0.5, 1.0, 2.5μg/ml culture.

The cultures were incubated for 72 hours in humidified atmosphere with five per cent carbon dioxide at 37°C before ^{14}C-thymidine addition (50 nCi/well, Amersham, UK). The cultures were harvested and counted (Packard, Tri-Carb) 20 hours after ^{14}C-thymidine addition. The mean number of cpm incorporated in the presence versus absence of steroid was expressed as the % suppression at each concentration. MP resistance of patient and control cultures in terms of the in vitro MP concentration that cause 50 per cent suppression (ED_{50}), was calculated from these dose response curves.

Statistics

A non-paired t-test was used to compare group means. Values of $p < 0.05$ were considered significant.

Results

Figure 1 shows the PHA (left) and Con A (right) responses in cpm of CAPD, HD and control cultures of PBL. The ^{14}C-thymidine uptake in cpm of unstimulated

231

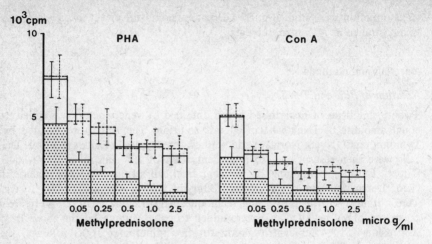

Figure 1. The PHA and Con A responses of peripheral blood lymphocytes (PBL) from controls, CAPD patients, and HD patients. Ordinate: ^{14}C-thymidine uptake in cpm x 10^3. Abscissa: concentration of MP in μg/ml culture. ——— Controls, n = 11. ------- CAPD patients, n = 11. Dotted area: HD patients, n = 11. The SEM values are indicated

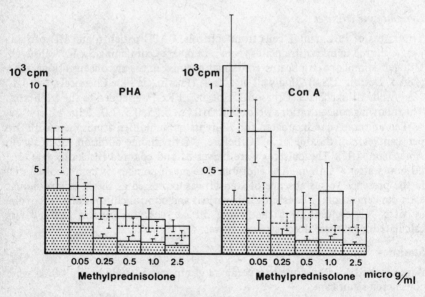

Figure 2. The PHA and Con A responses of T lymphocytes from controls, CAPD patients, and HD patients. Ordinate: ^{14}C-thymidine uptake in cpm x 10^3. Abscissa: concentration of MP in μg/ml culture. ——— Controls, n = 11. ------- CAPD patients, n = 11. Dotted area: HD patients, n = 11. The SEM values are indicated

232

cultures (not shown) was 3–10 per cent of mitogen stimulated cultures. The mitogen responses of CAPD and control cultures without MP (left bars) were similar, and significantly higher than that of the HD cultures (p<0.05). This difference was found throughout the concentration range of MP. Steroid resistance in terms of ED_{50} values were similar in CAPD and control cultures (PHA: 0.38μg/ml, 0.35μg/ml and Con A: 0.28μg/ml, 0.23μg/ml, respectively), but higher than in HD cultures (PHA: 0.07μg/ml and Con A: 0.1μg/ml).

Figure 2 shows the T lymphocyte PHA (left) and Con A (right) responses. The CAPD T cell responses were higher than the HD T cell responses and the difference was significant in the Con A stimulated T cell cultures without MP as well as in the MP suppressed cultures (p<0.05). The T cell resistance to steroid was higher in the CAPD and control cultures than in the HD cultures. The ED_{50} values were; PHA: 0.11μg/ml, 0.13μg/ml, and 0.04μg/ml and Con A: 0.02μg/ml, 0.05μg/ml, and 0.005μg/ml, respectively.

The relation between age and PBL response to PHA stimulation was studied in HD patients and normal controls. There was no relationship between age and PHA response in the control group (r = −0.19, p>0.05, n = 74). In the HD group, however, there was a significant trend of lower PHA responses with increasing age (r = −0.40, p<0.05, n = 32).

The relationship between the duration on HD and PHA transformation response is shown in Figure 3. The PHA responses are not significantly lower after several years on HD (r = −0.28, p>0.05, n = 32).

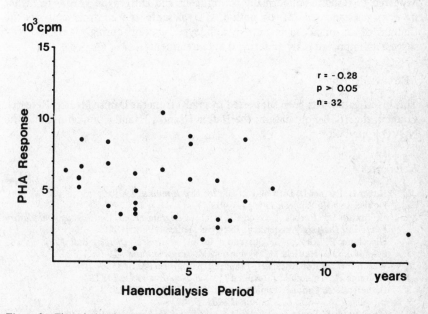

Figure 3. The relation between the duration of the period on haemodialysis and the PHA response of peripheral blood lymphocytes (PBL) from 32 patients. Ordinate: ^{14}C-thymidine uptake in cpm x 10^3. Abscissa: duration of haemodialysis period in years

233

Discussion

In chronic uraemia the in vivo cell mediated immune response is depressed and in vitro mitogen transformation decreased [1, 2, 6]. However, the mechanism by which uraemia impairs the T cell function remains obscure, although several factors, e.g. serum factors, have been suggested [7]. More recently a significantly increased E-rosette formation has been observed during CAPD treatment [4]. Serum factors blocking sheep cell receptors have been suggested to be selectively removed through the peritoneum during CAPD treatment [8]. The OKT$^+$4/OKT$^+$8 ratio has been reported to be within the normal range in CAPD patients [8]. In vivo evidence of enhanced delayed hypersensitivity skin reactions has been reported [4].

In the present study PHA and Con A responses of both PBL and T cells from CAPD patients, HD patients and control subjects were compared. In general both PBL and T cells from CAPD patients responded like the controls with significantly improved responses compared to the PBL and T cell responses of the HD patients. One reason could be patient selection i.e. 'best risk patient' would be on CAPD. In this study all patients were clinically well. The HD group was slightly older than the CAPD group but the present findings and previous reports [9, 10] have demonstrated mitogen responses to be almost unaffected by age, except at age extremes [9]. As shown in Figure 3 the slightly longer period of dialysis of the HD group compared to the CAPD group was not likely to explain the normal mitogen response of the CAPD patients, who being uraemic would be expected to respond subnormally to mitogens and antigens in vitro. The higher in vitro resistance to MP of both CAPD patients and controls supports the findings of an enhanced in vitro lymphocyte function during CAPD and may suggest an improved dialysis during CAPD treatment.

Acknowledgments

This investigation has been supported by grants from the Danish Medical Research Council, the 1870 Foundation, the Hafnia-Haand i Haand Foundation, and the NOVO Foundation.

References

1   Huber H, Pastner D, Dittrich P et al. *Clin Exp Immunol 1969; 5:* 75
2   Dobbelstein H. *Nephron 1976; 17:* 409
3   Goldsmith HJ, Forbes A, Gyde HB et al. In Legrain M, ed. *Continuous Ambulatory Peritoneal Dialysis.* Amsterdam: Excerpta Medica. 1980: 302
4   Giacchino F, Alloatti S, Quarello F et al. *Peritoneal Dialysis Bull 1982; 3:* 165
5   Schmidtke JR, Hatfield SM, Ferguson RM. *Transplantation 1979; 27:* 319
6   Wilson WEC, Kirkpatrick CH, Talmage DW. *Ann Int Med 1965; 62:* 1
7   Touraine JL, Touraine F, Revillard JP et al. *Nephron 1975; 14:* 195
8   Giangrande A, Cantù P, Limido A et al. *Proc EDTA 1982; 19:* 372
9   Birkeland SA. *J Clin Lab Immunol 1981; 5:* 47
10   Charpentier B, Fournier C, Fries D et al. *J Clin Lab Immunol 1981; 5:* 87

Open Discussion

GOLDSMITH (Chairman) May I congratulate you on your very nice paper. In view of what we know about biological (circadian) rhythms in lymphocytes, were all the samples taken at the same time of the day in the different patient groups?

LANGHOFF All the samples were taken at the same time of the day from both the controls, the haemodialysis group, and the CAPD group.

BINSWANGER (Chairman) Would you like to speculate on the clinical importance of your findings in respect to transplantation of different patient groups?

LANGHOFF Theoretically this question may be of some importance, but I do think that in the transplanted group this difference might disappear because of the heavy immunosuppression.

SCHREIBER (Cleveland, USA) If one considers there exists a multipotent stem cell population, did you attempt to correlate your results of T-cell suppression with erythropoiesis. Were the haematocrits in the patients which had good T-cell responses increased in comparison to those patients who were on haemodialysis or CAPD, thus looking for a common underlying stimulatory factor for multi-stem cell development?

LANGHOFF We did not find a relation between improved erythropoiesis and an improved lymphocyte transformation in vitro.

SCHREIBER Were you able to reverse this response by any changes in regard to crossing patients over from CAPD to haemodialysis or using some addition of dialysate or serum to inhibit these responses?

LANGHOFF We have not had the opportunity yet of following patients who are changed from CAPD to haemodialysis treatment.

SCHREIBER So you don't really know what regulates this response?

LANGHOFF The whole explanation is probably not a toxic plasma factor since uraemic plasma from patients on haemodialysis does not seem to change a normal lymphocyte response to a uraemic lymphocyte response.

SEVERE ABDOMINAL COMPLICATIONS IN PATIENTS UNDERGOING CONTINUOUS AMBULATORY PERITONEAL DIALYSIS

J Rottembourg, G M Gahl, J L Poignet, E Mertani,
P Strippoli, P Langlois, P Tranbaloc, M Legrain

Groupe Hospitalier Pitié Salpétrière, Paris, France

Introduction

Since 1977 continuous ambulatory peritoneal dialysis (CAPD) has been proposed as an effective maintenance therapy for patients with end-stage renal disease (ESRD). Many studies dealing with a large number of patients, often in a high risk population, have now been reported with encouraging results [1–3]. Nevertheless drop-out rates including deaths and transfers remain high and peritonitis is still a major problem. This study outlines the severe abdominal complications encountered in one large centre.

Patients and methods

Patients

From August 1978 to February 1983, 143 patients (93 males, 50 females) were trained for CAPD. Their ages ranged from 17 to 83 years with a mean age of 61.2 ± 16.3 years. One hundred and six patients were exclusively treated by CAPD, 25 were transferred from chronic haemodialysis to CAPD and 12 from intermittent peritoneal dialysis to CAPD, for various medical reasons in 31 and personnal convenience in six. Sixty-five patients (49%) were older than 65 years at start of treatment by CAPD. The causes of ESRD were chronic glomerulonephritis 37, insulin-dependent diabetic nephropathy 34, chronic interstitial nephropathy 25, polycystic kidneys 13, nephroangiosclerosis 7 and nephropathy of various or unknown origin in 27.

The total experience on CAPD was 198 patient-years with a mean period on CAPD of 16.8 months per patient (range 1–48 months). At the end of the study, 59 patients were still on CAPD, 40 were transferred to chronic haemodialysis, three received a kidney transplant, two recovered renal function and 39 died.

Methods

CAPD was conducted through a double cuff Tenckhoff catheter with a preferential use of the curled type [4]. Most patients performed four exchanges daily using routinely three two litre bags with 1.5 per cent dextrose concentration during the day and one two litre bag with 4.5 per cent dextrose overnight.

Four types of dialysates were used: Dialysate from the Pharmacie Centrale des Hôpitaux de Paris in 74 patients, from Aguettant (Lyon, France) in 24 patients, from Travenol (Deerfield, USA) in 40 patients, and from Frezenius (Oberursel/Taunus, FRG) in five patients. Twelve patients initially dialysed with bags from the Pharmacie Centrale des Hôpitaux de Paris were transferred to Travenol Dianeal in eight cases and to Aguettant dialysate in four cases. Dialysates from Pharmacie Centrale des Hôpitaux and Aguettant Lab contained sodium acetate while Travenol and Frezenius dialysates contained sodium lactate as buffer; the concentration of acetate and lactate was similar: 35mmol/L.

Until October 1981 all peritonitis episodes were treated by continuous lavage using a cycler; treatment required lavage with 24–36 litres daily of an acetate buffered dialysate for two to five days. Since October 1981, peritonitis episodes were treated without lavage. In all cases antibiotics and heparin (2,500 units per two litre bag) were administered intraperitoneally.

Results

The following abdominal complications were observed: 244 acute peritonitis episodes, eight perforated peritonitis, nine sclerosing encapsulating peritonitis, and two necrotising enteritis. Such complications led directly to death in 20 cases (50% of all deaths) and required transfer in 27 cases (67% of all transfers).

Peritonitis

Peritonitis developed in 110 patients (77%), one week to 22 months after starting CAPD. Two hundred and forty-four episodes were observed with an overall rate of one episode every 9.7 patients-months. The prevalence of peritonitis decreased after the first year of treatment from one episode every 8.2 patient months to one episode every 13.2 patient-months. Thirty-three patients were never affected by peritonitis. Sixteen patients had more than four episodes, 10 more than five episodes and eight patients from 6–12 episodes.

Bacteria and fungi were grown from the peritoneal fluid in 198 (81%) of the 244 episodes, Gram-positive organisms in 146 episodes (60%), Gram-negative in 37 episodes (15%), fungi in 15 (6%). Cultures were negative in 46 episodes (19%).

Perforated peritonitis

Two traumatic bowel perforations occurred in two diabetic patients aged 68 and 53 once during a catheter replacement and once during a peritoneal lavage with an overheated dialysate due to the malfunction of the heater of the cycler. A

237

stercoral peritonitis resulted in a rapid death in these two high risk patients.

Six spontaneous perforation of a colonic diverticulae occurred in six patients, four males and two females with a mean age of 63 years (range 50–72) leading to death in two cases. Two patients were known from a previous routine barium enema to have diverticulae. All patients consumed low doses of aluminium containing phosphate binders. None had suffered a clinical acute diverticulitis episode. Peritoneal catheters were curled in four cases and straight in two cases. Prior to the perforation 19 peritonitis epsodes during a cumulative period of 116 months were observed. Organisms found in the dialysate were all Gram-negative (two Coliforms, two Pseudomonas, one Serratia, one Klebsiella). The three perforations occurred in a free peritoneal cavity with faecal material in the dialysate and this justified immediate surgery. Semi-elective colectomy with external colostomy was performed in all cases. One patient survived, two died during the early postoperative period. Spontaneous perforation in a closed cavity occurred in three cases. The complication was suspected on clinical symptoms of peritonitis with various or successive Gram-negative organisms and signs of sub-obstruction. The diagnosis was confirmed by water soluble contrast enema. Medical treatment included starvation diet, prolonged parenteral nutrition, general and peritoneal administration of antibiotics as well as prolonged peritoneal lavage. The three patients were transferred to haemodialysis. They all survived.

Necrotising enteritis

Two patients, one male 52 years old, one female 66 years old, treated by CAPD for 14 and 36 months respectively with three and four previous episodes of peritonitis suddenly developed high fever (40°C), anorexia, profound vomiting, severe abdominal pain and cardiovascular collapse with positive blood culture (Gram-negative). Dialysate effluent was not cloudy. During laparotomy extensive necrotising enteritis was found. Enterectomy was considered impossible. The two patients died early in the postoperative phase from sepsis and shock.

Sclerosing encapsulating peritonitis (SEP)

Nine patients (four males, five females) aged from 32–72 years (mean age 55.5 ± 13 years) treated during a mean period of 21.3±12.5 months (7–42 months) by CAPD developed SEP. The buffer of the dialysate used was exclusively acetate in seven cases, lactate and acetate in two cases. Thirty-four acute peritonitis episodes occurred during CAPD treatment (one episode every 5.7 patient-months). Organisms were Gram-positive in 25 cases, Gram-negative in six cases, fungi in one, and unknown in two. Symptoms suggesting SEP appeared during CAPD treatment in seven cases, but also after a symptom-free interval of 9.6 months (range 6–12 months) following discharge from CAPD in two patients. The major symptoms were: a decreasing ultrafiltration rate in six patients, anorexia, nausea and vomiting in seven patients, recurrent abdominal pain in eight patients, malnutrition in five and intermittent sub-obstructive episodes in six patients. Diagnosis was established either during

238

surgery for obstruction in five cases or during an attempt to implant a new catheter in four cases. At operation findings were similar in all cases: the entire peritoneal surface was opaque, markedly thickened and sclerotic, numerous adhesions were encountered. The entire small bowel was covered with a thick shaggy membrane. During surgery no attempt was made to separate the loops because of the danger of bowel perforation. One patient died on CAPD treatment. Eight were transferred to haemodialysis: four are still dialysed 5–30 months after transfer, four died 9–15 months after transfer of malnutrition and recurrent obstructive episodes.

Biopsy specimens from the visceral and parietal peritoneum were obtained in three cases. Light microscopy showed increased peritoneal thickness due to proliferation of the fibro-connective tissue, increased vascularity, infiltration with inflammatory cells, mostly mononuclear, and dilated lymphatics. No foreign bodies or debris were detected on light microscopy.

Discussion

Peritonitis, even though most episodes are benign and efficiently treated at home without lavage [5], remains a major limitation in considering CAPD as a true alternative to haemodialysis. Long-term follow-up of a large group of patients [6], as in our series, outlines the occurrence of some severe abdominal complications which are life-threatening and require a long and costly hospitalisation.

The prevalence of colonic diverticulosis increases with age and the disease is certainly frequent among the older age population treated by CAPD. Constipation, frequent among patients on CAPD, aggravated by the consumption of aluminium gels, possibly increases the risk of perforation. The presence of the dialysis fluid may explain the high rate of perforation in a free peritoneal cavity. The consequences of excluding from CAPD treatment older patients with asymptomatic diverticulosis remains to be evaluated. At present we exclude from CAPD only those patients with a history of diverticulitis and we do not perform routine evaluation for diverticulosis [7] in asymptomatic patients. Our two cases of necrotising enteritis with septicaemia occurred in the absence of acute peritoneal infection, but following a peritonitis episode treated by broad spectrum antibiotics given intraperitoneally and orally including exclusively tobramycin, cephalothin and cefotaxime. Although the exact cause of such a dramatic and exceptional complication remains unknown the conditions in which the complications occurred and the anatomical findings are similar to what has been observed in some neonates [8].

Sclerosing encapsulating peritonitis (SEP) is the most distressing abdominal complication encountered in our series because of its frequency, nine cases, and severity, five deaths. Our observations are clinically and anatomically similar to those reported among patients treated by intermittent peritoneal dialysis in 1980 by Gandhi et al [9] and more recently by Slingeneyer et al [10]. In France a recent survey among centres treating patients by CAPD has identified more cases to be reported in the coming months. The disease can progress slowly and remain asymptomatic for a long period. Symptoms can occur eventually

239

several months or even years after transfer of the patient either to other forms of dialysis or transplantation. However in some cases the peritoneal thickening process can extend to the total surface of the visceral and parietal peritoneum in a few weeks as demonstrated in one recent case by two laparotomies performed at six week intervals.

The main symptoms are membrane failure with impairment of the ultra-filtration rate without decrease of peritoneal clearances, abdominal pain with nausea, vomiting, and repetitive subacute obstructive episodes. Gastrointestinal transit problems and losses of protein through the drainage fluid can induce severe malnutrition and life threatening conditions.

The factors involved in the genesis of SEP are still not clearly defined. A history of recurrent peritonitis is encountered in many cases and the thickening of the membrane could be favoured by recurrent inflammation of the perito-neum [6, 9]. Indeed the rate of peritonitis episode in patients with the syndrome was higher (one every 5.7 patient-months) than in the entire population series (one every 9.8 patient-months), but six patients out of nine have only encountered one to three peritonitis episodes. The cases reported by Slingeneyer et al [10] occurred despite a very low rate of peritoneal infection. Moreover, many patients with severe recurrent peritonitis do not develop the syndrome. If infection is a contributing factor it does not seem alone to be the real cause of the disease.

A thorough comparative study of the records of all our cases with or without sclerosing peritonitis was unable to detect any risk factor such as age, sex, original disease, modalities of treatment of peritonitis, drugs including beta-blocking agents administered into the peritoneal cavity or through other routes with only one exception or the composition of the dialysate. All patients with the disease had been dialysed exclusively (seven cases) or at least for a certain period (two cases) with an acetate buffer solution and this was also true of the patients with the disease who had been treated by intermittent peritoneal irrigation [9, 10]. Until now, none of our 37 patients dialysed exclusively with a lactate solution have developed the syndrome. The potentially toxic role of acetate remains to be proven. Acetate salts could react directly with the peritoneum or with the containers and tubing but they are perhaps only an index of other toxic factors present either in the solution or the containers. It should be stated that the complication occurred in patients dialysed with various brands of acetate solutions and that the origin and the fabrication of the plasticisers are different. For these reasons we have made the decision from now on to dialyse all our patients with lactate solutions.

In conclusion in a large experience dealing with 143 patients treated by CAPD since August 1978 (198 patient-years) we have encountered various severe abdominal complications including nine cases of sclerosing encapsulating perito-nitis. Such complications remain the major cause of death and transfer of patient from CAPD. Better evaluation and detection of risk factors including the compo-sition of the dialysate, containers and tubing and the prevention of peritonitis through improved technology are required if CAPD is to be considered as an alternative to haemodialysis for long-term treatment of patients with end-stage renal disease.

References

1   Gokal R, Francis DMA, Goodship THS et al. *Lancet 1982; ii:* 1388
2   Kramer P, Broyer M, Brunner FM et al. *Proc EDTA 1982; 19:* 4
3   Nolph K, Boen F, Farell P, Pyle K. *Kidney Int 1983; 23:* 3
4   Rottembourg J, Jacq D, Agrafiotis A et al. In Gahl GM, Kessel M, Nolph KD, eds. *Advances in Peritoneal Dialysis.* Amsterdam: Excerpta Medica. 1981: 185–187
5   de Groc F, Rottembourg J, Jacq D et al. *Nephrologie 1983; 4:* 24
6   Heale WF, Letch KA, Dawborn JK. In Atkins RC, Thomsom NM, Farrell PC, eds. *Peritoneal Dialysis.* Edinburgh: Churchill Livingstone. 1981: 284–290
7   Mion C. *Proc EDTA 1981; 18:* 91
8   Walker WA. *Pediatrics 1976; 57:* 901
9   Gandhi VC, Humayn HM, Img TS et al. *Arch Intern Med 1980; 140:* 1201
10   Slingeneyer A, Canaud B, Mourad G et al. *Trans ASAIO 1983; Abstract:* 66

Open Discussion

VERGER (Pontoise, France) I would like to make a comment and ask two questions. We recently performed in France a multicentre study with eight different centres concerning more than 400 patients commencing CAPD since 1979. Only 1.2 per cent of them were proven or suspected of developing a sclerosing peritonitis. Patients who developed this complication had in common a history of prolonged peritonitis, previous use of acetate or, when using lactate, peritonitis had been treated with continuous lavage with acetate containing solution, sometimes there was loss of filtration. On the other hand we have never observed sclerosing peritonitis in patients who always used only lactate even those who had severe peritonitis and/or loss of filtration. I heard that in Italy some author had been using acetate for four years without encountering this kind of complication so it seems that not only acetate causes loss of filtration but maybe a special combination of causes are responsible for this sclerosing peritonitis. I would like to have your opinion about that, and do you have any preliminary data about the multicentre study which is being undertaken on the filtration follow-up with acetate versus lactate?

ROTTEMBOURG I don't think that loss of ultrafiltration is obligatory in cases of sclerosing peritonitis. Not all of our patients were showing a degree of loss of ultrafiltration at the time of diagnosis of sclerosing peritonitis, but we must be aware about this problem and with Professor Nolph, Professor Legrain and Professor Mion a multicentre study investigating the loss of ultrafiltration comparing acetate and lactate is now ongoing. This study showed that there is increased absorption of glucose by the peritoneal membrane when you use acetate than when you use lactate and there is less ultrafiltration capacity of the peritoneal membrane when you use acetate than when you use lactate.

HAMILTON (Glasgow) We have had five serious cases of sclerosing obstructive membranous peritonitis (SOP) in our Unit and we have used lactate exclusively in the dialysate. Three patients have died following surgery for obstruction but

241

we diagnosed the other two before obstruction occurred using ultrasound and barium studies to detect the membrane. At that stage elective surgery is possible, and the membrane separates by a natural line of cleavage from the small bowel and can be dealt with ahead of this very serious complication of obstruction. I wondered if you had any experience with ultrasound in these cases?

ROTTEMBOURG No, we haven't this experience. I am very surprised because in my opinion these would be the first cases of sclerosing peritonitis with lactate. Were your patients never treated on acetate even for their peritonitis episodes, or even after the initial insertion of the catheter?

HAMILTON No, we believe the membrane is a consequence of chronic inflammation.

MION (Montpellier) Just a brief comment to confirm that we have had a rather similar experience with five cases of sclerosing peritonitis but also to confirm what was just said that acetate is certainly not the only responsible agent. It is multifactorial and we have had at least two cases since our first publication to the ISAO*, which have been reported to us and who have never had any contact with acetate whatsoever. My question concerns necrotising enteritis as we don't feel that this is a specific complication of CAPD. We have seen at least six such cases in haemodialysis patients and one other case in an IPD patient. Did your two cases have a very low blood pressure?

ROTTEMBOURG I agree with you that necrotising enteritis is also observed in haemodialysis patients but we reviewed all our severe abdominal complications in CAPD and this one was very severe. These two patients were not hypotensive patients and their protein value was in the normal range for CAPD patients.

* Slingeneyer A, Mion C, Mourad G et al. *Trans ASAIO 1983; 29:* In press

MULTICENTRE STUDY OF PHYSICAL ACTIVITY AND EMPLOYMENT STATUS OF CONTINUOUS AMBULATORY PERITONEAL DIALYSIS (CAPD) PATIENTS IN THE UNITED STATES

J A Fragola, Shirley Grube, Linda Von Bloch, E Bourke

Allegheny Professional Building, Pittsburgh, USA

Introduction

Nothing approaching the detailed annual reports on dialysis by the EDTA is presently available in the United States. One recent study of rehabilitation in 2481 haemodialysis (HD) patients (about 4% of the HD population in the US), although acknowledged by its authors to be biased in sampling, does provide important baseline data on some of the limitations of this modality of therapy as currently practiced in this country [1]. It is to be anticipated that the CAPD Patient Registry, sponsored by the National Institutes of Health, will soon produce data comparable to the European reports. Meanwhile the information gap in this area prompted the present multicentre study of factors related to physical activity and employment status in CAPD patients.

Methods

All dialysis centres listed in the Health Care Financing Administration's Dialysis Directory were sent questionnaires containing 17 questions about demography, peritonitis, physical activity (modified Karnofsky scale [2] as adapted by Gutman et al [1]), employment status and perceptions of CAPD. Also enclosed was a return card stating the centre's participation in the study and the number of questionnaires distributed. The completed questionnaires were returned anonymously. One hundred and twenty-five centres participated and 1303 questionnaires were returned representing more than 80 per cent of those distributed and approaching 20 per cent of the CAPD population of the US. One thousand and seventy-six were suitable for analysis.

Results

The mean age of non-diabetics was 52.3 years (range 10–87), the mode decade was the sixth and 34 per cent were 60 or older. The mean age of diabetics was 46, the mode decade was the fourth and 18 per cent were 60 or more. The

TABLE I. Distribution of 1,076 CAPD patients according to selected characteristics

Characteristics	Percentage distribution
Male:Female	55:45
White: Black: Other	86.5: 9.8: 3.7
Married: Single: Widowed: Divorced	71.7: 10.4: 8.4: 9.5
Live alone: With others: Health facility	12.9: 86.9: 0.2
Education in years 0–8: 8–12: >12	15: 58: 27
Diabetes present: Absent	20: 80
Duration of CAPD training in days	
0–5: 6–10: 11–15: >15	48: 26: 22: 4
Prior modality of therapy*	
HD: None: >One: IPD: Home HD: CCPD	45: 20: 20: 9: 5: 1

* >One indicates more than one prior modality of therapy
IPD = Intermittent PD, CCPD = Continuous cyclic PD

mean duration on CAPD was the same for diabetics (11.8 ± 2.5 months) and non-diabetics (12.0 ± 1.8). Demographic characteristics are summarised in Table I. When the duration of training was analysed in relation to level of education by Chi square measure of association, more of those who had attended college or high school completed training within five days than did grade school attenders (p<0.01) a trend that was still apparent between college attenders and grade school attenders in the six to 10 day period (p<0.05). A clear difference emerged in the number of patients requiring assistance to perform CAPD between diabetics (30.6%) and non-diabetics (8.8%, p<0.01). This is partly attributable to visual impairment since 10 per cent of diabetics could only see objects and shadows at best.

Peritonitis was experienced by 55.4 per cent of non-diabetics on an average of 2.1 ± 0.2 occasions, the first episode occurring 2.7 ± 0.1 months after starting CAPD. The corresponding figures for the diabetics were remarkably similar at 56.6 per cent, 2.2 ± 0.1 occasions and 3.1 ± 0.2 months. The level of education was not related to the incidence of peritonitis but the duration of initial training was. Those who took longest to train (>15 days) were the most likely to develop peritonitis (p<0.01). Those with the lowest incidence of peritonitis trained in six to 10 days (p<0.01). Age may have been a factor in this latter finding since age did have an inverse bearing on the development of peritonitis. The mean age of non-diabetics who had not experienced peritonitis (55.0 years) was significantly more than those with more than two attacks per year (41.7 years, p<0.01). A significant negative correlation was observed between mean age and peritonitis rate (r = −0.96, p<0.01).

The data from the Karnofsky scale of physical activity [2] were regrouped into broader categories (Table II) since the studies of Hutchinson et al [3] suggest more reproducible results in dialysis patients by so doing and also such groupings permit comparisons with the HD patients of Gutman et al [1]. Significantly more non-diabetics than diabetics were capable of more physical

TABLE II. Comparison of modified Karnofsky physical activity scale[1] and work/employment scale in CAPD patients and HD patients[2]

| | | CAPD | | Haemodialysis[2] | |
		Non-diabetics	Diabetics	Non-diabetics	Diabetics
Karnofsky scale[1]					
80–100		585[3]	106	1315[4]	67[4]
		(68%)	(48%)	(59%)	(23%)
70–79		168	51	460	72
		(20%)	(23%)	(21%)	(25%)
1–69		103[3]	64	438[4]	147[4]
		(12%)	(29%)	(20%)	(51%)
Work scale					
Total (<59 years)	Before	428	106	1206	
	After	197	44	445	
		(46%)	(41%)	(37%)[5]	
Semi/unskilled[6]	Before	201	55	562	
	After	68	11	131	
		(34%)	(20%)	(23%)[5]	
Skilled[7]	Before	227	51	644	
	After	129	33	315	
		(57%)	(64%)	(49%)	

[1] (80–100) indicates capable of more activity than required for care of oneself, (70–79) only able to carry out self care, (1–69) requires assistance to care for bodily needs.

[6] Includes farm workers.

[7] Skilled blue collar, trained white collar, minor managerial to executive/professional.

[2] Data from Gutman et al [1].

[3] Different from the corresponding diabetic group ($p < 0.01$).

[4] Different from the corresponding CAPD group ($p < 0.01$).

[5] Different from the corresponding CAPD group ($p < 0.05$).

activity than that required for self care (Karnofsky score 80–100) ($p < 0.01$). Conversely, significantly less non-diabetics were incapable of complete self care (Karnofsky score 1–69) than diabetics ($p < 0.01$). When compared with HD patients, significantly more CAPD patients had a Karnofsky score 80–100 amongst both non-diabetics ($p < 0.01$) and diabetics ($p < 0.01$).

There was a substantial decline in the number of people working outside the home and in the number of hours which CAPD patients worked compared to values prior to commencing dialysis (Table III). The decline was more marked amongst semi/unskilled workers than skilled workers ($p < 0.01$). An increase in

TABLE III. Occupations of patients before dialysis and after starting CAPD expressed as percentages

| | Before | | After | |
	Non-diabetic	Diabetic	Non-diabetic	Diabetic
Working*	71.1	69.2	27.1†	26.6†
(>30h/week)	(64.7)	(60.9)	(11.4)†	(10.4)†
(<30h/week)	(6.4)	(8.3)	(15.7)†	(16.2)†
Homemaker	14.3	12.2	18.2†	14.3
Student	3.0	1.5	2.3	1.5
Disabled/retired	10.5	13.5	16.7†	15.9
Unemployed	1.1	3.6	35.7†	41.7†

* Refers to work outside the home.
† Significantly different from the corresponding values before dialysis (p<0.01).

homemakers was predominantly attributable to women who had worked outside the home prior to dialysis. When the work scale of the CAPD patients was compared to HD patients the trend was again better but the differences were less impressive than for the physical activity data (Table II). Thus the work record of semi/unskilled non-diabetic CAPD patients under 59 years was not statistically significantly different from similarly grouped HD patients and in the category of skilled worker the CAPD patients fared only marginally better ($\chi^2 = 4.4$, p<0.05).

The main advantages of CAPD as perceived by the patients were freedom, independence and/or the ability to be more in the home (57%), improved health status (20%), liberalisation of diet (10%) and an end to less pleasant recollections of haemodialysis (10%). Disadvantages included none (29%), a more frequent answer among those who had previously been on another modality of therapy, various aspects of the endless routine (27%), peritonitis or fear of it (18%) and various aspects relating to body image (16%). To the question "Would you recommend CAPD to another renal patient?" over 98 per cent responded "Yes".

Discussion

The higher proportion of whites than in the National Registry of CAPD patients [4] (78%) may have resulted in part from more questionnaires needing discarding from minorities due to errors attributable to lower educational attainment. The demography was otherwise remarkably similar to the Registry. Of interest was that 74 per cent completed CAPD training within 10 days with some positive correlation between the rapidity of training and level of education and the fact that only four per cent required more than 15 days to complete training and this group was at increased risk of developing peritonitis. More unexpected was the significant inverse relationships between peritonitis and age, an observation requiring further exploration.

The results indicate that diabetics were not at increased risk of peritonitis, that 69.4 per cent of them performed CAPD without assistance, that amongst skilled workers as many diabetics as non-diabetics resumed work and that they were more physically active than diabetics on HD. (Selection of less diabetics with blindness and severe neuropathy for CAPD may explain this.) The fact that diabetics generally fared less well than non-diabetics was nonetheless apparent.

The better physical activity scale of the non-diabetic CAPD patients compared to HD patients could also in part be a consequence of patient selection. Selection notwithstanding, however, the consistency of apparent improvement in their physical activity and their clearly articulated sense of greater independence, improved health status and "freedom from the machine", was not reflected in a better employment status for CAPD patients. Only 27 per cent were gainfully employed and 11 per cent worked more than 30 hours per week. This conclusion was despite keeping the questionnaire anonymous due to the recent suggestion that many dialysis patients are employed "off the books" [5]. The employment status was only marginally better than HD patients despite all the cited advantages. The influence of social, economic and labour market conditions on the return to work and the possibility that the Social Security System may represent a "barrier to rehabilitation" as reported elsewhere [6] deserves consideration.

This has been a retrospective analysis of demographic, socio-epidemiologic and 'quality of life' assessments. Lack of prospective experimental design with random allocation of patients to CAPD or HD requires caution in interpreting the above conclusions. An additional conclusion which impressed us was the high response rate amongst patients who received the questionnaire — a potentially valuable population group for future surveys.

Acknowledgments

We would like to thank the many centres throughout the United States for their co-operation in making this study possible. We are also most grateful to the patients who completed the questionnaires.

References

1 Gutman RA, Stead WW, Robinson RR. *N Engl J Med 1981; 303:* 309
2 Karnofsky DA, Burchenal JH. In Macleod CM, ed. *Evaluation of Chemotherapeutic Agents.* New York: Columbia University Press. 1949; 191
3 Hutchinson TA, Boyd NF, Feinstein AR. *J Chronic Dis 1979; 32:* 661
4 Nolph K, Pyle KW. *NIH CAPD Registry 1982; 15 April:* 3
5 Neff MS, Slifkin RF, Eiser AR. *N Engl J Med 1981; 305:* 646
6 Tews HP, Schreiber WK, Huber W et al. *Nephron 1980; 26:* 130

Open Discussion

GOLDSMITH (Chairman) CAPD seems to be like driving, as you get older you get a bit safer. Can you tell us, in relation to the tedium expressed by some of the patients, do you use four exchanges per day normally or have you tried reducing to three?

FRAGOLA We did not ask that question in our questionnaire, so we do not have that data.

GOLDSMITH Well it does seem possible to treat quite a high proportion of patients with three bags a day even if one sometimes needs more than two litres in the bag.

BINSWANGER (Chairman) I was surprised to see your data on the decreasing rate of peritonitis with age. I suggest that when you pass a certain age it might increase again, that's at least our experience. What do you think of this?

FRAGOLA The only other analysis I could find on that was in the initial NIH report by Nolph* of 514 patients in 1981 limited to 14 centres. This was in contrast to European reports which suggest that, in Europe at least, the incidence of peritonitis increases with age. In the Nolph report however there was no statistical significance, I suspect because of the small number of patients comprising people over a certain age group. I think we have to interpret our data with caution but it's something that merits further study.

MAHER (Bethesda, USA) Could you comment on how comparable your groups were in terms of duration of dialysis, whether one group might have been more disadvantageous? Secondly, do you have any answer as to whether a switch from CAPD to haemodialysis or vice versa influences the rehabilitation status?

FRAGOLA Are you referring to haemodialysis patients, or to diabetics or non-diabetics?

MAHER No, between the haemodialysis and the peritoneal population. Haemodialysis has a 20 year plus history and CAPD only four years, therefore you might have some very long-standing patients who are now unemployed on haemodialysis and that would be a very unfair comparison.

FRAGOLA It was impossible, obviously, because of the length of time that haemodialysis has been around as a treatment for the patient groups to be exactly comparable. The aim of our study was to (a) confirm or refute that physical rehabilitation has anything to do with returning to work and (b) to try to compare that to the only study we know that has been recently published regarding haemodialysis patients. Obviously the average duration of dialysis on Gutmann's† study was longer. Looking at return to work, if there was a difference,

---

*   Nolph KD. *Dialysis Transplant 1981; 10:* 744
†   Gutmann RA, Stead WN, Robinson RR. *N Engl J Med 1981; 304:* 309

it was only marginal. Even though rehabilitation was fair it did not influence the return to work in our patients. In answer to your second question, we could not ask that of our patients because our questionnaire was strictly addressed to CAPD patients.

BARTOVA (Prague) Have you noticed the difference between the number of peritonitis episodes between male and female patients, and if you have, what would you suggest could be the reason? We have noticed this difference in our Centre where we have more peritonitis episodes in male patients than in females.

FRAGOLA No, in our study, and I have to remind you of this point, that the peritonitis was reported by the patients, although we feel fairly confident that it is accurate information due to the fact that it agrees with present statistics in the United Sates. In our study, and in other studies that I'm aware of there has not been any difference in incidence but I have no idea why that should be.

PART VI

GUEST LECTURES – TRANSPLANTATION

Chairmen: R A Sells
              D N S Kerr

Proc EDTA (1983) Vol 20

EFFECTS OF BLOOD TRANSFUSIONS ON RENAL TRANSPLANTS: CONSIDERING EXCLUSIVE BLOOD PRODUCTS AND DONOR RELATIONSHIP

Sondra T Perdue, **P I Terasaki**

UCLA School of Medicine, University of California, Los Angeles, USA

Introduction

The efficacy of pretransplant blood transfusions in improving graft success in cadaveric donor renal transplantation has been confirmed by a myriad of studies [1]. However, controversy still abounds regarding the optimal protocol for transfusions, particularly with very small numbers of units, and regarding the effects of transfusions with non-cadaveric donors. We present here the analysis on results of small numbers of transfusions with particular blood products based on a relatively homogeneous patient subpopulation. We also evaluate the effectiveness of transfusions in living related transplants using the 'preventable fraction' of graft failures as a measure of effect in comparing the various recipient groups, and present a multicentre evaluation of donor-specific transfusions.

Methods

Data base

Transplants reported to the UCLA Transplant Registry that were performed after 1977 were considered in this study. More than 120 transplant centres, primarily in the United States and Canada, co-operated in reporting all cases to the Registry. All cases with complete information on the variables of interest were included in the subsets described below. Approximately 70 per cent of the transplants performed in the United States annually are reported to the UCLA Registry.

Statistical analyses

Survival rates were computed as actuarial estimates from cohort life tables [2]. The calculation of 'preventable fraction' is $(S_T-S_{NT})/(1-S_{NT})$ where S_{NT} is the estimated survival proportion of the nontransfused recipients and S_T is the survival proportion in the comparison transfusion category.

Results

Effect of transfusion by unit

Effectiveness of transfusion is shown with transfused units increasing by single units from zero (Figure 1). This subset of non-diabetic Caucasian recipients receiving first cadaveric donor transplants was selected to be relatively homogeneous across transfusion categories with respect to other major known risk

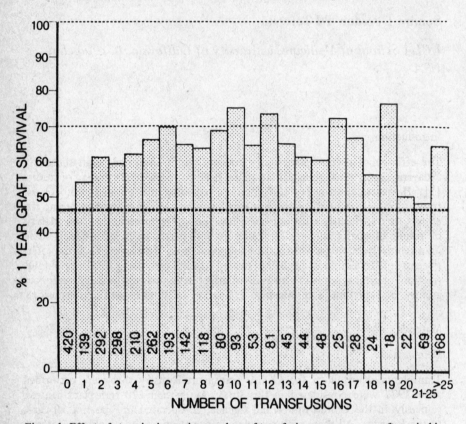

Figure 1. Effect of stepwise increasing numbers of transfusions on one-year graft survival in non-diabetic Caucasian recipients receiving first cadaveric donor transplants from 1979 to 1983. The number of cases in each transfusion category is noted on the lower part of each bar

factors. Data from 1979 to 1983 were selected to control for the increasing overall graft survival rates since the mid-1970s [3]. Even a single transfusion increases graft survival at one year. This effect increases with additional transfusions until approximately five units, is fairly steady until approximately 13 units, and then shows some trend towards decreasing effectiveness although there are fluctuations.

Effectiveness of transfusion by type of unit

The same patient subset was divided further into patients who had received only one type of blood product during their transfusion course (Table I, Figure 2).

TABLE I. Preventable fraction of graft failure in nontransfused cases by pretransplant transfusions (1st cadaveric transplants, non-diabetic Caucasian recipients, 1979–1982)

Exclusive blood product	1st transfusion		2−5 transfusions		6−10 transfusions	
	Number of cases	PF*	Number of cases	PF*	Number of cases	PF*
Whole blood	20	0.33	107	0.25	54	0.33
Packed cells	73	0.08	742	0.32	373	0.45
Washed cells	36	0.22	93	0.13	38	0.48
Frozen cells	9	−0.25	40	−0.14	26	0.05

* PF = preventable fraction using number of specific units of exclusive blood product as compared to zero pretransplant transfusions

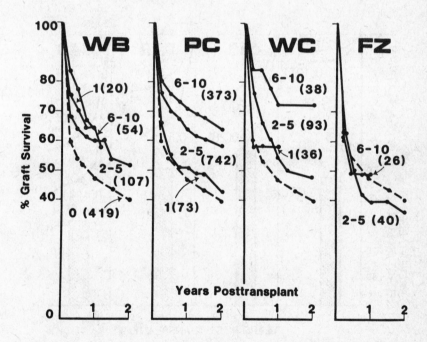

Figure 2. Graft survival in patients receiving an exclusive blood product by number of pretransplant transfusions (WB = whole blood, PC = packed cells, WC = washed cells, FZ = frozen cells). The number of cases is shown in parentheses following the number of transfusions. Non-diabetic Caucasian recipients of first cadaveric grafts from 1979 to 1983 are included

Clearly, the single-unit patients can be classified by transfusion type, but there were also patients with up to 10 units who received transfusions with such a limited protocol. Packed cells (PC) was the most likely blood product to be used in this way, followed by whole blood (WB), and next by washed cells (WC). A small number of patients were transfused with frozen cells (FZ) only.

The two-year survival curves for each group are shown compared to the nontransfused group (Figure 2). The effect of small numbers of units varies considerably with the blood product used. The measure that we have used for evaluating the transfusion effect in greater detail is the 'preventable fraction' at one-year post-transplant (Table I). The preventable fraction (PF) is interpreted as the proportion of nontransfused cases failing by one year that would have been prevented by transfusion.

Whole blood seems to be the most effective transfusion if a single unit is given (PF of 33%), and in fact no further benefit is shown with higher numbers of whole blood units. On the other hand, single transfusions of packed cells prevent only about eight per cent of failures, but packed cells equal the whole blood effect with two to five units and rise to a PF of 45 per cent with six to 10 packed cell transfusions. Exclusive use of washed cells seems to require six to 10 transfusions to be consistently effective even though the PF here for a

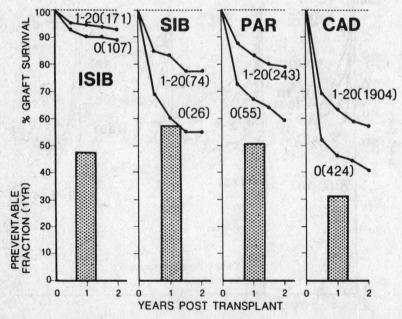

Figure 3. Effect of (1–20) blood transfusions compared to zero (0) transfusions on graft survival by donor relationship for glomerulonephritis patients receiving first grafts during 1978 to 1982. Both two-year survival curves and preventable fraction at one year by transfusion are given. The number of cases for each category is given in parentheses following the number of transfusions.

256

single transfusion is about 22 per cent. Frozen cells do not produce the transfusion effect, although the number of available cases is small.

Transfusion effect in related donor transplants

The transfusion effect by donor relationship is shown for all glomerulonephritis (GN) patients receiving first grafts between 1978–1982 (Figure 3). This is the largest recipient original disease group, and was used to control effects of disease on graft outcome. Survival curves for zero transfusions and one to 20 transfusions are plotted for two years post-transplant, and the PF at one year for each donor category is shown. Although baseline survival rate for zero transfusions is much higher for identical siblings (91% at one year), the PF measure of 48 per cent demonstrates clearly the strong effect of transfusions even in this class of transplant. The one-year PF is 31 per cent for cadaveric donor grafts, and ranges from 48 per cent to 58 per cent for related donor grafts.

Preliminary multicentre results for donor-specific transfusions indicate that these transfusions may be more effective than random transfusions in sibling transplants (Figure 4). The improvement in these cases was also apparent when only five or more transfusions were compared, and were thus probably not an effect of blood product differences between donor-specific and random transfusions.

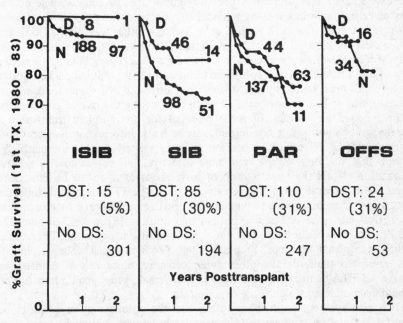

Figure 4. Comparison of donor-specific transfusions (DST; D) and random donor transfusions (No DS; N) by donor relationship. Number of cases with follow-up at one and two years post-transplant are given. All transfused first transplant cases from 1980 to 1983 are included

257

Discussion

In this study we have investigated the role of the type of blood in relation to the number of transfusions which might be optimal. In updating our overall figure for the number of transfusions over our previous studies [4,5], there has been relatively little change despite the accumulation of more patients and analysis of a more homogeneous subset. A single transfusion continues to have a significant effect. We introduce here the concept of preventable fraction in this context which can be used to compare the relative effects of the different blood products.

Data in Figure 2 show that efficacy of a single transfusion may be dependent on blood product, and this may explain part of the differences in conflicting reports regarding single transfusions. The effectiveness of one transfusion has been reported by a group using primarily washed cells [6], whereas a group using mainly packed cells found fewer than five units ineffective [7].

Although the numbers of cases are small in some categories, the preventable fraction results by single types of transfusions may imply that prophylactic transfusion can be effective with one or two whole blood transfusions. If the transfusion effect is mediated by leucocytes, we might expect that a single transfusion would be most effective with whole blood. Packed cells would be expected to have the next most leucocytes, followed by washed cells. Although we did not see that a single unit of packed cells was more effective than a single unit of washed cells, there was a strikingly greater effectiveness of two to five transfusions with packed cells than with washed cells. Stated another way, packed cells and whole cells are most effective with more than five units of blood, although these may be rather inefficient ways in which to transfuse leucocytes. Potential sensitisation of one whole blood unit compared to more than five units of packed cells or washed cells must be considered. Clearly, exclusive use of frozen blood, at least for 10 units or less, is not justified when considering the risk of graft failure.

In general, the efficacy of some protocol for pretransplant transfusion is widely agreed upon for cadaveric donor transplants. Information is much more sparse regarding effects of transfusion in living related donor transplants. We believe that the PF measure is a more effective tool for evaluating relative transfusion effects than comparison of survival curves when the baseline (zero transfusion) survival levels vary greatly. In fact, the PF for related donors is even higher than for cadaveric donors. The apparent effect seen by comparison of survival curves of one-haplotype matched kidneys [8] is verified here, but the PF comparison illustrates that the effect is equally strong in the 278 identical sibling transplants reported. Proportionately fewer identical sibling recipients are transfused than for any other donor category. Since risk of sensitisation against an HLA-identical sibling must be quite small, prophylactic transfusions should be considered for all types of recipients.

It is also apparent from these studies that the optimal way in which blood transfusions can be used is still not completely known. Although transfusions have a marked effect, at least used in the standard fashion, they do not result in 100 per cent survival. Other trials with various products are needed to optimise the transfusion effect.

Acknowledgments

This work was supported in part by the National Institute of Arthritis, Diabetes, Digestive, and Kidney Diseases Grant AM 02375-24.

References

1 Opelz G, Terasaki PI. *Transplantation 1980; 29:* 153
2 Miller RG. *Survival Analysis.* New York: Wiley & Sons. 1981
3 Terasaki PI, Perdue ST, Sasaki N et al. *JAMA* (in press)
4 Opelz G, Terasaki PI. *N Engl J Med 1978; 299:* 799
5 Horimi T, Terasaki PI, Chia D, Sasaki N. *Transplantation 1983; 35:* 320
6 Persijn GG, van Leeuwen A, Parlevliet J et al. *Transplant Proc 1981; 13:* 150
7 Fehrman I, Rigden O, Möller E. *Transplantation 1983; 35:* 339
8 Solheim BG, Flatmark A, Halvorsen S et al. *Transplantation 1980; 30:* 281

Open Discussion

SELLS (Chairman) Did I see in one of the slides evidence that one centre in the States, doing in excess of 200 transplants per year, is getting a one year survival rate of 35 per cent? I was racking my brains to try and think which centre that would be, but may be I misinterpreted the slide.

TERASAKI You did see those numbers correctly, but I am certainly not going to tell you which centre it was.

WING (London) I can appreciate the enormous amount of work and data collection and analysis that goes into that data you have given us today and I want to thank you very much for it. The question I have for you is concerning the effect of transfusion. One aspect of this is that it may make, by sensitisation, certain patients on the recipient waiting list effectively untransplantable and they are thereby excluded. I would like your comment on the statistical implication of that. What effect is that having on the survival curves? I would also like to know the proportion of recipients who might otherwise have been transplanted who are excluded by our transfusion policies.

TERASAKI It is an important problem that transfusions, although they do not have immunosuppression side effects, and patients do not develop infections, have no complications as with Cyclosporin A or excess azathioprine and so on and they are the most innocuous and the most specific kind of immunosuppression that we have to date, unfortunately have the side effect of sensitising some patients. This will have long-term implications for the patients on a transplant waiting list. We used to argue that it was better for patients to be detected as responders following blood transfusion rather than to go ahead with the transplant and subsequent rejection. The experience of having a transfusion and making antibody is a lot easier to take than going through a kidney transplant and rejecting it. This is certainly not the best answer for the future and this is why we and others have been trying to see if there is a way of transfusing

259

TERASAKI We have been gathering data from various transplant centres and I must admit I do not myself know exactly what criteria the different centres have used in transplanting diabetic patients. All we know is that everybody seems to be having better results. One of the possibilities is that people are less timid about transplanting diabetic patients and actually transplanting them earlier. The problem in the old days may have been that they waited too long and tried to transplant such patients when they were on their last legs. I think it is important to catch them as soon as they have kidney failure and once that is done their survival rate is almost the same as any other patient.

KURUVILA (Denver, Colorado) Could you comment on the relationship between transfusions and the acquired immune deficiency syndrome?

TERASAKI Although I come from the home of AIDS and where there are a number of cases, I must admit we have ourselves not done very many studies on that. I am not able to comment at all.

KURUVILA Do you have any data on plasma exchange for patients who have developed cytotoxic antibodies?

TERASAKI That too we have neglected to collect. As more and more centres perform plasma exchange we would like to start collecting data to see how effective it is in stopping rejection.

BROYER (Paris) Have you ruled out any effect of minor blood group mismatches, especially from the Lewis sub-group?

TERASAKI No, we have certainly not ruled out the effects of minor blood group mismatches. We have been unable to do a good study on the so-called minor antigens. It is quite possible that antigens, such as Lewis, are important in transplantation. As you know, Oriol* in France has studied the effect of Lewis and has reported that it is important. Subsequent studies have had some difficulty in confirming that and so we still have not ruled out the possibility that something like Lewis is very important. We know that Lewis antibodies occur in grafted patients, that they are present on lymphocytes and just like the HLA antigens they may have a small effect and therefore it would take many cases and a well controlled study in order to show its effects.

ANDREUCCI (Naples) You said that blood transfusion is innocuous, but we have always the danger of viral infection. When you talk about blood transfusion are you referring to whole blood transfusion?

TERASAKI Yes, I am sorry that I have not had time to give details of a study where we showed the effect of different types of blood products. Most of our data is based on what is called 'packed cells'. A very small fraction of the patients

* Oriol R, Cartron J, Yvart J et al. *Lancet 1978; i:* 574

without getting the sensitisation and this is the experience we have described to you. We happen to think that the best way is to give azathioprine, which we know is relatively innocuous, together with the transfusions and in this way we might be able to reduce the sensitisation rate. Now Dr Salvatierra* in San Francisco has done about 50 cases of donor specific transfusions giving three transfusions together with azathioprine, and his sensitisation rate is about 10 per cent. The same kind of sensitisation rate has been obtained by Dr Belzer in Wisconsin using azathioprine together with the transfusions. We think that it is possible to reduce the sensitisation rate by using azathioprine. However, if you give too much azathioprine you might also lose the transfusion effect and so this is another complication which eventually we may have to deal with.

SELLS The work you quoted was donor specific transfusion. Is anybody giving third party blood with immunosuppressives, as that would seem a rather important experiment to do?

TERASAKI Yes, there are already some groups doing that, but unfortunately the number of cases is not large enough to report as yet.

GABRIEL (London) Would you now recommend that azathioprine is given routinely at the time of pretransplant blood transfusion or is that going beyond your data? Secondly, would you like to speculate on the mode of action of azathioprine in these circumstances?

TERASAKI With regard to your first question, I doubt that it will become universal, nothing that we have advocated has been accepted by everybody, but we hope that more people would use this approach so that the percentage of sensitised patients will be decreased. Others have advocated using like HLA-matched blood and some have advocated using stored blood in an effort to decrease sensitisation.

With regard to your second question, we are not too sure but it does seem that azathioprine inhibits humoral antibody synthesis. We are hoping that in this situation we would inhibit the cytotoxic antibody formation and at the same time not inhibit whatever else the transfusion is doing to enhance the graft. There seem to be two effects: one is the production of antibody and second is the production of tolerance or enhancement. We think that if you give too much azathioprine you would cut off the formation of cytotoxic antibody but in addition also the formation of enhancing antibodies.

SODAGAR (Tehran) As you know, there have been reports concerning better results of transplantation in diabetic patients if undertaken earlier. In other words, the earlier you transplant diabetic patients the better the results. I would like to know your experience and criteria for transplanting diabetic patients?

* Salvatierra O. Am J Kidney Dis 1981; 1: 119

have been transfused with whole blood but we feel that whole blood seems to be the most effective. The least effective seems to be frozen blood. It is possible that this is directly related to the number of white cells in blood. The whole blood contains the most white cells, the frozen blood probably contains the least amount of white cells.

Proc EDTA (1983) Vol 20

IMMUNOLOGICAL MONITORING OF VIRAL INFECTIONS IN RENAL TRANSPLANT RECIPIENTS

B Brando, G Civati, C Grillo, G Busnach, G Colussi, M L Broggi, L Minetti

Niguarda-Ca'Granda Hospital, Milano, Italy

Summary

Twelve viral episodes occurred in 54 antilymphocyte globulin-treated renal transplant recipients (two primary cytomegalovirus, seven cytomegalovirus reactivations, one chickenpox, two influenza). In 11 of 12 cases the ratio between peripheral T4 and T8 subsets fell (from 1.698 to 0.986, p<0.01) due both to a reduction of T4$^+$ and to an increase of T8$^+$ cells. T10$^+$ and 5/9 subsets also increased. Suppressor T-cell function, as measured by two simultaneous assays, was enhanced. In antibody-negative CMV patients the reversal of T4/T8 ratio preceded the appearance of specific IgM. T4/T8 ratios rapidly returned to normal in mild episodes, but remained reverted in symptomatic CMV patients for several months, despite a reduction in the immunosuppressive regimen. Symptomatic viral episodes displayed marked imbalances in T cell subset numbers and function, while in asymptomatic cases the changes were less evident.

Introduction

Viral infections are a major cause of morbidity in renal transplant recipients. Cytomegalovirus (CMV) and other herpes viruses are most commonly involved as opportunistic agents in the first months after grafting [1, 2]. In such patients the spectrum of the virus-associated diseases may range from a fever of unknown origin to a severe multiple organ involvement and death.

A primary or reactivated viral infection may raise difficult diagnostic problems during clinical follow-up, since some features may be similar to rejection or bacterial infection.

Direct demonstration of the virus by extensive culturing is difficult and time-consuming, therefore it is hardly suitable as a routine investigation. Indirect evidence of viral infection can be accomplished by several methods, including demonstration of various specific antibodies in serum, histological and cytological features and by the appearance of a spectrum of clinical syndromes. In recent years a great deal of research has been undertaken on the immunological abnormalities associated with viral infections [1-4]. Thus, some immunological features, such as T cell subset imbalances or depressed cell-mediated responses, may be considered as further indirect markers of viral infection both in the normal and the immunocompromised host. Moreover, many reports indicate a role of viruses in determining immunomodulation in various conditions [3-6].

The present study was undertaken to assess the patterns and the clinical value of multiple cellular immunological monitoring coupled with serological assays in renal transplant patients with viral infections.

Patients and methods

During the clinical and immunological follow-up of 54 renal transplant recipients from cadaver donors 12 episodes defined as viral infections occurred. All patients were given prophylactic antilymphocyte globulin (ALG), azathioprine and tapering prednisone. Routine immunological monitoring was performed by determining serially blood T-cell subsets defined by the T3, T4, T8, T10 monoclonal antibodies (Ortho), B-cells and mitogenic response to ConA and PWM. In some cases the 5/9 antibody was also employed (kind gift of Dr G Corte, Genoa). Suppressor cell function was studied by the Concanavalin-A enhancement test (ConAE) and the OKT8-DEP PWM test [7] and the results were expressed as per cent suppressor index (SI). Serological studies were performed by measuring the anti-CMV and anti-Herpes Simplex (HSV) IgM and IgG titres with a solid phase ELISA method (Enzygnost-Behring Institut). Viral inclusions in urinary sediment cells were investigated by conventional staining techniques.

Viral infection episodes were defined by clinical criteria (unexplained fever, upper respiratory tract symptoms, pneumonia, hepatic dysfunction, leucopenia, thrombocytopenia, specific skin lesions) and/or by serologic changes (a four-fold increase of IgG titres in antibody-positive patients or the appearance of specific IgM). Twenty-four additional patients who were chronic carriers of HBs Ag were also studied. Student's t-test was employed for statistical analysis.

Results

There were 12 viral episodes, two primary non-fatal CMV infections, two were symptomatic and five asymptomatic CMV reactivations, one chickenpox and two influenza-like syndromes. The time of onset was 5-41 weeks after grafting (mean 12.1). In 11 of the 12 viral episodes the T4/T8 ratio decreased, due both to a reduction of T4$^+$ subset and to a rise of T8$^+$ cells. T10$^+$ subset sharply increased, and the 5/9$^+$ cells showed a slight but constant increase (Table I). No changes were observed in T3 and B populations. The SI, as determined by both the suppressor cell assays significantly increased, mostly in primary and symptomatic CMV episodes (Figure 1) while mitogenic responses were only occasionally depressed (data not shown). In primary CMV infections the T4/T8 reversal preceded the appearance of specific IgM by 6-10 days. The T4/T8 ratios persisted significantly lower than controls for 8-18 months in symptomatic and some asymptomatic CMV reactivations, despite a reduction in immunosuppressive therapy and clinical recovery. In contrast, patients with non-CMV infections showed only transient immunological changes, and returned

266

TABLE I. T-cell subset changes during 12 viral episodes in transplant recipients. Data at onset and after seven days are indicated. p values are calculated from quiescence data

	T3	T4	T8	T4/T8	T10	5/9
Quiescence before	63 ± 14.5	43.4 ± 10.6	26.5 ± 6.6	1.698 ± 0.45	7.9 ± 2.8	5.5 ± 1.3
Viral episode	58.8 ± 15.5	28.5 ± 11.1 ***	32.4 ± 12	0.986 ± 0.46 ***	17.8 ± 7.9 **	8.2 ± 3.3
One week after	65.2 ± 9.7	37.3 ± 10.9	37.5 ± 10.8 **	1.056 ± 0.49 ***	20.9 ± 9.2 *	8.4 ± 2.2 *

* p<0.05; ** p<0.025; *** p<0.01

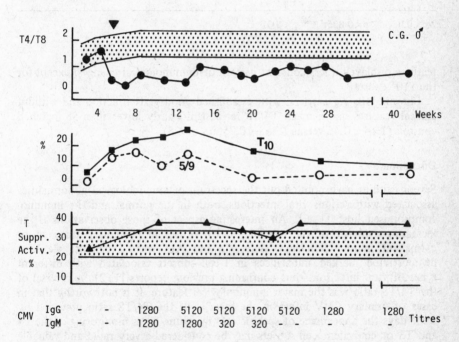

Figure 1. Immunological patterns during a primary CMV infection. The triangle at the upper left denotes the onset of symptoms. Dotted areas indicate the normal ranges

to normal in 6–15 days. Cellular inclusions were occasionally found in the urine of patients with high CMV IgG titres. Results were subsequently analysed according to the presence or absence of clinical symptoms (Table II). Symptomatic patients showed marked and significant changes in T-cell subsets. On the other hand patients in whom viral reactivation was assessed only by serological

TABLE II. T-cell subset changes in symptomatic and asymptomatic viral episodes. Asymptomatic cases were five silent CMV reactivations. Similar patterns were evident one week after onset

	T4	T8	T4/T8	T10
Symptomatic patients (7 cases)				
Quiescence before	44.2 ± 11.8	27 ± 7.1	1.724 ± 0.56	8.6 ± 4.1
Viral episode	27.2 ± 12 **	36.4 ± 13 *	0.815 ± 0.33 ***	22.4 ± 10 *
Asymptomatic patients (5 cases)				
Quiescence before	44.2 ± 9.9	25.8 ± 6.5	1.680 ± 0.36	7 ± 1.4
Viral episode	31.3 ± 11	29.4 ± 9.5	1.256 ± 0.58	15.5 ± 2.8 ***

* $p < 0.05$; ** $p < 0.025$; *** $p < 0.01$

features displayed a less constant pattern of immunological changes, except for the $T10^+$ subset.

Chronic HBs Ag carriers, with established good graft function and without clinical features had a mean T4/T8 ratio significantly lower than 58 matched controls (1.14 ± 0.46 versus 1.765 ± 0.75, $p < 0.025$).

Discussion

Several studies have pointed out the spectrum of immunological abnormalities associated with various viral infections, both in the normal and the immuno-compromised host [1–6]. An interesting aspect of those observations is the increasing evidence of the role played by viruses in promoting transient or permanent immunodeficiency states. In our ALG-treated patients we have demonstrated marked imbalances in T-cell subsets associated with different types of viral infection, thus confirming previous reports [1, 2]. A reversal of the T4/T8 ratio was the major immunological feature. It is noteworthy that in cases of primary CMV infection the reversal of the T4/T8 ratio preceded by some days the appearance of specific IgM in serum. Thus monitoring of the T4 and T8 or equivalent cell subsets may be considered a very rapid and valuable tool for the indirect diagnosis of primary CMV episodes [2].

Patients with symptomatic CMV episodes showed a long lasting imbalance, which may account for a permanent immunodeficiency state and an increased risk of opportunistic infections [1, 2, 6]. Similar changes were evident also in chronic HBs Ag carriers [8].

Long-term morbidity due to viral infections was not observed, perhaps due to the short follow-up. Only one case of frank CMV-induced graft dysfunction [2] was observed in an antibody positive subject. The different immunological behaviour between symptomatic and asymptomatic patients deserves some comment. Patients who experienced clinically symptomatic episodes, whatever the virus, showed marked and constant T-cell subset patterns. On the contrary, in asymptomatic reactivations the changes of immunological parameters appeared to be less evident [2]. This could be partly explained by the association between CMV viraemia and clinically important syndromes, both in antibody positive and negative subjects [9]. Moreover, CMV is known to induce T-cell proliferation in antibody positive patients only. Antibody-dependent and natural antiviral mechanisms can also occur in these subjects, possibly leading to different patterns of reactivity [10]. Furthermore, the increase of the $T10^+$ subset was a prominent feature in our study. $T10^+$ cells have been shown to be high in EBV mononucleosis and homosexual males with AIDS [5, 6]. Since increased numbers of $T10^+$ and $5/9^+$ cells may be found in acute rejection episodes, these findings must be considered as non-specific markers of immune activation.

The enhanced suppressor cell activity associated with low T4/T8 ratios that we have demonstrated mainly in symptomatic CMV episodes confirms that the virus-induced hyporesponsiveness may be due, at least in part, to an active mechanism [3–5]. It is still unclear how CMV may induce increased T-suppressor function, since direct infection of specific lymphocyte subsets has not been documented [4]. Accessory phenomena possibly associated with $T8^+$ cell reaction against self class I HLA antigens as an anti-viral defence may be postulated [10]. However monocytes may also play a role as suppressor cells in various diseases both in vivo and in vitro [4, 7]. At present it is not yet entirely clear how the $T8^+$ subset can be dissected into suppressor and cytotoxic cells. The appearance of Ia and T10 antigens on a part of activated $T8^+$ cells may partly help to explain some controversies.

Lastly, the ELISA assay used to detect HSV and CMV IgM and IgG antibodies proved to be a very sensitive and rapid tool to monitor the dynamics of serologic response. However, in some CMV reactivations with very high IgG titres, some cross-reaction may occur with HSV antigens.

It is concluded that a multi-assay immunological monitoring of the transplanted patient may yield valuable information for the differential diagnosis between viral infections and other episodes, and provide evidence for a better insight into the immune system of the abnormal host.

References

1   Rubin RH, Tolkoff-Rubin NE. *Proc EDTA 1982; 19:* 513
2   Schooley RT, Hirsch MS, Colvin RB et al. *N Engl J Med 1983; 308:* 307
3   Reinherz EL, O'Brien C, Rosenthal P et al. *J Immunol 1980; 125:* 1269
4   Carney WP, Rubin RH, Hoffman RA et al. *J Immunol 1981; 126:* 2114
5   De Waele M, Thielemans C, Van Camp BKG. *N Engl J Med 1981; 304:* 460
6   Gottlieb MS, Schroff R, Schanker HM et al. *N Engl J Med 1981; 305:* 1425
7   Brando B, Civati G, Nova ML et al. *Transplant Proc 1983; 15:* 776
8   Carella G, Chatenoud L, Degos F et al. *J Clin Immunol 1982; 2:* 93
9   Rubin RH, Cosimi AB, Hirsch MS et al. *Transplantation 1981; 31:* 143
10   Quinnan GV, Kirmani N, Rook AH et al. *N Engl J Med 1983; 307:* 7

Open Discussion

BARNES (Chairman) I wasn't quite sure about the type of immunosuppression you were giving these patients, and the relationship of the ALG to the observations that you were making. Perhaps you could give us a little more detail.

BRANDO All the patients received prophylactic ALG, azathioprine and steroids but none were on ALG at the time of infection. The timing of infection ranged from 5–40 weeks that is in the period of time when normally ALG had been stopped. However, a cluster of CMV reactivations was observed after adjuvant immunosuppression courses due to rejection.

BARNES Were they on azathioprine and prednisone at the time you were making these observations? How could the immunosuppression regimen account for artifacts?

BRANDO Yes, the dotted areas in the figures show the normal trend for uncomplicated patients and most of the cases were in the normal area before the crisis. The immunosuppressive regimen may account for a number of artifacts, especially in patients on Cyclosporin A. We have only very preliminary results about this but I feel that it will be difficult to interpret immunological features of patients with viral infection on Cyclosporin A, since many patients on Cyclosporin A have low T4/T8 ratios.

BARNES None of your patients had such medications?

BRANDO None of the cases reported were on Cyclosporin A.

BAHIER (Chicago) When you talk about asymptomatic patients do you mean patients who have viraemia but no fever or leucopenia?

BRANDO We cannot rule out viraemia but we consider the symptoms such as fever, leucopenia, pneumonia, thrombocytopenia, skin rash, hepatitis and so on. We have studied many cases in which seroconversion was observed only on routine determinations while the patients were totally asymptomatic.

BAHIER So you are talking basically just about patients who seroconverted?

BRANDO Yes, actually the asymptomatic patients that I described were all secondary CMV reactivations.

Proc EDTA (1983) Vol 20

HYPERIMMUNE IMMUNOGLOBULIN THERAPY FOR CYTOMEGALOVIRUS INFECTIONS IN RENAL TRANSPLANT PATIENTS

C B Brown, A J Nicholls, N Edward*, B Cuthbertson†, P L Yap‡, D B L McClelland‡

*Royal Hallamshire Hospital, Sheffield, *Aberdeen Royal Infirmary, Aberdeen, †Protein Fractionation Centre, Edinburgh, and ‡South-East Scotland Blood Transfusion Service, Edinburgh, United Kingdom*

Summary

Eleven renal transplant patients with CMV infection have been treated by passive immunisation, one with high-titre anti-CMV plasma and 10 with fractionated hyperimmune anti-CMV immunoglobulin. All were pyrexial for at least seven days before treatment with typical clinical and laboratory features of CMV infection. Seven of the 11 patients treated showed a striking and sustained response within 24–48 hours of therapy, with lysis of fever, resolution of pneumonitis, a rise in white cell count and improvement in renal function and liver function tests.

Introduction

The current treatment of cytomegalovirus (CMV) infections after renal transplantation is unsatisfactory. The illness usually comprises a syndrome of prolonged high pyrexia, leucopenia and/or atypical lymphocytosis, abnormal liver enzymes, lung infiltrates, and failing graft function occurring 4–10 weeks after transplantation [1]. It may be due to primary infection from the transplanted kidney or reactivation of a latent infection. Secondary lung infections with fungi, Pneumocystis carinii and Pseudomonas sp. are well recognised complications, and frequently lead to the death of the patient [2, 3].

In the absence of an effective therapeutic agent [4], we have administered CMV antibody-rich material in the form of plasma or hyperimmune globulin as a form of passive immunisation to 11 patients with CMV infection after renal transplantation.

271

Patients and methods

High-titre anti-CMV plasma

Plasma from randomly selected blood donations was screened for CMV antibody by an indirect fluorescent antibody (FA) system described previously [5]. High titre anti-CMV plasma was collected from the 3.5 per cent of blood donors with CMV titres of 1:32 or greater.

Hyperimmune anti-CMV immunoglobulin

Antibody-rich plasma obtained as above was subjected to cold ethanol fractionation to produce a hyperimmune anti-CMV immunoglobulin preparation. More than 95 per cent of the total protein in this product is IgG. Its FA titre is 1:900 compared with 1:64−1:256 found in Normal Human Immunoglobulin manufactured by the Scottish National Blood Transfusion Service.

Patients and treatment schedule

Eleven patients (five male, six female, aged 16−51) were treated on the basis of a clinical diagnosis of severe CMV infection 31−128 days after renal transplantation. The diagnosis of CMV infection was confirmed by culture at the time of treatment in three patients, and by serology retrospectively in the remainder (see below). Several other patients, not reported here, received antibody therapy, but the clinical diagnosis of CMV was not confirmed. Ten patients were taking conventional immunosuppression with prednisolone and azathioprine, while one was on cyclosporin A alone. Four patients had had previous splenectomy. The first patient received 900ml of hyperimmune plasma with a mean FA titre of 1:48. The other 10 patients received 25ml of CMV immunoglobulin, 12.5ml being administered intraperitoneally and a further 12.5ml being administered by slow subcutaneous infusion.

Virology

For each patient, serological studies were undertaken in order to confirm the clinical diagnosis of a CMV infection. Serum samples taken at the onset of illness and at intervals thereafter were assayed for CMV antibody titres by the complement fixation (CF) test and by an indirect FA test for CMV-specific IgG and IgM antibodies (data to be published elsewhere). Confirmation of primary CMV infection was made on the basis of sero-conversion from a CMV titre of <1:16−1:64 or greater. Secondary infection (reactivation) was confirmed by at least a four-fold rise in titre from a pre-onset CMV antibody titre of >1:20. Attempts were made to culture CMV from the urine of nine patients, (cases 3−11).

Results

CMV was isolated from the urine of three patients (cases 8, 9 and 11), while the diagnosis of CMV was supported by serology alone in the other eight patients.

272

TABLE I. Clinical features of the illness and CMV serology

| Case number | Pyrexia (days) | Overall clinical severity | Clinical features | | | | Pre- and post-illness anti-CMV titres (reciprocal) | Probable CMV status |
			Hypoxaemia/ Lung infiltrates	Leucopenia 3.0 x 10⁹/L	Raised liver enzymes	Deteriorating renal function		
1	12	Life-threatening	+	+	+	-	<16;256	I°
2	19	Moderate	-	-	+	-	NA;320	?
3	11	Life-threatening	++	(lymphocytosis)	+	+	<16;128	I°
4	7	Mild	-	-	+	-	40;160	II°
5	10	Life-threatening	++	+	+	-	<10;160	I°
6	7	Severe	+	+	+	+	40;320	II°
7	13	Life-threatening	++	+	+	+	<10;160	I°
8	11	Life-threatening	+	-	+	+	< 8;256	I°
9	16	Life-threatening	++	+	+	-	32;256	II°
10	14	Severe	-	+	+	+	<16;256	I°
11	13	Moderate	-	+	+	-	NA (positive culture)	?

Hypoxaemia + indicates pO$_2$ <9.5 kPa on air;

++ indicates profound hypoxaemia requiring oxygen enrichment and/or ventilation;

NA indicates data not yet available

273

Of these 11 patients, full serological data was available for nine, being consistent with primary infection in six patients and secondary infection in the other three. Table I lists the clinical and serological details of these 11 patients and Table II summarises the response to antibody administration. Seven patients responded to therapy. A typical pattern of response to hyperimmune immunoglobulin is shown in Figure 1. A response did not depend upon the presence or absence of a spleen, nor whether the patient had primary or secondary infection (Tables I and II).

TABLE II. Response to antibody therapy

Case number	Response	
1	Cure:	Pyrexia abolished within 48 hours; slow rise in white cell count; normal liver enzymes; improved respiratory and clinical state within 24 hours.
2	Cure:	Pyrexia abolished within 24 hours; rapid and total clinical recovery.
3	Cure:	Pyrexia abolished within 24 hours; improved oxygenation; improved renal function; decreased lymphocytosis; rapid and total clinical recovery; liver enzymes unchanged (Figure 1).
4	No Effect:	Pyrexia persisted for 25 days in total, settling after vidarabine therapy.
5	No Effect:	Concomitant pseudomonas and fungal pneumonia; ventilated; eventual slow recovery after drainage of empyema.
6	Cure:	Pyrexia abolished within 24 hours; white cell count normalised; normal liver enzymes; normal blood gases; improved renal function; total rapid clinical recovery.
7	Cure:	Normal blood gases within 48 hours; CXR improved; rise in white cell count; improved renal function; fever settled 12 days later when concomitant cotrimoxazole therapy stopped.
8	Cure:	Pyrexia 37.5°C within 48 hours; improved respiratory function; improvement in renal function; slow rise in white cell count; normal liver enzymes.
9	No Effect:	Transient loss of pyrexia for 48 hours. Died 14 days later from pneumonia.
10	Cure:	Pyrexia abolished within 48 hours; rise in WBC; improved renal function and liver function. Recrudescence of illness six days later on re-introduction of azathioprine.
11	No Effect:	Slow spontaneous recovery in one to two weeks.

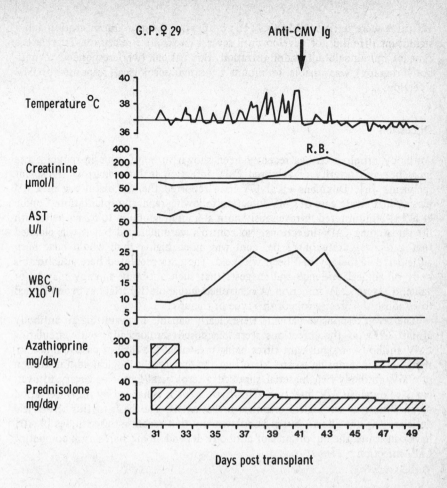

Figure 1. Case 3: Typical response to anti-CMV immunoglobulin in life-threatening primary CMV infection. Clinical picture included hectic fever, bilateral lung infiltrates, profound hypoxaemia, deteriorating renal function, raised aspartate aminotransferase (AST), and extreme lymphocytosis (total WBC 20–25 x 10^9/L, 80–90 per cent lymphocytes) despite stopping azathioprine. Renal biopsy (RB) on day 43 showed tubular vacuolation and giant cells, but no significant rejection

It is notable that one of the treatment failures (case 4) had only a relatively mild clinical illness, and was the least sick of the patients treated. A further unresponsive patient (case 5) had already developed a secondary Pseudomonas and Candida lung infection at the time of administration of hyperimmune immunoglobulin, but recovered after a long and stormy illness.

Of interest is that, at the time of immunoglobulin administration, patient 3 had significant antibody titres as assessed by the FA test, with an IgG titre of 1:32 and an IgM titre of 1:8. This contrasts with an anticipated IgG titre of 1:2 which would be induced by 25ml doses of CMV immunoglobulin. However,

275

CF titres were undetectable (<1:16) both pre- and post-administration and a significant titre did not develop until several weeks after remission. Thus, at the time of immunoglobulin administration, this patient (who responded to antibody therapy) was unable to mount a normal serological response to CMV infection.

Discussion

Antibody prophylaxis has recently been shown to be of value in reducing the incidence and severity of acquired CMV infection in bone marrow transplant recipients [6]. Dijkmans et al [7] have reported the successful use of CMV plasma in a single case of CMV infection following renal transplantation. Condie et al [8] administered intravenously normal immunoglobulin to 52 patients with life-threatening CMV infections. No controls were included but it was claimed that a recovery rate of 71 per cent was much higher than would have been anticipated if therapy had been withheld. The data presented here adds to this body of clinical evidence and suggests that such antibody therapy may be of value in severe CMV infection. A controlled, collaborative trial has been planned to establish the precise role of this type of therapy.

The seven responsive patients were clearly capable of mounting an antibody against CMV as the infections were diagnosed serologically, with circulating CMV antibody at significant titres being present at the time of passive immunotherapy. It is tempting to speculate that the apparently illogical administration of CMV antibody-rich material supplied a serological factor necessary to overcome fulminant CMV infection. This hypothesis is enhanced by the observation of an abnormal serological response in Patient 3. The basis of this serological deficiency is not known but it is noteworthy that recent mouse studies [9, 10] have confirmed the importance of antibody-dependent mechanisms in combating CMV infection.

Acknowledgments

We should like to thank Dr C C Smith, Infectious Diseases Unit, City Hospital, Aberdeen, for first suggesting that such treatment might be of value; many members of the West of Scotland BTS, the South-East Scotland BTS and the Protein Fractionation Centre for collaboration in the production of the CMV immunoglobulin; Mr J Watt, Director, Protein Fractionation Centre, SNBTS, for supplies of antibody-rich materials used; Dr J D Cash, Director, SNBTS, for advice and support; Mr M Fox, Consultant Transplant Surgeon, Royal Hallamshire Hospital, Sheffield, for allowing us to report cases 2–6; Miss C Evans and Mr R Sells, Royal Liverpool Hospital for data from case 7; Dr J Walls, Mr P Veitch and Dr A Flower, Leicester General Hospital for data from case 8; Dr A Davison, St James's University Hospital, Leeds, for data from case 9; Dr G Catto, Aberdeen Royal Infirmary, for data from case 10; and Dr J F Moorhead and Mr O Fernando, Royal Free Hospital, London, for data from case 11.

References

1   Peterson PK, Balfour HH, Marker SC et al. *Medicine 1980; 59:* 283
2   Rubin RH, Cosimi AB, Tolkoff-Rubin NE et al. *Transplantation 1977; 24:* 458
3   Simmons RL, Matas AJ, Rattazzi LC et al. *Surgery 1977; 82:* 537
4   Nicholls AJ, Brown CB, Edward N et al. *Lancet 1983; i:* 533
5   Cuthbertson B, Hart W, Sommerville RG. *Ann Clin Res 1980; 12:* 105
6   Winston DJ, Pollard RB, Ho WG et al. *Ann Intern Med 1982; 97:* 11
7   Dijkmans BAC, Versteeg J, Kauffman RH et al. *Lancet 1979; i:* 820
8   Condi RM, Hall BL, Howard RJ et al. *Transplant Proc 1979; 11:* 66
9   Shanley JD, Jordan MC, Stevens JG. *J Infect Dis 1981; 143:* 231
10 Manischewitz JE, Quinnan GV. *Infect Immun 1980; 29:* 1050

Open Discussion

OGG (Chairman)   Can I start off by asking you your indications for treating people? I imagine this serum is in very short supply, it's only available from one blood transfusion centre and they have to go through an elaborate process of selection of donors and purification of their serum, and I can't imagine that Edinburgh want us all on the 'phone every time we see a patient at six weeks with a temperature we can't explain. Which patients should be treated?

NICHOLLS   In particular we have been trying to select the patients who from the end of the bed appear to be very sick and toxic. These were all patients with prolonged fevers, and in particular we were worried about neutropenia, lung infiltrates and declining renal function. We have for the purposes of our proposed trial defined certain entry criteria. These comprise prolonged fever of at least five days with no response to any other therapy, together with either pneumonitis or declining renal function.

NEILD (London)   You seem to leave out the most interesting patients, that is to say the people with clinical CMV who presumably you treated as well but then subsequently you excluded because they presumably did not seroconvert. Can you expand on this group of patients?

NICHOLLS   Well they were a group of patients with, for example, fever, declining renal function or abnormalities in their white cell count who were shown subsequently to have a variety of other problems. One had infarcted her graft with no evidence of CMV infection. It is difficult if you just have a clinical suspicion of CMV infection and you cannot grow the virus and the patients don't seroconvert. One can't say what they are suffering from.

NEILD   How many responded to the therapy?

NICHOLLS   None.

NEILD   When you did your lung biopsy in your first anecdote did that show CMV?

NICHOLLS No, it didn't show the characteristic owl-eye lesions but it was a very small fragmentary transbronchial biopsy.

BRANDO (Milan) Since the natural occurring antibodies are ineffective in preventing relapses in CMV infection would you suggest that your kind of hyperimmune serum may be useful for reactivation and primary infection as well? In my opinion your immune serum is very interesting for pretransplant antibody positive patients.

NICHOLLS I think there are two fundamental problems here. The first one relates to the whole host of different classes and specificities of antibodies that the body raises to CMV. There are probably at least a dozen assay systems for CMV, for example by complement fixation, by fluorescent antibody testing or by neutralisation testing, and then there are too a variety of class-specific antibodies. Although many of these antibodies have diagnostic significance it is not clear what virological role they have in immunity. The second problem is that CMV has extreme heterogeneity as far as strain is concerned and one may have protection against certain strains but not against others. This is exemplified by the trial of Towne-125 CMV vaccine which was effective in preventing infection by that single strain but was ineffective in preventing infection against other strains. I think the virological problems are extremely complex.

PUGSLEY (Adelaide) Can you tell us why you arrived at that particular dose and that particular route of delivery?

NICHOLLS This happened after a telephone discussion! In the first case I presented we had success with 900ml of immune plasma and a similar volume of immune plasma was used by Dijkmans in 1979*. We chose a volume of hyperimmune immunoglobulin which would contain a similar amount of antibody to that found in approximately one litre of immune plasma. We also wanted to give it in the most readily assimilated form. Now normal human immunoglobulin preparations cannot be given intravenously and therefore we either had to give the dose intramuscularly, subcutaneously or intraperitoneally, and the kinetics of an intraperitoneal infection are most closely related to those of an intravenous injection. In some animal work showing the value of antibody therapy the intraperitoneal route has been used so we chose to give half the dose intraperitoneally and half subcutaneously thus we would achieve a high peak level and then a more sustained effect. So far as the proposed trial is concerned, there is now an intravenous preparation available both from the Scottish National Blood Transfusion and also from Elstree, we are not going to have this problem of route of administration.

BARNES (Chairman) In your failures was this related to whether they were reactivation or primary infections?

* Dijkmans BAC, Versteeg J, Kampfman RH et al. *Lancet 1979; i:* 820

NICHOLLS No, that's an important point. The various factors that might have been thought to play a role, such as whether it was primary or secondary infection or whether the patient had a splenectomy, did not appear to influence the response to therapy.

PROGNOSTIC FACTORS AT THE TIME OF RENAL RETRANSPLANTATION

B Frisk, L Smith, L Sandberg, H Brynger

Sahlgren's Hospital, Gothenburg, Sweden

Summary

One hundred and eighty-two patients with a second cadaver (CD) transplant performed during 1969–80 showed similar patient and graft survival to that of 535 recipients of first CD grafts. Loss of the first graft after 12 months resulted in a significantly higher second graft survival (GS II) than loss in early acute rejection within three months, 71 per cent vs 34 per cent at one year (p<0.01). A high frequency of presensitised patients was observed (53%) which negatively influenced the GS II, at one year 55 per cent vs 40 per cent for patients without and with antibodies (p<0.01). A good HLA-A, B match and absence of antibodies positively influenced GS II. Blood transfusions prior to the first transplantation did not influence survival of the second graft.

Introduction

Retransplantation after loss of a primary grafted kidney, has been a frequent procedure in our centre, providing the patient was willing and the medical condition was acceptable. We have previously shown that even repeated retransplantations in many cases were followed by a good long term function [1].

The aim of this retrospective investigation of a large single-centre experience was to study the outcome of secondary transplantation with cadaver donor kidneys (CD) in the following respects: patient survival (PS II) and graft survival (GS II) after secondary transplantation, influence of time of rejection of graft I, influence of HLA-A, B matching and presence of lymphocytotoxic antibodies.

Patients and methods

Between 1969 and 1980 1033 transplantations were performed in our institution, of which 29 per cent were retransplantations. Five hundred and thirty-five primary and 204 secondary transplantations were performed with CD kidneys.

One hundred and eighty-two of the latter were included in this study while 22 early cases were excluded due to incomplete data. The studied 182 retransplanted patients had a median age of 42 years at retransplantation. The cause of end-stage renal failure was chronic glomerulonephritis in 41 per cent, chronic pyelonephritis in 27 per cent, polycystic kidney disease in 13 per cent, diabetic glomerulosclerosis in five per cent and other diseases in 13 per cent.

In 26 patients (14%) the first graft originated from a living related donor and 156 (86%) from a cadaveric donor. Lymphocytotoxic antibodies were detected in 96 patients (53%) before the second transplantation. One hundred and eleven patients (61%) had received blood transfusions before the primary transplantation. At the second transplantation almost all patients had been transfused. The immunosuppressive regimen used during the period was based on azathioprine and prednisolone. Anti-rejection therapy, HLA-matching criteria and blood transfusion policy varied during the studied period.

In 1969–72 59 patients received a second renal graft. Small intravenous prednisolone doses (100mg/day, 1–3 days) plus Actinomycin C were used as anti-rejection therapy. Only one HLA-A, B mismatch was accepted except for a few cases. Most patients were transfused before the primary transplantation.

During 1973 to March 1977, 82 patients received a second graft. The anti-rejection therapy consisted of intravenous methylprednisolone in bolus doses (Ig, 0.5g, and 0.5g over three days). No attention was paid to HLA-matching. There was a very restrictive blood transfusion policy prior to the primary transplantation.

During April 1977 to December 1980 41 patients received their second CD grafts. For anti-rejection therapy intravenous methylprednisolone was still used but the doses reduced to half of those given during the preceding period. Two HLA-B mismatches were avoided but otherwise no attention was paid to HLA-A, B matching. A deliberate transfusion protocol was employed for non-transfused patients.

Mantel's test [2] was used for calculation significance of differences in survival. Only rejection was noted as graft loss in the calculations while other causes of graft loss were considered as 'lost to follow-up'.

Results

The actuarial PS II was 82 per cent and 65 per cent at one and three years, respectively. PS II was very close to PS after primary transplantation (PS I).

The one and three year GS II was 46 per cent and 33 per cent. These figures were not significantly different from the corresponding figures for GS I (52% and 37%, respectively). The GS II was calculated separately for 1969–72, 1973–77 and 1977–80, but no significant differences were found. The one and three year GS II for the three periods were 52 per cent and 38 per cent, 44 per cent and 28 per cent and 53 per cent and 41 per cent, respectively. These figures did not differ from GS I during the first two periods, but in the last period 1977–80 there was a higher GS I than GS II (65% vs 53% at one year). The patients were divided into three groups according to length of function of the first graft. Graft loss within three months was followed by

a GS II at one and three years of 34 per cent and 29 per cent. The GS II, following graft loss after three to 12 months and after 12 months were 49 per cent and
30 per cent and 71 per cent and 53 per cent, respectively (Figure 1). The difference was significant between the first and the last group (p<0.01). Twenty-three

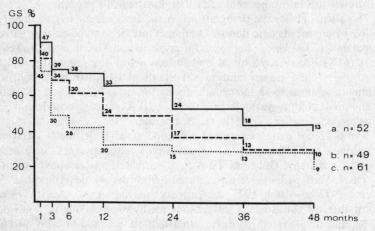

Figure 1. Graft survival of second grafts according to time of rejection of first graft. a: first
graft rejected after >12 months; b: first graft rejected after 3–12 months; c: first graft
rejected within three months. a vs b NS; a vs c p<0.01; b vs c NS

patients of the last group, who lost their first graft after more than three years
had a GS II of 83 per cent at one and three years. Twenty-one patients who lost
their primary grafts within three months for other reasons than rejection had a
better GS II than those who lost their grafts in rejection during the same period,
the one and three year GS II being 48 per cent and 42 per cent for this group
compared to 34 per cent and 29 per cent.

HLA-A-B matching influenced GS II. One hundred and three patients with
well-matched kidneys (0 or 1 incompatibility) had a superior GS II compared
with 79 patients with poor matches (two to four incompatibilities). The one and
three year GS II was 52 per cent and 37 per cent and 40 per cent and 27 per
cent, respectively. The difference did not quite reach statistical significance
(p=0.07).

Patients without lymphocytotoxic antibodies at secondary transplantation
had a significantly better GS II than patients with antibodies (p<0.01) (Figure 2).
The one and three year GS II was 55 per cent and 39 per cent compared to
40 per cent and 28 per cent for patients without and with antibodies, respectively.

The GS II in patients without antibodies and with a well-matched kidney
was 61 per cent and 43 per cent at one and three years, while patients with
antibodies and a poorly matched kidney did significantly worse, 36 per cent
and 23 per cent, p<0.05).

The GS II was studied in patients transfused and not transfused before
their first transplantation. No significant difference was found. However, in

282

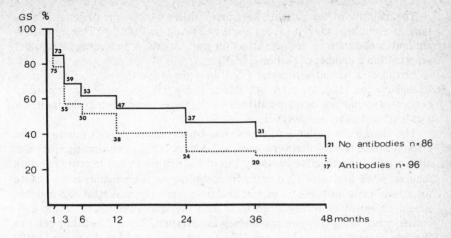

Figure 2. Graft survival of second graft according to existence of preformed lymphocyto-toxic antibodies (p<0.01)

48 transfused patients who did not develop lymphocytotoxic antibodies prior to the second transplantation, the GS II at one and three years was 66 per cent and 49 per cent compared with 42 per cent and 38 per cent in 33 non-transfused patients who developed antibodies prior to the second transplantation (NS).

Discussion

Patients who are offered a second transplantation consist of a selected group, having survived their first transplantation in the first place. And secondly, those in bad medical condition are not accepted for retransplantation. Against this background it might not be surprising that PS II was as high as PS I. Similar observations have been made both in a large multicentre and a single-centre study [3,4]. Data on second graft survival are conflicting, some authors reporting similar results for first and second grafts [3–5] while others find an inferior second graft survival [6]. In the present study, no differences were found during the two earlier periods, while in the last period there was a strong tendency for an inferior survival of second grafts, mainly due to an improved prognosis for first grafts attributed to an active transfusion policy.

The cause of loss of the primary renal grafts was of greatest importance for GS II. The primary grafts lost due to chronic rejection, after more than one year, or for other reasons than rejection, the prognosis for the second graft was better compared with that in patients losing primary graft function early due to acute rejection. This is in accordance with several other reports [4,7,8].

The effect of matching in retransplantation, is still a matter of dispute. However, in the present study, grafts with good HLA-A-B matches had a superior survival compared with poor matches which is in accordance with the findings of Fine et al [9] and Opelz and Terasaki [3].

283

The majority of the patients were presensitised at the time of retransplantation, as a result of previous failed grafts and blood transfusions. The presence of antibodies had a strong negative effect on graft survival, which confirms previous reports from a number of authors [3,5,9].

Persijn et al found a superior GS II in patients transfused prior to primary transplantation [10]. We were not able to verify this, but found that transfused patients who did not develop antibodies either after transfusion or failure of the first graft had a favourable GS II.

The chance for patients to survive and obtain adequate graft function after a second renal transplantation is good and does not differ significantly from that after primary transplantation. Early loss of the first transplant in acute rejection reduces, while loss after 12 months from chronic rejection augments the chance for a favourable outcome of second cadaveric graft. Optimal HLA-A-B matches should be aimed especially at patients with preformed lymphocytotoxic antibodies, when using conventional immunosuppression. Blood transfusion prior to the first transplantation does not influence the prognosis for the second graft.

References

1   Frisk B, Ahlmén J, Brynger H et al. *Proc EDTA 1980; 17:* 462
2   Mantel N. *J Am Statist Assoc 1963; 58:* 690
3   Opelz G, Terasaki PI. *Transplantation 1976; 21:* 483
4   Marni A, McMaster P, Evans DB, Calne RY. *Proc EDTA 1979; 16:* 352
5   Salvatierra O, Feduska NJ, Cochrum KC et al. *Ann Surg 1977; 186:* 424
6   Brynger H, Brunner FP, Chantler C et al. *Proc EDTA 1980; 17:* 45
7   Ascher NL, Ahrenholz DH, Simmons RL, Najarian JS. *Transplantation 1979; 27:* 30
8   Opelz G, Terasaki PI. *N Engl J Med 1978; 299:* 369
9   Fine RN, Malekzadeh MH, Pennisi AJ et al. *Pediatrics 1979; 95:* 244
10   Persijn GG, Lansbergen Q, D'Amaro J, van Rood JJ. *Transplantation 1981; 32:* 392

Open Discussion

BARNES (Chairman) Did you find any difference in the response to the second graft if the first graft had failed for technical reasons rather than immunological reasons?

FRISK The results shown were only results after the loss of the first graft from rejection.

BARNES They were not technical ones?

FRISK No, they were all lost in rejection. There were 21 patients who lost their kidney for reasons other than rejection, including technical failures, and they had a survival curve intermediate between the best and the worst survival curve.

OGG (Chairman) Did you find that there was any effect from the different periods patients spent on dialysis between the transplants? In other words, if they had their second transplant promptly after the failure of the first did they do worse or better than if there was a delay of a year or two between the two grafts?

FRISK There was actually a very short time between the first and second transplant in most cases. According to our policy, when patients lost their first grafts they were almost immediately, retransplanted. Therefore we can't analyse the effect of the time interval.

BARNES Did you remove the first graft in all cases or did you leave the first graft in, particularly in those who failed after a long time?

FRISK When patients lost their grafts in chronic rejection or after a long time most of them had their grafts left in situ, while most of the patients who lost their grafts in acute rejection had them removed.

BARNES Some people have claimed that you have to remove the graft to get a true indication of antibody status in patients.

FRISK Yes but we have not done that.

DIFFERENT PREDNISOLONE PHARMACOKINETICS IN CUSHINGOID AND NON-CUSHINGOID KIDNEY TRANSPLANT PATIENTS

H Bergrem, J Jervell, A Flatmark

Rikshospitalet University Hospital, Oslo, Norway

Summary

Prednisolone pharmacokinetics have been compared in 16 Cushingoid and 46 non-Cushingoid long term kidney transplant recipients. The Cushingoid patients had a significantly ($p<0.05$) higher peak concentration, a longer elimination half-time, a greater area under the time-concentration curve of total and free prednisolone, and a lower total body clearance of prednisolone. It is suggested that prednisolone pharmacodynamics may be influenced by pharmacokinetic differences, and that differences in renal function may be an important contributing factor.

Introduction

Prednisolone is used almost universally in kidney transplantation. Little is known about optimal dosages, and patients taking similar prednisolone doses may develop different degrees of side-effects. The purpose of the present study was to elucidate the possible connection between some Cushingoid side-effects and prednisolone pharmacokinetics.

Patients and methods

Sixty-two long-term (mean 62 months) kidney transplant recipients taking prednisolone 10mg/day gave their informed consent to participate in the study. Sixteen patients (mean age 56yr, 11 female) were classified as Cushingoid and 46 (mean age 44yr, 11 female) as non-Cushingoid by a combination of Cushingoid facial features and skin atrophy. There was no difference in liver function tests or serum protein concentration. Creatinine clearance was significantly ($p<0.02$) lower in the Cushingoid patients (90 ± 31 vs 67 ± 25ml/min).

After an overnight fast, each patient received two 5mg prednisolone tablets orally. Food was allowed after one and a half hours. Blood samples were drawn at appropriate intervals of 14 hours. Serum prednisolone concentrations were measured by radioimmunoassay [1]. The apparent in vivo concentrations of free pednisolone were calculated by non-linear regression analysis of the free prednisolone concentrations obtained by equilibrium dialysis [2]. Pharmacokinetic parameters were calculated by model independent methods [2]. Statistical analysis was by the Wilcoxon test.

Results

The Cushingoid patients had a nine per cent higher ($p<0.05$) peak prednisolone concentration (C_{max}), and 11 per cent longer ($p<0.05$) elimination half-time ($t_{1/2}$), a 20 per cent larger ($p<0.01$) area under the time-concentration curve (AUC) of total prednisolone (AUC_{tot}), a 15 per cent larger ($p<0.05$) AUC of unbound prednisolone (AUC_{free}), and a 17 per cent lower ($p<0.01$) total body clearance (Cl_t) of prednisolone than the non-Cushingoid patients. There was no statistically significant difference in time of peak concentration (T_{max}), volume of distribution (VD), or proportion of free prednisolone (P_{free}, $\frac{AUC_{free}}{AUC_{tot}} \times 100$) (Figure 1).

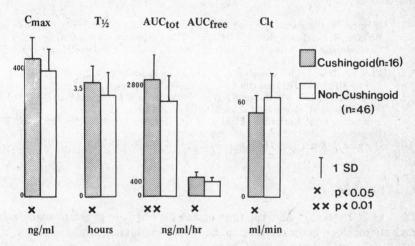

Figure 1. Prednisolone pharmacokinetics in transplant patients (prednisolone 10mg/orally). C_{max} = peak prednisolone concentration. $T_{1/2}$ = prednisolone elimination half-time. AUC_{tot} = area under the time-concentration curve of total (bound + free) prednisolone. AUC_{free} = AUC of free prednisolone. Cl_t = total body clearance of total prednisolone

Discussion

These results suggest that differences in prednisolone pharmacokinetics may influence prednisolone pharmacodynamics. Two previous studies have compared prednisolone pharmacokinetics in Cushingoid and non-Cushingoid kidney transplant patients [3,4]. Gamertoglio et al [3] found a prolonged elimination

287

half-time in Cushingoid patients, and a significantly lower Cl_t. Frey et al [4], however, were not able to demonstrate such differences. In both studies, results may have been influenced by administration of different steroid doses, as prednisolone pharmacokinetics are dose dependent [5,6]. The present Cushingoid group contained more females and had a higher mean age than the non-Cushingoid group, factors which may have influenced the degree of Cushingoid appearance. However, the pharmacokinetic differences are unlikely to be due to these factors, but more likely to differences in renal function, which may influence both renal [7] and total body prednisolone clearance [8,9,10].

The present results indicate that decreased prednisolone Cl_t may increase steroid side-effects, and suggest that the clinical use of prednisolone might be improved by monitoring serum concentrations, especially in patients with markedly reduced renal function.

Acknowledgment

This study was supported by grants from the Norwegian Council for Science and the Humanities and the Norwegian Medical Depot.

References

1   Bergrem H, Djøseland O, Jervell J et al. *Scand J Urol Nephrol 1981; Suppl 64:* 167
2   Bergrem H, Grøttum P, Rugstad HE. *Eur J Clin Pharmacol 1983; 24:* 415
3   Gambertoglio JG, Vincenti F, Feduska NJ et al. *Clin Endocrinol Metab 1980; 51:* 561
4   Frey FJ, Amend WJC, Lozada F et al. *Eur J Clin Pharmacol 1981; 21:* 235
5   Pickup ME, Lowe JR, Leatham PA et al. *Eur J Clin Pharmacol 1977; 12:* 213
6   Rose JQ, Yurchak AM, Jusko WJ et al. *J Pharmacokin Biopharmaceut 1981; 9:* 389
7   Woo J, Floyd M, Master G et al. *Ann J Clin Pathol 1980; 73:* 804
8   Gambertoglio J, Holford N, Lizak P et al. *Clin Pharmacol Therap 1983; 33:* 264
9   Bergrem H. *Acta Med Scand 1983:* in press
10   Bergrem H. *Kidney Int 1983:* in press

Open Discussion

DE VECCHI (Milan)   At what time of the day do your patients usually take their steroid dose, in the morning, in the afternoon, or randomly?

BERGREM   About 30 months after transplantation the patients take a single dose of 10mg prednisolone in the morning.

DE VECCHI   At what time did you perform your experiments?

BERGREM   Starting early in the morning at around 8.00 a.m.

HÄYRY (Helsinki)   I understand that your age and sex distribution was biased in these two groups. Have you run normal healthy controls with a corresponding age and sex distribution?

BERGREM No, the purpose of the study was to compare Cushingoid and non-Cushingoid patients and I agree that the two groups are different. We have done a lot of studies on prednisolone pharmacokinetics in normal controls and there is some variation in the pharmacokinetic parameters. We have also done studies in non-transplanted patients with impaired renal function and they have a prolonged elimination half-time and decreased clearance of prednisolone.

HÁYRY Do you really think that these extremely small differences would explain the very dramatic effects that you see in the patients?

BERGREM If you assume that the biological action is due to the free drug, and if you look at the amount of free prednisolone in a dosage interval there can be about a four-fold difference. Following a dose of 10mg one patient will have only one-fourth of the free drug compared to another patient and I think that, probably, this has an effect. I also think having a high concentration towards the end of the day when the body is geared to not having glucocorticoids probably increases this effect.

McGEOWN (Belfast) One of the difficulties about a study like this is the division of your patients into the Cushingoid and non-Cushingoid. I'd like more details as to how you decided who was Cushingoid and non-Cushingoid? For instance, obese patients may sometimes look fairly similar to Cushingoid patients if you don't take other factors into account. The reduced clearance in the patients with Cushingoid changes, who had impaired renal function, may be due to oedema as waterlogging can affect the clearance of prednisolone.

BERGREM Regarding the selection of the patients, this was done by two relatively experienced nephrologists who selected these patients on a subjective basis. We did not look at body weights, we decided to make it practicable and therefore we decided to get an impression of the degree of Cushingoid appearance and to look at the extremes of this population. We know that it is very difficult to make a fair selection but we did it that way and looked at the extremes.
  For your second question, one of these patients was oedematous.

KOPP (Munich) Have you any idea about salt balance or hypertension with relation to Cushingoid appearances in your patients?

BERGREM We have the data but we haven't looked at them.

BARNES (Chairman) One of the notable things about transplant patients is that they take an awful lot of tablets. Did you control the other tablets that these patients were taking or were they only taking prednisone and azathioprine?

BERGREM No, a lot of them used frusemide and hypotensive drugs, but I can say that there was no difference in blood pressure and certainly there was no difference in the distribution of these drugs between the two groups.

289

GABRIEL (London) Your paper is stimulating and provocative but don't you feel you should have done this study on these patients before they were transplanted to look at the kinetics before they were fouled up by varying doses of prednisolone and all the awful things that happen to transplant patients?

BERGREM I think that would be very difficult because at that time they would be practically anephric and they would have a very very long elimination half-time which would not relate to the time after a successful transplant.

GABRIEL It is still perfectly possible to produce AUCs and other pharmaco-kinetic data on single dose basis with or without renal function.

BERGREM Well, we didn't do that.

BAHIER (Chicago) In the US most people use prednisone which requires particular metabolism to become prednisolone. Do you think this could be a factor in determining whether certain patients become Cushingoid?

BERGREM Prednisone is a biologically inactive pro-drug of prednisolone and there have been some papers in the past in patients with markedly impaired hepatic function indicating that they have incomplete conversion to prednisolone. There is one study in kidney transplant patients from Gambertoglio* in San Francisco who finds no difference in prednisolone bioavailability from prednisone or prednisolone. I think practically speaking there is not much difference but certainly when you give prednisolone you know what you are giving and you don't have to worry about the hepatic conversion.

---

* Gambertoglio JG, Frey FJ, Nicholas HG et al. *Kidney Int 1982; 21:* 621

Proc EDTA (1983) Vol 20

RENAL ALLOGRAFT SURVIVAL IN PATIENTS TRANSFUSED PERIOPERATIVELY ONLY

W Fassbinder, U Frei, E H Scheuermann, P-B Bechstein, R Raab,
G Dathe, D Jonas, M Knöner, P Hanke, W Schoeppe

University Hospital, Frankfurt/Main, FRG

Summary

We investigated in a prospective study the effects of perioperative blood transfusions on the outcome of renal transplantation. All patients (n = 105)
receiving their first cadaveric renal allograft were transfused perioperatively
(i.e. 0–6 hours before transplantation) with two units of non-washed, unfiltered
packed red cells. Forty-eight were transfused perioperatively only; 57 patients
had received blood earlier and thus were transfused pre- and perioperatively.
Graft survival one and two years post-transplant was 79 per cent at both time
intervals in the group transfused perioperatively only, and 85 per cent and 74
per cent in the pre- and perioperatively transfused group. No adverse effects
were observed concerning perioperative transfusions. In patients transfused
perioperatively only, acceptable graft survival rates are obtainable. In these
patients the risk or presensitisation is avoided, and thus their chance of successful
transplantation increased.

Introduction

The positive effect of blood transfusions on kidney graft survival, originally
reported by Opelz et al [1], is now generally accepted. However, the optimal
timing of transfusions is still controversial [2]. Four groups, specifically
investigating this subject, found a beneficial effect of transfusions given shortly
before or during transplantation [3–6], while others could not confirm this
[7–9].

Van Es et al [10] demonstrated in Rhesus monkeys, that a single blood
transfusion, given 0–12 hours before transplantation, resulted in prolonged
graft survival. This observation prompted us to investigate prospectively
the effects of perioperative blood transfusion in human recipients of renal
allografts.

291

Patients and methods

Patients

All patients receiving their first cadaveric renal transplant between 1979 and 1982 (n = 105) were included in this prospective study; no exclusions were made for any reasons. No patient was lost from observation.

Transfusion history

Forty-eight patients had never been transfused previously; 57 patients had received at least one unit of blood (for reasons unrelated to the planned transplantation) earlier.

Organs

All kidneys were obtained under the auspices of Eurotransplant. Following the selection criteria of this organ exchange organisation, recipients were given ABO-compatible grafts optimally matched for the HLA-A, -B and -DR antigens. A negative crossmatch (standard microlymphocytotoxicity test) with donor lymphocytes and the recipient's most recent serum sample was mandatory.

The transfusion protocol

When suitable donor organs became available, all patients (both groups) were transfused with two units of packed red cells 0—6 hours before transplantation, i.e. perioperatively. These units were not washed and unfiltered. Blood donors were not selected on the basis of HLA-typing.

Immunosuppression

Prophylactic antirejection regimen consisted of azathioprine (2—4mg/kg body weight/day) and prednisone only. The prednisone therapy started at 100mg/day (irrespective of body weight), tapering down to 25mg/day after six months and 25mg every second day after 12 months. Immunosuppressive therapy was started after the administration of the perioperative blood transfusion.

Rejection crises

Rejection crises were initially treated with 6-methylprednisolone pulse therapy 1g i.v. repeated two to five times per rejection, and never exceeding a total dose of 15g per patient. If rejection was not reversed by methylprednisolone, graft biopsy was performed. Plasma exchange therapy was instituted, when vascular rejection was found histologically, whereas ALG (10 x 30mg/kg body weight/day) or ATG (10 x 3mg/kg/day) was administered, when interstitial rejection was diagnosed.

Patient and graft survival

Patient and graft survival were calculated using the life table method. Graft failure was defined as patient's death or return to dialysis irrespective of cause. This report deals with our experience up to May 1983.

Results

Table I shows a comparison of the two groups. By Student t-test there were no significant differences concerning mean age, duration of dialysis and HLA-matching. Eight patients in the group with pre- and perioperative transfusions had been immunised by their pre-operative transfusions and developed cytotoxic antibodies, which contributed to the 12.8 months longer waiting period on dialysis in this group. No patient developed new cytotoxic antibodies due to perioperative transfusions.

TABLE I. Comparison of the two groups concerning various parameters at the time of transplantation

| | Transfusions | | |
	Pre- and perioperative		Perioperative only
Number of patients	57		48
Diabetes mellitus	2		2
> 50 years old	3		8
Cytotoxic antibodies	8		0
Age (years)			
Mean ± SD	35.7 ± 10.8	NS	39.3 ± 9.2
Range	11 – 59		16 – 61
Time on dialysis (months)			
$\bar{X}$ ± SD	57.0 ± 42.1	NS	44.2 ± 32.4
Range	5 – 185		8 – 129
Number of HLA-compatibilities			
HLA-A	1.22 ± 0.54	NS	1.25 ± 0.53
HLA-B	1.05 ± 0.39	NS	1.04 ± 0.62
HLA-DR	1.17 ± 0.66	NS	0.98 ± 0.69

No patient died in the group transfused perioperatively only, resulting in a 100 per cent patient survival at all time intervals in this group. Five patients died in the group transfused pre- and perioperatively. Causes of death were:

myocardial infarction (2), liver failure (2) and cytomegalovirus-infection (1). In the two patients dying from liver failure, preoperative blood transfusions might well have contributed to the fatal outcome by inducing chronic liver disease. Cumulative patient survival in the group transfused pre- and perioperatively was 93 per cent one year and 89 per cent two and three years post-transplant.

In the group transfused perioperatively only, there appeared to be a slightly higher incidence of irreversible graft rejection in the early postoperative period, whereas in the other group graft losses seemed to occur more frequently during later periods. However, when analysed statistically, there were no significant differences at any time interval. Additional analysis by cumulative log rank test also failed to show a significant difference between the groups. Actuarial graft survival of both groups is shown in Figure 1.

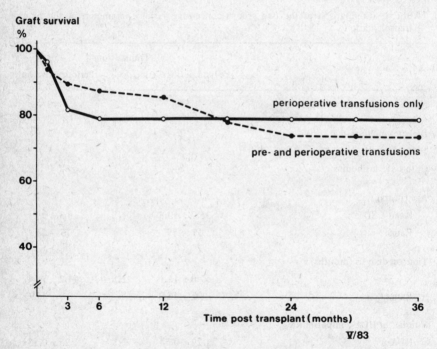

Figure 1. Actuarial kidney graft survival in 57 patients with pre- and perioperative transfusions, and in 48 patients with only perioperative transfusions (2 x 250ml not washed, unfiltered packed red cells)

To evaluate possible differences in immunosuppressive therapy, and in frequency or severity of rejection episodes, we compared steroid dosages, incidence of ALG-, ATG- or plasma-exchange therapy and serum creatinine concentrations in those 65 patients, who retained their grafts for more than

294

TABLE II. Comparison of the two groups concerning immunosuppressive therapy and graft function. Means ± SD are shown

| | Transfusions | |
	Pre- and perioperative	Perioperative only
Number of patients observed with functioning graft > 12 months	37	28
Oral prednisone dosage (mg/day)		
3 months	29.3 ± 7.3	32.2 ± 6.6
6 months post-transplant	22.0 ± 5.9	22.3 ± 3.0
12 months	15.4 ± 4.2	15.5 ± 5.0
Total methylprednisolone dosage (g)	4.6 ± 3.7	5.5 ± 3.2
Number of patients with:		
ATG/ALG	6	6
Plasma-exchange	4	5
Serum creatinine concentration (mg/100ml)		
3 months	1.38 ± 0.43	1.57 ± 0.77
6 months post-transplant	1.42 ± 0.54	1.41 ± 0.43
12 months	1.37 ± 0.49	1.44 ± 0.57

No significant difference was found in any parameter investigated

12 months. As shown in Table II, immunosuppression was similar in both groups, and graft function did not differ significantly.

Discussion

Our data show, in a prospective study, that patients transfused perioperatively only do no worse than those with previous blood transfusion. Our results confirm the findings of Williams et al [4], the only other authors who also studied prospectively the effects of perioperative blood transfusions on graft survival in previously non-transfused renal allograft recipients. They found in their smaller series with 13 patients a one year graft survival of 85 per cent.

It has been well established, that one year graft survival in non-transfused recipients of cadaveric renal transplants is consistently less than 50 per cent and often less than 40 per cent [1—5, 7—9]. We therefore did not study a non-transfused control group for ethical reasons.

The mechanisms whereby blood transfusions improve graft survival are still unknown. Opelz et al [7] discuss two possibilities. One is the induction of a state of immune unresponsiveness, the other is the elimination of highly immune responsive patients, who are identified by their production of cytotoxic antibodies. Our data are in favour of the first hypothesis, and make the second one unlikely, as the responder status of the patient remains unknown, when the interval between transfusion and transplantation is only six hours or less.

In vitro experiments also support the hypothesis that blood transfusions improve kidney graft survival by inducing a state of immune unresponsiveness rather than by selecting out highly responsive patients. There is reduced reactivity of lymphocytes against mitogenic stimulation following blood transfusions and we have demonstrated, using the MLC-technique, an immediate decrease of lymphocyte-reactivity against third-party donor cells following perioperative blood transfusions [6]. From these studies [6], it seems reasonable to assume that blood transfusions produce an immediate non HLA-specific immunosuppressive effect in man. Since the duration of this immunosuppressive effect is unknown, it may be advantageous to administer blood transfusions shortly before transplant surgery.

Multiple blood transfusions given deliberately prior to kidney transplantation do have an inherent number of risks for the patient, mainly transmission of hepatitis, iron overload and the possibility of sensitisation. About 30 per cent of patients produce cytotoxic antibodies after blood transfusions [7], and at least those patients with antibodies reacting with more than 50 per cent of a random donor cell panel become difficult candidates for transplantation. Their chance of being grafted is significantly decreased.

The policy not to transfuse patients during the waiting period unless there are strict medical indications and to prepare them for a cadaveric graft only perioperatively with two units of packed red cells given shortly, i.e. 0–6 hours before transplantation has thus major advantages: it minimises the patient's risk concerning post-transfusion hepatitis and increases his chance of receiving a suitable kidney transplant early by avoiding the possibility of presensitisation. According to our data perioperative blood transfusions are not associated with any harmful effects or with reduced graft survival. We therefore intend to continue our minimum transfusion policy.

References

1   Opelz G, Sengar DPS, Mickey MR, Terasaki PI. *Transplant Proc 1973; 5:* 253
2   Opelz G, Mickey MR, Terasaki PI. *Transplant Proc 1981; 13:* 136
3   Stiller CR, Lockwood BL, Sinclair NR et al. *Lancet 1978; i:* 169
4   Williams KA, Ting A, French ME et al. *Lancet 1980; i:* 1104
5   Hunsicker LG, Oei LS, Freeman RM et al. *Arch Surg 1980; 115:* 737
6   Fassbinder W, Frei U, Persijn GG et al. *Transplant Proc 1982; 14:* 164
7   Opelz G, Graver B, Terasaki PI. *Lancet 1981; i:* 1223
8   Opelz G, Terasaki PI. *Transplantation 1981; 31:* 106
9   Glass NR, Felsheim G, Miller DT et al. *Transplantation 1982; 33:* 430
10   Van Es AA, Marquet RL, van Rood JJ, Balner H. *Transplantation 1978; 26:* 325

Proc EDTA (1983) Vol 20

A NEW MECHANISM OF HUMORAL IMMUNODEPRESSION IN CHRONIC RENAL FAILURE AND ITS IMPORTANCE TO DIALYSIS AND TRANSPLANTATION

P K Donnelly, B K Shenton, A M Alomran, D M A Francis, G Proud, R M R Taylor

Royal Victoria Infirmary, Newcastle-upon-Tyne, United Kingdom

Summary

Whilst chronic renal failure (CRF) patients are known to have an impaired immune response the explanation is unclear. We investigated the immuno-suppressive effect of plasma from CRF patients on an in vitro assay of normal lymphocyte function.

One hundred and sixty regular dialysis patients had significantly greater plasma suppressive activity (PSA) than that of normal healthy subjects. PSA decreased after haemodialysis but increased after blood transfusion. Renal allograft recipients with low PSA were more likely to have accelerated rejection.

Assay of the functional capacity of plasma for inhibiting protease (e.g. plasmin, thrombin, trypsin) suggest that high PSA is associated with the excess formation of protease-inhibitor complexes and liberation of immunoregulatory peptide (<10,000 daltons).

Introduction

Although it has long been recognised that plasma from chronic renal failure (CRF) patients contains non-cytotoxic leucocyte blocking factors which are increased after blood transfusion and which relate to graft survival [1], the mechanism of this effect remains unclear. Whilst specific immunoglobulin related blocking factors [2] are undoubtedly involved there is abundant evidence that other naturally occurring non-specific humoral immunosuppressive substances, particularly α-globulin and glycopeptide, are related to a degree of anergy associated with CRF [3] and other acute and chronic conditions [4, 5, 6].

Our aim was (i) to investigate the clinical significance of this patient plasma suppressive activity (PSA) [5]; and (ii) to propose and test a possible mechanism of its effect.

297

Materials and methods

Patients studied

One hundred and sixty patients with CRF, all of whom had been previously transfused and required regular dialysis (aged 7–62, median 38 years, M:F 1.9:1), and 30 normal healthy subjects (aged 19–69, median 35 years, M:F 1.7:1) were studied. In addition 10 CRF and previously non-transfused patients were studied prior to and at monthly intervals after elective blood transfusion, consisting of four units of packed cells given over a four-week period.

Tests employed

PSA was determined as the titration volume (μl) of heparinised plasma required to produce 50 per cent suppression of response to recall antigen (PPD, Tuberculin) of lymphocytes from a panel of normal healthy subjects. Lymphocyte response was assayed in a rapid cytopherometric test [3]. This method of determining PSA was such that a *small* plasma volume (5μl) corresponded to a high degree of suppressive activity [5]. Lymphocytotoxicity was identified as described previously [5]. Plasma was fractionated on Sepharose S300 and each protein fraction tested for its percentage suppression (inhibition) of control lymphocyte-PPD response. Specific protein depletion was achieved by affinity chromatography [3].

α_2-Macroglobulin ($\alpha_2 M$) was quantified nephelometrically in plasma and in protein fractions by immunoelectrophoresis using rabbit antihuman antisera (Dako) [6]. The functional capacity of $\alpha_2 M$ for binding protease ($\alpha_2 MBC$) (trypsin) was estimated using esterolytic substrate (BAPNA) (Sigma) as previously [6], and expressed as mg of trypsin bound per unit weight (100mg) of $\alpha_2 M$.

Results

The plasma of 160 CRF patients was significantly ($p < 0.01$) more suppressive (PSA median 4.6μl, range 1.0–34.5) than that of 30 normal subjects (PSA median 37.0μl, range 22–41.4). The suppressive activity of 10 CRF patients prior to four hours haemodialysis (PSA median 9.1μl, range 2.4–12.8) was significantly greater ($p < 0.05$) than that taken postdialysis (PSA 9.8μl, range 2.4– 17.2).

Elective blood transfusion of 10 previously non-transfused CRF patients caused a rapid increase in PSA which was maximal within two months of transfusion (Figure 1). Patients were defined as having low PSA if the volume of their plasma required for 50 per cent lymphocyte suppression exceeded 5μl.

Of 146 consecutive transfused renal transplant recipients 138 had PSA estimated immediately prior to transplantation and before immunosuppressive therapy. During follow-up 17 grafts failed for non-immunological reasons [5] and of the remaining patients those with low PSA were at greater risk of accelerated rejection (Figure 2). Less than 10 per cent of the plasma tested were lymphocytotoxic to one or other of the normal lymphocyte donors but the concentration for cytotoxicity was considerably greater than that for PSA.

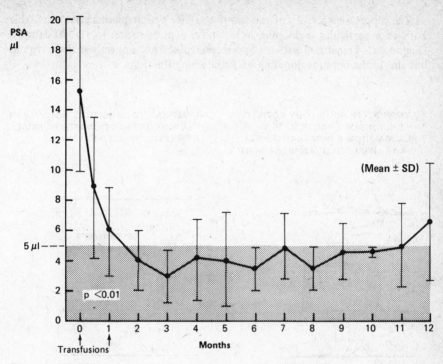

Figure 1. The effect of packed cell transfusion on the PSA of renal failure patients (n = 10)

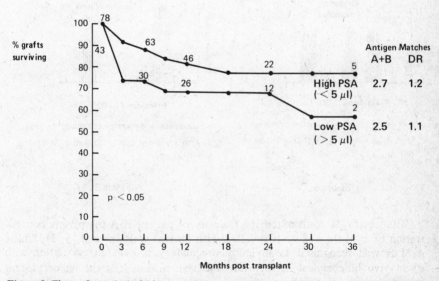

Figure 2. The graft survival of 121 consecutive renal transplants (non-immunological failures excluded) with high and low PSA

The suppressive activity of non-transfused CRF patient plasma was attributable both to a particular α-globulin, α_2M, and a peptide region (<10,000 daltons) (Figure 3a). Transfused patients had increased activity not only in these regions but also in the immunoglobulin (IgG) containing fractions.

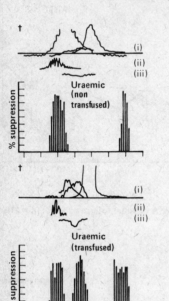

LYMPHOCYTE INHIBITORY ACTIVITY IN REGIONS OF FRACTIONATED PLASMA FROM A NON TRANSFUSED & A TRANSFUSED URAEMIC PATIENT

Fractions 21—90

† Fused rocket immunoelectrophoresis
(i) Anti-all human sera (ii) Anti α_2M
(iii) Anti IgG

Figure 3a

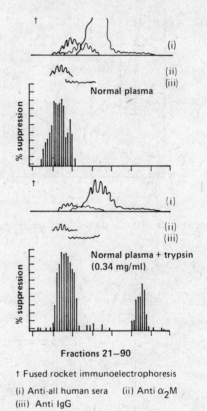

LYMPHOCYTE INHIBITORY ACTIVITY IN REGIONS OF FRACTIONATED NORMAL & TRYPSIN TREATED PLASMA

Fractions 21—90

† Fused rocket immunoelectrophoresis
(i) Anti-all human sera (ii) Anti α_2M
(iii) Anti IgG

Figure 3b

Although α_2M contributed the majority of patient PSA the plasma concentration of α_2M showed no correlation with PSA or graft survival [3, 5]. Whilst α_2M is well recognised as an immunoregulatory protein an association with its in vivo biochemical activity has not been shown. It is the major protein responsible for inactivating excessive amounts of protease (proteolytic enzyme) released by homeostatic and disease processes [6].

300

We compared the PSA, the quantity and the functional activity of $\alpha_2 M$ between CRF patients and normal subjects (Figure 4). Although PSA was greater in the renal patients there was no difference in $\alpha_2 M$ concentration. However, CRF patient plasma had significantly less $\alpha_2 MBC$ than that of normal subjects (Figure 4), and the difference was greatest ($p < 0.05$) for those patients with high PSA.

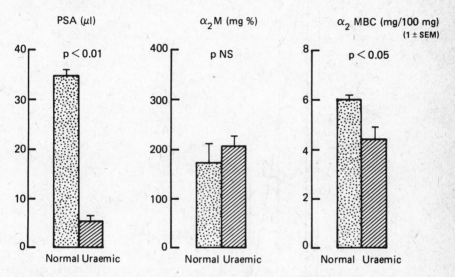

Figure 4. PSA, $\alpha_2 M$ concentration and $\alpha_2 M$ protease binding capacity ($\alpha_2 MBC$) in normal subjects (n = 16) and renal failure patients (n = 14)

In studying the effect of adding a protease (trypsin) on the suppressive activity of normal plasma (Figure 5) relatively small amounts of protease caused a marked increase in PSA. Changes in $\alpha_2 M$ functional activity ($\alpha_2 MBC$) corresponded closely with changes in PSA (Figure 5).

Gel fractionation of normal and trypsin-treated plasma (Figure 3b) showed that increased suppression was due both to an increase in the $\alpha_2 M$ region and also to the abnormal appearance of a peptide region of molecular weight <10,000 daltons similar to that of the peptide previously described in uraemic patients.

In vitro studies of purified $\alpha_2 M$ have shown that protease binding to $\alpha_2 M$ causes increased immunosuppressive activity due both to the complex itself and to the release of a peptide [7] of molecular weight <3,000 daltons.

Discussion

These results confirm earlier reports [1–3, 5] that CRF plasma has lymphocyte suppressive activity which is increased after blood transfusion and is of prognostic significance for graft survival. The timing of this beneficial effect suggests that blood transfusion may exert an effect by reducing accelerated rejections

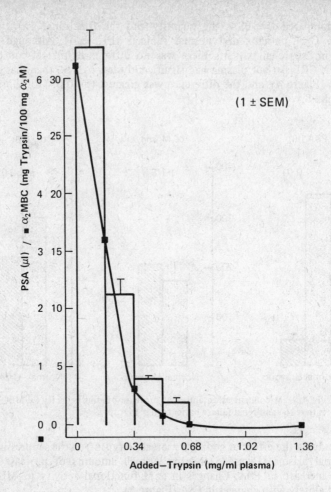

Figure 5. Effect of increasing protease (trypsin) complex formation with α_2M in a normal plasma and PSA on lymphocytes from normal subjects (n = 5)

[8]. Whilst this study confirms that the IgG region [2] contributes to the lymphocyte blocking effect of plasma from transfused subjects a major part of the suppressive activity was attributable to the α_2M and peptide fractions. Although high PSA was not quantitatively related to α_2M, patients with high PSA had qualitative differences from normal associated with reduced α_2MBC.

In vitro studies indicated that the suppressive activity of normal plasma could be made to closely resemble that of CRF plasma by the addition of subsaturation amounts of protease. We, therefore, suggest a hypothesis to explain impaired immunity exhibited by CRF patients (Figure 6). During the activation of humoral and cellular defence mechanisms due to the disease process, excessive amounts of protease are released which produce α_2M-complexes

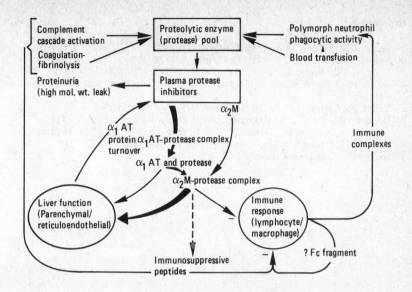

Figure 6. A mechanism of non-specific humoral immunoregulation in chronic renal failure

and liberate immunoregulatory peptide. Normally α_2M-complex is cleared by receptor-mediated uptake by the reticuloendothelial system (RES). Blood transfusion to diseased subjects may contribute to this endogenous plasma suppressive activity by providing foreign cells (both red and white) which compete for clearance by the RES [9] and directly contribute by their sub-cellular elements [6] to the body's protease pool (Figure 6). Since α_2M is the 'final common pathway' for protease clearance it accepts protease non-specifically and irreversibly from the other major inhibitor α_1-antitrypsin (α_1AT). Alteration in α_1AT turnover or loss as proteinuria may influence α_2M-complex metabolism. Although an immunosuppressive peptide has been derived from purified α_2M, it is probable that in plasma immunoregulatory peptides are derived from a number of protease cleaved substrates (Figure 6).

Our study raises the possibility of there being sensitive biochemical markers of immune response in the plasma of renal patients and a possible therapeutic application to transplantation of naturally occurring immunoregulatory peptide generated from plasma protease inhibitors.

Acknowledgments

The authors would like to give special thanks to the clinical staff of the Renal Unit, Royal Victoria Infirmary; to Mr P Trotter, Mr M White and Mrs P Chambers for technical assistance; and to Mrs E Shenton for secretarial help. This work was supported by a grant from the Northern Regional Health Authority and the Nothern Counties Kidney Research Fund.

303

References

1   Sengar DPS, Pelz G, Terasaki PI. *Transplant Proc 1973; V(1):* 641
2   Fagnilli L, Singal DP. *Transplant Proc 1982; XIV(2):* 319
3   Shenton BK, Proud G, Smith BM, Taylor RMR. *Transplant Proc 1979; XI(1):* 171
4   Cooperband SR, Nimberg R, Schmid K, Mannick JA. *Transplant Proc 1976; VIII(2):* 225
5   Veitch PS, Shenton BK, Proud G, Taylor RMR. *Br J Surg 1980; 67:* 703
6   Donnelly PK, Shenton BK, Alomran A et al. *Proc NY Acad Sci 1983:* In press
7   Alomran A, Shenton BK, Donnelly PK et al. *Proc NY Acad Sci 1983:* In press
8   Terasaki PI, Perdue S, Ayoud G et al. *Transplant Proc 1982; XIV(2):* 251
9   Keown PA, Descamps B. *Lancet 1979; i:* 20

Proc EDTA (1983) Vol 20

PRETRANSPLANT ANTIBODIES AND RENAL ALLOGRAFT SURVIVAL

A M MacLeod, R J Mason, D A Power, N Edward, K N Stewart, G Shewan, G R D Catto

University of Aberdeen and Blood Transfusion Service, Aberdeen Royal Infirmary, Aberdeen, United Kingdom

Summary

Fc receptor blocking antibodies directed against autologous lymphocytes were present in pretransplant sera from only one of a group of 24 cadaver donor renal transplant recipients. Such antibodies were present in recipient sera against B lymphocytes from the donor in 11/24, against normal B lymphocytes in 12/24 and against leukaemic B lymphocytes in 15/24 cases. There was a significant correlation between EA inhibiting antibodies directed against donor ($p<0.01$), normal ($p<0.05$) and leukaemic B lymphocytes ($p<0.001$) and improved one year allograft survival. No autolymphocytotoxic antibodies were detected. Fc receptor blocking antibodies detected by the Erythrocyte Antibody Inhibition assay may thus have a beneficial effect on graft outcome but do not appear to be autoantibodies.

Introduction

The presence of antibodies in recipient sera is generally thought to have a deleterious effect on transplant survival. In the standard crossmatch test, for example, the presence of recipient anti-donor lymphocytotoxic antibodies correlates with almost inevitable graft rejection. In the mid 1970s, however, sera from certain recipients were shown to contain cytotoxins directed against their own, as well as donor lymphocytes [1,2], and in these cases transplantation was successfully carried out. Subsequent larger studies confirmed the harmless nature of these autoreactive antibodies [3,4] and further work [5] showed that allograft survival was slightly, although not significantly, better in those with a positive B lymphocyte crossmatch due to autoantibodies than in those with a negative crossmatch. These antibodies were shown to react with normal panel lymphocytes but not with leukaemic (CLL) lymphocytes [5] and to be most active at $5°C$ [6].

In a previous study we showed that the presence of Fc receptor blocking

305

antibodies to B lymphocytes in pretransplant serum (detected by the erythrocyte antibody inhibition assay) correlated with improved allograft survival [7]. In this study, therefore, we aimed to determine whether such antibodies were autoantibodies.

Materials and methods

Sera were obtained from 24 recipients of cadaver donor renal transplants within the 12 hours prior to transplantation. All patients had been transfused with at least four units of blood prior to transplantation. An aliquot of each serum was heat inactivated at 56°C for 45 minutes and a further aliquot was absorbed with pooled human platelets. The sera were ultracentrifuged at 100,000g for one hour prior to use.

The target cells used were B lymphocytes from a) the transplant recipient, b) the transplant donor, c) 12 normal panel members and d) 12 patients with chronic lymphatic leukaemia (CLL).

Lymphocytotoxic antibodies were detected by the standard long NIH lymphocytotoxicity assay at 5°C, 23°C and 37°C [8]. EA inhibition was performed by a modification of the rosette technique [7].

Statistical analysis was performed using Fisher's exact test for four-fold tables.

Results

No lymphocytotoxic antibodies were detected in any of the 24 untreated or treated sera when the recipient's own B lymphocytes were used as targets and the assays were carried out at 5°C, 23°C and 37°C. B lymphocytotoxic antibodies were however present in two cases against donor B lymphocytes, in

TABLE I. Outcome at one year of transplants performed
with and without pretransplant EAI

Target cell		Success	Failure	Total	
Recipient B lymphocytes	EAI positive	0	1	1	
	EAI negative	14	9	23	
Donor B lymphocytes	EAI positive	10	1	11	p<0.01
	EAI negative	4	9	13	
Normal Panel B lymphocytes	EAI positive	10	2	12	p<0.05
	EAI negative	4	8	12	
CLL Panel B lymphocytes	EAI positive	13	2	15	p<0.001
	EAI negative	1	8	9	

nine cases against normal panel B lymphocytes and in 14 cases against CLL panel B lymphocytes. There was no statistically significant correlation between the presence of such lymphocytotoxic antibodies in pretransplant sera against any of the types of target cells used and allograft survival (Table I).

EA inhibiting antibodies directed against the recipient's own lymphocytes were detectable prior to transplantation in sera from only one recipient; they were not removed by platelet absorption and the graft failed within three months of transplantation. EA inhibition was not present against donor lymphocytes in this case. In the group of 24 patients as a whole, however, EA inhibiting antibodies were detected in 11 cases against donor, in 12 cases against normal panel and in 15 cases against CLL B lymphocytes. The presence of EA inhibition against donor normal and leukaemic B lymphocytes correlated significantly with improved allograft survival ($p < 0.01$, $p < 0.05$, and $p < 0.001$ respectively).

Discussion

This study shows that Fc receptor blocking antibodies in pretransplant recipient sera (detected by the EA inhibition assay) were found in only one case when autologous lymphocytes were used as target cells, and in that case the graft failed. The sera, however, did contain such antibodies directed against the donor in around 50 per cent of cases and against panel lymphocytes even more frequently, and the correlation with improved allograft survival previously shown [7] was maintained.

Anti-donor cytotoxic antibodies, as occur in a positive crossmatch test, are harmful to allograft survival whereas similar antibodies which are also cytotoxic to autologous lymphocytes, particularly B lymphocytes, appear harmless [3,5]. They occur in the IgM fraction of serum [5] and since they react with normal panel B lymphocytes but not with leukaemic B lymphocytes (both of which possess HLA-A, -B, -C, and DR antigens) they are thought not to be directed to the products of the MHC. The Fc receptor blocking antibodies, however, which we have demonstrated occur in the IgG fraction of serum as shown by DEAE column chromatography and can react both with normal panel and leukaemic lymphocytes. We have shown that, as well as being indicative of favourable graft outcome, they are generated by blood transfusions [9] and therefore may represent a possible mechanism for the blood transfusion effect in renal transplantation. Antibodies detected by EA rosette inhibition has also been demonstrated in the sera of primigravid women but not in the sera of women undergoing spontaneous abortion [10]. Family studies using sera from primigravidae suggested that these antibodies were directed against HLA-linked antigens. They therefore have very different properties from previously determined autoantibodies.

Fc receptor blocking antibodies detected by the EA inhibition assay

a)   are rarely directed against autologous B lymphocytes
b)   correlate with improved allograft survival when present in pretransplant serum
c)   are generated by blood transfusion, and
d)   may be HLA-linked.

307

References

1   Cross DE, Greiner R, Whittier FC. *Transplantation 1976; 21:* 307
2   Stastny P, Austin CL. *Transplantation 1976; 21:* 399
3   Reekers P, Lucassen-Hermans R, Koene RAP, Kunst VAJM. *Lancet 1977; i:* 1063
4   Ting A, Morris PJ. *Lancet 1977; ii:* 1095
5   Morris PJ, Ting A. *Tissue Antigens 1981; 17:* 75
6   Park MS, Terasaki PI, Bernoco D. *Lancet 1977; i:* 465
7   MacLeod AM, Mason RJ, Stewart KN et al. *Transplantation 1982; 34:* 273
8   Bodmer JG. *Br Med Bull 1978; 34:* 233
9   MacLeod AM et al. *Lancet 1982; ii:* 468
10 Power DA, Mason RJ, Stewart KN et al. *Transplant Proc 1983; 15:* 890

T CYTOTOXIC/SUPPRESSOR CELLS AND T HELPER CELLS IN FINE NEEDLE RENAL ALLOGRAFT ASPIRATES DURING DIFFERENT PHASES OF REJECTION

D Taube, P Hobby, K Welsh

Renal and Tissue Typing Laboratories, Guy's Hospital, London, United Kingdom

Introduction

Although the identity and function of the mononuclear cells infiltrating human renal allografts has been extensively studied [1–3], little is known about the early cellular events of human renal allograft rejection, since these cells have almost always been obtained from irreversibly rejected allografts after transplant nephrectomy. However, with the development of fine needle aspiration (FNA) [4] of human renal allografts in situ, it has become possible to study rejection throughout its evolution and its response to treatment.

This paper describes the nature and function of the lymphocytes identified by monoclonal antibodies aspirated from human renal allografts during the first month post transplantation.

Patients, methods and materials

Patients

Tables I and II show that 72 FNAs and 56 samples of peripheral blood were simultaneously examined from 24 patients (mean age 43.5, range 17–73 years) during the first month after cadaveric renal transplantation. The patients were immunosuppressed with prednisolone and azathioprine and treated for rejection with methyl prednisolone as previously described [5]. Allograft rejection was diagnosed using standard clinical criteria, which included radionuclide scanning and on occasions, conventional needle biopsy.

The three day period preceding the diagnosis and treatment of rejection was defined as the pre-rejection (PR) period; the three days during which rejection was diagnosed and treated was defined as the during-rejection (DR) period and the three days following this was defined as the post-rejection (PoR) period. Allograft aspirates and peripheral blood were also examined outside this nine day period when there was no evidence of rejection (NR).

309

TABLE I. TH and TCS cells in allograft aspirates during different phases of rejection

Clinical state	Number of observations	Mean % TH cells ± 1SD	Mean % TCS cells ± 1SD	Mean ratio TH:TCS ± 1SD
Not rejecting	18	41.38±10.42	38.49±11.78	1.19±0.65
Pre-rejection	31	27.44±11.57	48.20±14.66	0.64±0.32
During-rejection	8	28.81±10.81	39.0 ±12.82	0.73±0.29
Post-rejection	16	32.03±11.19	38.67±12.78	0.90±0.52

TABLE II. TH and TCS cells in peripheral blood during different phases of rejection

Clinical state	Number of observations	Mean % TH cells ± 1SD	Mean % TCS cells ± 1SD	Mean ratio TH:TCS ± 1SD
Not rejecting	14	43.31±14.88	39.98±15.86	1.18±0.41
Pre-rejection	22	28.89±12.15	41.74±14.70	0.81±0.49
During-rejection	8	30.81±15.57	29.71±11.54	1.49±0.76
Post-rejection	12	35.04± 7.68	40.05±14.99	1.04±0.37

Methods and materials

The lymphocytes from the aspirates and peripheral blood were separated on Ficoll/Hypaque gradients. Monoclonal antibodies (Leu 3a and Leu 2a (Becton Dickinson)) directed against helper (TH) T cells and cytotoxic/suppressor (TCS) T cells respectively were used to define the nature and function of these lymphocytes. After incubation with monoclonal antibody, the lymphocytes were mixed with Biotin conjugated anti-mouse antibody (Miles Laboratories Ltd), washed and then treated with Avidin-FITC (Miles Laboratories Ltd). The appropriate controls were similarly set up. The number of fluorescence labelled cells were counted under an incident light fluorescence microscope. A minimum of 100 cells per antibody was counted.

Statistical analysis

Statistical analyses were performed using Wilcoxon's Rank Sum Test.

Results

Tables I and II and Figures 1 and 2 show the percentages and ratios of TH and TCS cells during the different phases of rejection in the patients' allograft

% TH cells in blood and aspirate during different phases of rejection

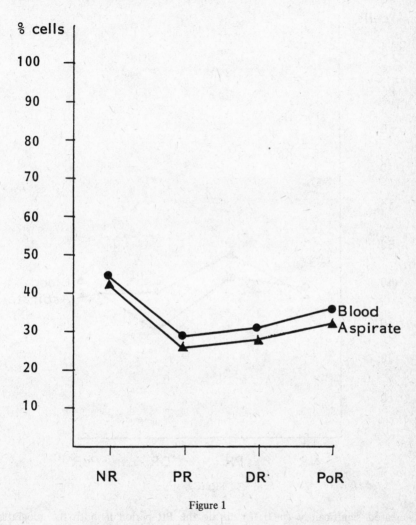

Figure 1

aspirates and peripheral blood. During the PR period, the number of TH cells in both the allografts and peripheral blood decreased significantly ($p < 0.01$) when compared with the number of TH cells in the allografts and peripheral blood during the NR period. There was a significant increase ($p > 0.02$, $p < 0.05$) in the number of TCS cells in the allografts, but not peripheral blood during the PR period when compared with the NR period. The ratio of TH:TCS cells

% TCS cells in blood and aspirate during different phases of rejection

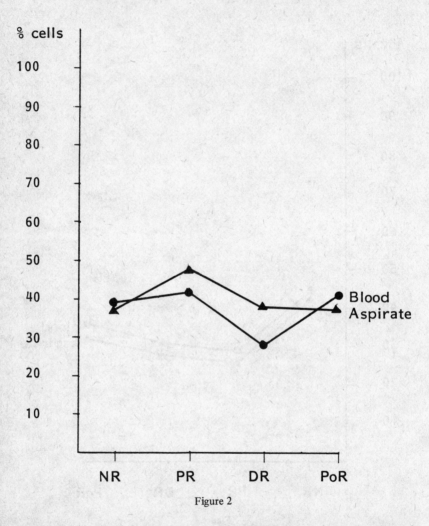

Figure 2

decreased significantly (p<0.01) during the PR period in both the allografts and peripheral blood when compared with the NR period. During the DR and PoR periods, there was a return in the numbers of TH and TCS cells to values approximating those found in the NR period. However, when the FNAs performed during the PoR period are examined further (Figure 3), the group of patients who have a poor prognosis (i.e. graft loss or further rejection within five days), have a persistently low TH:TCS cell ratio (p<0.01) when compared

312

Aspirate TH : TCS ratio in post rejection
phase and prognosis

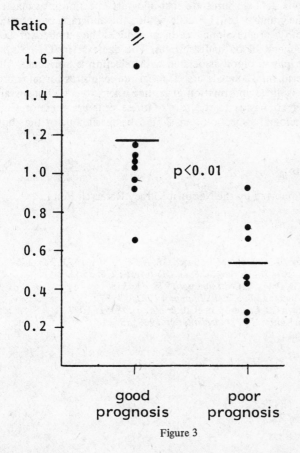

Figure 3

with the FNAs from the patients who have a good prognosis. TH:TCS cell ratios in the peripheral blood from these patients do not show this difference.

Discussion

Our data show that it is possible to diagnose renal allograft rejection before the clinical signs of rejection and deterioration of graft function occur. The diagnosis of 'pre-rejection' can be accomplished by either examination of allograft FNAs or peripheral blood with these monoclonal antibodies. Furthermore, by sequential examination of the numbers of TH and TCS cells in the allografts, it is possible to predict in the post-rejection phase, which allografts are going to do badly. Therefore, by early diagnosis and thus pre-emptive treatment of allograft rejection, it may be possible to reduce the severity of the rejection episode. By identifying, in the post-rejection period, which allografts are going to do badly after initial treatment, it may also be possible to save these allografts by early, more aggressive treatment.

In addition, our data demonstrate that allograft rejection is associated with an increase in the number of TCS cells within the allograft, but not the peripheral blood. Methyl prednisolone treatment reduces the numbers of TCS cells in both the peripheral blood and aspirates. The decrease in TH cells in both allografts and peripheral blood associated with rejection is intriguing. Although TH cells in experimental animals are essential pre-requisites for allograft rejection [6], there is little information regarding their role in human allograft rejection. Further studies as to the role of these cells are therefore indicated in human renal allograft rejection and should be feasible using the above described techniques.

Acknowledgments

This study was supported by the National Kidney Research Fund.

References

1 Strom TB, Tilney NL, Carpenter CB, Busch GB. *N Engl J Med 1975; 292:* 1257
2 Busch GJ, Schamberg JF, Moretz RC et al. *Lab Invest 1976; 35:* 272
3 Von Willebrand E, Hayry P. *Cell Immunol 1978; 41:* 358
4 Hayry P, Von Willebrand E. *Scand J Immunol 1981; 13:* 87
5 Papadakis J, Brown CB, Cameron JS et al. *Br Med J 1983; 1:* 1097
6 Loveland BE, McKenzie IFC. *Transplantation 1982; 33:* 217

DETECTION OF LYMPHOCYTE SUBSETS IN RENAL GRAFT BIOPSY BY MONOCLONAL ANTIBODIES

A Vangelista, G Frascà, A Nanni-Costa, V Bonomini

St Orsola University Hospital, Bologna, Italy

Summary

Monoclonal antibodies were used to study infiltrating cell subpopulations in 12 graft biopsy specimens taken from 12 patients during rejection episodes. A preponderance of T lymphocytes in the renal interstitium was observed in most cases, with a higher percentage of suppressor/cytotoxic cells. No correlation was documented between the type and severity of rejection and the percentage of the various infiltrating cells.

Introduction

An infiltration of mononuclear cells in the interstitium occurs typically in renal allograft rejection. Identification of the nature of the infiltrating cell populations could result in a better understanding of the mechanisms of rejection. The present report deals with the composition of the mononuclear cell infiltrates as determined by monoclonal antibodies applied to renal biopsy specimens taken from 12 transplanted patients during rejection episodes.

Material and methods

Twelve renal biopsies from 12 patients were examined. The age of the patients, time from transplantation, previous rejection episodes, and histological diagnosis at graft biopsy are shown in Table I. Cryostat sections of graft biopsy specimens were tested by the indirect immunofluorescence technique [1] using murine monoclonal antibodies directed against pan-T-cells (OKT3), T-helper/inducer cells (OKT4), T-suppressor/cytotoxic cells (OKT8), monocytes/macrophages (OKM1), natural killer/cytotoxic cells (Leu 7), B-cells (Leu 10). Ethidium bromide (1:5,000) was used to stain nuclei [2] and thus allow cell count. Graft tissue sections were examined with a Zeiss Universal Microscope in epifluorescence at magnification 400 X. Interstitial cells were counted in each of

315

TABLE I. Characteristics and histological diagnosis of the patients studied

Patient number	Age	Time from Tx number	Previous rejection	Renal Biopsy			Diagnosis
				Infiltration	Fibrosis	Vascular damage	
1	31	46 days	1	+ + +	0	+ + +	Acute irreversible
2	33	6 years	0	+ +	+ + +	+ +	Chronic
3	20	7 months	0	+ + +	+	+	Acute severe
4	35	2 months	0	+ +	0	0	Acute moderate
5	41	15 days	0	+ + +	0	+ + +	Acute irreversible
6	34	10 months	1	+ + +	+	+	Acute severe
7	21	28 days	0	+	0	0	Acute mild
8	26	27 days	0	+ + +	0	0	Acute moderate
9	20	9 months	1	+ +	+	+	Acute moderate
10	31	7 months	1	+ +	+	+	Acute moderate
11	52	12 days	0	+ +	0	+ + +	Acute irreversible
12	15	32 months	1	+ + +	+ + +	+ + +	Chronic

20 to 40 fields. Positive cells were expressed as a mean percentage of the total nuclei counted.

At time of biopsy, 20ml of heparinised venous blood was taken from each patient to evaluate peripheral cell subpopulations by means of the same monoclonal antibodies used for biopsy tissue.

Results

Indirect immunofluorescence provided good identification of infiltrating cell subpopulations (Figures 1 and 2). In all cases (Table II) the major component of the infiltrates was represented by T lymphocytes (OKT3), except in case 1, where OKM1 positive cells predominated. A preponderance of suppressor/cytotoxic cells (OKT8 positive) was observed, as compared to helper/inducer cells (OKT4 positive). The OKT4/OKT8 ratio was lower in renal tissue than in peripheral blood (Table III). Leu 7 positive cells (natural killer/cytotoxic) were present in 11 of the 12 biopsy specimens; their percentage ranged from seven to 32 per cent. The OKT8/Leu 7 ratio in renal tissue was higher than in peripheral blood (Table III). OKM1 positive cells were present in all cases, ranging from two per cent to 32 per cent. The percentage of Leu 10 positive cells varied from 0 to 16 per cent.

No correlation was observed between the percentage of T-cell subpopulations and the type and severity of rejection. A lower percentage of Leu 7 positive cells was observed in the presence of severe vascular damage. A higher percentage of OKM1 and Leu 10 positive cells was present in acute irreversible and chronic rejection.

316

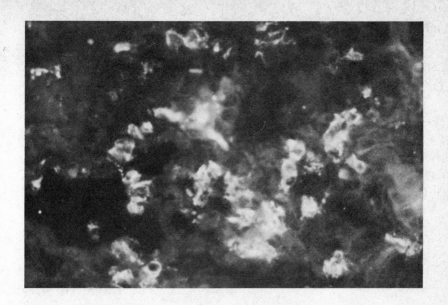

Figure 1. OKT3 positive cells in graft biopsy tissue

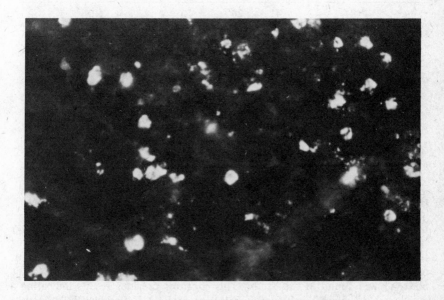

Figure 2. OKT8 positive cells in graft biopsy tissue

TABLE II. Infiltrating cell subpopulations identified by monoclonal antibodies in renal tissue

Patient number	OKT3 %	OKT4 %	OKT8 %	Leu 7 %	Leu 10 %	OKM1 %	T4/T8 ratio	T8/Leu 7 ratio
1	23	2	18	1	16	25	0.1	18
2	46	5	38	12	12	32	0.13	3.1
3	54	11	42	32	9	4	0.26	1.3
4	32	7	23	15	0	5	0.3	1.5
5	38	9	31	14	15	12	0.3	2.2
6	52	6	48	26	4	3	0.1	1.8
7	67	14	41	9	0	2	0.34	4.5
8	73	6	64	19	ND	7	0.09	3.3
9	64	11	54	7	6	2	0.2	7.7
10	49	7	46	14	8	5	0.15	3.2
11	37	5	34	16	12	29	0.14	2.1
12	43	12	32	11	14	21	0.37	2.9

TABLE III. Lymphocyte subpopulations identified by monoclonal antibodies in peripheral blood

Patient number	OKT3 %	OKT4 %	OKT8 %	Leu 7 %	T4/T8 ratio	T8/Leu 7 ratio
1	55	41	20	ND	2.1	ND
2	82	52	33	36	1.6	0.9
3	79	43	10	8	4.3	1.2
4	60	35	12	19	2.9	0.6
5	66	44	28	ND	1.6	ND
6	68	38	23	ND	1.6	ND
7	81	48	19	12	2.5	1.5
8	62	42	16	17	2.6	0.9
9	93	38	22	27	1.7	0.8
10	62	32	17	7	1.9	2.4
11	66	37	26	ND	1.4	ND

Discussion

Our study confirms that the use of monoclonal antibodies applied to biopsy specimens may contribute by identifying the nature and type of the infiltrating cells in renal allograft rejection [3]. Regardless of the type and severity of rejection, a preponderance of T cells in the interstitium (most of them OKT8 positive) was found in this study. This confirms previous results indicating a deficiency of helper-T cells within rejecting grafts [4]. Besides OKT8 positive cells, Leu 7 positive cells were present in all but one biopsy specimen. These findings suggest that mainly cells of the cytotoxic type (either T lymphocytes or natural killer cells) are responsible for the graft lesions during rejection episodes [5]. The analysis of the percentage of infiltrating cells did not afford identification of different patterns in acute or chronic rejection. However, a trend towards a higher proportion of OKM1 and Leu 10 positive cells, was documented in renal biopsy specimens from patients with acute irreversible or chronic rejection. The presence of these cells seems to correlate with the severity of vascular damage.

This report outlines the validity of the use of monoclonal antibodies to identify infiltrating cells in renal biopsy tissue during allograft rejection. Further extensive study, however, is needed to clarify both the importance and the role of infiltrating cell subpopulations in determining the various lesions which occur in different types of rejection.

References

1 Hammer C, Land W, Stadler J et al. *Transplant Proc 1983; 15:* 356
2 Platt JL, LeBien TW, Michael AF. *J Exp Med 1982; 155:* 17
3 Franklin WA, Locker JD. *J Histochem Cytochem 1981; 29:* 572
4 Hancock WW, Thomson NM, Atkins RC. *Transplant Proc 1983; 15:* 352
5 Häyry P, Soots A, Willebrand E et al. *Transplant Proc 1979; 11:* 785

Proc EDTA (1983) Vol 20

EARLY DETECTION OF OBSTRUCTED URETER BY ULTRASOUND FOLLOWING RENAL TRANSPLANTATION

D L McWhinnie, J A Bradley, J D Briggs, D J Galloway, K F Kyle, D N H Hamilton, B J R Junor, S G Macpherson, Patricia Morley

Western Infirmary, Glasgow, United Kingdom

Summary

Serial ultrasound examinations were carried out following 144 renal transplants. Eleven patients (8%) required surgery for ureteric obstruction and in all cases the ultrasound correctly identified the obstruction at an early stage. One false positive result was obtained with the ultrasound and this compared favourably with both the intravenous urogram (IVU) and isotope renogram. There were false positive and false negative results with both the IVU and renogram in addition to which neither of these techniques, particularly the IVU, is as simple or atraumatic for the patient as the ultrasound. Serial ultrasound examinations have a useful role in the detection of ureteric obstruction as well as being of value in the detection of perinephric fluid collections and acute rejection.

Introduction

Ureteric obstruction following transplantation may occur at an early stage due to technical factors or after several months or years as a result of ischaemic fibrosis of the ureter at its lower end. A wide range in incidence has been reported with a figure as high as eight per cent in some series [1]. The intravenous urogram (IVU) and isotope renogram have been the two investigations used most commonly in the diagnosis of this complication but, particularly when renal function is poor, they may yield only equivocal results. This study assesses the value of serial ultrasound examinations in the diagnosis of ureteric obstruction.

Patients and methods

Between January 1980 and March 1983, 176 renal transplants were performed on 169 recipients. At least three ultrasound examinations were performed following 144 (86%) of these transplants and it is these serial examinations which form the basis of this study. They were usually performed at two week intervals for the first two months, and thereafter at six months and then annually. The number of examinations per patient ranged from three to 15. The other 32 transplants failed at an early stage mostly as the result of acute rejection. An IVU was usually performed at two to three months and at one year and isotope renography using [123] I Hippuran only when a complication such as ureteric obstruction was suspected.

Results

Of the 144 patients undergoing serial ultrasound examinations, 11 (8%) subsequently required surgery for ureteric obstruction. The ultrasound correctly identified all 11 of these obstructions usually at an early stage before renal function had deteriorated. Figure 1 illustrates the ultrasound appearance of a normal renal transplant. In the presence of ureteric obstruction, dilatation of the calyces and usually also the renal pelvis can usually be clearly identified (Figure 2).

In seven of the 11 cases, ureteric obstruction was first detected on routine ultrasound examination before significant deterioration of renal function had occurred. In the other four cases, ureteric obstruction was suspected as a possible explanation or contributory factor for poor or deteriorating renal function and

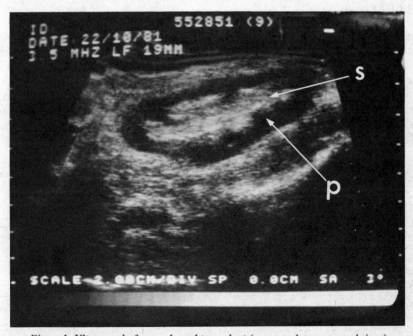

Figure 1. Ultrasound of normal renal transplant (p=parenchyma, s=renal sinus)

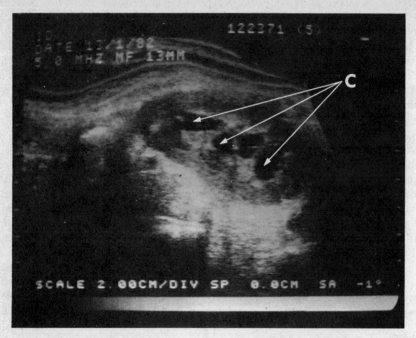

Figure 2. Ultrasound of transplant in patient with ureteric obstruction showing dilated calyces (c=calyces)

the diagnosis was confirmed by ultrasound. In addition to these patients who all had serial ultrasound, ureteric obstruction was correctly diagnosed within the first week following transplantation by ultrasound examination in two further patients.

The relative diagnostic accuracy of the ultrasound, IVU and isotope renogram is shown in Table I in relation to graft function. An IVU and isotope renogram were carried out in only four of the seven patients whose creatinine clearance was less than 15ml/min in view of the poor renal function. In two of

TABLE I. Diagnostic accuracy of imaging techniques in the detection of ureteric obstruction in relation to graft function

| Renal function | CORRECT DIAGNOSIS | | |
	IVU (n=8)	Renogram (n=7)	Ultrasound (n=11)
Poor renal function: (creatinine clearance <15ml/min) (n=7)	2 of 4	4 of 4	7 of 7
Good renal function: (creatinine clearance >30ml/min) (n=4)	4 of 4	2 of 3	4 of 4

TABLE II. The sensitivity and specificity of the three imaging techniques in detecting ureteric obstruction

Diagnostic techniques	Number of patients	False +ve results	False −ve results
Ultrasound	144	1	0
IVU	63	1	2
Renogram	21	2	1

the four, evidence of obstruction was not apparent on the IVU. The overall accuracy of the three diagnostic techniques is shown in Table II. Only one false positive ultrasound result was obtained in the 144 patients. In this patient, the IVU showed the anatomical variant of an intra-renal pelvis.

Discussion

The results of this study show that ultrasound is an accurate method of diagnosis of ureteric obstruction after renal transplantation. To avoid false positive results a repeat examination should be carried out after voiding as a distended bladder can be associated with pelvi-calyceal dilatation in the absence of ureteric obstruction [2]. In addition to its accuracy, the ultrasound can be repeated as often as required, is free from any risk to the patient, and can, if necessary, be carried out at the bedside. As well as providing evidence of ureteric obstruction, it has a useful role in the detection of perinephric fluid collections [3] and the diagnosis of acute rejection [4]. Finally obstruction can be confirmed and its site defined by percutaneous antegrade pyelography using ultrasound to localise the distended calyces.

Previously used methods of diagnosing ureteric obstruction have been the IVU and isotope renogram. The IVU, even with a high dose of contrast medium, may outline inadequately the calyces of a poorly functioning kidney and it has also been suggested that the contrast medium may have an adverse effect on an already damaged kidney although there is no proof of this [4].

The isotope renogram is a sensitive indicator of changes in the transit time of solutes through the kidney. However, it is non-specific in that it cannot differentiate between obstruction to urine flow and other causes of a prolonged transit time. Also its diagnostic value diminishes as renal function deteriorates.

In conclusion, the ultrasound combines the advantages of being non-invasive and totally safe for the patient with accuracy in the diagnosis of ureteric obstruction and the ability also to detect other complications, namely perinephric fluid collections and acute rejection. The results of this study suggest that it is useful to carry out serial ultrasound examinations following renal transplantation even if there is no biochemical evidence of deterioration in renal function.

References

1 Mundy AR, Podesta ML, Bewick M et al. *Br J Urol 1981; 53:* 397
2 Balchunas WR, Hill MC, Isikoff MB, Morillo G. *J Clin Ultrasound 1982; 10:* 221
3 Morley P, Barnett E, Bell PRF et al. *Clin Radiol 1975; 26:* 199
4 Cruz C, Hricak H, Eyler WR et al. *Proc EDTA 1980; 17:* 413
5 Peters C, Delmonico FL, Cosimi AB et al. *Surg Gynecol Obstet 1983; 156:* 467

CAPTOPRIL-INDUCED DETERIORATION OF GRAFT FUNCTION IN PATIENTS WITH A TRANSPLANT RENAL ARTERY STENOSIS

W J van Son, F J van der Woude, A M Tegzess, A J M Donker, M J H Slooff, L B van der Slikke, S J Hoorntje

State University Hospital, Groningen, The Netherlands

Summary

We evaluated nine captopril-treated patients with transplant renal artery stenosis. Captopril treatment always resulted in a dramatic decrease in renal function; in two patients complete anuria developed. Only in two patients with a stenosis in one out of two renal arteries was a satisfactory fall in blood pressure achieved. The mechanisms which may lead to these remarkable results will be discussed.

Introduction

Hypertension has a high prevalence among recipients of renal allografts and is still considered to be one of the major clinical problems in these patients [1, 2]. The cause of this hypertension is believed to be multifactorial in nature, but in the vast majority the hypertension is related to the recipient's native kidneys [3, 4]. There is, however, also the possibility of a transplant renal artery stenosis.

The use of captopril for hypertension after renal transplantation is no longer an exception since it has been shown that captopril provides anti-hypertensive properties which overshadow the results obtained with other available therapeutic regimens [5]. Recently, Curtis et al [6] described four patients with transplant renal artery stenosis in whom an acute loss of renal excretory function developed when captopril was added to the anti-hypertensive regimen.

We observed acute oliguric renal failure, not attributable to a fall in systemic blood pressure, after captopril treatment in two patients with transplant renal artery stenosis. This prompted us to look retrospectively at our transplant patients who had received captopril. Seven other patients with transplant renal artery stenosis had been treated with captopril in the past four years. This was always associated with a pronounced deterioration in graft function, in most cases without a satisfactory blood pressure response.

Patients and methods

All nine patients had an angiographically proven transplant renal artery stenosis (for details see Table I). Stenosis in the renal artery was defined as more than 60 per cent reduction in vessel diameter. All patients had hypertension (diastolic blood pressure ≥95mmHg) and a systolic murmur over the graft at the time captopril treatment was initiated. In five patients this murmur had been absent at the time when renal function had reached its maximum after transplantation.

TABLE I

Patient number	Age (years)	Sex M/F	Captopril dosage	Clinical course
1	41	M	50mg q.i.d.	Surgical reconstruction: BP 140/90 (metoprolol 50mg b.i.d.) GFR 81ml/min
2	29	M	12.5mg q.i.d.	Surgical reconstruction: BP 140/95mmHg GFR 73ml/min
3	47	M	50mg q.i.d.	Surgical reconstruction: BP 140/80mmHg GFR 82ml/min
4	39	M	50mg q.i.d.	Before captopril treatment: homogenous ^{99m}Tc-DMSA scan after captopril: defect lower pole
5	44	F	25mg t.i.d.	After surgery and discontinuation captopril: BP 180/115mmHg GFR 18ml/min
6	44	M	25mg q.i.d.	Situation accepted, captopril continued
7	48	M	25mg t.i.d.	Surgical reconstruction: BP 190/105mmHg GFR 116ml/min
8	16	F	25mg t.i.d.	Transplant nephrectomy: ischaemic graft
9	32	M	50mg t.i.d.	Discontinuation of diuretics and augmentation salt intake: BP 140/100mmHg GFR 77ml/min

BP: Blood pressure
GFR: Glomerular filtration rate

The underlying kidney diseases leading to renal failure before transplantation were adult polycystic disease (2), chronic pyelonephritis (2), chronic glomerulonephritis of unknown origin (3), membranous glomerulopathy (1) and renal hypoplasia (1). These patients (Table I: numbers 4, 6 and 9) were normotensive during the pretransplant period. The other six patients (Table I: numbers 1, 2, 3, 5, 7 and 8) had been treated with beta-blockers for mild hypertension.

A variable number of nephrectomies had been performed before transplantation. No nephrectomy had been performed in patients 1, 2 and 7, one nephrectomy in patients 4, 5, 6 and 8, and bilateral nephrectomy in patients 3 and 9 (Table I).

All recipients received a cadaveric graft. Machine preservation was never used. Of seven right kidneys four were placed in the right and three in the left iliac fossa. Two left kidneys were grafted equally to both sides. In seven patients a patch was used for the arterial anastomosis. A graft with two renal arteries was transplanted into three patients (Table I: numbers 4, 6 and 9). Later on, in two of them (numbers 4 and 6), only one of these two arteries appeared to be stenotic.

All grafted patients were initially treated for their hypertension with a diuretic (frusemide or hydrochlorothiazide), a beta-blocker (metoprolol or atenolol) and a vasodilator (hydralazine or minoxidil). Table I shows the added captopril dosage.

The nadir of renal function was defined as the moment when serum creatinine reached its highest point after start of captopril treatment. Glomerular filtration rate (GFR) was determined using ^{125}I-iothalamate as previously described [7]. If a GFR determination was not performed, creatinine clearance was calculated from the values of creatinine in serum and urine (24-hour collection). Values were not corrected to standard body surface area.

Results

The effects of captopril treatment on mean arterial pressure (MAP) and GFR are shown in Figure 1. The dotted lines indicate the two patients with two renal arteries and one stenosed.

Renal function deteriorated markedly in all nine patients. In four patients (numbers 1, 2, 4 and 8) the graft murmur disappeared. Two patients (numbers 1 and 8) developed anuria. Patient 1 became anuric seven days after starting captopril, blood pressure remained high (150/105mmHg) and the anuria necessitated haemodialysis. During the anuric period the murmur over the graft disappeared. A ^{131}I-hippuran scan however, was perfect, suggesting a highly viable graft with sustained blood flow. After withdrawal of captopril and the institution of minoxidil, renal function recovered (creatinine clearance 50ml/min) and the graft murmur reappeared. Although a former angiographic study had failed to reveal a transplant renal artery stenosis, a strong suspicion for a stenosis remained and the angiography was repeated. This time the angiographic study was performed in various positions. A posterior oblique view revealed a severe transplant artery stenosis which had been obscured on previous angiograms by the iliac artery. The patient underwent a successful surgical reconstruction which resulted in a return to normal of the blood pressure on only 50mg metoprolol b.i.d., and a further improvement of renal function (creatinine clearance 81ml/min).

In patient number 8 an ischaemic graft was found at transplant nephrectomy.

An optimal blood pressure response was observed in patient number 4 and 6. These patients had a stenosis in only one of two renal arteries (dotted lines in

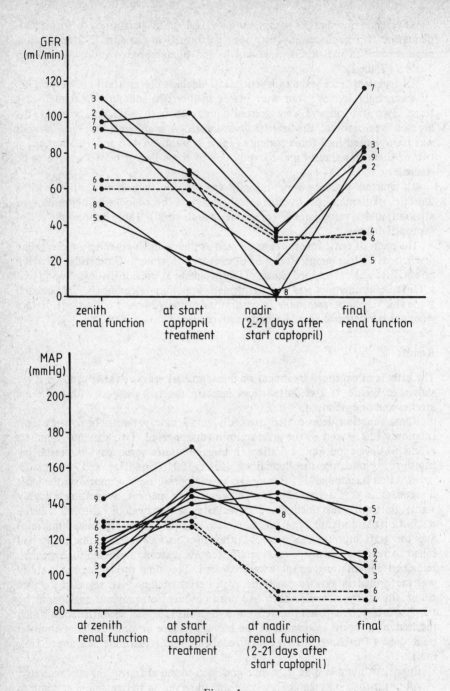

Figure 1

Figure 1). In patient number 4 the effect of captopril on filtration was also documented by repeated ^{99m}Tc-DMSA scans. Captopril administration produced a defect in the lower pole supplied by the stenotic artery.

In five patients (numbers 1, 2, 3, 5 and 7) a surgical reconstruction was attempted and only in patient number 5 was unsuccessful. Creatinine clearance in this patient recovered to about the pre-captopril value but the blood pressure remained high. In the other four patients, surgery restored graft function and normal blood pressure without anti-hypertensive medication in two patients (numbers 2 and 3).

Finally, in patient number 9 graft function could be partly restored by discontinuation of the diuretics and augmentation of the sodium intake. This patient is still on captopril treatment but a normal blood pressure has not been achieved.

Discussion

Hypertension in renal transplant recipients is generally related to patients' native kidneys [3, 4]. Nevertheless, in patients with a systolic graft murmur and/or rapidly developing hypertension after transplantation, an angiogram imaging the renal arteries should be performed, especially when the murmur was absent before. This investigation should always be extended to different views to minimise the risk of overlooking a stenosis and to facilitate subsequent surgery. This rather aggressive approach is warranted by the 'risks' of captopril in this particular group of hypertensive patients and by the possibility of successful surgical correction of a transplant renal artery stenosis as documented in this study.

In patients with essential hypertension, angiotensin I converting enzyme inhibition results in a blood pressure fall, an increased renal blood flow and a maintained GFR [8]. The effect on renal function has been explained by a reduction in endogenous angiotensin II generation and/or by alterations in intra-renal kinin and prostaglandin metabolism. In essential hypertension the renal response to captopril does not depend on salt intake.

In our particular patient group a direct relationship between the fall in blood pressure and the loss in renal function is not likely, although it is known that patients with renal vascular hypertension can develop renal function loss during the combination of salt depletion and captopril treatment [9]. Only in two of our nine patients captopril treatment resulted in a pronounced blood pressure fall. However, these two patients represented a subgroup, since a stenosis was present in only one of two renal arteries. In the other seven patients blood pressure reduction was small or did not occur (Figure 1), indicating that systemic blood pressure did not depend on circulating angiotensin II. Moreover, treatment with the non-specific vasodilator minoxidil resulted in an even more pronounced blood pressure fall in patient number 1 and did not interfere with the restoration of renal function after discontinuing captopril treatment. Thus, a direct relation between the loss in renal function and the drop in blood pressure is not probable. Comparable observations have been made recently by Hricik et al [3] and by Curtis et al [6] in patients with

329

bilateral renal artery stenosis or in patients with a solitary kidney.

The effects of captopril on blood pressure and renal function seems to be identical in patients with transplant renal artery stenosis, with renal artery stenosis in a solitary kidney and with bilateral renal artery stenosis. In all these situations the functioning renal mass is located distal to the stenosis. Glomerular filtration in a kidney with a stenosis of the renal artery appears to be dependent on the intrarenal effect of angiotensin II. Angiotensin II causes constriction responses in efferent, not in afferent arterioles [10]. Blocking of the intrarenal angiotensin II generation then will lead to efferent dilatation, a fall in hydrostatic filtration pressure in the stenotic kidney and consequently to a striking renal function loss in solitary kidneys, as in our patient group.

We conclude that captopril treatment in patients with transplant renal artery stenosis can lead to a dramatic loss in graft function. This loss in renal function, even to complete anuria, can be explained by the mode of action of angiotensin I converting enzyme inhibitors in general, and appears not to be a special side-effect of captopril. Converting enzyme inhibitor induced loss in renal function, and the possibility of successful surgical reconstruction, both stress the importance of detecting such stenosis in hypertensive renal transplant recipients.

In the situation of a stenosis in one of multiple renal arteries, captopril can be used to lower blood pressure, although it might induce a functional amputation of a part of the renal parenchyma.

References

1   Polline J, Guttman RD, Beaudoin JG et al. *Clin Nephrol 1979; 11:* 202
2   Ypersele De Strihou C van, Vereerstraaten P, Wauthier M et al. *Actualités nephrologiques de l'hospital Necker 1982; 12:* 43
3   McHuygh MI, Tanboger H, Marcen H et al. *Q J Med 1980; 196:* 393
4   Ingelfinger JR, Grupe WE, Levey RH. *Clin Nephrol 1981; 15:* 236
5   Prins EJC. *Converting Enzyme Inhibition. Thesis, University of Groningen, 1979*
6   Curtis JJ, Luke RG, Whelchel JD et al. *N Engl J Med 1983; 308:* 377
7   Donker AJM, Hem GK van der, Sluiter WJ, Beekhuis H. *Neth J Med 1977; 20:* 97
8   Hoorntje SJ. *Thesis, University of Groningen, 1981*
9   Hricik DE, Browning PH, Kopelman R et al. *N Engl J Med 1983; 308:* 373
10   Edwards RM. *Kidney Int 1983; 23:* 243

PREVENTION OF OSTEONECROSIS FOLLOWING RENAL TRANSPLANTATION BY USING VITAMIN D$_2$ (ERGOCALCIFEROL)

D Scholz, M Mebel, I Töpelmann, I Grossmann, J Scholze, H Mrochen

Charité, Humboldt-University, Berlin, GDR

Summary

Osteonecrosis is a frequently disabling complication of renal transplantation. Thirty-one of 244 patients (12.7%), who received cadaver renal transplants from 1968 to 1978 developed an osteonecrosis. An analysis of 14 possible risk factors suggested that only the following were significantly more frequent in the osteonecrosis group: >3 pulse doses of 1.2g prednisolone, serum creatinine >133μmol/L, steroid-induced diabetes mellitus and second and subsequent transplantation.

An important decline in the incidence of osteonecrosis (26.7 per cent to 6.5 per cent) was seen with prophylactic vitamin D$_2$ treatment and the onset of osteonecrosis was on average one year later. Dangerous side effects of the large doses of vitamin D$_2$ were minimal. Hypercalcaemia due to overdosage with vitamin D$_2$ during simultaneous prednisolone therapy was usually mild and returned to normal in a few days by dose reduction.

Introduction

The incidence of avascular necrosis, osteonecrosis, in renal transplant patients from earlier studies varies from three to 41 per cent. The pathogensis of osteo-necrosis is not known but various factors have been proposed: the duration of uraemia and the dialysis time, the use of phosphate-binding antacids [1] and hypophosphataemia, secondary hyperparathyroidism, ligation of the hypogastric artery, bone ischaemia due to fat embolism, osteopenia [2] and microfractures, hyperuricaemia, corticosteroids [1, 3], weight gain after trans-plantation and the bone status at the time of renal transplantation [2].

The mechanism by which corticosteroids cause osteonecrosis has not so far been established with certainty. In 1968 it was shown that prednisone caused a rapid turnover of vitamin D$_3$ and a diminished production of a biologically active vitamin D metabolite leading to a decrease in the intestinal absorption of calcium [4]. The effect of corticosteroids on intestinal calcium absorption appears to be dose-related [5–7] and its combination with uraemia increases the need for $1,25(OH)_2D_3$ seven to tenfold to maintain normal serum calcium values [8]. It is well established that pharmacological doses of $1,25(OH)_2D_3$ [7] and $1\alpha(OH)D_3$ [9] increases calcium absorption in patients receiving corticosteroids and in haemodialysis patients [10]. This study was started before the most important synthetically produced vitamin D metabolites were available. Vitamin D_2 (ergocalciferol; calciferol; Dekristol®) is the oldest of all the available vitamin D preparations. The present study was undertaken to find out whether vitamin D_2 can be used in renal transplant patients for prevention of skeletal complications with particular regard to osteonecrosis.

Patients and methods

Between 1968 and the end of 1982, 616 renal transplants were performed at the kidney transplantation centre in Berlin, GDR. Of the 616 patients, 406 with functioning grafts were studied. Forty-nine patients had osteonecrosis (49/406: incidence 12.07%). The incidence at any time (1968–1982) varied between 28.6 per cent and 3.3 per cent (Table I). The time between transplantation and onset of osteonecrosis was 0.5–9.1 years (median 1.5 years; mean ± SD 2.1 ± 1.8 years).

TABLE I. Incidence of osteonecrosis by transplant years

Years of transplant	Number of transplant (CD-grafts)	Number of patients studied	Incidence of osteonecrosis*	
			Number	%
1968–1970	19	11	3	28.6
	7 (LD)	3	1	
1971–1973	88	64	16	25.0
1974–1976	147	96	14	14.6
1977–1979	170	112	11	9.8
1980–1982	185	120	4	3.3
TOTAL	616	406	49	12.07 (49/406)

CD = cadaver; LD = living donor
* Occurrence at any time after transplant

Because of possible late manifestation of osteonecrosis the study of the influence of vitamin D_2 therapy can only be estimated on patients transplanted up to 1978. We examined the incidence of osteonecrosis in a group of 244 cadaver renal transplant patients and analysed the possible risk factors in 31 affected patients. For the analysis of factors contributing to the development of

332

osteonecrosis each patient with osteonecrosis was matched with the following patient without osteonecrosis. There were no statistically significant differences between the two groups for age, sex, nature of renal disease, corticosteroid therapy, duration of dialysis before transplantation, and the HLA-A-B-match. The investigative methods included serial biochemical estimations of serum creatinine, serum lipids, calcium and phosphorus (serum and urine), alkaline phosphatase, ASAT, ALAT and creatinine clearance. The number of rejection episodes was assessed in all patients.

After transplantation and yearly thereafter each patient underwent both bone mineral content analysis using the ^{125}J photon absorptiometric method with the Norland bone mineral analyser and radiographic skeletal surveys (chest, shoulders, spine, pelvis, femurs, knees, hands, feet).

The total dosage of prednisolone received by each patient in the time between transplantation and onset of osteonecrosis was estimated for study and control groups. There were no statistically significant differences between the groups. Acute rejection crises were treated with an average bolus of 1.2g prednisolone (4 x 5mg/kg at 48 hours).

The approximate total dosage of prednisolone was 2.25g in the first month, 6.31g in the first six months, and 9.05g in the first year.

Parathyroidectomy was performed for hyperparathyroidism in four patients: two before and two after transplantation.

One hundred and sixty-nine patients were treated with vitamin D_2 (15,000–20,000 IU in oil daily; Dekristol®) and 75 patients without. Age, sex, HLA-A-B-match, status of renal function, corticosteroid-dosage, and the time of renal transplant of the treated and untreated patients were matched. There was no significant difference between the two groups.

Statistical methods

The results are presented as the arithmetic mean and the standard deviation or as median and the largest and smallest values. For the comparison of individual means in the two groups the Student's t-test was used. In the studies of possible risk factors for osteonecrosis, the two groups were tested by chi-square analysis, by the Fisher test or by the median test.

Results

Since the introduction of vitamin D_2 prophylaxis the incidence of osteonecrosis has steadily fallen from 28.6 per cent (1968–1970) to 3.3 per cent (1980–1982) despite unchanged doses of prednisolone (Table I).

The distribution of possible risk factors in the osteonecrosis and control groups showed that only four of 14 studied factors were significantly more frequent in the osteonecrosis group. Steroid-induced diabetes mellitus and second and subsequent transplantation are thought to be closely related to the number of bolus prednisolone doses (Table II). Patients in the osteonecrosis group received significantly more frequent boluses of prednisolone (4–8; p<0.001) before onset of complications (Table III).

TABLE II. Distribution of possible risk factors in osteonecrosis and control groups

Possible risk factors	Osteonecrosis group (n = 31 patients)	Control group (n = 31 patients)	p
Serum creatinine $>133\mu$mol/L	20	9	$<0.025*$
>3 x bolus of prednisolone as antirejection therapy	12	1	$<0.001**$
Steroid diabetes mellitus	16	7	<0.02
Retransplantations (second and third grafts)	5	0	$<0.05**$
Hypertension	26	19	NS
Bilateral nephrectomy	11	9	NS
Hypercholesterolaemia	15	9	NS
Skeletal changes of secondary hyperparathyroidism	10	5	NS
Proteinuria >5g/day	5	2	NS**
Age of recipient >40 years	7	2	NS**
>20 min warm ischaemia	9	3	NS**
Chronic liver pathology	14	13	NS
Hyperuricaemia	7	8	NS
Weight gain >10kg after renal transplantation	10	13	NS

(x^2 test; **Fisher test; *Median test/Contingency Table Analysis)

TABLE III. Comparison of distribution of bolus prednisolone therapy

Number of bolus prednisolone therapy*	Osteonecrosis group (n = 31 patients)	Control group (n = 31 patients)
0	4	9
1	9	7
2	3	11
3	3	3
4	4	1
5	3	
6	0	
7	4	
8	1	

$p<0.001**$

* One bolus prednisolone = 1.2g prednisolone; ** Fisher test

334

The frequency of simultaneously occurring risk factors out of the first eleven factors under study (Table II) was twice as high in the osteonecrosis group (4.5 ± 1.7) than in the control group (2.2 ± 1.1).

Bone mineral content of the osteonecrosis group compared with control group (90.5 ± 10.4% and 91.6 ± 13.5% respectively, corrected for age and sex; $p > 0.05$) was not significantly different. The most frequent site of osteonecrosis was the femoral head (27/31). In 22 per cent (7/31) another site was affected (Table IV). The incidence of osteonecrosis in the vitamin D_2 group (n = 169 patients) at 6.5 per cent was significantly lower ($p < 0.0001$) than in the group without prophylaxis (26.7%) (Figure 1).

TABLE IV. Localisation of osteonecrosis after transplant (n = 31 patients)

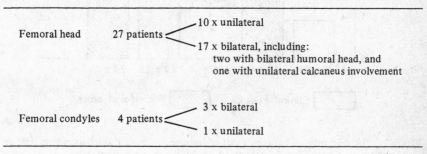

Femoral head   27 patients   10 x unilateral

17 x bilateral, including:
two with bilateral humoral head, and
one with unilateral calcaneus involvement

Femoral condyles   4 patients   3 x bilateral

1 x unilateral

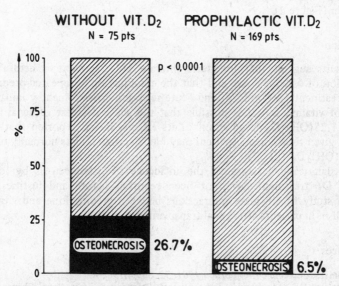

Figure 1. Influence of vitamin D_2 therapy on the incidence of osteonecrosis after renal transplant (n = 244 patients)

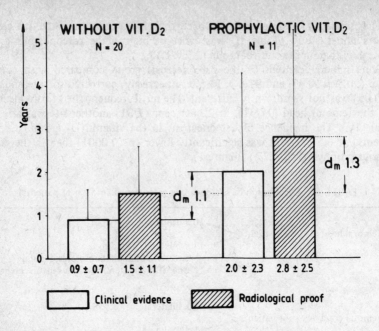

Figure 2. The time interval between onset of osteonecrosis and transplantation in relation to vitamin D_2 therapy (n = 31 patients; d_m = difference of mean values)

During vitamin D_2 prophylaxis the osteonecrosis developed on average one year later (Figure 2).

Discussion

The results suggest that long-term vitamin D_2 treatment is helpful in the prevention of osteonecrosis, and that the combination of repeated prednisolone bolus treatment (>3 x 1.2g) and acute rejection crises somehow impaired the action of vitamin D_2. It is possible that the acute decrease of renal function blocks $1,25(OH)_2D_3$ production or its effects. It was reported that corticosteroids given to a uraemic patient may block certain effects normally produced by $1,25(OH)_2D_3$ [8].

The significant decrease of the incidence of osteonecrosis by long-term vitamin D_2 treatment have not been reported before and justifies further detailed study to elucidate interactions between prednisolone and vitamin D_2 metabolism in patients after renal transplantation.

References

1   Elmstedt E. *Acta Orthop Scand 1981; 52, Suppl 190:* 1
2   Nielsen HE, ed. *Uremic Bone Disease Before and After Renal Transplantation.* Aarhus: Laegeforeningens forlag. 1981: 1–26

3   Park WM. In Davidson, ed. *Aseptic Necrosis of Bone.* Amsterdam: Excerpta Medica. 1976: 213–269

4   Avioli LV, Birge SJ, Lee SW. *J Clin Endocrinol 1968; 28:* 1341

5   Hahn TJ, Halstead LR, Haddad JG. *J Lab Clin Med 1977; 90:* 399

6   Pierides AM, Aljama P, Kerr DNS et al. *Nephron 1978; 20:* 203

7   Klein RG, Arnaud SB, Gallagher JC et al. *J Clin Invest 1977; 60:* 253

8   Wong EG, Siemsen AW, Sugihara JG, Coburn JW. *Contrib Nephrol 1980; 18:* 152

9   Graf H, Stummvoll HK, Kovarik J et al. *Proc EDTA 1980; 17:* 736

10   Davison AM, Peacock M, Walker GS et al. *Clin Endocrinol 1977; 7:* 91S

Proc EDTA (1983) Vol 20

TRANSFUSION-INDUCED ANERGY: SKIN TEST AS AN INDEX FOR PRETRANSPLANT TRANSFUSIONS

F Valderrábano, F Anaya, R Pérez-García, E Olivas, F Vasconez, R Jofre

Hospital Provincial de Madrid, Spain

Summary

Cell-mediated immunity in vivo was studied by delayed cutaneous hypersensitivity (DCH) to seven antigens in 156 chronic haemodialysis (HD) patients, using a disposable multipuncture device. Anergy was found in 46.8 per cent of patients, and a positive correlation was seen between anergy and female sex, time on HD, glomerulonephritis as primary renal disease, younger age and previous blood transfusions (BT).

The effect of BT on DCH was studied prospectively in 29 responsive patients. A significant decrease in DCH response was seen. The transfusion-induced anergy remained for a variable time. The pretransplant BT policy suggested by our data would be to periodically undertake skin tests and to transfuse only responsive patients, thereby avoiding the adverse effects of multiple BT.

Introduction

Depression of cell-mediated immunity in chronic renal failure (CRF) is well known. By studying delayed cutaneous hypersensitivity (DCH) to different antigens previous studies have demonstrated that reactions are weaker and less frequent in uraemic patients [1].

Several authors have shown a relationship between the outcome of renal transplantation and the degree of depression of cell-mediated immunity measured by DCH to dinitrochlorobenzene (DNCB) [2–5].

In addition, the beneficial effect of pretransplant blood transfusions (BT) on kidney graft survival is well documented [6], but the possible influence of BT on DCH has not been reported.

The purpose of the present study is to evaluate the response to DCH recall antigens in a population of CRF patients using an easy and reproducible test, attempting to define those factors which might determine the depression of cell-mediated immunity and also its spontaneous evolution. Finally, the effect of BT on DCH was studied prospectively.

Patients and methods

A group of 156 stable chronic haemodialysis (HD) patients were studied. There were 86 males and 70 females with an age range from 12–70 years. All patients were dialysed for four to five hours three times weekly.

In those patients and in 51 healthy controls we tested DCH to seven recall antigens using a disposable plastic device containing a 70 per cent glycerinated solution of the antigens ready to use by multipuncture application (Multitest®).

The antigens were tetanus (550,000 Mérieux units/ml), diphtheria (1,100,000 Mérieux units/ml), streptococcus (2,000 Mérieux units/ml), tuberculin (300,000 IU/ml), candida (2,000 Mérieux units/ml), tricophyton (150 Mérieux units/ml) and proteus (150 Mérieux units/ml), while a 70 per cent glycerin dilution was provided as a negative control.

Multipuncture was performed in an area of the forearm and the reaction (diameter of induration to each antigen) was measured at 48 hours, by the same person, considering positive 2mm or more of induration, and total score the sum of positive reactions in millimetres.

According to the score patients were classified: anergic (less than 5mm); responsive (more than 10mm); and intermediate (between 5 and 10mm).

The results of the skin tests were correlated with several variables including age, sex, time on HD, primary renal disease, previous BT, ABO blood group, HLA tissue typing, haematocrit, total serum proteins, serum albumin and transferrin, HBs antigen, HBs and HBc antibodies, lymphocytotoxic antibodies and previous maximum lymphocytotoxic antibody titre.

To study the effect of BT on DCH, 29 responsive patients received one unit of packed red cells and skin tests were carried out again after one month. Seventeen of these patients were also tested six and 12 months after BT. Five patients received several BT (2–5 units) and skin tests were repeated after each BT.

A control group of 19 responsive patients did not receive BT and were followed up for a six month period.

The spontaneous evolution of DCH during six and 12 months was studied in a group of 40 patients with different scores (anergic, responsive and intermediate) that did not receive any BT.

During the study, 16 tested patients were grafted from cadaver donors, and the outcome was evaluated in relation with the score. Seventeen patients previously grafted were also tested at different times after transplantation.

Statistical analysis was by the χ^2 test, paired and unpaired t test and Dunnet test.

Results

Table I shows the distribution of healthy controls and patients according to the DCH reaction, and its relationship to patient's sex, age, primary renal disease, time on HD and previous BT.

339

TABLE I. Absolute number and percentage of controls and chronic renal failure patients according to the delayed cutaneous hypersensitivity response

| | Healthy controls | Chronic renal failure patients | | | | | | | | | | | | | | |
| | | Total | Sex | | Age (years) | | Primary renal disease | | | | | Time on HD | | Previous BT | |
			M	F	<40	>40	GN	PN	CRD	RVD	AU	<1 year	>1 year	Yes	No
Anergic															
Number	3	73	30	43	38	37	33	23	7	8	6	23	58	63	10
(%)	(5.8)	(46.8)	(34.8)	(61.4)	(60.3)	(39.7)	(67.3)	(48.9)	(33.3)	(30.7)	(50)	(43.3)	(56.3)	(54.7)	(24.3)
Intermediate															
Number	9	32	18	14	11	20	10	6	4	8	2	4	17	19	13
(%)	(17.8)	(20.5)	(21)	(20)	(17.4)	(21.5)	(20.5)	(12.8)	(19.1)	(30.8)	(20)	(11.4)	(18.4)	(16.5)	(31.7)
Responsive															
Number	39	51	38	13	14	36	6	18	10	10	4	22	24	33	18
(%)	(76.4)	(32.7)	(44.2)	(18.6)	(22.3)	(38.8)	(12.2)	(38.3)	(47.6)	(38.5)	(30)	(45.3)	(25.3)	(28.8)	(44)
TOTAL	51	156	86	70	63	93	49	47	21	26	12	53	103	115	41
	$p<0.0001$	$p<0.01$			$p<0.05$		$p<0.01$					$p<0.05$		$p<0.01$	

GN   Glomerulonephritis
PN   Pyelonephritis
CRD Congenital renal disease
RVD Renal vascular disease
AU   Aetiology uncertain
HD   Haemodialysis
BT   Blood transfusions

340

Normal controls

Only three (5.8%) controls were anergic, whereas 39 (76.4%) were responsive and nine (17.8%) intermediate. All the male controls were responsive, but only 63.6 per cent of females.

CRF patients

Seventy-three patients were anergic (46.8%), 51 responsive (32.7%) and 32 intermediate (20.5%) (p<0.0001 compared to the normal controls).

The mean number of positive antigens was 3.2 ± 0.06 in the responsive patients, and 0.3 ± 0.06 ($\overline{X}$ ± SEM) in the anergic patients (p<0.0005).

Anergy was more frequent in female (61.4%) than in male patients (34.8%) (p<0.01), and in patients younger than 40 years (p<0.05). A higher incidence of anergy was also found in relation with glomerulonephritis as primary renal disease (p<0.01) and time on HD. The mean score decreases as time on HD increases (Figure 1), and there was statistical difference in the score of patients on HD during more than one year (p<0.05).

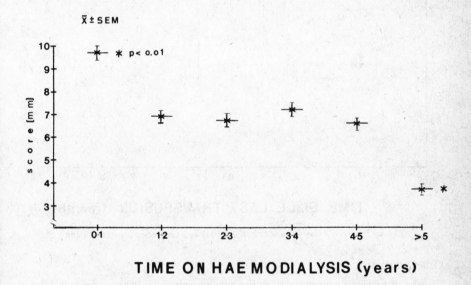

TIME ON HAEMODIALYSIS (years)

Figure 1. Score ($\overline{X}$ ± SEM) according to time on haemodialysis

Previous BT

Anergy was significantly more frequent in previously transfused than in non-transfused patents (p<0.01). Otherwise, the mean number of blood units

341

received by all the anergic patients was greater ($\overline{X}$: 7.5 ± 1.1) than that received by responsive ones ($\overline{X}$: 3.4 ± 0.6, $\overline{X}$ ± SEM) (p<0.005).

Figure 2 demonstrates the relationship between score and time since previous transfusion. Mean score was lower in patients who received their last transfusion within four months before test. When skin tests were done after five or more months from the last transfusion the scores were higher and with greater variation.

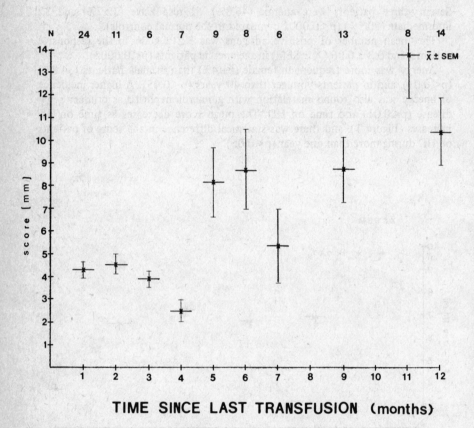

Figure 2. Relation between score ($\overline{X}$ ± SEM) and time since last transfusion

Other parameters

There was no significant correlation between anergy and ABO blood group, HLA tissue typing (A, B or DR), haematocrit, total serum proteins, serum albumin and transferrin, HBs and HBc antibodies, and HBs antigen, although nine out of 15 (60 per cent) Hbs positive antigen patients (carriers) were anergic.

There was no difference in the lymphocytotoxic antibody value, but the maximum previous value was higher in anergic than in responsive patients (17.3 ± 3.9% versus 4.4 ± 1.9% ($\overline{X}$ ± SEM) p<0.01).

342

Effect of BT on DCH

Figure 3 shows the decrease of the score in all responsive patients that prospectively received one unit of packed red cells. Mean score fell from 17.3 ± 1.3mm before BT to 5.2 ± 0.6mm ($\overline{X}$ ± SEM) one month later (p<0.0001). Sixteen became anergic, 10 intermediate and three remained responsive, but showing a marked decrease in the score.

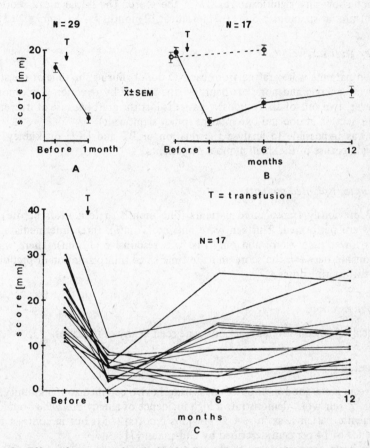

Figure 3. Effect of one unit of packed red cells on the score. A: decrease at one month in 29 responsive patients (p<0.0001). B and C: follow-up at one, six and 12 months after transfusion in 17 responsive patients (B: $\overline{X}$ ± SEM. Open circles: control group of 19 non-transfused responsive patients)

Follow-up at six and 12 months showed an increase in the mean score, although some patients remained anergic at one year, while others recovered a responsive state at six months.

343

No change in the score was observed in the control group of 19 non-transfused responsive patients at six months (Figure 3 B).

Patients who received repeated BT showed a different decrease in the score after each BT.

Spontaneous evolution of DCH

The follow-up at six and 12 months of DCH tests in 40 non-transfused patients did not show any significant change in the score. The initial mean score was 5.4 ± 1mm, at six months 5.5 ± 0.7mm and at 12 months 4.4 ± 1.1mm ($\overline{X} \pm$ SEM).

Kidney graft survival

Sixteen patients were grafted from cadaver donors during the time of the study. Ten were anergic and none of them lost the kidney by rejection at six months. However, two out of six responsive patients lost the graft because of irreversible acute rejection at one and two months (p not significant).

It was impossible to analyse the relation of BT and DCH on kidney graft survival because of the small number of patients.

DCH in transplanted patients

In 17 previously transplanted patients (one month to four years before) skin tests were performed. Thirteen were anergic (76.4%), three intermediate with scores lower than 8mm, and only one was responsive (12mm). There was no relationship between the score and the time since transplantation or prednisone and azathioprine doses.

Adverse reactions

No local or general adverse reactions were seen in any of the cases.

Discussion

Skin tests are a good method of measuring in vivo cell-mediated immunity. The results of our work demonstrate a high incidence of anergy in a wide population of uraemic patients, as in several previous reports[2—5], but in contrast to an incidence of 14 per cent described by Guttmann [7].

The main factors related to the anergic state were in our experience female sex, time on HD, glomerulonephritis as primary renal disease, younger age and previous BT. Higher incidence of anergy in female sex has also been reported in normal controls [8] and CRF patients [1, 5, 7]. Time on HD increases the incidence of anergy as has been shown by Watson et al [5] and Guttman et al [7]. The latter author pointed out the association between anergy and age in contrast with our data.

The relationship of anergy and previous BT has been stressed by Watson et al [4] in a retrospective analysis. We have confirmed this observation in retrospect, and this fact prompted us to make a prospective study of the effect of BT on DCH.

All our patients were in a stable clinical situation, and no correlation was seen between anergy and haematocrit or serum proteins. We have not studied DCH in malnourished patients, a situation which probably may affect DCH. No relation was seen with ABO groups, HLA tissue typing and HB markers, although anergy is predominant in HBs antigen carriers.

A higher maximum lymphocytotoxic antibody activity observed in anergic patients suggests a relationship with the greater number of BT received by these patients.

The multipuncture test used in this work has been shown to be a simple, safe and reproducible method. Non-transfused patients keep the same score up to one year and no adverse reactions were seen.

Some authors emphasise the advantage of DNCB over other antigens because it is a new antigen and the test does not measure the patient's immunological memory [4, 5]. However, some severe adverse reactions have been reported [9].

The multipuncture test used in this study has a wide number of antigens, is easier to use and more reliable than intradermal tests.

The main conclusion of our work is that DCH can be modified by transfusions, and responsive patients converted to anergic. This means that in a good nutritional state DCH is not a stable parameter. Immunosuppression depresses DCH also, as may be suggested from our data.

The change in the immune response induced by BT could be in relation to the beneficial effect of pretransplant BT on renal allograft survival. Weak response to skin tests is correlated with the outcome of kidney transplantation as shown by different authors [2–5], and our results are suggestive in this sense.

Our data demonstrate that transfusions induce anergy, but a high number of cases are necessary to differentiate the effect of spontaneous and transfusion-induced anergy on graft survival. However, the results reported by Watson et al [5] suggest that the beneficial effect of BT is independent of the influence of the anergic state on the outcome of renal transplantation.

In this way we conclude that DCH is a good index for transfusion requirements in patients awaiting kidney transplantation. The controversy concerning the optimum number of BT and the optimum interval between BT and transplantation may be explained by our results. Transfusion-induced anergy persists during a variable time, and some patients convert to a responsive state early while others remain anergic one year after BT. According to that, the pretransplant BT policy would be to perform DCH tests periodically and to transfuse only to responsive patients. This may avoid the adverse effects of BT in CRF patients [10].

References

1   Traeger J, Touraine JL, Navarro J et al. *Proc EDTA 1980; 17:* 375
2   Rolley RT, Sterioff S, Parks LC et al. *Transplant Proc 1977; 9:* 81
3   Diamondopoulos AA, Hamilton DNH, Briggs JD. *Proc EDTA 1978; 15:* 283
4   Watson MA, Briggs JD, Diamondopoulos AA et al. *Lancet 1979; ii:* 1323

5   Watson MA, Hamilton DNH, Briggs JD et al. *Proc EDTA 1981; 18:* 387
6   Opelz G, Terasaki PI. *Transplantation 1980; 29:* 153
7   Guttmann RD, Meakins JL, Morehouse DD et al. *Kidney Int 1981; 20:* 275
8   Dabouis G, Degroix G, Fiere A et al. *Med Oncology, Abstr 5th Annual Meeting Med Oncology Soc, Nice, December 1979.* Berlin: Springer-Verlag. Abstract number 89, 23
9   McDaniel DH, Blatchley DM, Welton WA. *Arch Dermatol 1982; 118:* 371
10 Moore SB. *Mayo Clin Proc 1982; 57:* 431

Open Discussion

HAMILTON (Glasgow) We have extensive experience of the dinitrochlorobenzene skin test in the same situation as you have described. In our data from the year before deliberate blood transfusion studying the effect of blood given on clinical grounds, we also noticed the transfused patients had a lower DNCB skin reactivity which we, in fact, interpreted very cautiously as being some common effect on the marrow. I congratulate you on your bold alternative explanation of your findings. Since Professor Terasaki is the Chairman my question is, did your reactive patients show any increased incidence of antibody formation during the deliberate blood transfusion?

VALDERRÁBANO No, we have seen no correlation between cytotoxic antibody titre and the skin test, but analysing the highest titre of cytotoxic antibody we have seen that in anergic patients it is higher than responsive patients, but we feel that this is related to the greater number of transfusions received by anergic patients.

TERASAKI (Chairman) Following up on that question, you mention that you had six patients that were responsive, were those six patients transfused?

VALDERRÁBANO Well some of these patients were previously transfused and others not. The number of transplanted patients was small, only 16 and really it is impossible to differentiate the effect of spontaneous and transfusion-induced anergy. I feel that we need a larger number of patients to differentiate this effect.

TERASAKI Yes but I was wondering if these patients were responsive and despite transfusion did not lower their immune response. You mention that patients who are transfused have a lower response, they are anergic, but it is possible that these six patients after transfusion did not respond.

VALDERRÁBANO One of the patients who rejected the kidney was transfused and the other was not.

TERASAKI The others were not transfused and were responsive from the beginning.

346

VALDERRÁBANO Yes, anergy induced by transfusion is variable from one patient to another. In some patients we have made repeat transfusions and we have seen a different decrease in the score after each transfusion.

TERASAKI So does that then mean that possibly your failure is due to the fact that those patients were not transfused, not because they were responsive. If you say that your responsive patients were not transfused then it's possible that you divided your patients only according to whether they had been transfused, those are the non-responsive, and the patients who were not transfused, those were your responsive patients.

VALDERRÁBANO In both groups (anergic and responsive) we have patients transfused and non-transfused and at different times before transplantation.

BARNES (Birmingham) I was interested you were using seven different antigens. Was there any difference in the discriminating value one against the other or was it necessary to use quite as many as that? Could you have got the same result by just using two antigens?

VALDERRÁBANO I feel that in our area we have a high incidence of tuberculine positive reactions. One of the advantages of this method is the fact that using seven different antigens we obtain good information about the immune response of the patient, and not only the immunological memory.

BARNES Have you analysed any difference between any of the antigens? Are they all necessary or could you dispense with one or two of them?

VALDERRÁBANO No, we have only analysed the score of the patient.

PERDUE (Los Angeles) You showed a quite dramatic effect with the single packed cell transfusion in 29 responsive patients. Had those patients received this as an initial transfusion or had some or all of them had transfusions prior to this responsive state?

VALDERRÁBANO No, none of these patients were transfused in the one year before, but some patients had received transfusion more than one year before.

WILLIAMS (Chairman) You did not mention pregnancy as a possible factor influencing your findings in your tests. Did you look at this in the female patients?

VALDERRÁBANO Well we analysed the high incidence in the female sex but there was no relation with previous pregnancies.

PERAINO (Houston) I believe you showed that blood transfusion and time on haemodialysis was associated with an increasing precentage of anergy. Are they additive or can you account for one in terms of the other?

VALDERRÁBANO I think that transfusions are an additive factor to time on haemodialysis.

INTERLEUKIN-2 PRODUCTION AFTER BLOOD TRANSFUSIONS IN PROSPECTIVE KIDNEY TRANSPLANT RECIPIENTS

J C Gluckman, D Klatzmann, F Triebel, J Rottembourg, C Foucault, E Brisson, U Assogba, F Metivier*

*U.E.R. Pitié Salpétrière, *Hôpital Broussais, Paris, France*

Summary

We have investigated whether suppression of the allogeneic response after blood transfusion (BT) could be due to inhibition of the production or activity of Interleukin-2 (IL-2), a soluble mediator involved in T lymphocyte proliferation. Reduction of IL-2 production after BT was less frequent than, but significantly associated with, non specific MLR suppression. However, MLR suppressor cells did not inhibit the release of IL-2 from autologous pre-BT lymphocytes. In addition, post-BT soluble suppressor factors of the MLR did not affect the ability of IL-2 to promote cell proliferation. Thus, although MLR suppression after BT is associated with reduced IL-2 production, this is not a major mechanism involved in this effect.

Introduction

Blood transfusion (BT) in uraemic patients can induce the generation of mixed lymphocyte reaction (MLR) suppressor cells [1], some of which may act through the production of soluble suppressor factors (SF) [2]. Such a mechanism might explain the beneficial effect of prior BT on kidney graft survival [3]. It has recently been shown, in experimental models, that suppression of the response to conventional antigens [4] or to alloantigens [5] could be mediated by the regulation of Interleukin-2 (IL-2) production or function. IL-2, a lymphokine which is released by sensitised T cells, is considered the second signal in T cell activation [6], inducing the proliferation only of antigen- (or lectin-) preactivated helper and cytolytic T cells. Therefore its activity is required in those immunological responses where T cell proliferation takes place.

This study investigates whether suppression of the allogeneic response after BT in man could be due to inhibition of IL-2 production and/or activity.

Patients and methods

Eighteen previously non-transfused uraemic patients awaiting kidney transplantation received two or three transfusions of packed blood from different donors, given at three to four week intervals.

Lymphocytes were obtained from each donor. They were collected sequentially from the patients prior to and after each BT. They were cryopreserved in liquid nitrogen and all samples from a given patient were assayed in single retrospective experiments to eliminate test-to-test variations. One-way MLR was performed with stimulating cells from each of the blood donors and from a control lymphocyte pool of 10 unrelated subjects [1].

For IL-2 production, lymphocytes were adjusted to 1×10^6 cells/ml in Culture Medium and stimulated by 1% PHA-M (DIFCO) as previously described [7]. Supernatants were collected after 48 hours. In some experiments, supernatants were obtained from patients cells which had been specifically stimulated for two to six days by cells from one of the donors.

Culture supernatants were assayed for IL-2 activity by a microtitration technique on an IL-2 dependent, PHA-unresponsive, cultured human T cell line (CTC) [7]. IL-2 concentration in an unknown sample was measured by the mitogenic activity of serial dilutions on CTC in a 72 hour ^{3}H-Thymidine incorporation assay. Units were calculated by comparison with the activity of a standard preparation containing by definition 1U/ml, as previously described [7].

Results

Immune responsiveness before BT

Lymphocyte reactivity of the patients prior to BT did not differ significantly from that of normal donors in the MLR against pooled allogeneic cells (Log_{10} cpm = 4.88 ± 0.32 versus 4.79 ± 0.36) or in the mitogenic response to PHA (Log_{10} cpm = 4.98 ± 0.21 versus 5.06 ± 0.11). There was a very wide variation in the production of IL-2 by the patients as well as by the control group, but the values observed in both were similar (0.81 ± 0.40 U/ml and 0.81 ± 0.50).

A significant correlation was observed in both populations between IL-2 production and the intensity of the MLR to the control pool (r = 0.501, p<0.05 and r = 0.563, p<0.01), but not with responsiveness to PHA. However, supernatants from two to six day MLR were consistently negative for IL-2 activity. This finding confirms previous observations in man and it is best explained by the fact that MLR-activated T cells express receptors for IL-2 and can therefore adsorb the IL-2 synthesised [8].

IL-2 production and MLR response after BT

Seventy-nine post-BT lymphocyte samples were tested in parallel for IL-2 production and MLR and compared to pre-BT values. MLR was non-specifically reduced in 11 out of 17 samples (65%) with decreased IL-2 production (p<0.01),

TABLE I. Non-specific suppression of the MLR after blood transfusion (BT) is not IL-2 related

Responder cells	Modulating cells	MLR to stimulators from: 1st blood donor net cpm[1]	1st blood donor % suppression[2]	2nd blood donor net cpm	2nd blood donor % suppression	IL-2 production U/ml	IL-2 production % suppression[3]
(1) Pre-BT	–	76.0		64.8		0.85	
(2) Pre-BT	Pre-BT*[4]	52.3		41.9		1.25	
(3) Pre-BT*[5]	–					1.45	
(4) Post-BT	–	25.8	67	42.9	34	0.80	6
(5) Pre-BT	Post-BT	46.6	39	38.1	41	0.70	15
(6) Pre-BT	Post-BT*	33.1	37	21.8	48	1.00	5
(7) Post-BT*	–					1.05	26

[1] net cpm = (cpm allogeneic – cpm control) x 10^{-3}

[2] % suppression = (1 – net cpm test/net cpm control) x 100. Lines (4) and (5) versus line (1), line (6) versus line (2)

[3] % suppression line (4) = (1 – (4)/(1)) x 100
(5) = (1 – (5)/[(1) + (4)/2]) x 100
(6) = (1 – (6)/[(1) + (7)/2]) x 100
(7) = (1 – (7)/(3)) x 100

[4] *indicates 20 Gy irradiated modulating cells

[5] *indicates 12 Gy irradiated responder cells

351

TABLE II. Supernatants from specifically stimulated post-BT lymphocytes, with reduced MLR, express unmodified IL-2 production and do not inhibit growth of PHA-activated pre-BT lymphocytes

Experiment

$(RnxD_2*)$

	3 days		2 days		6 days	
	Supernate + R_0*^2 + PHA $\rightarrow$ IL-2		Supernate $\rightarrow$ IL-2			
	$(RnxD_2*)$ + PHA					
Assay :	:		:		: MLR	
Lymphocyte[1] sample	U/ml	% suppression[3]	U/ml	% suppression	net cpm[4]	% suppression
R_0	2.05		4.45		174.8	
R_2	2.05	0	4.35	2	87.4	50
R_3	1.95	5	4.70	-5	135.7	24
R_6	2.15	-5	4.25	4	110.2	37
R_7	1.85	10	4.90	-10	151.2	13

[1] Lymphocyte samples: R_0 = before BT, R_2 = 30 days after the 1st BT, R_3 = 10 days after the 2nd BT, R_6 = 30 days after the 3rd BT, R_7 = 90 days after the third BT. D_2* = 20 Gy irradiated stimulating cells from the second donor.

[2] * indicates 12 Gy irradiated cells.

[3] % suppression as in Table I.

[4] net cpm x 10^{-3}

352

unchanged in 21 of 23 samples (64%) with unmodified IL-2 production (p<0.05), and augmented in nine of 10 samples (90%) with increased IL-2 production (p<0.001).

However, post-BT lymphocytes which could suppress the MLR of autologous pre-BT lymphocytes when mixed in three-cell experiments had no suppressive effect on IL-2 production (Table I).

These results indicate that MLR variations after BT cannot exclusively be ascribed to modifications of IL-2 production.

MLR supernatants from post-BT lymphocytes and IL-2 activity

It is currently assumed that immunological suppression results from the activation of a circuit of suppressor T cells. In one of the proposed models [4], antigen-specific suppressor T cells produce antigen-specific suppressor factors which arm acceptor T cells, and these latter liberate a non-specific inhibitor of IL-2 production.

To test this hypothesis we examined whether supernatants of post-BT lymphocytes specifically stimulated in vitro by cells of a blood donor, and whose own allogeneic proliferation was reduced, had decreased IL-2 production when compared to similarly treated pre-BT cells (Table II). Therefore patient lymphocytes were co-cultured with irradiated donor cells. After a three day incubation the supernatant was collected and replaced with fresh medium containing PHA so as to obtain detectable IL-2 activity. This supernatant was collected after a two day incubation and tested for IL-2 activity. Neither modification of IL-2 production nor inhibition of its production from PHA-activated pre-BT lymphocytes could be noted under these conditions.

However SF released by suppressor cells might act as IL-2 inhibitors [9] which could block the action, but not the production, of IL-2. To exclude this possibility, SF, which had been prepared exactly as previously reported [2] were added to CTC in the presence of the standard (1U/ml) IL-2 preparation. In these experiments proliferation of CTC was not affected by those SF that clearly inhibited (approximately 40%) the MLR.

Discussion

Uraemia is known to impair the immune response, but this concept has never been critically analysed. The data presented here are at variance with other reports [10] although they confirm our previous findings [1,3] that at least proliferation to mitogens and to alloantigens is in the normal range prior to blood transfusion. It is thus unlikely that a previously deficient reactivity interferes with the BT effect [3].

We have recently demonstrated the occurrence of suppressor cells in the peripheral blood of uraemic patients who had received prospective blood transfusions [1,2]. Two different types of suppression have been suggested: one appears to be alloantigen non-specific whereas the other seems to be specific for HLA-DR antigens. In this study we tested, therefore, whether suppressor cells had any effects on the release of IL-2 from in vitro activated lymphocytes.

353

The first observation was that non-specific MLR suppression after BT was associated with, but could not be exclusively due to, low production of IL-2. Moreover, suppressor cells did not inhibit the release of IL-2 from specifically sensitised producer lymphocytes. In addition SF had no detectable effect on the growth promoting activity of IL-2 or CTC. Thus MLR suppression must act through another, still unknown, mechanism since it cannot be explained either by inhibition of IL-2 production or by interference with the functional interaction of IL-2 with receptor T cells.

As suggested by our findings when comparing IL-2 production and response to PHA, a dissociation between the ability to synthesise IL-2 and to respond to it is possible under some conditions. Diminished responses could be due to a selective defect in the response to IL-2. Indeed such responsiveness is acquired, after lymphocyte activation, through the expression of a surface receptor, and suppression could prevent these cells from becoming responsive to IL-2 by modulating the expression of this receptor. Further investigations aimed at studying this hypothesis by absorption experiments [8] or with anti-receptor specific monoclonal antibodies, when they are available, have to be undertaken before ruling out inhibition of IL-2 action as a mechanism of the BT effect.

Acknowledgments

This work was supported by INSERM (CRL 81 50 35) and by the Ministère de la Recherche et de l'Industrie (contrat No. 82 L 1313).

References

1   Klatzmann D, Gluckman JC, Foucault C et al. *Transplantation 1983; 35:* 332
2   Klatzmann D, Bensussan A, Gluckman JC et al. *Transplantation:* in press
3   Klatzmann D, Gluckman JC, Foucault C et al. *Proc EDTA 1982; 19:* 453
4   Malkovsky M, Asherson GL, Stockinger B et al. *Nature 1982; 300:* 652
5   Kramer M, Koszinowski U. *J Immunol 1982; 128:* 784
6   Coutinho A, Larsson EL, Grönvik KO et al. *Eur J Immunol 1979; 9:* 587
7   Azogui O, Gluckman E, Fradelizi D. *J Immunol:* in press
8   Bonnard GD, Yasaka K, Jacobson D. *J Immunol 1979; 123:* 2704
9   Hardt C, Röllinghoff M, Pfizenmaier M et al. *J Exp Med 1981; 154:* 262
10 Birkeland SA. *Scand J Immunol 1976; 5:* 107

Open Discussion

SELLS (Liverpool)   I wonder if you have studied IL-2 production in lymphocytes from patients on Cyclosporin A?

GLUCKMAN   No, I have not studied patients on Cyclosporin A, but I think that it is reduced. It has been previously demonstrated that IL-2 production in patients treated by Cyclosporin A is reduced.

354

POZUANSKI (Frankfurt) What time after blood transfusion did you take the blood from the patient?

GLUCKMAN The blood was drawn 10 days and one month after each transfusion.

POZUANSKI Did you try to make the MLR just right after the blood transfusion?

GLUCKMAN No.

TERASAKI (Chairman) Would you say, in the first instance, that blood transfusions produced suppressor cells?

GLUCKMAN Yes.

TERASAKI That's definite, would you say?

GLUCKMAN It is what we have observed.

TERASAKI Secondly, would you say that IL-2 production is not affected by transfusion?

GLUCKMAN No, I think that approximately 65 per cent of patients who have reduced IL-2 production after blood transfusion have reduced MLR. There is a relationship certainly between IL-2 production and blood transfusion but the reduction of IL-2 production cannot be ascribed to the suppressor cells. Each time that we did three cell co-culture experiments which we felt would suppress the MLR we could not show suppression of IL-2 production. If IL-2 is reduced after blood transfusion I don't know the mechanism but it is not the suppressor cells of the MLR.

Proc EDTA (1983) Vol 20

DIFFERENTIAL DIAGNOSIS OF CYCLOSPORIN A NEPHROTOXICITY VERSUS REJECTION BY FINE NEEDLE ASPIRATION BIOPSY

P Häyry, E von Willebrand, J Ahonen

University of Helsinki, Helsinki, Finland

Summary

Twelve transplants with signs of graft failure and five with good function on CyA, were aspiration biopsied and analysed for (a) the presence of inflammation, (b) morphological changes in the graft parenchymal cells and (c) by indirect immunofluorescence for the presence of CyA in the renal tubular cells. Four reaction patterns were recorded: (i) good transplants with a normal serum creatinine, no evidence of inflammation, no parenchymal cell changes and no deposits of CyA in the graft; (ii) patients with elevated serum creatinine, no inflammation but distinct parenchymal cell changes and massive deposits of CyA (i.e., nephrotoxicity); (iii) patients with elevated serum creatinine, distinct inflammation in situ, modest tubular cell changes and no CyA in the graft (i.e., rejection); and (iv) patients with elevated serum creatinine, distinct inflammation in situ, distinct tubular cell changes and concomitant deposits of CyA (i.e., nephrotoxicity and rejection). CyA deposits in the graft had only a marginal relationship to drug dose and concentration of the drug in serum. When the dose was reduced, the deposits rapidly disappeared and tubular cell changes resolved. We recommend the FNAB for differentiating between nephrotoxicity and rejection in renal transplants.

Introduction

Among the practical difficulties in the clinical use of Cyclosporin A (CyA) are the nephrotoxic and hepatotoxic effects of this drug. These difficulties are even more pronounced when a differential diagnosis of rejection must be made, especially if the transplant is complicated by prolonged acute tubular necrosis (ATN). Although some investigators have claimed that specific histological changes are recorded in renal biopsies [1,2] others have failed to confirm this [3,4].

Fine needle aspiration biopsy (FNAB) is an atraumatic method of assessing intragraft events in parenchymal organ transplantation in man [5,6]. In this study we have analysed 27 consecutive aspiration biopsies performed on human renal allografts in cases of suspected Cyclosporin toxicity, rejection and quiescence. In addition to analysing the cytological changes in graft parenchymal cells, we have analysed the deposition of CyA in the grafts by indirect immunofluorescence and correlated these changes to the serum creatinine, dose of CyA and serum concentration of the drug.

Materials and methods

Thirteen of the 27 patients received initially only CyA (10mg/kg/d) i.v. adjusted to produce a plasma concentration of approximately 200–300ng/ml after i.v. administration for three days; the remaining also received initial methylprednisolone (MP), 3.6mg/kg/d tapered to 0mg in nine days. All rejection episodes were treated by elevating the oral dose of MP to 3.6mg/kg/d until inflammatory cells disappeared from the aspirates. Repeated episodes necessitated routine administration of approximately 0.1–0.5mg/kg/d of MP for basic immunosuppression to 24 of these patients from the third week onwards.

Plasma concentrations of CyA were determined by radioimmunoassay, using the standard Sandox RIA-kit nr. 031180 (Sandoz Pharmaceuticals, Basle) [7].

Fine needle aspiration biopsies were performed as previously described [6], and several cytocentrifuged cell preparations were made from these specimens. One of the preparations was stained with May-Grünwald-Giemsa [6] to quantify the morphological changes in the graft parenchymal component and to assess, if any, the inflammatory events in the graft.

One or more duplicate FNAB specimens were fixed with cold acetone for 15 min, treated with 1:1000 diluted rabbit anti-Cyclosporin serum (courtesy of Sandoz Co), and subsequently with 1:20 diluted FITC-conjugated swine anti-rabbit IgG (Dakopats, Copenhagen). The antiserum has been reported to be specific for CyA and to a number of (still unidentified) split products of this drug [7]. Occasionally indirect PAP-peroxidase technique was used instead of immunofluorescence. The frequency and amount of CyA in the graft parenchymal cells was assessed from coded FITC-stained specimens mixed with normal rabbit serum treated control specimens by scoring the intensity of reaction from 0 to 3+.

On three occasions, a concomitant needle and/or open biopsy was performed. Part of the biopsy was snap-frozen in liquid nitrogen, cut and immunoperoxidase or immunofluorescence evaluation was performed from the frozen section specimens as above.

Results

In good grafts, with entirely normal serum creatinine, there was no inflammation in the graft, no or only very modest tubular cell changes and no or only faint deposits of CyA demonstrable by immunofluorescence.

Four different patterns of alterations were delineated in cases of elevated serum creatinine (Table I).

The first pattern consisted of no inflammation, distinct though not extreme

TABLE I. Differential diagnosis of renal transplant failure by FNAB

S-creat	FNAB			Explanation
	Inflammation	Tubular cell changes	CyA deposits in graft	
Normal	-	±	±	Good graft
Elevated	-	++	-	ATN
Elevated	-	+++	+++	CyA toxicity
Elevated	+++	+	-	Rejection
Elevated	+++*	+++	+++	Rejection *and* CyA toxicity

*The possibility that CyA deposits occasionally induce some inflammation, is not entirely excluded. (From von Willebrand and Häyry, Transplant Proc 1983; In press)

tubular cell changes and no CyA deposits in the graft. All these cases fell within the postoperative period, and because they coincided with the clinical signs of postoperative acute tubular necrosis, they were interpreted as being due to ATN.

In the second pattern distinct changes, including swelling, vacuolisation and inclusions, were recorded in the tubular cells. This pattern was associated with distinct deposits of CyA in the graft but no inflammation in the specimen. These cases were interpreted as being due only to CyA toxicity.

In the third pattern, the biopsy was dominated by pronounced inflammation with modest tubular cell changes and no CyA deposits in the graft. These cytological alterations entirely coincided with those described previously for acute renal allograft rejection.

In the final pattern, distinct tubular cell changes were associated with CyA deposits in the graft and, in addition to this, a marked inflammation in situ containing T and B blast cells, lymphocytes and mononuclear phagocytes. On these occasions, an inflammatory response of rejection was apparently going on in the graft in spite of maximal cyclosporin therapy.

CyA deposits in the graft had no correlation to the drug dose and only a marginal correlation ($p > 0.05$) to the concentration of CyA in the serum.

In the concomitantly obtained immunofluorescence and immunoperoxidase specimens, deposits of CyA were also seen particularly prominent in the proximal tubular cells.

Discussion

Our results demonstrate that deposits of CyA are invariably seen in a renal allograft during episodes of clinical Cyclosporin nephrotoxicity. Similar deposits have been seen in the liver and kidney of liver transplant recipients and in the kidney of bone marrow transplant recipients during CyA therapy. In general, the kidney rather than the liver seems to be the more sensitive organ and a limiting factor for the administration of CyA.

Cyclosporin deposits in the kidney are associated with marked changes in the graft tubular cells and more modest changes in the vascular endothelial cells. These changes are, as expected, non-specific in nature and similar though more modest changes, are seen, e.g., during acute tubular necrosis and in advanced rejection. Thus direct demonstration of CyA in a renal transplant, is the only clear-cut method of assessing the deposition of this drug in the transplant.

Deposition of CyA is not followed, per se, by any inflammation. This is clearly seen in cases where serum creatinine is strongly elevated, extreme deposits of CyA are seen in the kidney while no inflammation is present in the graft. This observation makes it possible to differentiate between the three most commonly encountered clinical disorders: acute tubular necrosis, rejection and CyA toxicity.

Acknowledgments

Supported by grant 1RO1 AM26882-03 from the National Institutes of Health, Bethesda, Maryland and grants from the Sigrid Juselius Foundation, and the Association of Finnish Life Insurance Companies, Helsinki, Finland.

The authors thank Ms Leena Saraste for secretarial help.

References

1   Marbet UA, Graft U, Mihatsch JM et al. *Schweiz Med Wschr 1980; 110:* 2017
2   Shulman H, Striker G, Deeg HJ et al. *N Engl J Med 1981; 305:* 1392
3   Calne RY, Rolles K, White DJG et al. *Lancet 1979; ii:* 1033
4   Keown PA, Stiller CR, Ulan RA et al. *Lancet 1981; i:* 686
5   Häyry P, von Willebrand E. *Scand J Immunol 1981; 13:* 87
6   Häyry P, von Willebrand E. *Ann Clin Res 1981; 13:* 288
7   Beveridge T, Grathwohl A, Michot F et al. *Curr Ther Res 1981; 30:* 5

Open Discussion

WILLIAMS (Chairman) Did you do a control in which you put a rabbit serum, or rabbit immunoglobin on the cell to prevent it having antibody specificity?

HÄYRY Absolutely, yes.

TAUBE (London) I wonder if you have looked at the mononuclear cell infiltrates in your graphs in which you showed rejection, and Cyclosporin A toxicity, with monoclonal antibodies directed against helper and cytotoxic suppressor cells?

HÄYRY   Yes, we have been analysing that, you mean the composition of infiltrates during rejection under Cyclosporin?

TAUBE Yes, if you've analysed individual episodes of rejection.

359

HÄYRY As most people have found, in most rejection episodes the suppressor killer T-cells infiltrate the graft predominantly. To my knowledge there is one single exception to this rule. This is a paper by Tusveson in Uppsala. They claim that the T-helper cells predominate. We found that in eight out of 10 cases there is a clear suppressor cytotoxic T-cell predominance in the graft regardless of whether we are treating the patient with Cyclosporin or with azathioprine. However, in the remaining two of 10 cases we have found cases where the helper T-cells predominate the infiltrate. Most of these cases were on Cyclosporin, and most of those ended up in irreversible rejection.

Secondly, you asked about the mononuclear cell infiltrates under Cyclosporin. It is a very strange thing, but we see mononuclear phagocyte and lymphocyte dominated inflammatory episodes regularly but very late under Cyclosporin therapy. These may or may not be related to Cyclosporin deposits in the kidney. We don't know if these episodes finally represent a reaction to Cyclosporin, or if they are a strange uncommon type of reaction.

DE VECCHI (Milan) In our experience in several cases of Cyclosporin A toxicity white blood cells in the renal infiltrate have a foamy aspect in their cytoplasm just like that observed in tubular cells. Do you confirm my still small and pre-liminary experience? What is the time interval between Cyclosporin A dose reduction and improvement in renal tubular cell damage?

HÄYRY To answer the first question, our findings are exactly similar. We can also demonstrate similar changes in really severe cases by classic histology or by frozen section histology. We have seen the foamy tubular cells you have seen and in addition mononuclear phagocytes which also incorporate Cyclosporin.

With regard to the second comment, if you reduce the Cyclosporin dose these deposits disappear in a couple of days, in other words extremely quickly. However, about half of the kidneys where you decrease the administration of Cyclosporin end up in rejection. The rejections you can see by the appearance of inflammatory blast cell and lymphocytes as well as mononuclear phagocytes into the graft. That may complicate at least sometimes, the post-reduction course. If you have a clean case with no episode of rejection after reduction of Cyclosporin dose, the serum creatinine level falls rapidly.

ZAZGORNIK (Vienna) Can you give us a comment about the differential diagnosis of Cyclosporin A nephrotoxicity versus rejection in patients with graft tubular damage caused by prolonged warm or cold ischaemia and primary transplant insufficiency?

HÄYRY It is in these situations where we have found aspiration cytology most informative and important. You can easily recognise the changes related to acute tubular necrosis in the graft tubular cells and these changes disappear when the graft resumes its normal function. If you, during this period of time, see inflammatory cells appearing in the graft, this is a rejection. In these cases, in the lack of clinical signs, we treat the inflammation. If you find Cyclosporin deposits in the kidney you know that it is a sign of nephrotoxicity and you must reduce the dose of Cyclosporin. These different patterns make the differential diagnosis very easy. Another thing related to your comment is that there is no difference between initially functioning and non-functioning kidneys to Cyclosporin A. Both do exactly as well or as badly under Cyclosporin therapy.

IMPROVED GRAFT PROGNOSIS BY TREATMENT OF STEROID RESISTANT REJECTIONS WITH ATG AND PLASMAPHERESIS

W Fassbinder, E-H Scheuermann, H J Stutte, P B Bechstein, A Fürsch, W Ernst, W Schoeppe

University Hospital, Frankfurt/Main, FRG

Summary

Conventional therapy of acute rejection is almost exclusively based on increased steroid dosage, however, a considerable number of grafts undergo irreversible steroid resistant rejection (SRR). We investigated in a prospective study the effects of antithymocyte globulin (ATG) and plasmafiltration (PF) in cases of SRR. Acute interstitial rejections were treated with ATG, acute vascular rejections with PF. Thirty-nine of 42 (93%) cases of SRR were reversed by these forms of therapy. In 68 recipients of first cadaveric renal allografts actuarial one year graft survival has improved to 88 ($\pm$5) per cent since the introduction of ATG and PF for SRR. Severe side effects or increased mortality were not observed, none of the patients with either form of therapy died. Thus ATG and PF are valuable adjuncts in the treatment of SRR.

Introduction

Uncontrolled rejection is still the main cause of graft failure after cadaveric human renal transplantation. Therefore every effort should be made to reverse rejection and improve graft prognosis.

Conventional therapy of acute rejection is almost exclusively based on increased steroid dosage. However, a considerable number of grafts fail to improve with this form of therapy, and thereafter undergo irreversible steroid resistant rejection (SRR). In these cases alternative therapy is urgently needed. We decided to treat SRR with antithymocyte-globulin (ATG) or plasmafiltration (PF), and to study the effects of this experimental therapy prospectively.

Patients and methods

Patients Sixty-eight patients, who received their first cadaveric renal transplant between September 1980 and December 1982, formed the experimental group. In these patients SRR was treated with ATG or PF. Forty-four patients, who received their first cadaveric renal transplant between January 1978 and August 1980, in whom acute rejection episodes had been treated exclusively with methylprednisolone pulses, served as historical controls.

Prophylactic antirejection therapy   Our standard prophylactic antirejection therapy (azathioprine and prednisone only) and blood transfusion policy have been published in detail elsewhere [1]. These methods were not changed during both periods.

Diagnosis and therapy of rejection   Rejection was diagnosed, when serum creatinine concentration rose more than 0.5mg/dl within 48 hours, and other causes of deterioration of graft function could be ruled out. Rejection was initially treated with 2–4 1g methyl-prednisolone bolus doses given i.v. every day, or on alternate days in less severe cases. If the rejection was not reversed, a graft biopsy was obtained three to four days after the first pulse. The specimen was examined histologically on the same day. Nomenclature of Zollinger and Mihatsch [2] was used to define different types of acute transplant rejection. When focally accentuated interstitial infiltrates of mononuclear cells were found, *acute interstitial rejection* (AIR) was diagnosed. Here obviously activated T-cells play a predominant pathogenetic role, and therefore ATG therapy was begun on the same day. When signs of a proliferative vasculopathy were found, *acute vascular rejection* (AVR) was diagnosed. As humoral mechanisms may be involved in this type of rejection, cases of AVR were treated with plasmafiltration, which was started 24–36 hrs after graft biopsy, to avoid bleeding complications. After initiation of ATG and/or plasmafiltration no further boluses of methylprednisolone were administered, and oral steroid dosage was reduced to pre-rejection levels.

ATG-therapy   ATG-Fresenius, which is produced in rabbits immunised with a T-lymphoblast cell line [3], was given in a dosage of 3mg/kg/day slowly over a period of eight to 12 hrs i.v. for 10 days.

Plasmafiltration therapy   6 x 5L plasma were filtered within two weeks and replaced by 3.5 per cent Albumin-Ringer-Lactate solution. To prevent complications of severe antibody deficiency, 20g IgG were substituted i.v. after each plasmafiltration. Further details of the procedure have been described elsewhere [4].

Patient and graft survival   Patient- and graft-survival were calculated using the life table method [5]. No patient was excluded for any reason from analysis. Graft failure was defined as patient death or return to dialysis irrespective of cause. Cumulative log-rank-test was used, to compare survival data [5].

Results

In the 68 patients, who formed the experimental study group, a total of 112 acute rejection episodes occurred. Eight patients (11%) never had a rejection episode. Twenty-seven patients (40%) had only one, 21 patients (31%) had two, and 12 patients (18%) had three or more rejection episodes.

The incidence of steroid resistance rejection episodes increased significantly (χ^2 = 6.2; p <0.02) with the number of rejections a patient experienced. Twenty-eight per cent of first rejections, 55 per cent of second rejections and 75 per cent of third rejections were not reversed by bolus methylprednisolone. Graft histology revealed 20 AIR, 19 AVR, and four cases where both types of lesions were found concomitantly (Table I). Experimental therapy, as indicated by the histological type of rejection, was instituted after a mean (± SD) methylprednisolone dosage of 3.4 ± 2.3g/case.

TABLE I. Final outcome of 43 steroid resistant rejection episodes treated with ATG and/ or plasmafiltration (PF)

Type of rejection	Number of cases	Therapy	Reversal of rejection		Serum creatinine concentration (mg/dl; $\overline{X}$ ± SD)			
			yes	no	Before rejection	Peak	2 weeks after rejection	6 months after rejection
AIR	20	ATG	19	1	2.3±0.9	4.8±3.1	2.1±0.8	1.6±0.4
AVR	19	PF	18	1	2.1±0.9	4.5±2.1	2.5±1.4	1.6±0.6
AIR + AVR	4*	ATG+PF†	2	1	1.2±0.4	5.8±3.2	1.4	1.1
Total	43*		39	3				

* One graft lost due to spontaneous rupture before change of therapy; † n = 3

Rejection was reversed in 39 of 42 cases (93%) by experimental therapy. As shown in Table I, serum creatinine concentrations returned to values approximating those before rejection about two weeks after initiation of successful ATG and/or plasmafiltration therapy, and declined further during the next months, thus indicating long-term salvage of the grafts.

Both forms of therapy had acceptable rates of side effects.

ATG: The initial dose(s) of ATG frequently induced fever (up to 40°C) possibly as a sort of 'physiological' response to lymphocytolysis. Continuation of therapy was generally well tolerated and fever reached only lower grades during subsequent infusions. Leucopenia and thrombocytopenia occasionally necessitated interruption of therapy for one or two days during the later course. Phlebitis at the injection site and arthralgia were observed in some cases.

PF: In patients treated with PF clotting of the av-fistula was observed in two cases. This was probably due to antithrombin III deficiency induced by this form of therapy. Other side effects or antibody deficiency syndromes were not observed, as immunoglobulins (20g) were substituted i.v. after each treatment.

Fifteen patients experienced recurrence of acute rejection episodes at various time intervals ranging from two weeks to three months after reversal of SRR, and 11 of these rejection episodes again were steroid resistant. Five patients, in whom recurrence of AIR occurred, received a second course of ATG without particular problems.

The introduction of ATG and/or plasmafiltration as treatment of steroid resistant rejection episodes has significantly improved our graft survival rates (Figure 1). Actuarial graft survival in the actively treated group was 88 (±5) per cent and 85 (±9) per cent one and two years post transplant, whereas it had been 71 (±7) per cent and 64 (±7) per cent at the same time intervals in the historical controls. ATG or plasmafiltration did not increase mortality. Patient survival two years post-transplant was 96 per cent in the actively treated group, while it had been 95 per cent in the historical controls. None of the four patients, who died after the introduction of ATG and plasmafiltration, had received either form of therapy.

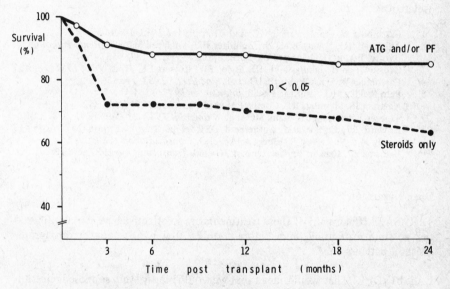

Figure 1. Actuarial kidney graft survival in 44 patients, where acute rejections were treated with steroid only, and in 68 patients, where steroid resistant rejection episodes were treated with ATG and/or plasmafiltration

Discussion

Two different strategies may improve graft survival rates after human cadaveric renal transplantation. One is the prophylactic use of ALG or ATG additional to standard immunosuppressive therapy in order to prevent rejection; this has been proposed by several groups [3,6,7]. The other strategy is, to reserve this and further types of immunosuppressive measures for those patients who do not respond to standard immunosuppressive therapy, as suggested by others [8–10]. The latter policy has obvious advantages, if it is able to reverse the majority of rejections. It maximises the benefit/risk ratio of alternative forms of antirejection therapy, and limits more aggressive modes of immunosuppression to those patients, who urgently need it, whereas immunological low-responders are not put at increased risk.

We found, that ATG and plasmafiltration are highly effective in reversal of steroid resistant rejection, one for acute interstitial rejection, the other for acute vascular rejection. ATG and/or plasmafiltration have to be instituted early, i.e. three to five days after onset of rejection. Neither form of therapy induced predictable long-term tolerance of the graft. Re-rejections of the same or other type do occur, and are then susceptible to reinstitution of ATG or plasma-filtration, as indicated by the histological type of rejection. No severe infections and no added mortality were observed. Thus ATG and plasmafiltration are valuable adjuncts in the treatment of steroid resistant rejection.

References

1   Fassbinder W, Frei U, Persijn GG et al. *Transpl Proc 1982; 14:* 164
2   Zollinger HU, Mihatsch MJ. In Zollinger HU, Mihatsch MJ, eds. *Renal Pathology in Biopsy.* Berlin, Heidelberg, New York: Springer-Verlag. 1978: 565–587
3   Grosse-Wilde H, Jakubowski HD, Eigler FW, Kuwert EK. *Proc EDTA 1981; 18:* 481
4   Fassbinder W, Ernst W, Stutte HJ et al. *Proc EDTA 1982; 19:* 536
5   Peto R, Pike MC, Armitage P et al. *Br J Cancer 1977; 35:* 1
6   Najarian JS, Simmons RL, Condie RM et al. *Ann Surg 1976; 184:* 352
7   Traeger J, Touraine JL, Malik MC et al. *Kidney Int 1983; 23 (Suppl 14):* S74
8   Howard RJ, Condie RM, Sutherland DER et al. *Transplantation 1977; 24:* 419
9   Hardy MA, Nowygrod R, Elberg A, Appel G. *Transplantation 1980; 29:* 162
10   Hoitsma AJ, Reekers P, Kreeftenberg JG et al. *Transplantation 1982; 33:* 12

Open Discussion

TERASAKI (Chairman) If these treatments are so effective have you considered the possibility of using them before steroids, that is not doing it on steroid-resistant patients only?

FASSBINDER That would mean that we would biopsy every supposed rejection and I think, that there are no particular problems with transplant biopsy, but maybe to biopsy every case of suspected rejection would be dangerous.

GUTSCHE (Kiel, FRG) If you encountered mixed forms of rejection i.e. cellular and vascular rejection in the same patient, what kind of treatment should be given when both forms are about equally severe?

FASSBINDER We found mixed rejection in four of 42 cases (10%), and we then put these patients on both forms of therapy, plasma filtration first and afterwards ATG. Three cases were treated like that.

TAUBE (London) I wonder if you could tell us how you actually make the diagnosis of acute vascular rejection. I appreciate you make some sort of diagnosis on the biopsy, but I wonder if you go through the biopsy and look at 10 vessels or 20 vessels and decide what proportion of the vessels show signs of rejection. Do you have any sort of way of grading your biopsies?

FASSBINDER There have to be at least two or three small vessels which show the typical features of acute vascular rejection. Two or three affected vessels are sufficient for our diagnosis.

TAUBE If you don't get any vessels in the biopsy do you re-biopsy?

FASSBINDER Yes, we would perform a second biopsy.

HÄYRY (Helsinki, Finland) I'm not commenting on your study but I think it really is a beautiful piece of work. I would like to comment on the steroid resistant rejection episodes. We have now been treating systematically rejections that we can't overcome by steroids with a very short course of Cyclosporin A. We have found that even if given at this very late stage it is extremely efficient in reverting steroid resistant rejection episodes. The cytological pattern of inflammation that is responsive to CyA is acute blastogenic rejection that corresponds in your terms to the inflammatory pattern you see around the blood vessels in the so called vascular cuff, i.e. acute cellular rejection. I think that one should keep this alternative also in mind.

FASSBINDER Yes, Dr Markreiter from Insbruck has reported similar results.

BARNES (Birmingham, UK) It's a beautiful demonstration of very good results of transplantation. What you haven't shown is any specificity between the two. You have not treated any of your patients who have primary cellular changes with plasmapheresis and the other way round, so really you haven't yet demonstrated any specificity. Could it not be that these are alternative treatments irrespective of the histology?

FASSBINDER Well, from the theoretical point of view you are absolutely right that it could be that plasma filtration would help in cellular rejection and the other way round, but I think we have a rationale when we treat those rejections with ATG, which are obviously caused by T lymphocytes, and on the other hand to treat other rejections, vascular rejections with plasmapheresis which are said to be caused by antibodies directed against the vascular endothelium.

PART X

GUEST LECTURES — STONES

Chairmen: M Peacock
              W G Robertson

FORMATION OF RENAL STONES MAY BE PREVENTED BY RESTORING NORMAL URINARY COMPOSITION

C Y C Pak

The University of Texas Health Science Center, Dallas, Texas, USA

Introduction

Various changes in urinary composition have been identified in patients with nephrolithiasis. The exact alteration depends on the specific physiological derangement identified. Thus, hypercalciuria may result from an enhanced intestinal absorption of calcium, and hypocitraturia (low urinary citrate) from a defective renal acidification. There is substantial evidence that these bio-chemical disturbances in urine are pathogenetically important in stone formation, and that the restoration of normal urinary composition by appropriate treatment of physiological derangements may prevent formation of new stones.

I shall first describe various biochemical disturbances in urine and discuss their pathogenetic significance. The underlying physiological derangements in patients with stones will then be considered. I shall conclude by a critical evalu-ation of various treatment programmes, from the perspective of their ability to correct physiological derangements and biochemical alterations and to inhibit new stone formation.

Alteration in urinary composition in nephrolithiasis

Different forms of altered urinary composition may be categorised according to exaggerated renal excretion of stone-forming constituents — calcium, oxalate, uric acid, cystine and ammonium ion (Table I). These disturbances contribute to stone formation by creating a supersaturated urinary environment with respect to stone-forming salts.

Another common form of altered urinary composition is characterised by a reduced renal excretion of inhibitors of crystallisation of stone-forming salts. They include small molecular weight substances (citrate and pyrophosphate) as well as macromolecules (e.g. glycosaminoglycans). Finally, urinary composi-tion may be modified by passage of unusually acid or alkaline urine.

371

TABLE I. Altered urinary composition in nephrolithiasis

1. Excessive renal excretion of stone-forming constituents
   a. Hypercalciuria
   b. Hyperoxaluria
   c. Hyperuricosuria
   d. High urinary cystine
   e. High urinary ammonium

2. Reduced renal excretion of inhibitors
   a. Hypocitraturia
   b. Low urinary pyrophosphate
   c. Low urinary macromolecules

3. Altered urinary pH
   a. Low urinary pH
   b. High urinary pH

Pathogenetic significance of altered urinary composition

Hypercalciuria

The physicochemical environment of urine in patients with hypercalciuric nephrolithiasis may be conducive to the crystallisation of stone-forming calcium salts [1,2]. It is characterised by a supersaturated state with respect to calcium phosphate (brushite) and calcium oxalate, reduced limit of metastability (formation product ratio), and increased propensity for the spontaneous nucleation of these salts (assessed from formation product ratio-activity product ratio discriminant score [2] and permissible increment in calcium or oxalate [3]). That these characteristics are important determinants for stone formation is indicated by their uniqueness from normal urinary environment, the positive correlation found between the discriminant score of calcium oxalate and the severity of stone disease, and by the close association between changes in these parameters towards normal and the clinical improvement (inhibition of stone formation) following successful treatment [2].

Hypercalciuria may be responsible for some or all of the physicochemical derangements enumerated above. Urinary concentration of calcium has been shown to be directly correlated with urinary saturation and inversely with the formation product ratio of brushite and calcium oxalate. Moreover, a significant relationship has been found between urinary calcium concentration and discriminant scores or permissible increments [3]. In our preliminary study, the exaggeration or induction of hypercalciuria increases supersaturation and reduces the limit of metastability. The correction of hypercalciuria by appropriate treatment typically reverses much of the physicochemical disturbances toward normal [2]. Finally, when the computer program of Finlayson was used for the calculation of activity products, a rise in calcium concentration was equally as effective as the increase in oxalate concentration in raising the saturation of calcium oxalate [4].

Hyperoxaluria

That hyperoxaluria contributes to stone formation is supported by its identification as an important factor for stone formation, and by its frequent association with calcium nephrolithiasis. Hyperoxaluria probably facilitates stone formation by increasing urinary saturation of calcium oxalate.

Hyperuricosuria

The association of hyperuricosuria with calcium nephrolithiasis has long been recognised. Although concrete proof is lacking, there is substantive evidence that hyperuricosuria may have caused the formation of calcium stones. The following scheme has been proposed [5]: when the urinary environment may be supersaturated with respect to monosodium urate because of a high urinary content of uric acid and a favourable pH (>5.5) in which this urate phase is sparingly soluble. It has been suggested that either a colloidal or crystalline monosodium urate forms from such a supersaturated environment, and initiates formation of calcium stones by a direct induction of heterogeneous nucleation of calcium oxalate, or by adsorption of certain macromolecular inhibitors.

Hyperuricosuria may exaggerate the formation of uric acid stones. However, the stone formation is unlikely unless urinary pH is also reduced (<5.5), because of increased solubility of uric acid at a higher pH.

High urinary cystine

Cystine is sparingly soluble in urine. Its solubility is greater at a higher pH and is enhanced by electrolytes and macromolecules [6], however, it rarely exceeds 400mg/L. Cystine stones may form when urinary cystine concentration exceeds the solubility of cystine.

Hypocitraturia

The pathogenetic role of hypocitraturia in nephrolithiasis may be ascribed to the inhibitor activity of citrate. Citrate lowers urinary saturation of calcium oxalate by forming a soluble complex with calcium and lowering calcium activity. Moreover, citrate may inhibit crystal growth of calcium oxalate and calcium phosphate [7]. Certain trace metals may exaggerate this inhibitor action [8].

Low urinary pyrophosphate and macromolecules

Pyrophosphate, glycosaminoglycans and glycopeptides are potent inhibitors of the crystallisation of calcium oxalate and calcium phosphate. Inhibition of spontaneous precipitation, crystal growth and aggregation has been reported.

373

Altered urinary pH

The passage of unusually acid urine (pH<5.5) would favour the formation of uric acid stones, because of reduced uric acid solubility in such an environment. In contrast, a high urinary pH (neutral or alkaline) favours formation of calcium phosphate stones especially if urinary calcium concentration is high, because of the increased dissociation of phosphate and elevated concentration of trivalent phosphate ion. If there is a high concentration of ammonium ion present, struvite (magnesium ammonium phosphate) stones may form [9].

Identification of physiological derangement

Much of the alteration in urinary composition may be ascribed to specific physiological or metabolic derangements identified in patients with nephrolithiasis. Reliable diagnostic criteria have been established based on these derangements.

Hypercalciuria

Hypercalciuria may be resorptive, absorptive or renal, depending on whether the principal derangement is excessive skeletal resorption, enhanced intestinal absorption of calcium, or an impaired renal tubular reabsorption (renal leak) of calcium, respectively [10].

Resorptive hypercaliuria associated with nephrolithiasis is accountable almost entirely by primary hyperparathyroidism. In primary hyperparathyroidism, the primary derangement is excessive parathyroid hormone (PTH) dependent osteoclastic resorption. The intestinal calcium absorption may be increased secondarily from the PTH-dependent stimulation of the renal synthesis of 1,25-dihydroxyvitamin D (1,25(OH)$_2$D$_3$) [11]. Hypercalciuria often ensues, since the rise in the filtered load of calcium and the suppressive effect of hypercalcaemia on renal tubular reabsorption of calcium usually overcomes the opposing effect of PTH in enhancing renal calcium reabsorption. Hypercalciuria is therefore primarily resorptive and secondarily absorptive.

Absorptive and renal hypercalciurias constitute the two major variants of the condition termed idiopathic hypercalciuria [12]. As the term implies, the intestinal calcium absorption is presumed to be primarily increased in absorptive hypercalciuria. The resulting elevation in the circulating concentration of calcium, though typically occurring within the normal range, causes hypercalciuria by increasing the filtered load of calcium. The concurrent parathyroid suppression further contributes to the hypercalciuria by inhibiting renal tubular reabsorption of calcium.

There is sufficient physiological and practical basis for subdividing absorptive hypercalciuria into three types [13]. Absorptive hypercalciuria Type I represents the classic presentation, where intestinal hyperabsorption and excessive renal excretion of calcium are encountered during a high as well as during a low calcium intake. In the Type II presentation, hypercalciuria may be corrected by a low calcium diet, though manifested on a high calcium diet. In absorptive hypercalciuria Type III, the presumed primary impairment in the renal tubular reabsorption of phosphorus stimulates the renal synthesis of $1,25(OH)_2 D_3$ and accounts for the increased calcium absorption.

In renal hypercalciuria, the 'primary' impairment in the renal tubular reabsorption of calcium causes secondary hyperparathyroidism. The compensatory intestinal hyperabsorption of calcium, occurring from the PTH-dependent stimulation of $1,25(OH)_2 D_3$ synthesis, further contributes to the hypercalciuria.

Hyperoxaluria

Although primary hyperoxaluria is a rare cause of calcium nephrolithiasis, enteric hyperoxaluria, associated with an inflammatory disease of the small bowel or with intestinal bypass surgery, may be encountered in one to five per cent of patients with nephrolithiasis.

An increased intestinal absorption of oxalate is present and accounts for the hyperoxaluria in ileal disease [14]. Two influences probably combine to cause the intestinal hyperabsorption of oxalate. The intestinal transport of oxalate may be primarily increased from the action of bile salts and fatty acids on the permeability of intestinal mucosa to oxalate. The total amount of oxalate absorbed may also be increased because of an enlarged intraluminal pool of oxalate available for absorption. The intestinal fat malabsorption characteristic of ileal disease may exaggerate the soap formation with divalent cations, limit the amount of 'free' divalent cations to complex oxalate, and thereby raise the available oxalate pool.

Hyperuricosuria

Hyperuricosuria may be the only recognisable physiological abnormality in patients with calcium nephrolithiasis. Such an abnormality (hyperuricosuric calcium oxalate nephrolithiasis) comprises nine to 15 per cent of patients with renal calculi. Hyperuricosuria may coexist with various forms of hypercalciuria previously enumerated.

The cause for the hyperuricosuria in the majority of patients with hyperuricosuric calcium oxalate nephrolithiasis is probably the 'dietary overindulgence' with purine-rich foods. They give a history of a liberal intake of meat, poultry and fish. However, in the minority of patients with hyperuricosuric calcium oxalate nephrolithiasis, hyperuricosuria may be partly the result of uric acid overproduction.

High urinary cystine

High urinary cystine is encountered in cystinuria, an inborn error of metabolism characterised by a disturbance in renal and intestinal handling of dicarboxylic acids.

Hypocitraturia

Though largely ignored, hypocitraturia probably represents an important risk for the formation of calcium stones. Reduced citrate excretion has long been recognised in renal tubular acidosis, enteric hyperoxaluria, hypokalaemia, and in urinary tract infection. However, preliminary studies suggest that hypocitraturia may be present in other conditions (e.g. absorptive and renal hypercalciurias and 'no metabolic abnormality'), even in the absence of defective renal acidification [15].

The cause for the reduced renal excretion of pyrophosphate and macromolecular inhibitors is not known.

Altered urinary pH

Low urinary pH may be found in gouty diathesis, chronic diarrhoeal syndromes and ingestion of a high acid-ash diet. Neutral or alkaline pH in urine may be encountered in patients with renal tubular acidosis or infection with urea-splitting organisms. In renal tubular acidosis, urinary calcium may be high, if there is not a significant impairment of renal function. In infection, there is increased formation of ammonium ion in urine from the enzymatic degradation of urea by bacterial urease [9].

Therapeutic considerations

The above elucidation of biochemical and physiological derangements in nephrolithiasis has permitted formulation of effective treatment programmes. We ourselves have espoused the 'selective' treatment approach, where certain treatment is specifically chosen for its ability to correct the particular physiological derangement characterising that disorder [13]. This selective approach differs from the more randomised treatment programme in which the same drug may be used for several causes, even though its actions may be poorly defined. I shall review available data concerning the ability of selective treatments to restore normal urinary environment and inhibit new stone formation.

Absorptive hypercalciuria Type I [13]

Sodium cellulose phosphate (2.5–5g with each meal, 10–15g/day) was considered to be selective for absorptive hypercalciuria Type I, since it has been shown to correct the intestinal hyperabsorption of calcium (by binding calcium in the intestinal tract). It has been reported to restore the 'normal' physicochemical environment of urine, by reducing saturation of urine with respect to brushite and calcium oxalate, and by decreasing the propensity for the spontaneous nucleation of brushite and calcium oxalate [2]. However, the treatment may cause secondary hyperoxaluria [16] and reduced magnesium excretion. Thus, it has been our customary practice to impose a moderate oxalate restriction and to provide oral magnesium supplements (magnesium gluconate 1.0–1.5g twice/day separately from cellulose phosphate).

This treatment reduced the stone formation rate from 2.28 stones/patient year to 0.23/patient year (p<0.001 χ^2 test), caused remission in 77.8 per cent of patients and lowered individual stone formation rate in all patients [13].

Absorptive hypercalciuria Type II

The features of absorptive hypercalciuria Type II are identical to those of absorptive hypercalciuria Type I, except for normocalciuria (<200mg/day) on a diet of 400mg calcium and 100mEq sodium/day [17]. In addition, many patients show disdain for drinking fluids and excrete concentrated urine [17]. A low calcium intake (400–600mg/day) and high fluid intake (sufficient to achieve a minimum urine output of 2L/day) would seem ideally indicated [13], since normocalciuria could be restored by dietary calcium restriction alone, and increased urine volume has been shown to reduce urinary saturation of calcium oxalate, brushite and monosodium urate, and inhibit spontaneous nucleation of calcium oxalate [18].

In 24 patients so treated, stone formation rate decreased from 1.83 stones/

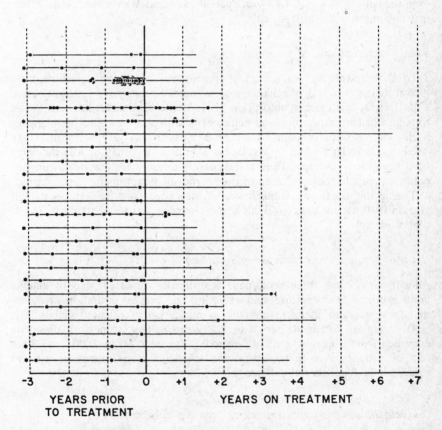

YEARS PRIOR TO TREATMENT

YEARS ON TREATMENT

Figure 1. Effect of high fluid intake and low calcium diet on renal stone formation in absorptive hypercalciuria Type II (AH-II). Each line represents study in a separate patient. Each circle represents a new stone episode (formation or passage). Asterisks indicate pre-existing stones when treatment started. Vertical line at zero represents time when treatment was initiated.

377

patient year to 0.38/patient year (p<0.001), 70.8 per cent of patients were in remission over a mean follow-up of 2.32 years/patient, and individual stone formation declined in 22 patients (91.7%) (Figure 1).

Absorptive hypercalciuria Type III [13]

Orthophosphate (neutral salt of sodium and potassium, 1.5–2.0g phosphorus in three divided doses/day orally) would seem to be the logical treatment because of its potential for the inhibition of $1,25(OH)_2D_3$ synthesis. Moreover, it has been shown to reduce urinary saturation of calcium oxalate, and to inhibit spontaneous nucleation of brushite and calcium oxalate [2].

This treatment lowered stone formation rate from 2.38 stones/patient year to 0.36/patient year (p<0.001), produced a remission in 62.5 per cent of patients over a mean follow-up of 4.13 years/patient, and caused a reduced stone formation rate individually in all patients.

Renal hypercalciuria

Thiazide represents an ideal treatment programme for renal hypercalciuria, since it corrects the renal leak of calcium, restores normal parathyroid function, serum $1,25(OH)_2D_3$ and calcium absorption [12]. Moreover, thiazide has been shown to reduce urinary saturation, and enhance inhibitor activity against spontaneous nucleation of both calcium oxalate and brushite [2]. Hypocitraturia may develop, particularly when hypokalaemia is present, and may oppose the beneficial response to therapy. Thus, it has been our customary practice to provide potassium supplementation even in the absence of symptomatic hypokalaemia.

During this treatment, stone formation decreased from 1.83 stones/patient year to 0.40/patient year (p<0.001), and remission was encountered in 75 per cent of patients.

Hyperuricosuric calcium oxalate nephrolithiasis

Allopurinol (100mg three times/day) is optimally indicated, since it inhibits urate synthesis, reduces uric acid excretion and urinary saturation of monosodium urate, and inhibits spontaneous nucleation of calcium oxalate [2].

Over a mean treatment period of 2.28 years/patient, stone formation rate decreased from 1.00 stone/patient year to 0.09/patient year (p<0.001), 83.3 per cent of patients were in remission, and individual stone formation rate was reduced in 95.8 per cent of patients (Figure 2).

Uric acid lithiasis and hypocitraturic calcium nephrolithiasis

In patients with uric acid lithiasis, potassium citrate (approximately 20mEq three times/day) effectively raises urinary pH to normal values at which uric acid is more soluble. In patients with hypocitraturic calcium nephrolithiasis, potassium citrate treatment restores normal urinary citrate, lowers urinary

378

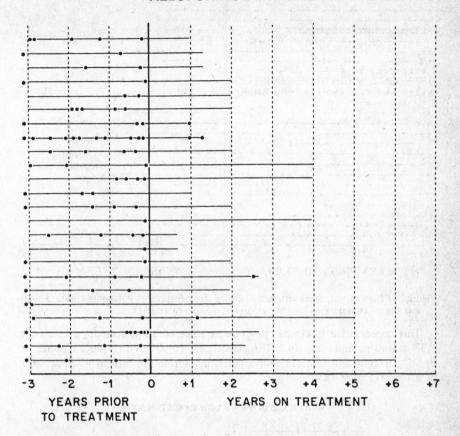

-3   -2   -1   0   +1   +2   +3   +4   +5   +6   +7

YEARS PRIOR   YEARS ON TREATMENT
TO TREATMENT

Figure 2. Effect of high fluid intake and low calcium diet on stone formation in no metabolic abnormality (NMA)

saturation and inhibits crystallisation of calcium salts [19].

This treatment has been shown to lower stone formation rate from 10.46 stones/patient year to 0.59/patient year (p<0.001), cause a remission in 79.2 per cent of patients and reduce individual stone formation rate in all 24 patients evaluated (Figure 3).

No metabolic abnormality

No metabolic abnormality constitutes the entity in which no clear-cut physiological derangement has been found. However, urine volume is often low, a finding suggesting that a disdain for drinking fluids may have contributed to stone formation [17]. A high fluid intake would appear logical for the same reasons stipulated above.

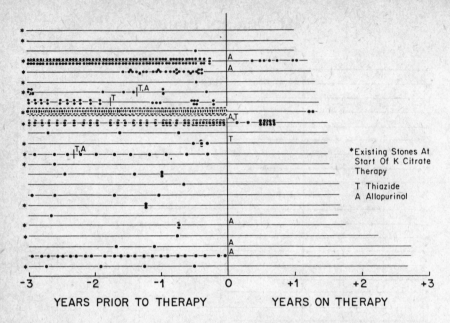

YEARS PRIOR TO THERAPY   YEARS ON THERAPY

Figure 3. Effect of potassium citrate therapy on stone formation. Potassium citrate therapy was begun at time zero. Some patients also took thiazide (T) and/or allopurinol (A)

This conservative treatment programme lowered stone formation rate from 1.33 stones/patient year to 0.18/patient year (p<0.001), produced remission in 75 per cent and reduced individual stone formation rate in 87.5 per cent of patients (Figure 4).

HIGH FLUID INTAKE + LOW Ca DIET IN NMD

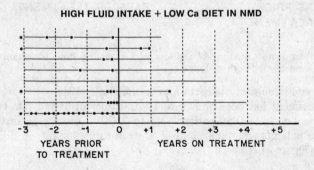

YEARS PRIOR   YEARS ON TREATMENT
TO TREATMENT

Figure 4. Effect of allopurinol treatment on stone formation

Critique of clinical trial

The favourable clinical response to selective treatment programmes described above supports, but does not prove, the validity of the concept of a selective treatment approach [19]. Since randomised placebo control groups were not included and as pre-treatment history was obtained retrospectively without benefit of direct care, non-specific influences associated with our close follow-up observation could have modified the clinical response to treatment. These non-specific effects probably include change in dietary habits and fluid intake, and improved patient compliance (from close follow-up). Positive 'placebo effect' on the course of nephrolithiasis is well known.

Although the need for the assessment of the placebo effect is clear, randomised trials with the inclusion of the placebo control are difficult to conduct because of the difficulty in disguising test medications. Most patients could tell that they were taking sodium cellulose phosphate, thiazide or neutral phosphate.

Despite the lack of randomised control studies, several lines of evidence indicate that selective treatments themselves had exerted a positive impact on the clinical course of stone disease [19,20]. The clinical improvement (reduced stone formation rate) produced by treatment was ·correlated with objective measures for the propensity of stone formation (reduced saturation of calcium salts in urine). Our preliminary study suggests that the decline in urinary saturation of calcium salts occurring during treatment with sodium cellulose phosphate of patients with absorptive hypercalciuria Type I resulted largely from the effect of treatment itself (reduction in urinary calcium) rather than from non-specific influences (change in urine volume). When patients with absorptive hypercalciuria who had been on sodium cellulose phosphate were placed on alternate treatments, 57.1 per cent of them had a relapse of stone formation (compared to 22.2 per cent during sodium cellulose phosphate treatment). Thirteen patients who relapsed (continued to form stones on thiazide, sodium cellulose phosphate, allopurinol or conservative therapy) under our care were found to have hypocitraturia. The addition of potassium citrate prevented new stone formation in all but three patients.

Finally, as previously discussed, a cogent argument may be made for a strong cause and effect relationship between various biochemical disturbances in urine and renal stone formation. All selective treatments chosen were effective in restoring normal urinary composition and in correcting much of the physico-chemical disturbances in urine.

The available evidence therefore strongly suggests that the restoration of normal urinary composition by appropriate correction of physiological derangements in patients with stones is effective in inhibiting new stone formation.

Acknowledgments

Supported by USPHS grants RO1-AM20543 and MO1-RR00633.

References

1   Pak CYC, Holt K. *Metabolism 1976; 25:* 665
2   Pak CYC, Galosy RA. *J Clin Endocrinol Metab 1979; 48:* 260
3   Nicar MJ, Hill K, Pak CYC. *Metabolism 1983:* in press
4   Pak CYC, Nicar MJ, Northcutt C. In Ritz E, Massry SG, eds. *Pathophysiology of Renal Disease. Contro Nephrol 1982; 33:* 136

5   Pak CYC, Holt K, Zerwekh JE. *Invest Urol 1979; 17:* 138
6   Pak CYC, Fuller CJ. *Invest Urol 1983:* in press
7   Meyer JL, Smith LH. *Invest Urol 1975; 13:* 36
8   Meyer JL, Thomas WC Jr. *J Urol 1982; 128:* 1376
9   Griffith DP, Musher DM. *Invest Urol 1973; 11:* 228
10   Pak CYC, Ohata M, Lawrence EC, Snyder W. *J Clin Invest 1974; 54:* 387
11   Kaplan RA, Haussler MR, Deftos LJ et al. *J Clin Invest 1977; 59:* 756
12   Pak CYC. *Am J Physiol 1979; 237:* F415
13   Pak CYC, Peters P, Hurt G et al. *Am J Med 1981; 71:* 615
14   Barilla DE, Notz C, Kennedy D, Pak CYC. *Am J Med 1978; 64:* 579
15   Nicar MJ, Skurla C, Sakhaee K, Pak CYC. *Urology 1983; 21:* 8
16   Hayashi Y, Kaplan RA, Pak CYC. *Metabolism 1975; 24:* 1273
17   Pak CYC, Britton F, Peterson R et al. *Am J Med 1980; 69:* 19
18   Pak CYC, Sakhaee K, Crowther C, Brinkley L. *Ann Int Med 1980; 93:* 36
19   Pak CYC. *J Urol 1982; 128:* 1157
20   Pak CYC. In Narins RG, ed. *Controversies in Nephrology and Hypertension.*
     New York: Churchill-Livingston: in preparation

Open Discussion

TSCHÖPE (Heidelberg) Dr Pak thank you very much for this really enthusiastic demonstration of therapy in stone disease. We could discuss many problems related to this, but I want to focus on one, the citrate problem. You know that the excretion of citrate and the plasma citrate levels are very sensible indicators of the acid-base status of the individual. It makes no difference whether you give these people potassium citrate, bicarbonate or lactate, all of which will increase urinary citrate. In other words the citrate you give these people by mouth is not the citrate that appears in urine. The urinary pH is increased by citrate therapy and so you might increase the risk of calcium phosphate stone disease which has been observed by some urologists giving patients, not in a very controlled fashion, potassium citrate and they had calcium oxalate concrements with a layer of calcium phosphate. Can you comment on this?

PAK I had a session with Dr Nancollas earlier about the possible uniqueness of potassium citrate from the sodium alkali. I really agree with you entirely that at the most alkali would have about the same effect in terms of increasing urinary pH and citrate excretion. We believe there is something unique about potassium preparation versus sodium preparation. Sodium citrate therapy increases urinary calcium in some patients, whereas potassium citrate therapy, even if given in sufficient amounts, typically lowers urinary calcium excretion. Urinary titration of sodium urate increases with sodium citrate therapy but not with potassium citrate therapy. You talked about the possible role of sodium urate in initiating calcium oxalate crystallisation, now the formation product, the measure of limit of metastability, increases with potassium citrate therapy but decreases with sodium citrate therapy. The reason why we went for potassium citrate treatment is precisely this finding and supplementary complementary clinical data showing that patients who took sodium bicarbonate for uric acid lithiasis presented to us with calcium stones, but ceased when substituted with potassium alkali.

ANDREUCCI (Naples) What is the dose of chlorothiazide you suggest to reduce hypercalciuria? Why don't you use amiloride to decrease potassium excretion since amiloride has been shown to also reduce calcium excretion?

PAK Concerning the thiazide dosage required to produce adequate hypocalciuric response there is sufficient data suggesting that hydrochlorothiazide 50mg twice a day orally should be able to lower calcium excretion in the majority of patients provided that they are not taking excessive sodium intake. I believe the comparable dose of tricrochloromethiazide is about 8mg per day, but many patients show adequate hypocalciuric response to 4mg per day. Chlorthalidone 50mg a day is equivalent in my experience to 50mg of hydrochlorothiazide twice a day. Tricrochloromethiazide and chlorthalidone may be given only once a day because of a long half life. Concerning amiloride therapy you are probably aware of Dr Maschio's* work published in the American Journal of Medicine several years ago. He suggested that the addition of amiloride might reduce the requirement for hydrochlorothiazide. In most of the patients who took 50mg of hydrochlorothiazide the addition of 5mg of amiloride per day produced the equivalent hypocalciuric response as that which had been reported with hydrochlorothiazide with 50mg twice a day orally. In our hands amiloride alone is capable of reducing calcium excretion in only a minority of patients (only two of seven in fact). However when amiloride is added to the hydrochlorothiazide therapy there appears to be a slight modest exaggeration of the hypocalciuric effect of thiazides.

WILL (Leeds) Can we pin you down on the fluid? I think it has been generally assumed that you have to drown people to try and lower their urinary saturation and that's why they object to it, but in fact if you look at the risk-index approach to urinary concentration and calculate how much water would be necessary to lower the distributions of excess mineral ions towards the normal ranges, it's not very great. Do you have any clues as to how much fluid volume might suffice?

PAK I can only give you my personal experience. My aim is to bring about a urine output on a persistent basis of two litres or more per day. It can be achieved if a person is not swelling by drinking 3,000 cc of water daily. I can tell you I have a very prominent stockbroker who happens to support my research programme, he used to put out 500mg of calcium and a modest amount of oxalate in the urine each day forming many stones but he refused to take any medication whatsoever. So I told him to drink lots of water and he took enough to drown himself, precisely four litres per day at least. He has not formed a single stone in the last 10 years.

FOURNIER (Amiens) I am seduced by your case for specific treatment according to the pathophysiology of renal stones. However I would like to have some

* Maschio G, Tessitore N, D'Angelo A et al. *Am J Med 1981; 71:* 623

more information for this justification. For example the use of phosphate in the absorptive hypercalciuria type III. You say that there is bone involvement, what data do you have to support that, and have you seen any improvement with phosphate therapy?

PAK That's an area that I'm kind of hazy on. Dr Bordier* has about the best paper addressing the issue that there is bone involvement in hypophosphataemia and I believe he provided some evidence that phosphate did help correct some of that abnormality. Personally, looking carefully at a very large number of patients, I have to say it is difficult to find a clear cut case of a patient who fits all of that. In my experience phosphate therapy, even those with hypophosphataemia, does not lower the intestinal calcium absorption even after five years of treatment.

FOURNIER Do you have specific clinical data as regards the risk of metastatic calcification with phosphate therapy, because I think in the literature there is no such data in humans?

PAK Yes there is one from Australia†, in patients with normocalcaemic renal calculi as well as in primary hyperparathyroidism. Neutral phosphate therapy caused calcification of conjunctivae and aortic calcifications.

FOURNER Do you think that an increase of bone mineral content is a serious side effect when you give thiazides to absorptive hypercalciuric patients?

PAK I'm not sure. The bone density was measured only at a distal third radius and not in the spine. I have seen a rise, on average, of about six per cent in bone density over a five year period but after then it seems to flatten out. I have yet to determine what the problem is, and I'm trying to answer this by looking at the spine.

CATTELL (London) Returning to the sodium story, you commented on its blocking effect on thiazide therapy, but do you accept that a very high sodium intake on its own may produce significant hypercalciuria as suggested by Muldowney‡ so that in your therapeutic approach you should counsel or investigate the patients as to their sodium intake prior to thiazide therapy?

PAK If you take large amounts of sodium you increase urinary calcium excretion even in hypercalciuric patients, but it is very difficult to induce fasting hypercalciuria in normal subjects. We have studied that very carefully. Now the second point is that when you increase urinary calcium by increased sodium intake while you increase the urinary calcium concentration you do not necessarily increase the saturation with respect to calcium salts because sodium content goes up as

* Bordier P, Ryckewart A, Guerls J, Rasmussen H. *Am J Med 1977; 63:* 398
† Dudley FJ, Blackburn CRB. *Lancet 1970; ii:* 628
‡ Muldowney FP, Freaney R, Moloney MF. *Kidney Int 1982; 22:* 292

well and activity coefficient falls. As a result the saturation may not change appreciably. However, the sodium loading appears to lower the limit of meta stability as measured by the formation product, a possible suggestion being sodium urate-induced calcium oxalate crystallisation.

FEEST (Exeter, UK) You have talked a lot about 24-hour urine calcium and oxalate, but have you looked at the enormous variation in concentrations of these substances during the 24-hour period? Have you possibly looked at the effect of the timing of your treatment and the timing of giving water?

PAK Yes I think that's a very good point and that's a subject that should be looked at. I have done only one study in that regard but essentially it magnifies your work by about eight times. I think that kind of work should be done but technically it has not been possible yet.

FEEST You haven't looked, for example, at the timing of drinking rather than the volume that people drink?

PAK No, I think that those are very valid points and certainly they should be addressed, but by someone with a large staff.

Proc EDTA (1983) Vol 20

THE MECHANISM OF FORMATION OF RENAL STONE CRYSTALS

G H Nancollas

State University of New York at Buffalo, Buffalo, New York, USA

Summary

Typical renal stone minerals such as the calcium phosphates and oxalate hydrates may nucleate, grow, or dissolve in the fluctuating concentration conditions of the urinary tract. A study has been made of the rates of formation of these minerals under conditions in which the concentrations of ionic species were maintained constant by the potentiometrically controlled addition of lattice ions. The kinetic studies were made under conditions of low supersaturation similar to those in vivo and, in the case of calcium phosphates, at least three solid phases have been shown to participate in the overall reaction depending upon factors such as pH, nature and concentration of supporting medium, supersaturation, ionic strength, temperature, and the presence of inhibitors of crystallisation. For the calcium oxalates, the mineralisation process may involve the initial precipitation of less stable hydrates before conversion to the most stable whewellite. Urinary stone inhibitors may have a considerable influence in stabilising thermodynamically less stable hydrates.

Introduction

Urine is normally supersaturated with respect to calcium oxalate hydrates [1,2], octacalcium phosphate ($Ca_4H(PO_4)_3$, OCP) [1], hydroxyapatite ($Ca_5(PO_4)_3OH$, HAP) [1], and sometimes dicalcium phosphate dihydrate ($CaHPO_4 \cdot 2H_2O$, DCPD) [3]. The degree of supersaturation is usually higher in patients with urinary stones [1–4] mainly because they tend to have higher urinary calcium [4]. Although the significance of such differences has been questioned, a recent analysis has indicated that they can be amplified by including magnesium analytical data in the assessment [5]. The importance of elevated calcium and oxalate concentrations in the renal papillae has also been emphasised [6]. Although there are many factors that must still be elucidated concerning the the control of nucleation of pathological concretions, the growth of such solid phases in vivo must be mediated by physical chemical principles governing the kinetics of crystallisation. At its simplest, the first stage of this process involves the formation of new centres, in a nucleation step, from which subsequent crystal growth can occur. The nucleation process may be homogeneous or, in the presence of suitable surfaces offering nucleating sites, heterogeneous nucleation may take place. In a moderately supersaturated homogeneous solution, crystals cannot form due to the instability of very small particles or embryos. In terms of classical nucleation theories, statistical fluctuations in these solutions result in the formation of ionic or molecular clusters through stepwise aggregation which can increase in size or dissociate according to the scheme.

$$A + A \rightleftharpoons A_2$$
$$A_2 + A \rightleftharpoons A_3$$
$$A_{n-1} + A \rightleftharpoons A_n \text{ (critical cluster)}$$

where A represents the single crystallising unit, A_2 the dimer etc.

The relatively short lived clusters are produced by stepwise bimolecular reactions involving the single ions or associated molecules and may be considered to be minute spherical droplets to which we can apply well established theoretical considerations relating to vapour condensation. Since the surface has to be created, cluster formation requires energy which is provided by the favourable free energy term due to the tendency of the supersaturation to deplete itself by depositing on the surfaces. Clusters larger than the critical size will tend to grow since the surface energy term becomes less important as the size increases. Once the critical size has been reached by aggregation, the supersaturation collapses and the crystallites which have been formed will tend to grow by a process of crystal growth. The rate of formation of the critical nucleus, A_n, is proportional to $(\ln S)^{-2}$ and is therefore extremely sensitive to changes in supersaturation [7]. This is shown in Figure 1 in which the rate of nucleation is plotted as a function of supersaturation $S = (\ [(Ca^{2+})(Ox^{2-})/K_{so}]\ ^{1/2})$. In this expression, round brackets enclose the activities of ionic species, Ox^{2-} represents the oxalate ion and K_{so} the thermodynamic solubility product of the

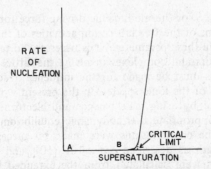

Figure 1. Nucleation rate plotted against supersaturation with respect to calcium oxalate

renal stone mineral (here, calcium oxalate). It can be seen that below the critical supersaturation, the nucleation rate is extremely small but once this value is reached, the rate increases very rapidly.

Many spontaneous precipitation experiments have been made at concentration values above the critical supersaturation. These results are very difficult to reproduce since the size and size distribution of the crystallites change continuously during the reactions. In most biological situations, the typical supersaturation range (AB in Figure 1) represents supersaturated solutions which may remain stable, for long periods of time. Since in biological systems, surfaces offering suitable sites for nucleating renal stone minerals may be present, it is probably more appropriate to use seeded crystal growth experiments as models for the mineralisation reactions.

The relatively large crystallites which are frequently observed in vivo may also be formed by aggregation and coagulation of particles formed initially in the supersaturated solutions. In these processes, the charge at the solid/liquid interface plays an important part since similarly charged particles will tend to remain dispersed in the aqueous phase due to electrostatic repulsion. Ions or molecules of opposite charge which may be adsorbed at the surface of these crystals may therefore reduce the surface charge and induce agglomeration or aggregation. Typically, the lattice ion in excess will determine the charge on the crystal surface but the proton in the solutions may also be a potential determining ion. Adsorption of polyanionic urine components at the crystal surfaces may influence both the size of the aggregates and the morphology of the grown crystalline phases. In addition, fluid shear forces and collisions between particles may produce secondary nuclei at a rate dependent upon the supersaturation and the fluid dynamics. The use of a mixed suspension mixed product removal crystalliser, frequently used in industrial crystallisation processes has been proposed by Finlayson in order to model crystallite formation in vivo [8]. In this technique, crystallisation and nucleation occur continuously as the solution flows into the crystalliser. At steady state, particle size analysis in the outflow can be used to estimate both the nucleation and growth rates under urine-like conditions [8,9].

Supersaturation

The supersaturation, S, or thermodynamic driving force for crystallisation must be expressed in terms of the free lattice ion activities of the crystallising phase. In order to calculate these parameters, it is necessary to take into account the formation of ion-pairs and complexes involving the lattice ions in solution. In addition, corrections must be made for the influence of ionic strength on the activity coefficients of the ionic species. In the present work, lattice ion speciation was elucidated by using mass balance and electroneutrality expressions together with the appropriate thermodynamic equilibrium constants for each complex species. The computations were made by successive approximation for the ionic strength as described previously [10], and activity coefficients of the ionic species were calculated from the extended form of the Debye-Hückel equation proposed by Davies [11]. For crystallisation experiments

388

made at constant ionic strength, appropriate conditional equilibrium constants are used in the calculations and activity coefficients, assumed constant, are incorporated into these parameters. The computations involve the solution of simultaneous non-linear equations by means of a generalised computer programme. In synthetic urine solutions, for which the extent of calcium complexing with each of the components has been measured, the free calcium concentration may be calculated with some confidence. In urines, however, complexing of calcium with the macromolecular components is ill-defined, although numerous attempts have been made to estimate the ionised calcium concentrations. Thus Robertson [12] measured the ionised calcium concentration in urines by spectrophotometric and potentiometric methods and compared the results with computer calculations. With approximately 50 per cent of the total calcium in the ionised form, good agreement was obtained between all three methods. Later, Marshall and Robertson [13] published a simple nomogram for estimating the saturation of urine with respect to each of the major constituents of urinary calculi. Other successful computational procedures for calculating free ion concentrations in simulated urines were developed by Finlayson [14]. The use of specific ion electrodes such as the calcium electrode for measuring the free calcium concentration in the biological fluids must be approached with caution since the electrodes will frequently respond to concentration changes of many of the urinary components.

Crystal growth

At its simplest, crystal growth must involve the following steps:

a) Bulk diffusion of lattice ions to the crystal surface.

b) Adsorption at the crystal surface. This step may also involve the formation of two-dimensional nuclei.

c) Partial dehydration of the adsorbed lattice ions.

d) Surface diffusion of growth units to energetically favourable sites.

e) Incorporation of growth units into the crystal lattice.

f) The dissolution process involving desorption of growth units.

The rate of reaction will reflect the slow step or steps in this reaction scheme. It is now generally accepted that the formation of a two-dimensional nucleus at the surface is unlikely to be a controlling step since it would require an appreciable supersaturation whereas crystals typically grow at supersaturations below one per cent. The rapid increase in the rate of nucleation with increase in concentration (Figure 1) suggests that if the formation of a nucleus is rapid, new layers may start before the development of the deposited underlying layer is complete. This multiplicity leads to polynuclear crystallisation [15] with many nucleation sites forming and developing simultaneously.

The observation that crystals grow at much lower supersaturations than those required for two dimensional surface nucleation led to the mechanism proposed by Frank and his co-workers [16] in which it was assumed that real crystals are imperfect and contain screw dislocations which emerge from the

389

surface. Since crystallisation takes place at energetically preferred sites offered by these ledges, growth spirals develop on the crystal surface. These spirals provide perpetual steps for crystallisation and avoid the necessity for additional surface nucleation. During crystallisation, the ion must penetrate the hydration layer at the crystal surface. As indicated above, dehydration or partial dehydration must also take place during the crystallisation steps. The kinetics representing a spiral growth mechanism can also be interpreted in terms of rate determining steps involving the removal of bound water molecules in order for the ions to approach those already integrated on the crystal surface. The energy needed for this dehydration is several times the thermal energy and will be larger for cations than for anions.

In step (a), although solute must be transported from the bulk solution to the crystal surface, if this process were rate determining, Fick's Law of Diffusion would require the crystallisation rate to be linearly proportional to the supersaturation expressed as, (= S-1). However, there is now considerable evidence that for many sparingly soluble inorganic minerals such as M_aX_b, the crystallisation rate is controlled by a surface process and follows Equation 1:

$$\text{Rate} = dn/dt = -k_g s \, K_{so}{}^P / \nu_\sigma{}^P$$

In Equation 1, n represents the moles of mineral phase precipitated, $\nu = (a + b)$, k_g is the rate constant for the surface controlled cyrstallisation, p is the effective order of the reaction, and s is the function of the surface area of the crystals. For many simple salts, the rate of crystallisation has been found to follow a parabolic rate law with p = 2 in Equation 1. At low supersaturation, this is consistent with a spiral growth mechanism. At higher supersaturations the rate of crystallisation may vary more strongly with supersaturation (p > 2 in Equation 1) indicating a polynuclear growth mechanism. However, it is clearly important to establish not only the dependence of crystal growth upon supersaturation but also the influence of solid/solution ratio, stirring dynamics and temperature. Thus for surface controlled processes, the activation energy, typically ~40 J mol^{-1} would be considerably greater than the value ~12 J mol^{-1} for bulk transport control. Since different mechanisms may prevail at different degrees of supersaturation, comparisons between natural biological growth inhibitors should only be made under carefully controlled values of these experimental parameters.

Calcium oxalate crystallisation

At least three calcium oxalate hydrates have been characterised with solubilities represented by Figure 2. In conventional crystallisation experiments, of these different hydrates, metastable supersaturated solutions (Figure 1) are inoculated with seed crystals and the rate of reaction is determined by measuring the decrease in concentration of calcium and oxalate ions as a function of time. It can be seen in Figure 2 that for crystallisation experiments made at relatively high supersaturation, different hydrate phases may form and subsequently dissolve as the lattice ion concentrations are allowed to decrease. Moreover, as the

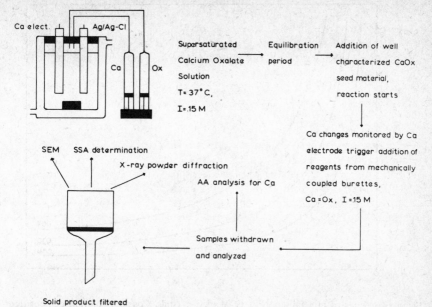

Ca elect.   Ag/Ag-Cl

Ca   Ox

Supersaturated   Equilibration   Addition of well
Calcium Oxalate   period   characterized CaOx
Solution   seed material,
T= 37°C,   reaction starts
I=.15 M

                                               Ca changes monitored by Ca
SEM   SSA determination   electrode trigger addition of
          X-ray powder diffraction   reagents from mechanically
                    AA analysis for Ca   coupled burettes,
                                               Ca =Ox, I =.15 M

                    Samples withdrawn
                    and analyzed

Solid product filtered

Figure 2.   The solubilities of calcium oxalate mono-(COM), di-(COD) and tri-hydrates (COT) at 37°C

reactions approach equilibrium with respect to calcium oxalate monohydrate (COM), the changes in lattice ion concentrations become too small to allow reliable estimates to be made of the rates of crystallisation.

These problems were overcome by using a technique in which the precipitation is studied under conditions of constant activities of ionic species [17]. Following the addition of seed crystals to metastable supersaturated solutions of calcium oxalate, the activities of crystal lattice ions are maintained constant by the simultaneous addition of titrant solutions containing calcium and oxalate ions from mechanically coupled burettes and controlled by a specific calcium ion electrode. A block diagram of the procedure is shown in Figure 3. It is significant that specific ion electrodes, which would not respond sufficiently rapidly to follow changes in concentrations, may be used in the stated mode in order to maintain the activities of the ionic species in the supersaturated solutions. Rates of crystallisation of the calcium oxalate hydrates could be determined with a precision (5%) unattainable by conventional seeded crystallisation experiments. A typical plot of titrant volume added as a function of time following the addition of COM seed crystals to metastable calcium oxalate supersaturated solutions is shown in Figure 4. It can be seen that the correction for increase in surface area of the COM crystals, assuming perfect spheres or cubes, results in excellent linearity of the rate plots, the slope of which reflect the rate of crystallisation. For the calcium oxalate hydrates, the value of p = 2

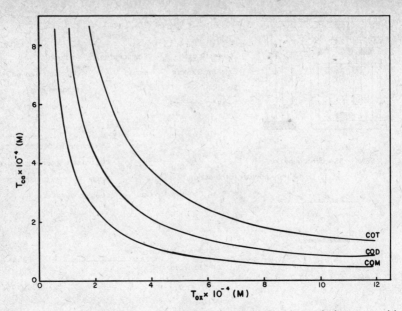

Figure 3. Rates of mineralisation of COM seed cyrstals. Constant solution composition method. (From DJ White. *A Constant Composition Study of the Kinetics of Crystallisation and Demineralisation of Calcium Oxalate: Application to Renal Stone Disease.* PhD Thesis, University of Buffalo, 1982)

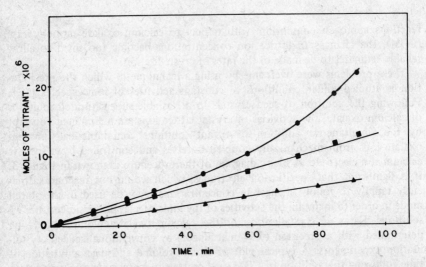

Figure 4. CC growth of COM at $37°C$. Plots of moles of titrant (as calcium oxalate) against time; 100% growth at 85 min. Supersaturated solutions, $T_{Ca} = T_{ox} = 4.0 \times 10^{-4}$ mol L^{-1}, seed concentration 0.0108g L^{-1}. ●: uncorrected rate plot; ■: corrected for change in surface area by multiplicative factor $(w/w_i)^{2/3}$ where w_i and w are the masses of solid phase initially and at time t, respectively; ▲: influence of added urine (1.1% dilution by volume)

392

in Equation 1 confirms the applicability of the parabolic rate law suggesting a spiral growth mechanism for crystallisation.

It has been shown that the constant composition method may be used as a reliable indicator of urine inhibitory potential [18]. A typical COM growth curve in the presence of urine is shown in Figure 4. In order to distinguish between relatively small changes in the rates of crystallisation in the presence of urine components, it is essential to ensure that the supersaturation is the same for each experiment. Moreover, the studies must be made at urine dilutions below that corresponding to adsorption saturation on the calcium oxalate seed crystal surfaces by the growth inhibitors [18]. Since calcium oxalate dihydrate (COD) is frequently observed as a urinary stone component, it is quite likely that urinary inhibitors may selectively prevent the crystallisation of the thermo- dynamically more stable monohydrate. Thus it has been shown that the transformation of COD to COM is markedly inhibited by the presence of traces of crystal growth inhibitors such as polyphosphate, phytate, pyrophosphate, and whole urine [19].

Studies of the kinetics of dissolution of COM at constant composition have indicated a striking change in the mechanism of the reaction as the under- saturation is reduced [20]. At high undersaturations, a first-order dependence of the rate on undersaturation points to a normal diffusion controlled dissolution reaction. At very low undersaturations, however, the reaction appears to be surface controlled. Moreover, the two regions of undersaturation show markedly different dependencies on changes in temperature hydrodynamics, and upon the addition of adsorbing molecules. It is interesting to note that the dissolution of calcium oxalate renal stones appears to be surface controlled at all under- saturations [20]. Different sensitivities to inhibitors such as those found in urine may have important implications in our understanding of stone dissolution in vivo.

Calcium phosphate

In the relatively wide range of urinary pH, the importance of calcium phosphate phases as stone forming minerals has long been recognised. Thus Pak has shown that the urines of patients with idiopathic hypercalciuria and calcium-containing renal calculi may be supersaturated with respect to DCPD [3]. It is now well established that kinetic factors are important in determining the nature of the calcium phosphate solids which form during the precipitation reactions [21] and the participation of these phases during crystallisation accounts, to a large extent, for the difficulties in elucidating the overall mechanism of the process. It is likely that in vivo, different mineralisation inhibitors may selectively reduce the formation of the thermodynamically most stable HAP, while having a much smaller effect on the crystal growth of DCPD and OCP. By carrying out crystal- lisation reactions at low constant supersaturation. it is possible to grow, exclusively, the thermodynamically most stable HAP without the participation of precursor phases such as DCPD and OCP. Thus it has been shown that the crystallisation of HAP is controlled by a spiral growth mechanism [22]. Although HAP is the most stable phase over a wide range of conditions, as the lower

393

urinary pH values are approached, HAP surfaces may be covered by a surface coatings of more acid calcium phosphates [3].

In terms of the Ostwald-Lussac Law of Stages [22], precipitation of calcium phosphate at pH 5.5 would be expected to commence with the formation of the most soluble, least stable, DCPD, before transformation to the thermodynamically more stable forms. At pH $\leqslant$ 5.6, DCPD is kinetically favoured and subsequent transformation is immeasurably slow. It is interesting to note that this phase was used as a urine saturation indicator [3] and has been proposed as a possible stone and HAP precursor [23]. The crystallisation rate of DCPD follows the kinetic Equation 1 with p = 2.

OCP may also be an HAP precursor phase [24] and the growth of OCP on OCP seed crystals has been demonstrated in the pH range 6.0 to 7.0. The constant composition method enables macroscopic amounts of pure OCP to be grown under these conditions. In the range of urinary pH, therefore, OCP is clearly a viable calcium phosphate phase which may grow for extended periods. Moreover, the rate of crystallisation of OCP is appreciably greater than that for HAP at comparable supersaturations. Urinary components may influence the growth of these calcium phosphate phases to different extents and these studies are underway in our laboratory.

Mixed phases

Many kidneys and bladder stones contain more than one mineral phase and frequently both calcium oxalate and calcium phosphate phases are present. Epitactic relationships between HAP and the hydrates of calcium oxalate have been examined from the crystallographic point of view [25] and a constant composition study in our laboratory has confirmed the growth of DCPD on COM seed crystals added to supersaturated solutions of calcium phosphate. Crystallisation of the new phase takes place after an induction period reflecting the initial heterogeneous nucleation step. Such heterogeneous nucleation reactions are facilitated if the substrate surfaces offer good crystal lattice matches to the substance being precipitated. The catalytic effect of the heteronuclei is to reduce the critical supersaturation (Figure 1) at which the rapid increase in nucleation occurs with concomitant catastrophic precipitation. In order for true epitaxy to occur, an immobile monolayer of regular atomic pattern must be formed on the substrate surface and the orientated overgrowth will take place where the atomic pattern and the orientation of the embryo are preserved throughout the entire lattice of the overgrowth. Although it is not possible to grow HAP crystallites sufficiently large to verify such lattice orientation in the mixed phases, there is evidence to suggest that COM will nucleate on the surface of DCPD seed crystals [26,27] and HAP has also been found to induce the heterogeneous nucleation of calcium oxalate both at 25°C [28] and at 37°C [27]. In general, the ease of heterogeneous nucleation of the new crystalline phase follows the theoretical predictions for epitaxial growth on the basis of matching lattice parameters. The constant composition method is ideally suited for studies of the growth of such mixed phases since conventional crystallisation experiments in which the lattice ion concentrations decrease with time, provide

394

insufficient extents of reaction for quantification. The ability to grow macroscopic amounts of new phase at relatively low supersaturation on the substrate surfaces enables physical chemical characterisation of these precipitates. Thus during the growth of HAP on calcium oxalate trihydrate crystal surfaces, the specific surface areas of the solids increase markedly reflecting the formation of microcrystalline HAP. It is likely that the presence of urinary components may influence the formation of intermediate phases to different extents.

Acknowledgments

We thank the National Institute of Arthritis, Diabetes, Digestive and Kidney Diseases for a grant (number 3RO1AM19048) in support of this work.

References

1   Robertson WG, Peacock M, Nordin BEC. *Clin Sci 1968; 34:* 579
2   Robertson WG, Peacock M, Marshall RW et al. *N Engl J Med 1976; 294:* 249
3   Pak CYC. *J Clin Invest 1968; 48:* 1914
4   Marshall RW, Cochran M, Robertson WG et al. *Clin Sci 1972; 43:* 433
5   Hartung R, Leskovar P, Riedel J et al. *Proc IV Int Symp Urol Res.* New York: Plenum Press. 1981: 28
6   Hautmann R, Lehmann A, Komor S. *J Urol 1980; 123:* 317
7   Garside J. In Nancollas GH, ed. *Biol Min and Demin.* Berlin: Springer-Verlag. 1982: 23
8   Finlayson B. *Invest Urol 1972; 9:* 258
9   Miller JD, Randolph AD, Drach GW. *J Urol 1977; 117:* 342
10 Nancollas GH. *Interactions in Electrolyte Solutions.* Amsterdam: Elsevier. 1966
11 Davies CW. *Ion Association.* London: Butterworths. 1962
12 Robertson WG. *Clin Chim Acta 1969; 24:* 149
13 Marshall RW, Robertson WG. *Clin Chim Acta 1976; 72:* 253
14 Finlayson B. In David DS, ed. *Perspectives in Renal Failure and Nephrolithiasis.* New York: John Wiley. 1977: 337
15 Nielsen AE. *Kinetics of Precipitation.* Oxford: Pergamon Press. 1964
16 Burton WK, Cabrera N, Frank FC. *Philos Trans Roy Soc Lond 1951; A243:* 299
17 Sheehan M, Nancollas GH. *Invest Urol 1980; 17:* 446
18 Lanzalaco AC, Sheehan ME, White DJ et al. *Invest Urol 1982; 128:* 845
19 Tomazic BB, Nancollas GH. *Invest Urol 1979; 16:* 329
20 White DJ, Nancollas GH. *J Crystal Growth 1982; 52:* 267
21 Tomazic BB, Nancollas GH. *J Coll Int Sci 1975; 50:* 451
22 Ostwald W. *Lehrbuch Allegm Chem.* Leipzig: Engelmann. 1896–1902: 444
23 Francis MD, Webb NC. *Calcif Tissue Res 1971; 6:* 335
24 Koutsoukos P, Amjad Z, Tomson MB et al. *J Am Chem Soc 1980; 102:* 1553
25 Koutsoukos P, Sheehan ME, Nancollas GH. *Invest Urol 1981; 18:* 358
26 Pak CYC. *J Crystal Growth 1981; 53:* 202
27 Meyer JL, Bergert JH, Smith LH. *Clin Sci Mol Med 1975; 49:* 369
28 Nancollas GH, Gardner GL. *J Crystal Growth 1974; 21:* 267

Open Discussion

ROBERTSON (Chairman) You have already been trying to identify the various inhibitors on the calcium oxalate crystallisation system. Have you any clues as to the identity of these?

NANCOLLAS We are now looking at different molecular weight fractions and looking at very low molecular weight substances such as magnesium, citrate and pyrophosphate which appear to count for something like 30 per cent of the inhibition. We are also now separating by Sephadex columns, molecular weight fractions of urine and we find significant inhibition of mineralisation of calcium oxalate by both very high molecular weights, which might be something like the Tam Horsfall protein, and the lower molecular weight fractions (up to 10,000).

KERR (Newcastle-upon-Tyne) Following on that question, would you care to speculate on the role of hyperuricosuria in calcium oxalate stone formation. Do you think it is an inhibitory effect of urate in absorbing inhibitors or does it act by nidus formation or by some other acceleration of calcium oxalate stone formation.

NANCOLLAS We have done some work in which we have been able to grow calcium oxalate monohydrate on sodium urate crystals, and nucleation on the surface is certainly facilitated: it is dangerous to talk about epitaxis but certainly heterogeneous nucleation occurs. If you measure the induction period, that delay period for nucleation, as a function of concentration it follows very closely the classical nucleation theory. In other words, the rate is inversely proportional to the log of the supersaturation squared. You can calculate the surface energy from these results. In the presence of urate of course calcium urate may also be a viable phase and it always surprises me that very little work has been done on calcium urate growth. It is certainly a very insoluble phase and it is certainly possible to form mixed phases of calcium urate oxalate in solution. Now what effects the urinary inhibitors have specifically on each of the phases is not yet determined to my knowledge.

WILL (Leeds) Could you comment from the scientific point of view on the stability of the so-called formation product, the concentration product at the point at which homogenous nucleation is supposed to occur. Is it just a facet of pure solution or can it have any real meaning in more complicated, for example urinary solutions?

NANCOLLAS It has a real meaning, because there is a relationship between the creation of surface and the release of supersaturation. You have an un-favourable creation of surface and a favourable release of supersaturation, so there is definitely a real supersaturation above which spontaneous precipitation takes place. This business of threshold is a rather nebullous one because if you wait long enough, and one cannot wait for geological time, then crystallisation would take place and you would go down to the solubility level. To determine the threshold concentration above which crystallisation takes place, depends very much upon the laboratory technique. Your technician may do it for years and get the same result, whereas another laboratory would find it very difficult to reproduce because it depends upon, very often, impurities in solution which might act as sites for nucleation, and so break down the supersaturation. I think that simply measurement of threshold concentrations is rather dangerous. This is why we always try to do seeded crystal growth rather than homogenous precipitation, because those are absolutely reproducible. You can look at the effects of inhibitors and so on, and you can find, for instance, that a Langmuir adsorption isotherm appears to explain how the inhibitors block sites for crystallisation. You can do threshold experiments, but they are dangerous to do. I do not know whether that answers your question.

WILL I think it does. What you said is that measured threshold depends on who measures it and how long they wait for crystallisation to occur.

TSCHOEPE (Heidelberg) We have read and heard much about the role of the so-called inhibitors. Can you tell us a little bit about the so-called role of the promoters which have been put forward for some time.*

NANCOLLAS There is no such thing as a promoter of crystallisation. There is a promoter of apparent precipitation in which case you form a different phase. For instance, in the calcium phosphate fluoride field, of great interest to dental researchers, fluoride is often touted as a promoter of precipitation. Indeed if you add fluoride precipitation occurs more rapidly, but you form a different phase, you form fluorapatite rather than hydroxyapatite which has a different solubility. The most rapid crystallisation of a homogenous phase is the phase itself because it is offering a perfect surface for crystallisation to take place. If you happen to mix up that phenomenon with an additional heterogenous nucleation process then it might appear to increase the rate of precipitation when in fact you will probably be forming a different phase. The whole question of a crystal in solution is an interesting one because if you change the surface of a crystal then the solution has seen a completely different phase. The solution may only be looking at a monolayer and that monolayer may be crucial for controlling the whole behaviour of the solid liquid interface.

*   Hallson PC, Rose AG. *Lancet 1979; i:* 1000

CRITICAL ROLE OF OXALATE RESTRICTION IN ASSOCIATION WITH CALCIUM RESTRICTION TO DECREASE THE PROBABILITY OF BEING A STONE FORMER: INSUFFICIENT EFFECT IN IDIOPATHIC HYPERCALCIURIA

P Bataille, A Pruna, Isabelle Gregoire, Geneviève Charransol*,
J-F de Fremont, B Coevoet, C Galy, A Fournier

*Service de Néphrologie, CHU Amiens, and *Institut d'Hydrologie,
CHU Pitié-Salpétrière, Paris, France*

Summary

The probability of being a stone former (PSF) was calculated according to the method of Robertson in three groups of idiopathic calcium stone formers (normocalciuria (NCa), dietary hypercalciuria (DH) and idiopathic hypercalciuria (IH)) during four conditions: on a free diet; on a calcium and oxalate restricted diet for four days and after an oxalate load (200g of spinach) while on a calcium unrestricted or calcium restricted diet. Combined calciuria (Ca) and oxaluria (Ox) restriction significantly decreased PSF only in NCa and DH whereas the decrease was not significant in IH because of a concomitant significant increase in oxalate excretion. Increase of PSF with the oxalate load was significantly greater on calcium restricted than on calcium unrestricted diets in all groups of patients (4-6-12 times greater in NCa, DH and IH respectively). This shows the critical role of oxalate restriction when calcium is restricted in order to decrease the PSF. Combined restriction is not sufficient in idiopathic hypercalciuric patients to decrease their probability of stone formation.

Introduction

Calcium and oxalate are the main risk factors in calcium stone formation [1]. Many therapeutic measures have been tried in an attempt to reduce these risk factors and a low calcium diet became a popular form of therapy since many authors outlined the high incidence of hypercalciuria in stone formers. Unfortunately, calcium restriction induces an increase in urinary oxalate excretion [2], which led investigators to pay attention to additional oxalate restriction in the diet [3, 4]. Galosy [5] found that a low calcium diet (400mg/day) associated with a moderate oxalate restriction prevents the increase of oxaluria consequent to calcium restriction. Conversely, Nordin [4] failed to confirm the efficacy of this double restriction (400mg/day for calcium, 60mg/day for oxalate). He observed that stone formation ceased completely in only 12 of 37 recurrent stone formers and that oxaluria increased significantly in spite of a low oxalate diet.

Because of these differing results, we have studied the effects of a low calcium-low oxalate diet in various groups of idiopathic stone formers classified according to calcium excretion. Because of the supposed opposite variations of oxaluria and calciuria, the final effect of this double restriction was determined by changes in the 'probability of being a stone former' (PSF) of Robertson [6]. Knowing that some foods with high oxalate contents may induce peaks in oxalate excretion [7], we have determined the potential danger of an oxalate load during a 1g calcium diet and during a restricted calcium diet.

Methods

Protocol

Forty-two patients with calcium urolithiasis, and without gastrointestinal disorders, were studied on an ambulatory protocol. They collected their 24 hour urine during four conditions: on a free diet, after four days of a low calcium-low oxalate diet, and after an oxlate load (200g of frozen spinach, i.e. 1g of oxalic acid [8]) while on a 1g calcium diet and on a calcium restricted diet. Oxalate restriction was obtained by exclusion in the diet of the following products: rhubarb, spinach, beet, parsley, turnip, sorrel, nuts, asparagus, haricot, celery, redcurrant, strawberry, chocolate, cocoa, tea, instant coffee, fruit juices, white wine and vitamin C supplements. Calcium restriction was obtained by exclusion of all dairy products and resulted in an intake of approximately 400mg/day.

In the 24 hour urine collections, creatinine, calcium, phosphate, sodium and oxalate were measured. Blood was analysed for calcium, phosphate, creatinine, alkaline-phosphatase and parathormone, to eliminate patients with specific causes of calcium-stone formation.

Calcium, phosphate and creatinine were determined by automatic colorimetry (Technicon auto-analyser) and oxalic acid by gas liquid chromatography. Parathormone was measured by C specific radioimmunoassay. Statistical differences were assessed by the Student t-test for paired data.

Determination of the probability of being a stone former

The PSF was determined by the method of Robertson [6] using our own control and patients' data. The frequency distribution curves of the 24 hour excretion of calcium and oxalate and the risk curves for oxaluria and calciuria determined by the ratio (α) of the (frequency of stone formers)/(frequency of normals) at each value of oxaluria (Ox) and calciuria (Ca) have been published elsewhere [9]. The PSF combining the risk factors αCa and αOx was calculated by using the equation:

$$PSF = \frac{\alpha Ca \cdot \alpha Ox}{1 + \alpha Ca \cdot \alpha Ox}$$

Then it was possible to determine for each patient the PSF during the four dietary conditions.

402

Results

Classification of the patients

With our control data published elsewhere [9], we classified the 42 idiopathic calcium stone formers. Eighteen were normocalciuric (NCa) (calciuria < 4mg/kg/day), seven patients who were hypercalciuric on a free diet, presented a diet

TABLE I. Values (mean ± SEM) of daily excretion (mg/day) of urinary calcium (UCa) and oxalate (UOx) and values of the PSF on free diet and on a low calcium-low oxalate diet, in the various calcium stone former groups (NCa: normocalciuric, DH: with dietary hypercalciuria, IH: with idopathic hypercalciuria)

Stone former groups	Free diet			Calcium and oxalate restricted diet		
	UCa	UOx	PSF	UCa	UOx	PSF
NCa (n = 18)	185 ± 13	39 ± 2	0.56 ± 0.05	114 ± 11 ***	44 ± 3	0.44 ± 0.05 *
DH (n = 7)	403 ± 71	42 ± 4	0.80 ± 0.08	166 ± 21 ***	40 ± 2	0.48 ± 0.6 **
IH (n = 17)	423 ± 26	33 ± 2	0.77 ± 0.04	282 ± 16 ***	39 ± 2 *	0.68 ± 0.06

Significance of the difference between free diet and low calcium-low oxalate diet:
* $p < 0.02$; ** $p < 0.01$; *** $p < 0.001$

TABLE II. Variations (mean ± SEM) of the daily excretion (mg/day) of calcium (ΔUCa) and of oxalate (ΔUOx) and variations of the PSF (ΔPSF) induced by oxalate load while on 1g calcium diet and on calcium restricted diet

Stone former groups	1g calcium diet			Calcium restricted diet		
	ΔUCa	ΔUOx	ΔPSF	ΔUCa	ΔUOx	ΔPSF
NCa (n = 18)	−5 ± 10	+6 ± 2 **	+0.08 ± 0.04	−13 ± 10	+25 ± 4 ***††	+0.28 ± 0.05 ***††
DH (n = 7)	+17 ± 32	+4 ± 2 **	+0.06 ± 0.05	−8 ± 21	+30 ± 4 ***††	+0.36 ± 0.06 **†
IH (n = 17)	−25 ± 36	+6 ± 2 **	+0.02 ± 0.05	+11 ± 16	+25 ± 4 ***††	+0.24 ± 0.05 ***††

Significance of the variations of these parameters after oxalate load:
*$p < 0.01$; **$p < 0.01$; $p < 0.001$

Significance of the difference between calcium restricted and 1g calcium as regards variations Δ: † $p < 0.01$; †† $p < 0.001$

dependent hypercalciuria (DH), a diagnosis based on the return to normal urinary calcium excretion after calcium restriction, when compared to controls on the same restricted diet (calciuria < 3mg/kg/day). Idiopathic hypercalciuria (IH) was found in 17 patients who were hypercalciuric on a free diet and on a restricted calcium diet (i.e. calciuria > 4mg/kg/day on a free diet, calciuria > 3mg/kg/day on calcium restricted diet).

Effects of a low calcium-low oxalate diet on calcium and oxalate excretion and on the PSF

Table I shows the values of the daily urinary excretion of calcium and oxalate, and the values of the PSF in the various groups of patients on free diet and on calcium and oxalate restricted diet. The PSF decreased in all groups but only significantly in normocalciuric patients and in patients with diet dependent hypercalciuria. In all groups there was a significant decrease of calciuria, whereas oxaluria increased significantly only in patients with idiopathic hypercalciuria.

Variation of oxaluria, calciuria and PSF after oxalate load on 1g calcium diet and on calcium restricted diet

Table II shows the variations of daily excretion of calcium and oxalate and the variations of PSF after oxalate load during a 1g calcium diet and a low calcium diet. In all groups oxaluria increased on the 1g calcium diet and on the calcium restricted diet, but the increase of oxalate was four times more marked during the calcium restricted diet than during the 1g calcium diet, so that the PSF increase was significant only when patients were on the calcium restricted diet.

Assuming that oxalate is not catabolised after absorption [10], the percentage of absorbed oxalate from the orally ingested oxalate-rich foods was calculated thus for each patient:

$$\frac{\frac{\text{24 hour urine oxalate excretion}}{\text{on oxalate rich food}} - \frac{\text{24 hour urine oxalate excretion}}{\text{on low oxalate diet}}}{\text{oxalate load }/24\text{ hour}} \; 100\%$$

The percentage of absorbed oxalate increased significantly on the calcium restricted diet in every group: in NCa (mean ± SEM) from 0.71 ± 0.2% to 2.36 ± 0.38% (p<0.001), in DH from 0.36 ± 0.2% to 2.74 ± 0.33% (p<0.001), in IH from 0.48 ± 0.18% to 2.32 ± 0.50% (p<0.001).

Discussion

Our data, based on a short-term study, disagrees with Galosy's results [5]. Oxalate restriction does not prevent the increase in urinary oxalate excretion induced by calcium restriction in idiopathic hypercalciuric stone formers. In normocalciuric patients, oxalate excretion increases moderately but not significantly. The discrepancy between our results and those of Nordin [4] who observed a significant increase of oxalate in 17 patients (normo- or hypercalciuric) after a three year's calcium and oxalate restriction, may be explained by the fact that our study was of a shorter term basis.

Our study was performed with 42 outpatients, classified according to their calcium excretion, while they were asked to avoid foods with high content of oxalate. The oxalate content in the diet was not measured, maintaining the usual recommendations to patients, in order to judge the practical efficiency of these recommendations. Therefore, our results are different from those of Marshall [3] who found that in eight hospital patients with a controlled diet, a calcium and oxalate restricted diet could reduce urinary calcium and prevent an increase of urinary oxalate. This opposite result may be explained by the difficulty in reducing dietary oxalate at home. Particularly in patients with hyperabsorption of calcium, as in idiopathic hypercalciuric patients, the small quantity of oxalate in the diet is not complexed by intraluminal calcium during a low calcium diet, and is therefore available for passive absorption in the colon. It must be pointed out too, as was demonstrated by Finch [7], that the percentage absorption of oxalate is higher on a low oxalate diet than on a high oxalate diet.

The influence of dietary calcium on oxalate absorption is supported by the effects of the oxalate load performed on high and low calcium diets. The increase of oxaluria, induced by the significant increase of oxalate absorption, is four times greater during low calcium diets than during a 1g calcium diet, and would be able to induce peaks in concentration and crystaluria as observed by Finch [7].

In conclusion, a low oxalate-low calcium diet reduces urinary calcium but does not effectively prevent the increase in oxalate excretion, particularly in idiopathic hypercalciuric patients, so that the PSF does not change significantly in this group. The dramatic increase of urinary oxalate observed in all patients after the oxalate load during calcium restriction, stresses the critical role of oxalate restriction. This must reinforce our dietary instructions to patients, and invite us to seek additional measures to lower urinary oxalate during a low calcium diet.

References

1   Robertson WG, Peacock M. *Nephron 1980; 26:* 105
2   Zarembski PM, Hodgkinson A. *Clin Chim Acta 1969; 25:* 1
3   Marshall BW, Cochran M, Hodkinson A. *Clin Sci 1972; 43:* 91
4   Nordin BEC, Barry M, Bu Lusu L, Speed B. In *Urinary Calculi. Int Symp Renal Stone Res., Madrid.* Basel: Karger. 1972: 170—176
5   Galosy R, Clarke L, Ward DL, Pak CYC. *J Urol 1980; 123:* 320
6   Robertson WG, Peacock M, Marshall BW et al. *Br J Urol 1978; 50:* 449
7   Finch AM, Kasidas GP, Rose GA. *Clin Sci 1981; 60:* 411
8   Kasidas GP, Rose GA. *J Hum Nutr 1980; 34:* 255
9   Bataille P, Charransol G, Fournier A et al. *J Urol.* In press
10   Elder TD, Wyngaarden JB. *J Clin Invest 1960; 39:* 1337

Open Discussion

ROBERTSON (Leeds) I think we would agree with your observations. If you reduce the urinary calcium far enough, however, the probability of being a stone former will decrease significantly. What was the lowest urinary calcium you managed to achieve on your low calcium, low oxalate diet?

BATAILLE The purpose of the study was to observe what happened after calcium restriction in patients.

ROBERTSON When we tried this as a therapy we found it was only really successful when we added a high fluid intake to the low calcium, low oxalate diet. The low calcium, low oxalate diet as Nordin* presented was not particularly successful, perhaps about 50 per cent of the patients responded but at least 50 per cent did not.

PAK (Dallas) The discrepancy between Nordin and Bataille is not perhaps too surprising because of the complex nature of the control of oxalate excretion from ingestion of different diets. Oxalate absorption and excretion from food is not only a function of oxalate content in the food, but of the bioavailability. In fact the percentage of oxalate which can be absorbed from food in general is substantially less than from soluble sodium oxalate and the bioavailability seems to vary from person to person.

McGEOWN (Chairman) Have you in any way controlled sodium intake during these experiments?

BATAILLE We checked the value of the sodium excretion before and after the low calcium, low oxalate diet and there was no significant difference.

---

* Nordin BEC, Robertson WG, Barry H et al. In Hioco D, ed. *Rein et Calcium.* Rueil-Malmaison: Sandoz Editions. 1974: 345

DIFFERENT EFFECTS OF ORAL GLYCINE AND METHIONINE ON URINARY LITHOGENIC SUBSTANCES

W Tschöpe, E Ritz, H Schmidt-Gayk, L Knebel

University of Heidelberg, FRG

Summary

Nine male healthy volunteers were examined during a control period, during an oral glycine load (45g/day, 600mmol) and oral methionine (6g/day, 40mmol). Glycine caused a significant increase of urinary oxalate above baseline (from 644 to 797μmol/day) without change in calciuria (4.74 vs 4.84mmol/day). In contrast methionine caused no change of oxaluria, but a significant increase in calciuria (from 4.74 to 6.9mmol/day). Alterations of lithogenic ions in urine after protein ingestion are mediated by different amino acids. The particular lithogenic risk of animal protein may be related to its high methionine/cystine and glycine content.

Introduction

The pandemic of nephrolithiasis in Western societies has been related to dietary factors, in particular to high animal protein consumption [1]. Both high urinary Ca and high urinary oxalate have been identified as important lithogenic risk factors [2]. While an increase of urinary Ca with protein ingestion is well documented [3–5], information on the action of dietary protein or amino acids on urinary oxalate is conflicting. Several recent communications failed to demonstrate an increase of urinary oxalate in response to glycine loads [6, 7].

The present study examines to what extent calciuria and oxaluria are affected by methionine (a calciuric sulphur containing amino acid and glycine (a putative oxalate precursor).

Probands and methods

Nine male healthy volunteers, physicians of the nephrological staff, age 31 ± 5 years, were examined under constant self-selected diet with known energy and protein content under ambulatory conditions. Studies were carried out during three metabolic periods of five days each with no study on the intervening weekends. After a control period the probands received in a second period glycine (45g/day, 600mmol) as three divided doses dissolved in distilled water taken together with meals. In a subsequent third period they received methionine (6g/day, 40mmol). Urine was collected in plastic bottles with thymol. Fasting morning plasma samples and 24 hour urinary samples were examined for: Plasma-SMA 12 Autoanalyser; RIA for PTH (carboxyterminal), glucagon, insulin, GH; urine-oxalate with isotachophoresis [8]; citrate (lyase method); pH; cAMP (RIA); electrolytes with emission or AA spectrophotometry; sulphate with indirect AAS.

Results

As shown in Table I, 600mmol/day, glycine increased urinary oxalate in seven of the nine probands by an average of 153μmol/day. This was not associated with any significant change of calciuria. A preliminary dose response curve in one single proband showed a dose-related increase of oxaluria (baseline 476μmol/day; 3 x 4g glycine: +239μmol/day; 3 x 8g: +354; 3 x 16g: +506).

TABLE I

	Control period	Oral glycine (600mmol/day)	Oral methionine (40mmol/day)
UV$_{oxalate}$ (μmol/day)	644 ± 155	797 ± 194*	598 ± 150
UV$_{Ca}$ (mmol/day)	4.74 ± 2.36	4.84 ± 1.19	6.90 ± 3.2**
UV$_{cAMP}$ (μmol/day)	4.0 ± 1.7	4.5 ± 0.79	4.25 ± 1.03

The values represent $\overline{X}$ ± SD for the average values of nine probands.

* p < 0.05 (Wilcoxon test for paired differences)
** p < 0.01

In contrast, oral methionine caused no significant change of oxaluria, but a consistent increase of calciuria in all probands, the mean increment being 2.16 mmol/day. Complete intestinal absorption was suggested by an increase of urinary sulphate above baseline of 36mmol/day and by a corresponding increase of urea generation rate (urinary excretion plus Δ plasma urea x space of distribution). No significant associated change of iPTH or urinary cAMP/GFR was noted.

Discussion

A precursor product relationship between glycine and oxalate has been demonstrated with ^{14}C-radioglycine in man [9], 0.027–0.081 per cent of oral radioglycine tracer being recovered as urinary radio-oxalate. Subsequent investigations

408

showed inconsistent or no increase of urinary oxalate after oral [10] or intravenous [6, 7] non-labelled glycine. This may be due to several factors: (a) interindividual heterogeneity, possibly related to pyridoxal status; such heterogeneity was also noted in our study with only 7/9 probands showing increased oxaluria; (b) difficulties of measuring urinary oxalate; or (c) differences in the protocol of glycine administration. In particular, intravenous infusion of glycine [6, 7] may not achieve equally high glycine concentrations in portal blood as does oral administration of glycine. This is of note since glycine-oxalate interconversion is restricted to hepatic tissue. Our finding of 0.025 per cent of administered oral glycine appearing as urinary oxalate is in good agreement with the oral radioglycine study [9]. Although a 40g glycine load is high in relation to the usual daily protein consumption of 70g, preliminary dose-response data suggest that extrapolations into the range of usual dietary intake are legitimate. For physicochemical reasons [2], even a minor diet related increase in oxaluria may be relevant for lithogenesis.

The increase in calciuria upon ingestion of protein [3–5] and sulphur containing amino acids is well known. Our results show that such calciuria is not associated with detectable changes if iPTH and cAMP. This casts some doubt on evaluating these indices in clinical studies on the mechanism of calciuria in nephrolithiasis. No change of oxaluria with methionine suggests that the oxaluric action of protein is restricted to individual amino acids.

The particular lithogenicity of animal protein consumption [1] may be due, amongst other factors, to its high content of sulphur containing amino acids and glycine (or possibly aromatic amino acids). This may explain why the risk of nephrolithiasis is related to animal protein, but not total protein consumption [1].

References

1   Robertson WG, Peacock M, Heyburn PJ et al. *Br J Urol 1978; 50:* 449
2   Robertson WG, Peacock M. *Nephron 1980; 26:* 105
3   Walker RM, Linksweiler HM. *J Nutr 1972; 102:* 1297
4   Anand CR, Linksweiler HM. *J Nutr 1974; 104:* 695
5   Allen LH, Oddoye EA, Margen S. *Am J Clin Nutr 1979; 32:* 741
6   Nordenvall B, Backman L, Larsson L. *Scand J Gastroenterol 1981; 16:* 395
7   Nordenvall B, Backman L, Larsson L. *Scand J Gastroenterol 1981; 16:* 389
8   Tschöpe W, Brenner R, Ritz EJ. *Chromatogr 1981; 222:* 41
9   Elder TD, Wyngaarden JB. *J Clin Invest 1960; 39:* 1337
10   Crawhall JC, Scowen EF, De Mowbray RR, Watts RWE. *Lancet 1959; ii:* 810

Open Discussion

PEACOCK (Leeds) Did you find any change in the glomerular filtration rate because some of the changes that one might see with protein feeding could be due to alteration in glomerular filtration rate?

TSCHÖPE We did not see any change in glomerular filtration rate: there was no increase in urinary creatinine. One explanation might be that we started from a normal dietary protein intake. The reports of an increase in glomerular filtration rate with protein intake started from a low protein diet (30–50g daily) and then added 100g protein and in these circumstances the glomerular filtration rate increases.

PARSONS (Chairman) Is there any significance between the fact that one of the amino acids was essential while the other was non-essential? Do you have any observations on other amino acids in similar studies?

TSCHÖPE No, to my knowledge these are the first studies showing these effects. There are several reports on the calciuric effect of dietary protein. The calciuric effect is associated with increased urinary excretion of uric acid, sulphate and probably with a negative calcium balance. It is possible that some of these patients consuming a high dietary animal protein are at risk of developing negative calcium balance and bone disease, and perhaps are those patients claimed by Dr Pak to have a renal leak.

ROBERTSON (Leeds) We can confirm at a lower dose the results you have obtained with methionine, in that we found an increased urinary calcium. As far as increases in urinary oxalate in response to a high animal protein diet, there are some other amino acids, other than glycine and tryptophan, which are present in higher concentrations in animal than vegetable protein. Perhaps hydroxyproline might be one of interest as other workers have shown this to increase urinary oxalate excretion. Have you looked at any other amino acids?

TSCHÖPE No, we have not looked at other substances. Before starting our experiments we would have anticipated no effect of oral glycine. The metabolic fate of glycine is very diverse and so the effect of a single dose of glycine is very difficult to assess. There is one explanation of how glycine might be capable of inducing hyperoxaluria. A marginal pyridoxine (Vitamin B_6) deficiency, not a deficiency in the true nutritional sense. It might be that some individuals do not exhibit clinical signs of pyridoxine deficiency, but are at risk for oxalate formation as the threshold for oxalate synthesis from glycine, in these individuals, might be lower than the threshold for developing clinical signs of pyridoxine deficiency. In German surveys the plasma pyridoxine concentrations in the general population tends to be lower than that recommended by the World Health Organisation.

410

DIETARY ANIMAL PROTEIN AND URINARY SUPERSATURATION IN RENAL STONE DISEASE

B Fellström, B G Danielson, Britta Karlström, H Lithell, S Ljunghall, B Vessby

University Hospital, Uppsala, Sweden

Summary

Eight stone-forming patients were given diets that were high (HPD) and low (LPD) in dietary animal protein, each for two weeks. Urines were collected by the end of each diet period. Urinary calcium, phosphate, urate and acids were increased on HPD whereas citrate and urine-pH decreased. The urinary super-saturation and thereby the risk of forming crystals and stones of uric acid and ammonium urate was increased on HPD. The supersaturation of calcium oxalate was unchanged, but the inhibition of calcium oxalate crystallisation may have become unfavourably affected.

Introduction

A dietary uptake of purine-rich animal protein has been claimed to be the basis for an increased incidence of urolithiasis in the western world [1,2]. The urinary excretion of calcium, the main cation in most renal stones, and oxalate has been reported to increase with dietary animal protein [3]. Urinary urate has also been related to dietary purine and protein [3,4]. As the risk of forming crystals and stones in the urinary tract is dependent upon a balance between supersaturation and an inhibitory activity against crystallisation in the urine, the object of the present investigation was to further elucidate the metabolic effects of a high dietary intake of animal protein, and to study the concomitant effects on the urinary composition and supersaturation of salts which may potentially crystal-lise in the urine.

Material and methods

Eight calcium stone-forming patients were admitted to a metabolic ward for four weeks. There were seven males and one female, who altogether had passed 78 stones in 85 patient years. The patients received a low protein diet (LPD) for

411

two weeks and a high protein diet (HPD) for two weeks. Four patients began with LPD followed by HPD and the other patients received the diets in reverse order.

The two diets were isocaloric and the nutrient contents were obtained from food tables. The diets contained equal amounts of fat and the difference in protein calories was balanced by carbohydrate. The LPD contained 12 per cent protein and 48 per cent carbohydrates whereas the HPD contained 29 per cent protein and 31 per cent carbohydrate. The amount of protein in LPD was 57g/2000kcal and in HPD 142g/2000kcal. The excess of protein in HPD was mainly animal protein. The two diets contained equal amounts of calcium and oxalate. There were no restrictions regarding the fluid intake.

The patients collected urine on two consecutive days by the end of each dietary period and analysis of electrolytes, organic acids and nitrogen compounds were made. Urine-pH was measured on freshly voided urine in the morning and in the evening on the same days. The mean values of these two consecutive urine collections are presented below. Calcium and magnesium were analysed by atomic absorption spectrophotometry, urate by a uricase method, citrate by a citrate lyase method and oxalate by a colorimetric procedure. Supersaturations, ionic activities and urinary complexes were calculated through solving the thermodynamic mass equations by using an iterative, computerised procedure (EQUIL) [5]. The limits of metastable ionic activity products, the solubility products and the formation products were adopted from Marshall and Robertson. Student's t-test (paired values) were used to compare differences of mean values on the two diets.

Results

The 24-hour excretion of calcium increased in all subjects from 5.55 ± 1.8mmol on LPD to 7.43 ± 2.7 ($p<0.02$) on HPD. Urinary phosphate also increased from 26 ± 6mmol/24hr on LPD to 43 ± 9 on HPD ($p<0.001$). Urinary magnesium did not differ on the two diets. Urinary citrate decreased from 4.3 ± 1.5mmol/24hr on LPD to 3.1 ± 1.2 on HPD ($p<0.001$). Urinary oxalate was unchanged.

There was a 90 per cent increase in urinary urate from 3.5 ± 0.4 to 6.6 ± 1.0mmol/24hr ($p<0.001$). The excretion of both titratable acid and ammonium ions increased on HPD compared with LPD and thereby an increase in the net acid excretion from 28 ± 10 to 81 ± 21mmol/24hr ($p<0.001$). The morning urine pH was 0.9pH-units lower ($p<0.05$) on HPD compared with LPD.

The calculated thermodynamic equilibrium of the urines disclosed an increase of the ionised fraction of calcium on HPD. Changes in soluble calcium complexes are shown in Table I. The calculated ion activity product (AP) of calcium oxalate was within the metastable limits on both diets. Taking into account only the partial contributions of the changes in urinary calcium, oxalate, citrate and urine pH, the AP of calcium oxalate would have increased, but this effect was counteracted by the changes in urinary sulphate, phosphate, sodium and urinary volume. The net effect on calcium oxalate supersaturation was not different on HPD compared with LPD. On the other hand the ion activity product of uric acid increased in all patients. The urines were all undersaturated

412

TABLE I. Ionised calcium (mmol/24hr), calcium complexes (mmol/24hr) and ion activity products (-log(AP)) on low protein (LPD) and high protein (HPD) diets (mean ± SD)

	Low protein diet	High protein diet	p
Ionised calcium	2.3 ± 1.0	3.7 ± 1.8	p < 0.02
Calcium complexes			
CaCit	1.70 ± 0.64	1.15 ± 0.62	p < 0.001
$CaSO_4$	0.42 ± 0.18	1.26 ± 0.40	p < 0.001
$CaHPO_4$	0.83 ± 0.42	0.57 ± 0.46	NS
$Ca(H_2PO_4)_2$	0.17 ± 0.14	0.59 ± 0.38	p < 0.01
Ion activity products			
Calcium oxalate (SP = 8.68, FP = 7.45)	7.93 ± 0.34	7.91 ± 0.15	NS
Uric acid (SP = 8.71, FP = 8.3)	9.66 ± 0.24	8.74 ± 0.38	p < 0.001
Ammonium urate (SP = 5.0, FP = 3.16)	4.81 ± 0.32	4.52 ± 0.19	p < 0.05
Sodium urate (SP = 4.34, FP = 2.9)	3.94 ± 0.27	3.86 ± 0.17	NS

FP = formation product
SP = solubility product

on LPD but supersaturated in five patients on HPD. The ion activity products of ammonium urate was within the metastable region on both diets, but a higher degree of supersaturation was seen on HPD. The sodium urate ion activity product was not different on the two diets (Table I).

Discussion

In the present investigation the overall patient compliance was good, as judged by the nitrogen balance. As in previous studies it was demonstrated that the urinary calcium and urate increased on purine rich animal protein diet [3, 4]. The reason for the induction of calciuria on HPD is believed to be a primary renal effect and not increased intestinal absorption [6]. The mechanism is probably a decreased tubular reabsorption of calcium complexes. A less specific effect on the tubular reabsorption of calcium may have occurred from the increased diuresis and natriuresis demonstrated in seven of the eight patients. This view is supported by the fact that the urinary excretion of cyclic AMP was higher on HPD than on LPD (not shown). The substantial increase in urinary urate is readily understood, as dietary purines become absorbed in the intestine,

413

further metabolised to urate and subsequently mainly excreted in the urine [7]. Because of a high content of ash acids in proteins the urinary content of titratable acid and ammonium ions increased profoundly on HPD. Despite an increase in the buffering capacity of the urine, there was also a decrease in the urine pH. Urinary citrate was in the high normal range on the LPD but decreased by 27 per cent on HPD. The degree of acidity in serum and in urine, induced on HPD, probably stimulated the renal oxidation of citrate causing a diminished excretion.

The propensity for crystal formation, growth and aggregation depends on the balance between urinary supersaturation and inhibitory activity. The validity of the method used here to calculate ionised fractions and complexes in the urine has previously been compared with direct measurements of ionised calcium and found to predict Ca^{++} accurately. The net effect on calcium oxalate supersaturation was not different on the two diets by the current method. On the other hand the risk of forming uric acid or ammonium urate crystals or stones was significantly higher on HPD than on LPD. Microcrystals of uric acid are weak promoters of calcium oxalate crystallisation [8] but may also under certain conditions interfere with naturally occurring macromolecular inhibitors of calcium oxalate crystal growth [9]. Furthermore the decrease in urinary citrate and pH on HPD may have an unfavourable effect on the inhibitory activity of calcium oxalate crystal growth [10].

It is concluded that the risk of forming uric acid or ammonium urate crystals or stones becomes increased on a high protein diet. Calcium oxalate supersaturation, on the other hand, is not different on the two diets but the inhibitory activity of calcium oxalate crystal growth and aggregation may become affected unfavourably.

Acknowledgments

The work was supported by the Swedish Medical Research Council (No. 2329, 5640, 6354), the Swedish Society of Medical Sciences and by the Tore Nilsson Foundation.

References

1   Andersen DA. In Cifuentes Delatte, Rapado, Hodgkinson, eds. *Urinary Calculi.* Basel: Karger. 1973: 130–144
2   Robertson WG, Peacock M, Heyburn PJ et al. In Brockis, Finlayson, eds. *Urinary Calculus.* PSG Publishing Company. 1981: 3–12
3   Robertson WG, Heyburn PJ, Peacock M et al. *Clin Sci 1979; 57:* 285
4   Coe FL, Moran E, Kavalach AG. *J Chron Dis 1976; 29:* 793
5   Finlayson B. In David, ed. *Calcium Metabolism in Renal Failure and Nephrolithiasis.* New York: John Wiley. 1977: 337–382
6   Allen LH, Bartlett RS, Block GD. *J Nutr 1979; 109:* 1345
7   Löffler W, Gröbner W, Zöllner N. In Rapado, Watts, de Bruyn, eds. *Purine Metabolism in Man.* New York: Plenum Press. 1979; III(122A): 209–214
8   Pak CYC, Arnold LH. *Proc Soc Exp Biol Med 1975; 149:* 930
9   Fellström B, Backman U, Danielson BG et al. *Cli Sci 1982; 62:* 509
10   Sheehan ME, Nancollas GH. In Smith, Robertson, Finlayson, eds. *Urolithiasis: Clinical and Basic Research.* New York: Plenum Press. 1981: 391–399

Open Discussion

RITZ (Heidelberg) Could you mention what sort of protein you added to your basal diet?

FELLSTRÖM The one diet contained an excess of animal protein in the form of meat, while the other one was more based on carbohydrates.

RITZ So the excess protein was animal protein?

FELLSTRÖM That's right.

PEACOCK (Leeds) Could you tell me what the average change in urine volume was in your study?

FELLSTRÖM There was an increase in urine volume from about 1,500ml to 1,700ml per day.

PEACOCK And what would your range be in these 24-hour urines; would any be in excess of three litres?

FELLSTRÖM No, I think the standard deviation on both diets was about 400, and I do not think any volume was greater than 2,500ml.

PEACOCK It is a little bit difficult to appreciate since you plot your data as activity products in some way, and you are not really correcting for the change in fluid volume.

FELLSTRÖM That has been included in the calculation.

PEACOCK If there is a rise in urine volume in these studies, this will offset any effect on the saturation level.

FELLSTRÖM Yes, it certainly did, but it was included in the calculations.

PAK (Dallas) Did I understand correctly that carbohydrate intake in the two diets varied substantially?

FELLSTRÖM Yes, it did.

PAK How about the phosphate intake: it must also have varied substantially?

FELLSTRÖM The phosphate intake was different: it was much higher on the high protein diet.

PAK So some of the effects you observed could have been, at least partly, attributable to the effect of carbohydrate or phosphate?

415

FELLSTRÖM It is possible, yes.

McGEOWN (Chairman) Did the sodium intake vary also?

FELLSTRÖM We did not have any restriction on the sodium intake. The sodium intake was just measured and accordingly there was no difference, but still the measured urinary excretion of sodium was higher on the high protein diet.

PAK Substantially higher?

FELLSTRÖM It did not mean that the patients had, without recording, taken more salt while on the high protein diet, which may be part of the explanation of the hypercalciuria.

McGEOWN Can I ask the stone experts present if they advise their patients to have a modest dietary protein reduction?

PAK Yes, but it is extremely hard to do that on dialysis, because in Texas there are a lot of cattle. I try to do it but it seems ineffective.

PEACOCK Yes, we have put the occasional patient onto a vegetarian diet, and certainly we have got data that the stone prevalence rate is less in vegetarians. It is an approach, particularly in patients willing to accept the diet, and some of them are quite happy to do that, and it may well be one other form of therapy we have at the present time in very difficult cases.

SMITH (Richmond, USA) Dr Peacock, I would not agree with you. The vegetarian Hopi have a high incidence of stones, and those are mostly ammonia acid urates.

McGEOWN Are you suggesting one form of stone might be exchanged for another?

SMITH I am suggesting that a stone former is a stone former regardless of the diet.

PEACOCK I would like to disagree with you.

SMITH That's legitimate.

Proc EDTA (1983) Vol 20

PYRIDOXINE THERAPY IN PATIENTS WITH RENAL CALCIUM OXALATE CALCULI

P Balcke, P Schmidt, J Zazgornik, H Kopsa, E Minar

University of Vienna, Vienna, Austria

Summary

In 12 patients with idiopathic calcium oxalate calculi pyridoxine was administered. Within six weeks mean daily oxalic acid excretion decreased from $480 \pm 122\mu$mol to $336 \pm 83\mu$mol. Glycolic acid excretion fell from $208 \pm 51\mu$mol to $153 \pm 26\mu$mol (normal range: oxalic acid $228-412\mu$mol/day, glycolic acid $130-290\mu$mol/day). The reduction of oxalic acid excretion seems to be beneficial in prevention of idiopathic calcium oxalate calculi.

Introduction

In patients with type I primary hyperoxaluria pyridoxine treatment is reported to be beneficial by decreasing urinary oxalic acid and glycolic acid excretion. The decrease has been shown to be due to a diminished synthesis of both substances [1]. As urinary oxalic acid concentration is also an important factor in the pathogenesis of idiopathic calcium oxalate stones [2], we studied the effect of pyridoxine administration on urinary oxalic acid and glycolic acid excretion in patients without any evidence of metabolic disease.

Patients and methods

Twelve patients with recurrent stone formation were studied. Chemical analysis of calculi obtained by surgical intervention or voided spontaneously, had proved calcium oxalate composition in all patients. Disorders with high incidence of renal calcium oxalate calculi such as primary hyperparathyroidism, primary hyperoxaluria, renal tubular acidosis and intestinal diseases were excluded by routine clinical and laboratory investigations. However, idiopathic hypercalciuria was noted in four patients. Pyridoxine was administered orally in a dose of 300mg/day. Urinary excretion of oxalic acid, glycolic acid and calcium were measured at the beginning and after six weeks pyridoxine administration.

Oxalic acid determinations in urine were performed according to the photometric method described by Krugers et al [3]. To improve the precision of oxalic acid determination the procedure suggested by Hodgkinson [4] was used, adjusting the urinary pH value to 1.0–2.0, to dissolve all crystals of calcium oxalate. While stirring the urine samples the pH was then adjusted to 7.4 and the samples diluted 1:20. Oxalic acid determinations were performed subsequently.

Glycolic acid concentrations were determined by an enzymatic method [5].

Urinary calcium concentrations were measured by ACA-Autoanalyser (Dupont).

Before initiation of pyridoxine therapy intra-erythrocyte glutamic-oxalo-acetic transaminase (GOT) acitivity was studied before and after addition of pyridoxal-5-phosphate, the active metabolite of vitamin B6, to haemolysed blood samples in vitro, according to the procedure described by Stone et al [6].

Results

Prior to pyridoxine administration mean oxalic acid excretion of all patients under investigation was 480 ± 122μmol/day being slightly higher than the

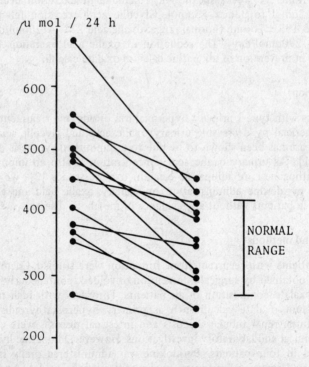

Figure 1.   Urinary oxalic acid excretion (μmol/day) in patients with idiopathic calcium oxalate calculi before (left) and after (right) 6 weeks pyridoxine administration

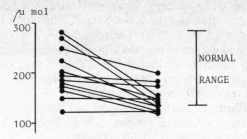

Figure 2. Urinary glycolic acid excretion (μmol/day) in patients with idiopathic calcium oxalate calculi before (left) and after (right) 6 weeks pyridoxine administration

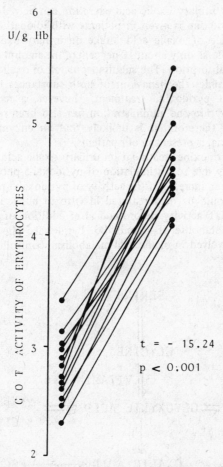

t = − 15.24

p < 0.001

Figure 3. Intra-erythrocyte glutamic oxaloacetic transaminase activity (GOT) in patients with idiopathic calcium oxalate calculi before (left) and after (right) addition of pyridoxal-5-phosphate in vitro to haemolysates

419

normal range (228–412μmol/day). When pyridoxine was administered mean oxalic acid excretion decreased to 336 ± 83μmol/day within six weeks (T-test for paired samples : t = 5.46, p <0.01 (Figure 1).

Mean glycolic acid excretion fell from 208 ±51μmol/24 hr to 153 ± 26μmol/ 24 hr (t = 3.16, p <0.05, normal range 130–290μmol/day) during the observation period (Figure 2). Urinary calcium values being 317 ± 179mg/day and 312 ± 128mg/day respectively remained unchanged.

Mean intra-erythrocyte GOT-activity increased by addition of pyridoxal-5-phosphate to haemolysed blood samples in vitro from 2.47 ± 0.3U/gHb to 4.63 ± 0.43U/gHb (t = −15.24, p <0.001) (Figure 3).

Discussion

Our data show that urinary oxalic acid excretion can be reduced by about 30 per cent when pyridoxine is given in patients with idiopathic calcium oxalate calculi. The influence of oxalic acid intake on urinary oxalic acid excretion seems to be negligible as only about 10 per cent of the amount normally excreted is due to intestinal absorption. The simultaneous fall of oxalic acid and glycolic acid excretion resembles the behaviour of both substances in type I primary hyperoxaluria under pyridoxine treatment. However, a reduction of oxalic acid excretion by pyridoxine administration has also been reported in normal volunteers [7] and therefore, it is unlikely that an enzyme disorder, as in primary hyperoxaluria, is present in our patients.

The effect of pyridoxine treatment on urinary oxalic acid and glycolic acid excretion is probably due to a stimulation of pyridoxal-5-phosphate dependent transaminases. Such an increase of the activity of pyridoxal-5-phosphate dependent transaminases could be demonstrated in vitro in our study measuring the intra-erythrocyte GOT activity before and after addition of pyridoxal-5-phosphate, the active metabolite of vitamin B6. Pyridoxal-5-phosphate dependent transaminases are involved in oxalic acid metabolism, controlling the conversion

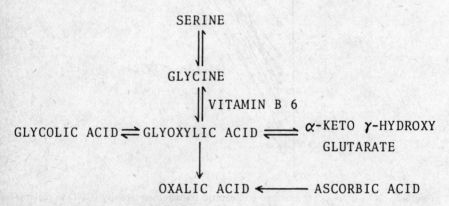

Figure 4. Pathways of oxalic acid formation [8]

of glyoxylic acid to glycine. It is therefore likely, that in our material, pyridoxine administration, by increasing the activity of pyridoxal-5-phosphate dependent transaminases, has caused an increased conversion of glyoxylic acid to glycine and thus a diminished synthesis of oxalic acid (Figure 4). Urinary oxalic acid concentration is mainly responsible for urinary calcium oxalate saturation [2], which, again is an important factor in urinary stone formation. Therefore, in patients with idiopathic calcium oxalate calculi the reduction of urinary oxalic acid excretion by pyridoxine treatment should be beneficial in preventing stone formation.

References

1   Will EJ, Bijvoet OLM. *Metabolism 1979; 28:* 542
2   Robertson WG, Peacock M, Heyburn PJ et al. *Br J Urol 1978; 50:* 449
3   Krugers Dagnaux PGLC, Olthuis FMFG et al. *Clin Chim Acta 1977; 75:* 123
4   Hodgkinson A. *Clin Chim Acta 1981; 109:* 239
5   Kasidas GP, Rose GA. *Clin Chim Acta 1979; 96:* 25
6   Stone WJ, Warnock LG, Wagner C. *Am J Nutr 1975; 28:* 950
7   Gershoff SN, Mayer AL, Kulczycki LL. *Am J Clin Nutr 1959; 7:* 76
8   Ribaya JD, Gershoff SN. *J Nutr 1979; 109:* 171

Open Discussion

BAKKALOGLLI (Ankara)   Have you estimated serum oxalic acid and glycolic acid concentrations? It is worthwhile estimating these substances in the serum.

BALCKE   We did not estimate serum oxalic acid and glycolic levels: it is very difficult to measure serum concentrations of these substances in whole blood in people with normal renal function.

BAKKALOGLLI   How about the urinary calcium excretion during the pyridoxine treatment?

BALCKE   We measured urinary calcium excretion during pyridoxine treatment and it was unchanged.

RITZ (Chairman)   Dr Balcke, do you attribute the effect of pyridoxine to a pharmacological action of the compound or do you assume that your patients were in latent vitamin B_6 deficiency? Unfortunately you did not present any data on Vitamin B_6 status.

BALCKE   We did not measure the pyridoxal I-phosphate concentrations in the serum, but I would say it is pharmacological.

RITZ   Do you have any evidence on erythrocyte morphology or iron kinetics to see whether there was any evidence of Vitamin B_6 dependence?

BALCKE   We have not studied this.

421

PLACEBO VERSUS ALLOPURINOL FOR RECURRENT URINARY CALCULI

M J V Smith

Medical College of Virginia, Richmond, Virginia, USA

Introduction

Many early workers noticed that hyperuricosuria and uricaemia were often associated with renal calculus disease [1,2]. In 1968, we reported our finding in a survey of recurrent active stone formers [3] and suggested that there was an association between these mild abnormalities. It was reported that 14 of 21 patients placed on allopurinol had stopped making stones [4]. This study was expanded and we were able to show that 63 per cent of patients improved [5]. It is well known that uric acid variation has been associated with progression in many disease processes. The marginal solubility of the undissociated and ionic forms of the molecule in blood and urine often present serious and special problems in man. Thus it seemed reasonable to see whether these abnormalities were associated with stone disease or perhaps were an unhappy relationship of two processes. This work was confirmed independently by Coe [6]. In the interim, a blind study of placebo versus allopurinol in the management of recurrent calcium oxalate stone formers was begun in 1970.

This report is the twelve year follow-up on this group of patients.

Materials and methods

All patients included in the study had undergone a full biochemical and uro-logical evaluation. They were not on any uricosuric drugs and had passed or had had a minimum of four renal calculi in the preceding three years, of which there must have been at least one crystallographic analysis confirming calcium oxalate. This preliminary evaluation had disclosed only that the serum uric acid was more than 6mg/dl. Some might or might not have had uricosuria but it was necessary for the serum concentration to be elevated for inclusion in the study.

The nature of the study was explained to the patient and an appropriate consent form was signed. The patient was then given a simple diet and advice about maintaining an adequate urine output. They also were given nitrazine paper and asked to record the pH of the urine voided in two, 24-hour periods. The patients then returned two weeks later with a 24-hour urine specimen and the serum studies were repeated. If no significant biochemical changes had occurred and the patient had demonstrated an ability to be interested in the therapy by recording the pH of the urine they were entered in the study.

The patient was then given a prescription for allopurinol 100mg t.i.d. for a week and then 100mg each morning. This prescription was only to be filled at our hospital pharmacy. The hospital pharmacy dispensed 100mg allopurinol tablets if the patient's hospital number ended in an even digit and a placebo tablet if it were odd. This information was not known to the investigator until June 1975. The prescription always called for more tablets than would be required. The patient was instructed to bring them with him and the number of remaining tablets was recorded before a new prescription was written.

All patients were instructed to maintain the urine alkaline (more than pH 6.5) by using sodium bicarbonate in varying doses, which was self-regulated by the use of nitrazine paper. This device was used for two reasons: 1) to prevent the theoretical iatrogenic formation of xanthine stones and 2) it was believed that by being allowed to regulate partially his own therapy the patient would be involved.

TABLE I

Years on study	Allopurinol			Placebo		
	No.	Improved	Lost	No.	Improved	Lost
7	31	8	10	1	2	40
8	28	4	12	1	2	33
9	19	4	13	1	2	29
10	18	3	7	1	1	24
11	14	3	9	1	0	16
12	9	1	6	1	0	7

The patients were followed at appropriate intervals, usually every month for three months and then at three monthly intervals. A patient was regarded as improved if there was a decrease in the number of calculi formed and/or passed, and the investigator as well as the patient thought that the therapy was helpful. No change in stone disease was defined as a patient who continued to have and/or to pass stones at the same rate as before treatment. No new stones was defined as no further stone formation even though the patient might pass stones that were documented to be present prior to initiation of therapy.

In 1975, the code was broken and the patients continued on their 'medicine'. Those who were on placebo were offered the opportunity to change to allopurinol, 300mg daily, and their results are also reported.

TABLE II

Placebo patients
Now on allopurinol 300mg daily

Years on study	No.	Improved	Lost
6	23	4	13
5	22	6	12
4	22	10	8
3	22	12	5
2	21	14	5
1	18	18	4

Results

The results of the years seven to 12 of this study are given in Table I and the six year follow-up of patients transferred from placebo to 'active' treatment are shown in Table II.

Discussion

It has become very clear that careful attention to 'treatment' details by both doctor and patient play a significant role in the management of renal calculus disease [7]. The use of urinary alkalinisation by all patients may have played a role in the good results we have achieved. This aspect of our work is under current study.

It is now important to realise that there are only a very small group of patients who will benefit from the use of allopurinol. These are patients in whom the urinary uric acid concentration in a twenty-four hour urine exceeds 40mg/100ml.

Excessive purine intake probably is a real factor in patients since this has far reaching effects on the urinary constituents and pH and dietary advice will help these patients. However, it is important to realise that the patients in this study received this advice *prior* to their entry and this hopefully the diet effect was eliminated.

References

1   Gutman AB, Yu TS. *Am J Med 1968; 45:* 756
2   Hall AP, Barry PE, Dawber TR, McNamara PM. *Am J Med 1967; 42:* 27
3   Smith MJV, Hunt LD, King JS Jr, Boyce WH. *J Urol 1969; 101:* 637
4   Smith MJV, Boyce WH. *J Urol 1969; 102:* 750
5   Smith MJV. *J Urol 1977; 117:* 690
6   Coe FL, Raisen L. *Lancet 1973; i:* 129
7   Pak CYC. *J Urol 1982; 128:* 1157

Open Discussion

EDWIN (New Orleans) Could you share with us your experience of adding allopurinol to other drugs in treating stones?

VERNON SMITH The statements that I am about to make are certainly somewhat biased by some of the recent findings particularly from this part of the world. It has always been my opinion that hydrochlorothiazide has a part to play in the management of patients. Sometimes it apparently will not work. One of the major things that we forget to look at is the urinary acid and sodium. Many of my patients defeat the action of the drug by increasing their salt intake after the introduction of hydrochlorothiazide to their diet and I might just as well have not placed them on it. They then become severely uricosuric and the only way I can manage them is to then add allopurinol. This does appear to have an effect but I stress again that we need to know what happens at five years because this is life long therapy that we're talking about.

KERR (Newcastle upon Tyne) First of all you said that you think the therapy works only in the patients who excrete an excess of uric acid in the urine but you did not define what an excess is. Do you have a value about which you prescribe allopurinol for an average size adult male?

VERNON SMITH I define what I regard as excess anything above 40mg per cent. That can be 40mg in 100cc or 800mg in 2,000cc and then my mathematics run out. In fact the definition is 40mg per cent because it's my experience, as many people in this room would agree with me, that most stone formers don't know a normal urine output.

KERR Is this measured on an early morning sample or what?

VERNON SMITH These are all measured on 24 hour specimens.

KERR Secondly, do you place any restrictions on alcohol intake in people who are taking allopurinol?

VERNON SMITH I live in the South, no!

KOPP (Munich) What was your average bicarbonate dose for your patients to bring the urine pH to 6.5?

VERNON SMITH The only commercial that I will give is one heaped teaspoon of Almond Hammer baking soda four times a day. That is approximately 60 grains four times a day.

AHMAD (Liverpool) I can just confirm the data that you presented. We recently completed our double blind study of allopurinol versus placebo and will be presenting our work tomorrow in the Workshop on renal stone disease. We did not find any difference between the two groups.

CAMERON (Chairman)   What are the reasons for giving bicarbonate? Can I challenge you on one of the reasons being that you prevent xanthine stones on allopurinol treatment by giving sodium bicarbonate. Unlike uric acid, which is remarkably pH sensitive in terms of its solubility within the physiological range of urine pH, xanthine and other insoluble purines like 2—8 dihydroxy-adamine are markedly insensitive. I don't think giving bicarbonate is going to make any difference to the risk of xanthine stones at all.

VERNON SMITH   I think that in today's world I probably would agree with you. I think my placebo effect may in part be due to the sodium bicarbonate I give these patients, who, as we all know, have remarkably acid urine. Originally my hospital in North Carolina would not allow me to give allopurinol alone or a placebo alone to this group and rather than spoil the study I kept going. I agree with your statements completely.

Proc EDTA (1983) Vol 20

ALTERNATIVE TREATMENT OF CYSTINURIA WITH α-MERKAPTOPROPIONYLGLYCINE, THIOLA®

T Denneberg, J-O Jeppsson, P Stenberg

University Hospital, Malmoe, Sweden

Summary

Sixteen patients with cystinuria have been treated with Thiola for 0.5—4 years. Only two of the patients had recurrence of stones because of initial inadequate dose. The excretion of free cystine and the mixed Thiola-cysteine disulphide in the urine has been measured on an automatic amino acid analyser. Thiola has less side effects than D-penicillamine with respect to bone marrow, kidney, liver, gastrointestinal tract and skin. No chelating properties on urinary excretion of copper and zinc were observed during Thiola treatment. We conclude that successful treatment will depend on determining an individual dose of Thiola for every patient and from monitoring free cystine and Thiola-cysteine disulphide in the urine.

Introduction

Cystinuria is an inherited metabolic disease which is characterised by the urinary excretion of abnormally high amounts of the amino acids cystine, arginine, lysine and ornithine. The aim of management in cystinuria is to keep the urinary cystine concentration less than supersaturation thereby preventing cystine precipitation and subsequent stone formation. This may be accomplished by reducing the concentration of cystine in the urine and/or by increasing its solubility. In severe cases specific treatment is necessary to prevent formation of cystine stones and the most common form of therapy is changing cystine to a chemically more soluble form, the mixed disulphide, with D-penicillamine.

Since Crawhall et al [1] introduced D-penicillamine treatment, several reports have confirmed this concept. However, as many as 50 per cent of patients develop one or more complication such as hypersensitivity reactions, haematological changes, abnormalities of taste and smell, nephrotoxicity, formation of abnormal antibodies, dermatopathy and connective tissue changes, as well as an antipyridoxine effect and chelating properties [2—4]. The signs of renal damage are described with slight to severe proteinuria, clinically as a nephrotic syndrome and 'penicillamine nephropathy', and immune-complex glomerulo-nephritis [5]. Thus clinical experience with D-penicillamine has shown that the drug has serious side effects which limits its application. For this reason new potential drugs, other than thiol derivatives, with better tolerance have been developed. Among the new compounds, α-merkaptopropionylglycine* has been selected because of its advantages compared with other thiols [6,7].

This report records our experience of Thiola and the value of cystine and Thiola-cysteine disulphide analysis in the urine. The determination of free cystine and its mixed disulphide makes it possible to determine individual treatment for cystinuric patients using Thiola as a safe and effective drug in preventing stone formation.

Material and methods

Of sixteen patients with homozygote cystinuria treated with Thiola, seven were female and nine male, aged 18–70. The observation period at treatment was 0.5–4 years. The cases were selected postoperatively for prophylactic purposes because of stone recurrence. The diagnosis of cystinuria was made by chemical analysis of the stones.

As a screening procedure cyanide-nitroprusside reaction (Brand's test) was used with a sensitivity for urine cystine $>300\mu mol/L$. All positive urines were run on high voltage electrophoresis at pH 1.9 and 6.4. Final quantitations of cystine, arginine, lysine and ornithine were performed on a Kontron Liquimat III amino acid analyser. During the Thiola treatment quantitative determinations of cystine and Thiola-cysteine disulphide were routinely made by an automatic 40 minutes programme of ion-exchange chromatography developed for this purpose (Figure 1).

Treatment with Thiola was started in hospital with a dose of 250–500mg given at night. After a few days the dose was increased to 750–1000mg. The patient was hospitalised for a 10-day period and was then followed up monthly or every second month as an outpatient. As the patients were treated conservatively prior to surgery with hydration and alkalinisation they were instructed to drink adequately, especially in the evening, to achieve an output of 2L/day or more. Previous sodium bicarbonate medication of 15–20g daily was reduced (3–6g) to maintain a urinary pH at approximately 6.5–7.0.

Results

Figure 2 summarises the clinical results of the sixteen patients treated with Thiola. The bars show 24-hour urine cystine excretion before treatment with Thiola and Thiola-cysteine disulphide during treatment with Thiola. The excretion of cystine before treatment varies between 1500–3800μmol/24 hours, and the excretion of Thiola-cysteine disulphide between 1000–5000μmol/24 hours. The dose of Thiola required (0.5–2.5g) was adjusted to achieve a urinary cystine excretion of less than 1200μmol/24 hours.

*Thiola, Santen Pharmaceutical Co Ltd., Osaka, Japan

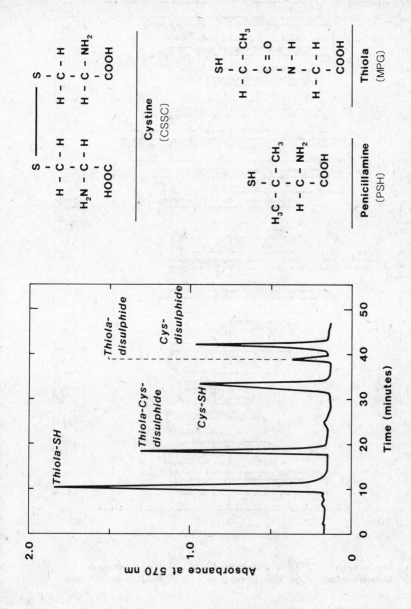

Figure 1. Analysis of cystine and related compounds on a Kontron Liquimat III amino acid analyser equipped with a Durrum DC-6A resin. The ninhydrinamino acid complexes were monitored at 570nm

429

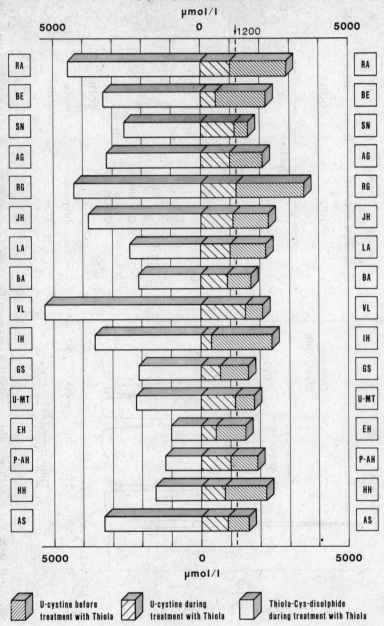

Figure 2

430

Only two of the patients (case AG and LA) had stone recurrence during treatment. All the other fourteen patients had no recurrence of stones or signs of further growth. Case AG was given a dose which was too low at the start of treatment and case LA had gastrointestinal side effects (gastritis). None of the other patients had side effects of skin rash or fever, but some of them had registered soft faeces and could accept the sulphurous smell of Thiola in the urine and faeces.

There was no evidence of bone marrow depression (granulocytopenia, thrombocytopenia or anaemia). The liver enzymes were normal and no proteinuria was found. No increased urinary excretion of copper or zinc, due to chelation, were observed during Thiola treatment which was in contrast with the massive excretion of copper and zinc in D-penicillamine treated patients.

Discussion

We have employed the Brand's test as a screening method for the early diagnosis of cystinuria and found it to be simple, rapid and reliable. The occurrence of a positive Brand's test in the urine and a radiopaque calculus was however not diagnostic of cystinuria. There is a need for further investigation before treatment with Thiola is started. The sensitivity limit of the Brand test is $300\mu mol/L$ and it is also positive in cases of heterozygote cystinelysinuria, isolated cystinuria, homocystinuria, β-merkaptolactatecysteine-disulfiduria and general aminoaciduria.

High voltage electrophoresis is a suitable medium for the identification of cystine and the other three dibasic amino acids. If the patient is homozygous, all four amino acids are represented in high concentration. The amount of cystine in a 24-hour urine should, if possible, be quantified by ion-exchange chromatography before treatment with Thiola. A specially designed programme on an amino acid analyser is of great value for sequentially following urinary cystine excretion. On our chromatography system the free cystine is eluted with the free Thiola and the Thiola-cysteine disulphide. Thus therapy could be monitored by periodic quantitation of free cystine and the Thiola-cysteine disulphide. The determination of the mixed Thiola-cysteine disulphide is a therapeutic control of the co-operation of the patient during the life-long treatment.

Our results are in agreement with other investigators [8–10] but we recommend the quantitation of Thiola and the Thiola-cysteine disulphide for careful follow-up of these high-risk patients. The results of the present study confirm the efficiency of Thiola in the prophylaxis of cystine stone formation. Only two of the sixteen patients had stone recurrence during treatment. Furthermore therapy with Thiola was not associated with any serious side effects and appears to be well tolerated, making it acceptable long-term therapy. This is a distinct advantage of Thiola over D-penicillamine which produces side effects of such severity necessitating that withdrawal is necessary in some patients.

References

1   Crawhall JC, Scowen EF, Watts RWE. *Br Med J 1963; 1:* 588
2   Lulle RG. *Postgrad Med J Suppl 1968; 44:* 21

3   McDonald JE, Henneman PH. *N Engl J Med 1965; 273:* 578
4   Henkin RJ, Keiser HR, Jaffe JA et al. *Lancet 1967; ii:* 1268
5   Jaffe IA, Treser G, Suzuki Y et al. *Ann Int Med 1968; 69:* 549
6   Kallistratos G, Timmermann A. *Naturwissenchaften 1968; 55:* 648
7   Kallistratos G, Malorny G. *Drug Res 1972; 22:* 1434
8   Hautmann R, Terhorst B, Stuhlsatz HW et al. *J Urol 1977; 117:* 628
9   Kallistratos G, Burchardt P, Freerksen P. *Folia Bioch et Biol Graeca 1978; 15:* 21
10   Miano L, Gallucci M, Petta S. *Eur Urol 1979; 5:* 265

Open Discussion

HALDIMAN (Sierre, Switzerland) An escape phenomenon to the effect of D-penicillamine has been observed in patients with cystinuria. Have you observed the same escape phenomenon to the effect of Thiola? Secondly, how many months of therapy are needed until the effect of D-penicillamine can be seen again?

DENNEBERG The first question about the value of Thiola and penicillamine is difficult to answer but we can't say as we have only a short experience of Thiola in comparison to penicillamine in dissolving stones, but we can say that it is a very good drug for the prophylaxis. From the literature we were a little ambivalent about the dose at which we should begin. I would say that you can start with a dose of 500mgs and increase very quickly and don't wait as we did in the beginning. We start treatment in hospital for 10 to 12 days because if you have side effects they will be manifest during this time.

HALDIMAN My question has not been completely answered. The escape phenomenon I am referring to is the fact that the patients will have an increase in the 24 hour urinary excretion of cystine and this has been described after a few months or a year of treatment. Have you seen this effect?

DENNEBERG No.

HALDIMAN Does anybody know how many months of therapy are needed until the full effect can be seen again?

CAMERON (Chairman) I don't know either.

MARANGELLA (Turin, Italy) This is just to confirm your results. We have presented in Williamsburg some data about patients with cystinuria who had been treated with 2HPG for a mean of 36 months. We haven't observed any escape phenomenon.

DENNEBERG Yes, I know of your work from Italy. There are, in fact three groups in Europe who have used this drug*. Some papers come from Japan† where this drug comes from.

*   Johansen K, Gammelgard PA, Jorgensen FS. *Scand J Urol Nephrol 1980; 14:* 189
*   Pavanello L, Rizzoni G, Dussini N et al. *Europ Urol 1981; 7:* 139
*   Dimopoulos C, Stokidis D, Kallistratos G et al. *J Urol (Paris) 1981; 87:* 265
†   Araki T, Tanahashi T, Ishito N et al. *Nippon Hinyokika Gakkai Zasshi 1981; 72:* 221

PAK (Dallas, USA) We have been conducting a multi-centre trial in the United States concerned with the question of whether penicillamine is more toxic than Thiola, or conversely whether Thiola is safer to use than penicillamine. To test this hypothesis we have taken patients who had developed clear cut toxicity to penicallamine and offered them instead Thiola. To date 45 per cent of the patients developed toxicity to Thiola suggesting that there is at least an element of cross reactivity of side effects.

CAMERON That's a very important comment.

GOLDSMITH (Liverpool) It may be impossible in a hot climate to procure the necessary high urine volumes to deal successfully with cystinuria in people with established stones. I have the impression that at least in this country most nephrologists simply use a very high fluid intake and adequate amounts of bicarbonate. Certainly this is true of one or two colleagues with whom I have discussed this. In my own practice, and in view of the toxicity of these drugs I would have thought that this should be the first line of approach.

CAMERON Would you like to comment on that Dr Denneberg, because I think the custom in Britain, which has been heavily influenced by the late Dr Giles Dent, was to exploit the physical chemistry of cystine in the urine to educate patients very carefully and very thoroughly with alkalinisation giving them pH papers. We use, for example, the British Drug Houses medium range pH paper to test their early morning urine. In addition to ensure a high fluid intake, and with this regime, as Dr Goldsmith said, one can achieve a great deal that one can achieve with either of the chelating drugs. You mention that you only use moderate diuresis and I wonder if you could tell us before the patients reach the Thiola and penicillamine treatment how intensively was diuresis or alkalinisation exploited, or was it not at all?

DENNEBERG I'm situated in the south of Sweden and the patients are coming from the urologists so they are operated on and sent to me afterwards. They are instructed to drink as much as four to five litres daily and with about 15 to 20 grams bicarbonate. So I reduce their drinking and reduce also their bicarbonate to about three to six grams daily.

ROBERTSON (Leeds) Just to come back on this question of giving bicarbonate for cystine stone formation. One of the problems is that you have to give fairly high doses of bicarbonate. The urine pH must go up well into the sevens to have any significant effect on the solubility of cystine. I think if you look in the literature on this form of therapy you will find several reports of calcium phosphate that precipitates being overlayered on the top of cystine stones. It is not entirely effective in every individual in preventing stone formation.

DENNEBERG Yes, this is described in the literature and is also our experience.

Proc EDTA (1983) Vol 20

CRITICAL EVALUATION OF VARIOUS FORMS OF THERAPY FOR IDIOPATHIC CALCIUM STONE DISEASE

M Marangella, A Tricerri, S Sonego, M Ronzani, B Fruttero, P G Daniele*, M Bruno, F Linari

Osp Mauriziano Umberto I di Torino, and
*Università di Torino, Torino, Italy

Summary

The results are presented of the dietary management, alone or in association with thiazides and/or allopurinol, evaluated in 143 idiopathic calcium stone formers after a mean follow-up of 18 months. Diet alone proved to be effective in the prevention of stone relapses. The addition of thiazide and/or allopurinol provided mild improvements of urine environment but seemed to give no further clinical benefits irrespective of underlying metabolic abnormalities.

Introduction

It is now widely agreed that idiopathic nephrolithiasis can be related to some risk factors whose influence on urine environment make it conducive to stone formation [1,2]. Increases in calcium, oxalate, uric acid excretions and decrease in urine volume have been suggested as the most frequent causative factors in this disease [3,4].

For the prevention of stone recurrence various therapies have been proposed which centre on the correction of underlying urine abnormalities [5,6]. Two general approaches are suitable in this regard: dietary management and the use of drugs such as thiazides and allopurinol.

These therapies have been employed for the prevention of stone recurrence in idiopathic calcium stone-formers who we have been observing in our stone-unit over the last four years. The aim of this paper is the critical evaluation of the results obtained after a mean follow-up of 18 months and a comparison of the effectiveness of the various forms of therapy.

Material and methods

One hundred and forty-three patients, 88 males and 55 females, which had had at least two stone episodes in the two years preceding the initiation of treatment

434

were considered for the study. Infra-red spectroscopy of passed stones or X-ray documentation of radiopaque calculi and clinical and laboratory findings were used as criteria for the diagnosis of idiopathic calcium stone-disease. Patients with persistent urinary-tract infection or with significant reduction of creatinine clearance were excluded.

All patients were then asked to increase urine volume by drinking at least 1.5–2.0 litres of fluids per day. Milk, dairy products, spinach, cocoa, rhubarb and beetroot were abolished from the patients' diets in order to lower calcium and oxalate intake. Some patients were encouraged to 'eat less' to achieve a body weight reduction.

They were then allocated into one of the following groups:

A. Thirty-eight patients (23 males); no drug was added to the dietary treatment.

B. Thirty-eight patients (26 males); allopurinol (ALP 300mg daily was given together with a diet.

C. Sixty-seven patients (39 males); hydrochlorothiazide (HCT) 50mg/day, sometimes in association with ALP (17 patients) were given with diet.

The allocation of a patient into one of the above groups depended in part on the metabolic presentation and in part on the patient's compliance to the drugs. Many patients were included in group A after they had to discontinue HCT and/or ALP because of side-effects. Patients with mild or border-line hypertension were always given HCT irrespective of other clinical and biochemical features. Patients with basal or HCT inducted hyperuricaemia were generally given ALP. Stone history, biochemical and physicochemical parameters were recorded before entering the treatment programme and during treatment. Well documented passages of gravel with renal colic were assumed as being stone-episodes.

Routine methods were used for calcium, magnesium, sodium, potassium, ammonium, zinc, citrate, sulphate, phosphate, chloride, creatinine, uric acid and pH determination in urine. Oxalate was determined by a modified colorimetric procedure [7]. Urine saturation with respect to calcium oxalate monohydrate and with brushite was calculated by an original equilibrium-based computer model system [8].

Results

The metabolic presentation in the overall series is reported in Table I, which shows that the percentages of patients with metabolic disorders are equally represented in each treatment group; a mild difference in the percentage of hypercalciuric patients has been found only between group B and group C.

The changes in biochemical and physicochemical parameters obtained during each treatment (means have been used when more than one value was available) resulted as follows: significant differences have been found for calcium excretion which decreased in all the three groups ($p < 0.01$ in group A; $p < 0.05$ in group B; $p < 0.001$ in group C). Uric acid excretion decreased only in group B ($p < 0.01$) and in group C ($p < 0.001$). Decreases in oxalate excretion were mild but not of treatment peaks of urine supersaturation with calcium salts disappeared in the majority of the patients.

The clinical course recorded before and during treatment is shown in Table II: an important reduction in the stone recurrence rate has been achieved in most of the patients and the differences of the treatment clinical parameters between groups were not significant.

Discussion

The improvement of the knowledge of the mechanisms which lead to the formation of stones in the urinary-tract and the recognition that certain features of urine composition may act as risk factors have been assumed as the basis for a modern therapeutic approach to the idiopathic stone-disease. A number of series have been reported in which thiazides and allopurinol alone or in association have proved to be effective in idiopathic calcium stone-formers [9,10].

Dietary management gave favourable results in Pak's patients who presented with no metabolic changes [6].

An extensive use of controlled diets has been made by us and the dietary regimen has been associated with ALP and/or HCT in some of our patients, whereas others did not receive any drug. Our data seem to show that the dietary management produces a satisfactory and significant decrease of stone recurrence rate. These results seem to be related to decreases in urine calcium excretion and oxalate concentration coupled with increase in urine volume and to the consequent disappearance of peaks of supersaturation with calcium salts.

When added to the dietary regimen ALP and HCT have induced, in our experience, mild improvements in urine environment, but this did not appear to increase clinical benefits. These results cannot be explained by the fact that we selected patients and specific treatment because the population of each group was homogeneous with respect to age, sex, severity of the disease and metabolic abnormalities. Moreover when we have compared the results obtained in patients presenting with similar metabolic abnormalities but allocated to different treatment groups we failed to find significant differences in the clinical course during treatment.

This leads us to suggest that the effectiveness of the diet alone could be independent of the underlying metabolic disorders and that patient's compliance to the different therapies could be the most important factor in the treatment choice.

This is likely to be the case when neither hypercalciuria, of the non-absorptive type, nor hyperuricosuria are present, but firm conclusions cannot be drawn from this study due to the small number of patients in the single treatment groups. Only a prospective study with random allocation to either dietary or drug therapy will answer this question. However, when drug induced side-effects or failure to obtain adequate results with HCT and/or ALP occur we suggest the discontinuation of drug therapy. A careful dietary management could give, in our opinion, a good chance of success even in patients presenting with those specific metabolic disturbances.

TABLE I. Percentages of patients with specific metabolic presentations in each treatment group (*p<0.05 for the difference of group B vs group C performed by Chi square)

Group	A	B	C	Total
Number of patients	38	38	67	143
No metabolic disorders	28.9	28.9	26.9	28
Hypercalciuria (uCa ⩾ 0.1mmol/24h)	26.3	13.2*	32.8	26
Hyperuricosuria (uUA ⩾3.6mmol/24h)	15.8	23.7	11.9	16
Hyperoxaluria (isolated) (uOx ⩾ 0.5mmol/24h)	13.2	15.8	11.9	13
Hypercalciuria + Hyperuricosuria	15.8	18.4	16.5	17

significant. Significant increases in urine volume were obtained ($p<0.05$) in the three groups. Ionic strength decreased only in group A ($p<0.05$).

Urine saturation with respect to calcium oxalate and brushite decreased mildly but not significantly in group A and B while the decrease was weakly significant in group C ($p<0.05$). It is noteworthy however that during each type

TABLE II. Clinical outcome in each treatment group. Means ± 1 SEM are shown

Group	A	B	C
Number of patients	38	38	67
Age (at presentation)	39.5 ± 2.0	40.9 ± 1.8	39.6 ± 1.6
PRETREATMENT			
Follow-up (months)	65.4 ± 10.4	92.3 ± 13.6	82.0 ± 7.7
Stones/patient	8.7 ± 2.1	12.7 ± 3.5†	7.5 ± 0.9
Stones/patient/year	1.47 ± 0.15	1.74 ± 0.29	1.43 ± 0.13
Cumulative stone-operations	20	19	33
TREATMENT			
Follow-up (months)	18.4 ± 1.4	17.5 ± 1.5	20.0 ± 1.5
Stones/patient/year	0.48 ± 0.11*	0.54 ± 0.15*	0.45 ± 0.08*
Cumulative stone-operations	–	–	1
Stones observed/predicted	26/93 (28%)**	30/91 (33%)**	38/120 (31.7%)**
Remission	55.3%	63.2%	58.2%
Reduction in stone recurrence	89.5%	92.1%	83.6%

* $p<0.01$ for the difference between pretreatment and treatment values assessed by paired t-test
** $p<0.001$ for observed vs predicted stone-events assessed by Chi square
† $p<0.01$ for the differences both vs group A and group C assessed by the variance analysis

1   Pak CYC. *Metabolism 1976; 25:* 665
2   Robertson WG, Peacock M, Marshall RW et al. *N Engl J Med 1976; 294:* 249
3   Robertson WG, Peacock M, Heyburn PJ et al. *Br J Urol 1978; 50:* 449
4   Coe FL. *Arch Intern Med 1978; 138:* 1090
5   Coe FL. *Ann Intern Med 1977; 87:* 404
6   Pak CYC, Peters P, Kadesky M et al. *Am J Med 1981; 71:* 615
7   Pellegrino S, Zaffino MC, Tondolo M et al. *Giorn It Chim Clin 1980; 5:* 171
8   Daniele PG, Marangella M. *Annali di Chimica 1982; 72:* 25
9   Yendt ER, Guay GF, Garcia DA. *CMAJ 1970; 102:* 614
10   Backman U, Danielson BG, Johansson G et al. *Br J Urol 1979; 41:* 175

Open Discussion

CAMERON (Chairman) Could I perhaps start the discussion by asking you what the calcium concentration is in the water in the area of Turin?

MARANGELLA It is quite low.

CAMERON This, of course, is a problem in some parts of Britain, including where we are now, when one tries to increase the intake of raw water. Should we give up and just talk to our patients getting them to drink. I can't believe that everyone is willing to accept that.

PEACOCK (Leeds) Could you speculate why you think the three forms of therapy were equally effective?

MARANGELLA I think this might have occurred because after treatment we obtained comparable values in the main biochemical and physiochemical parameters in the three treatment groups. We had a slight decrease of the saturation levels of calcium oxalate and brushite in patients treated by thiazides. This did not imply further benefits from a clinical point of view.

KERR (Newcastle upon Tyne) First a comment cn the Chairman's remark. I have seen Dr Rose from London present data on a number of occasions, which suggest that even London tap water is highly beneficial though the effect of the diuresis far outweighs the calcium content. My question to Dr Marangella, as some of your patients have had relatively few stone episodes, two I think was your criterion for inclusion, my concern is whether you can maintain compliance with a stringent dietary regime for longer than 18 months of your average period of follow-up. Do you find there is any reduction in compliance or any evidence that the urinary solutes are reverting to the pre-dietary advice stage?

MARANGELLA That is certainly a good question. The patients compliance to this kind of diet we found, at least in Turin, to be quite good. The control of the patients compliance to the diet was performed by determining the main biochemical parameters during treatment every three to six months. We found, however, that the most relevant problems, as far as compliance is concerned, was with the fluid intake.

GOGGIN (Canterbury) I would like to confirm Professor Kerr's observation about the value of increasing fluid intake in this part of the country. Down in Canterbury, with water I guess with an analysis very similar to London, we get some very good results in patients over five years, by just advising an increase in the fluid intake. If I could ask one question of the presenter, and that is does he think that his period of follow-up is long enough to make any observation about his data?

MARANGELLA No, I think that it isn't enough. However, we think that this study will be continued to achieve more certainty about these results.

RITZ (Chairman) I was surprised to see that the urine output in your patients increased by only about 20 per cent. If we are to devise strategies to treat patients with nephrolithiasis wouldn't it be much cheaper and with respect to long-term hazards less dangerous, to advise patients to increase their fluid intake? Fluid intake of about 1.5 litres per day in your patients is certainly inadequate. I am concerned about long-term hazards of thiazides, glucose intolerance, hyperlipidaemia etc. We should use them only when we have exhausted non-drug intervention.

Proc EDTA (1983) Vol 20

POLYANIONIC INHIBITORS OF CALCIUM OXALATE CRYSTAL AGGLOMERATION IN URINE

D S Scurr, A B Latif, V Sergeant, W G Robertson

*MRC Mineral Metabolism Unit, The General Infirmary,
Leeds, United Kingdom*

Summary

The excretions and relative potencies of various macromolecular inhibitors of the crystallisation of calcium oxalate (CaOx) were measured in the urines of idiopathic calcium stone-formers and normal subjects. The stone-formers excreted significantly less polyanionic macromolecules in their urine than did the normals, the difference being attributable to the lower excretions of glycosaminoglycans (GAGS), ribonucleic acid (RNA) and Tamm-Horsfall mucoprotein (THM), all of which are precipitable with alcian blue.

The relative potencies of the various inhibitors measured under 'whole urine equivalent' conditions using a batch crystallisation system, showed that the order of inhibitory activity towards CaOx crystal agglomeration was RNA > GAGS > THM > pyrophosphate (PP_i). This paralleled the order of ability of these inhibitors to produce a high negative zeta potential on the surface of CaOx crystals.

Introduction

There have been many articles in recent years on the subject of urinary inhibitors of calcium oxalate (CaOx) crystallisation [1-6]. In general, these have shown that certain polyanions present in urine are important as true inhibitors of crystallisation i.e. they act at low concentration by adsorbing to the surfaces of CaOx crystals where they alter the crystal growth and agglomeration properties of the crystals [7]. The polyanions of main interest in this respect are macromolecules including ribonucleic acid (RNA), glycosaminoglycans (GAGS) and non-polymerised Tamm-Horsfall mucoprotein (THM). The only low molecular weight polyanion of any note so far found in urine is pyrophosphate (PP_i). Other small ions, such as citrate and magnesium, may retard the observed growth rate of CaOx crystals but do so mainly by reducing the degree of supersaturation of urine with respect to CaOx through the complexing of calcium and oxalate ions respectively in urine. This paper concerns itself only with the first type of inhibitor.

The study consists of a comparison of the excretions of the main polyanionic inhibitors in the urines of idiopathic calcium stone-formers and their controls and the effect of these inhibitors on the degree of crystal agglomeration in a batch crystalliser in which CaOx crystals are generated in situ at degrees of supersaturation approximating those in the urines of recurrent CaOx stone-formers [8].

Methods

Twenty-four hour urine samples were collected in sterilised containers without preservative from 30 normal men, aged 23–57 (mean 34.1 years), and 21 recurrent, idiopathic calcium stone-formers, aged 28–74 (mean 39.5 years). The urines were analysed for alcian blue precipitable polyanions (ABPP) using a modification of the method of Whiteman, glycosaminoglycans by measurement of uronic acids, Tamm-Horsfall mucoprotein by protein assay and RNA by a modified orcinol method for measuring ribosyl groups [9].

In a separate study, the effects of various concentrations of RNA, GAGS and non-polymerised THM were measured on the rates of agglomeration of CaOx crystals generated spontaneously in a batch crystalliser [9]. Pyrophosphate was also studied as an example of a low molecular weight polyanion. The zeta potential produced by the inhibitors on the surface of CaOx crystals was measured using a Zeta Meter (Zeta Meter Inc., New York).

Results and discussion

Figure 1 shows the mean values (± 1 SEM) of the daily excretion of the ABPP and their constituent GAG, THM and RNA fractions in the urines of stone-formers and normals. The overall urinary excretion of polyanions (ABPP) was reduced in the stone-formers compared with the normals confirming our earlier finding [10]. The lower excretions of ABPP in the stone-formers was attributable to a reduction in the excretion of all three constituent polyanions but the reason for the reduction in the excretion of these structurally unrelated compounds is not yet clear. It may be that, for some reason, polymerisation of these macro-molecules is promoted in the urines of the stone-formers and this inactivates them as inhibitors or even causes them to act as mild promoters of crystallisation as noted in an earlier paper [9].

Figure 2 shows the measured inhibition of agglomeration produced by a number of inhibitors in a high supersaturation batch crystallisation system. In terms of molar concentration, the most active inhibitor tested was RNA. The order of inhibitory activity towards agglomeration of CaOx crystals was found to be RNA > GAGS > THM > PP_i. The last-mentioned was more active at pH 6.5 than 5.5 presumably because of its greater dissociation and higher negative charge at the more alkaline pH. Other studies, not reported here, show that the ability to inhibit crystal growth was in the order RNA > GAGS > PP_i > THM, the last-mentioned having virtually no effect on this process within the urinary range of concentration.

441

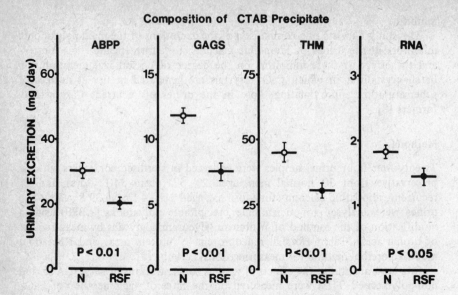

Figure 1. The 24-hour excretions of alcian blue precipitable polyanions (ABPP), glycosaminoglycans (GAGS), Tamm-Horsfall mucoprotein (THM) and ribonucleic acid (RNA) in the cetyl trimethyl ammonium bromide (CTAB) extracts of urines from normals (N) and recurrent stone-formers (RSF) (mean ± SEM)

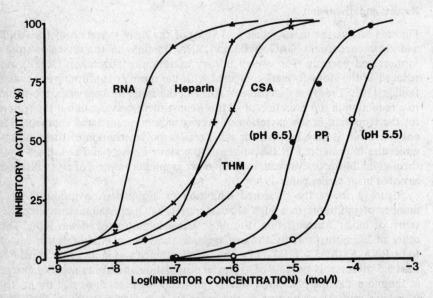

Figure 2. The percentage inhibition of agglomeration of calcium oxalate crystals produced by various inhibitors in a batch crystalliser at high supersaturation in relation to the concentration of inhibitor in solution

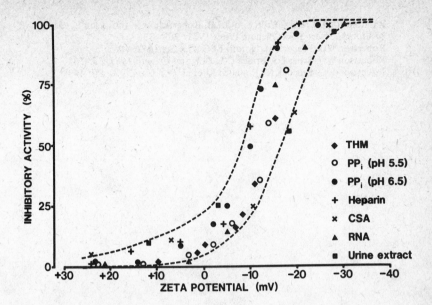

Figure 3. The percentage inhibition of agglomeration of calcium oxalate crystals in a batch crystalliser in relation to the zeta potential on the crystal surface produced by different concentrations of various polyanionic inhibitors and macromolecular extracts from urine

Figure 3 shows the inhibitory effect of various polyanions on the agglomeration of CaOx in relation to the zeta potential produced by these inhibitors on the crystal surface. This figure brings together a wide variety of polyanionic inhibitors of different structures, potencies and concentrations. Although other factors such as Van der Waal's forces and steric effects also play a role in determining the likelihood of agglomeration of crystals, clearly zeta potential must dominate the extent to which CaOx crystals will agglomerate in this system.

In conclusion, it would appear that, of the various urinary inhibitors of crystallisation so far suggested to be of possible importance in protecting the individual against calcium oxalate stone-formation, only the macromolecular polyanions significantly inhibit agglomeration within the urinary range of concentrations of these ions and these are the inhibitors which are reduced in stone-formers' urine. Further studies are required to establish the cause of this reduction, or apparent reduction, in the excretion of these polyanions.

References

1   Robertson WG, Peacock M, Nordin BEC. *Clin Chim Acta 1973; 43:* 31
2   Meyer JL, Smith LH. *Invest Urol 1975; 13:* 36
3   Fleisch H. *Kidney Int 1978; 13:* 361
4   Ryall RL, Harnett RM, Marshall VR. *Clin Chim Acta 1981; 112:* 349
5   Randolph AD, Drach GW. *J Crystal Growth 1981; 53:* 195
6   Sheehan ME, Nancollas GH. *Invest Urol 1980; 17:* 446

7   Randolph AD, Drach GW. In Smith LH, Robertson WG, Finlayson B, eds. *Urolithiasis*. New York: Plenum Press. 1981: 383–390
8   Robertson WG, Peacock M, Nordin BEC. *Clin Sci 1971; 40:* 365
9   Robertson WG, Scurr DS, Bridge CM. *J Crystal Growth 1981; 53:* 182
10 Robertson WG, Peacock M, Heyburn PJ et al. *Br J Urol 1978; 50:* 449

STUDY OF INHIBITOR AND NUCLEATOR ACTIVITIES IN CALCIUM STONE FORMERS

E Duranti, P Imperiali, M Badii, S Capiccioni, M G Masi, M Sasdelli

Ospedale di Arezzo, Arezzo, Italy

Summary

In 30 calcium stone formers urinary citrate, magnesium, calcium, phosphorus, uric acid and oxalate excretion were compared with the activity product ratios and formation product ratios of oxalate, brushite and monosodium urate.

A positive correlation was found between calcium and phosphorus excretions and APRox and APRbr; no correlation was found between oxalate, uric acid, citrate and magnesium excretion and APR or FPR.

Thus calcium and phosphorus contribute significantly to the increments of urine saturation; citrate and magnesium do not modify the inhibitor urinary activity, and oxalate and uric acid do not influence inhibition and saturation activities of urine.

Introduction

Currently three main factors are thought to be important in urinary lithogenesis: saturation of urine, inhibition and promotion of crystal formation and aggregation [1]. In stone formers an estimate of these factors is necessary, in order to single out all those physiochemical imbalances responsible for lithogenesis. Pak [2] has proposed the activity product ratio (APR) to assess the saturation of urine, and the formation product ratio (FPR) as an index of inhibitor and/or promoter activity which can also be investigated by measuring single inhibitors such as magnesium, citrate, pyrophosphates and glycosaminoglycans [1].

The aim of this work was to find, in a group of calcium stone formers, all the possible correlations between the estimates of urine saturation (APR) and the excretion of the single ions involved in lithogenesis; we also wanted to examine the possible correlations between the excretion of the principal urinary inhibitors and the total inhibitor activity as assessed by FPR.

Methods

Thirty patients aged from 18 to 72 years with primary renal calcium stone disease were studied. All had normal renal function. In all we evaluated: clinical

445

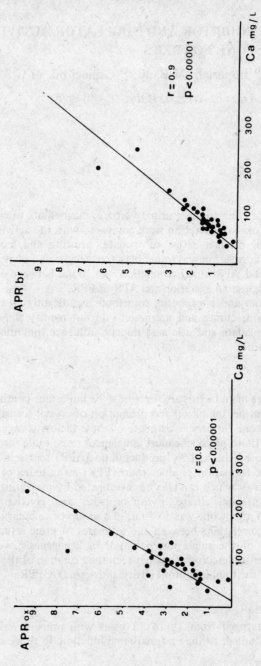

Figure 1. Correlations between urinary calcium, APRox and APRbr

history, chemical analysis of stone(s), 24hr urinary excretion of calcium, phosphorus, sodium, magnesium and uric acid (standard laboratory methods); urinary oxalate (colorimetric method from Hodgkinson-Williams) and citrate (Boehringer colorimetric method). We also evaluated APR and FPR of brushite (br), oxalate (ox) and monosodium urate (NaU) [2].

The relationships between the laboratory data were obtained by linear regression analysis using a computer program.

Results and discussion

Significant correlations were found between urinary Ca, APRox (y= −0.5+0.04x; r=0.8) and APRbr (y= −0.9+0.03x; r=0.9) (Figure 1). Urinary phosphorus (Figure 2) also correlated significantly with APRbr (y= −1.4+0.01x; r=0.7).

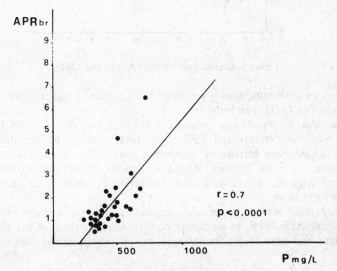

Figure 2. Phosphorus excretion and APRbr

Increased Ca excretion leads to a greater increment of APRox than APRbr, in fact 21 patients showed metastably supersaturated urines with respect to Calcium Oxalate (CaOx) while eight patients only had metastably supersaturated urines with respect to brushite for urinary Ca values ⩾100mg/litre.

This finding suggests that for high urinary Ca excretion, CaOx and brushite could play important roles in nucleation, while for low urinary Ca concentrations (<100mg/litre) only CaOx is likely to be the possible seed. Phosphorus excretion when compared with APRbr showed the same behaviour, even if only for high values (⩾400mg/litre) could the metastability limit be achieved.

A positive correlation was found between APRbr and APRox (y=1.3+1.1x; r=0.7) (Figure 3), confirming the importance of urinary calcium excretion [4], which, being the common ion of brushite and CaOx, can also increase the

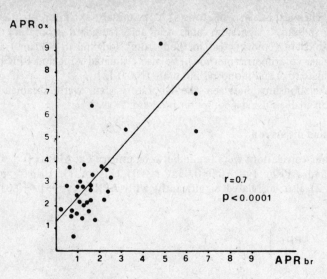

Figure 3. Correlations between APRbr and APRox

saturation of both salts, even if we found in all patients a higher urine saturation with respect to CaOx than brushite.

There was no significant correlation between the excretion of inhibitors (citrate and magnesium) and FPR. This finding could be explained either because the inhibitor activity on nucleation depends on other unknown factors or because, in stone formers, inhibitor excretion is not proportional to or correlated with the degree of urinary saturation in order to increase the risk of stone formation.

Finally there was no significant correlation between urinary oxalate and uric acid and APR–FPR, so we cannot confirm the hypothesis of the importance of oxalate and uric acid urinary excretions as lithogenic risk factors [5–7].

Conclusions

1. High Ca and P excretions increase the urinary saturation with respect to CaOx and brushite.

2. Citrate and magnesium excretions, in stone formers, do not seem to modify the inhibitor activity of urine on nucleation.

3. Oxalate and uric acid do not influence saturation and inhibition activities of stone formers' urine.

Acknowledgments

The authors would like to thank Mrs R Della Scala for the technical assistance and Professor B Bruni for statistical analysis.

448

References

1 Fleish H. *Kidney Internat 1978; 13:* 361
2 Pak CYC, Holt K. *Metabolism 1976; 25:* 665
3 Pak CYC. *J Crystal Growth 1981; 53:* 202
4 Pak CYC. *Disorders Min Metab 1981; 3:* 119
5 Pak CYC. *Proc Soc Exp Biol Med 1976; 153:* 83
6 Coe FL, Strauss AL. *Kidney Internat 1980; 17:* 662
7 Robertson WG, Peacock M. *Nephron 1980; 26:* 105

RENAL THRESHOLD PHOSPHATE CONCENTRATION IN PATIENTS WITH IDIOPATHIC NEPHROLITHIASIS: CORRELATIONS WITH TUBULAR FUNCTIONS, SERUM PARATHYROID HORMONE AND $1,25(OH)_2D_3$

R C Pabico, Barbara A McKenna, R B Freeman

University of Rochester Medical Center, Rochester, New York, USA

Summary

The renal handling of inorganic phosphate was measured in 17 idiopathic nephrolithiasis patients with normal glomerular filtration rate and effective renal plasma flow. Tm_{PO_4}/GFR was $<2.5mg/dl$ in nine subjects (Group I) and $\geqslant 2.5$ in eight (Group II). The former had serum PO_4 of $2.5 \pm 0.13mg/dl$ and the latter, $3.5 \pm 0.11mg/dl$ ($p<0.01$). Four in Group I and five in Group II were hypercalciuric. There was no significant difference in the serum parathyroid hormone and $1,25(OH)_2D_3$ between the two groups.

However, renal tubular functions were abnormal in both groups. The low Tm_{PO_4}/GFR in 53 per cent of the patients is another manifestation of tubular functional abnormality seen in idiopathic nephrolithiasis.

Introduction

In patients with calcium nephrolithiasis, hypercalciuria and normal serum calcium, the serum inorganic phosphate concentration tends to be lower than the values obtained from healthy control subjects [1–5]. Several studies have shown a 'renal phosphate leak' to be a common finding in idiopathic hypercalciuria [5–6]. The phosphaturia and hypophosphataemia may play a key role in idiopathic hypercalciuria: on the one hand, the phosphate depletion directly stimulates the synthesis of $1,25(OH)_2D_3$ which enhances intestinal calcium absorption leading to increased calcium delivery to the kidney and hypercalciuria; on the other hand, if hypercalciuria is the primary disorder, the continuing loss of calcium leads to stimulation of parathyroid hormone secretion; this secondary hyperparathyroid state stimulates the synthesis of $1,25(OH)_2D_3$ both directly and indirectly through the inhibition of tubular phosphate reabsorption leading to phosphaturia and hypophosphataemia. Thus, two possible clinical subsets of idiopathic hypercalciuria may exist: the first, a group of patients with elevated serum $1,25(OH)_2D_3$ and normal

450

or low serum parathyroid hormone, and the other with elevated serum concentrations of both $1,25(OH)_2D_3$ and parathyroid hormone [3–5]. It seems that phosphate metabolism has an important role in the idiopathic hypercalciuric syndrome. Indeed, abnormalities in phosphate transport outside of the kidneys may also be present, probably independent of parathyroid hormone [6].

However, there have been clinical studies of idiopathic hypercalciuria and nephrolithiasis where serum phosphate values have been normal [7]. Furthermore, at least half the patients with idiopathic calcium containing nephrolithiasis are normocalciuric, but they do have abnormalities in proximal and distal tubular functions [8].

We elected to study the renal handling of inorganic phosphate in patients with idiopathic nephrolithiasis and normal renal excretory function. Serum parathyroid hormone and $1,25(OH)_2D_3$ were also measured, and their possible role in relation to the phosphaturia was evaluated.

Subjects

Seventeen idiopathic nephrolithiasis patients, 14 men and three women, aged 23–60 years, with 1–30 years of renal stone history, were the subjects of this study. Their serum concentrations of urea nitrogen, creatinine, sodium, potassium, chloride, and CO_2 were normal. They had no urinary tract infection. At the time of the study, they were on no dietary or drug regimen. The protocol of study was explained in detail to each patient, and their consent was obtained.

Procedures

Seven to 10 days prior to admission to the short-term unit of our hospital, the patients were instructed to follow approximately a diet containing 400mg calcium per day. Complete 24-hour urine specimens were collected; blood specimens were drawn from non-occluded anticubital veins. Subsequently, measurements of glomerular filtration rate and effective renal plasma flow were made using the renal plasma clearance of Inulin and para-aminohippurate, respectively. Proximal tubular reabsorptive and secretory functions were determined using the tubular maximum reabsorption of glucose and tubular maximum secretion of para-aminohippurate, respectively. Distal nephron functions were evaluated by the determination of maximum urinary concentration and dilution as well as short-term urinary acidification. The procedures and laboratory techniques in performing these various studies have been published in detail in a previous communication from our laboratory [9].

Immunoreactive parathyroid hormone was measured in the serum by the radioimmunoassay technique using antibodies directed toward the carboxyl terminal. Plasma $1,25(OH)_2D_3$ was determined by the modification of the protein-binding technique.

Tm_{PO_4}/GFR was calculated from the normogram of Walton and Bijvoet [10].

451

The data are expressed as mean ± 1SE. Non-paired student t-test was used in the analysis of the data, and p values <0.05 are considered significant.

Results

In Table I are summarised the values of serum phosphate, calcium, PTH and $1,25(OH)_2 D_3$ as well as the urinary calcium excretion in 16 normal controls, Group I and Group II subjects. Note that patients with Tm_{PO_4}/GFR <2.5

TABLE I

	Normal (n=16)	Group I (n=9)	Group II (n=8)
Tm_{PO_4}/GFR (mg/dl)	>2.5	<2.5	>2.5
Serum PO_4 (mg/dl)	3.8±0.15	2.5±0.13*	3.5±0.11
Serum calcium (mg/dl)	9.9±1.2	9.7±1.5	9.7±1.3
Urine calcium (mg/dl)	205±31	149±45	228±35
Serum PTH (pg/ml)	1340±204	1550±170	1940±210
Serum $1,25(OH)_2 D_3$ (pg/ml)	30±5	32±3	36±7

*p<0.01 vs normal and Group II

have lower serum phosphate concentrations, when compared with normals and with Group II patients, the difference is significant. However, the rest of the variables are not significantly different in the three groups of subjects. Four patients in Group I and five patients in Group II are hypercalciuric (urinary calcium excretion >4.0mg/kg body weight/day). Although the mean values for serum PTH and $1,25(OH)_2 D_3$ are higher in Groups I and II when compared to normal controls, the values are not significantly different.

In Table II are summarised the renal haemodynamic and representative renal proximal tubular functions. Glomerular filtration rate and effective renal plasma flow in the normal and the two groups of patients with idiopathic nephrolithiasis are not significantly different. However, the proximal tubular reabsorption and proximal tubular secretory function in Group I and II patients are significantly lower than normal controls, but the values are not different between Group I and Group II patients.

452

TABLE II

	Normal (n=16)	Group I (n=9)	Group II (n=8)
GFR (ml/min/1.73m^2)	110±9	108±7	121±9
ERPF (ml/min/1.73m^2)	550±35	490±71	581±58
Tm$_{glucose}$/GFR	3.40±0.5	1.93±0.3*	1.82±0.3*
Tm$_{PAH}$/GFR	0.81±0.12	0.54±0.09*	0.58±0.05*

*p<0.05 vs normal

Discussion

In our patients with idiopathic nephrolithiasis (n=17), nine (53%) have low Tm$_{PO_4}$/GFR. Their serum PO_4 is significantly lower compared with the rest of the patients. Four of the nine phosphaturic patients (44%) are also hypercalciuric. Our initial concern that there may be elevation of serum PTH and/or $1,25(OH)_2D_3$ as previously described [5,6] proved not to be the case in our nephrolithiasis patients. Although serum PTH and $1,25(OH)_2D_3$ in both groups of patients are higher than in the normal controls, the difference is not significant. Furthermore, the actual values of serum PTH and $1,25(OH)_2D_3$ in the nephrolithiasis patients are within the normal range. It appears that neither an excess PTH nor an elevated $1,25(OH)_2D_3$ are playing a causative role in the metabolic abnormalities of our patients.

We have found in our recent study that proximal and distal tubular functions are abnormal in patients with idiopathic nephrolithiasis with normal GFR [9]. It may well be that the low Tm$_{PO_4}$/GFR, in our patients at least, represents another tubular functional abnormality. That not all have diminished Tm$_{PO_4}$/GFR implies that there are varying degrees of renal tubular functional aberrations in patients with idiopathic nephrolithiasis.

Acknowledgment

The authors wish to express their appreciation to the laboratory team of Consolidated Biomedical Laboratories of Columbus, Ohio for the determination of serum parathyroid hormone and Vitamin D metabolites, and to Mrs Lynn Carpenter for the preparation of this manuscript.

References

1   Hemmeman PH, Benedict PH, Forbes AP et al. *N Engl J Med 1958; 259:* 802
2   Edwards NA, Hodgkinson A. *Clin Sci 1965; 29:* 93
3   Coe FL, Canterbury JM, Firpo JJ et al. *J Clin Invest 1973; 52:* 134

4   Shen FH, Baylink DJ, Nielsen RL et al. *J Lab Clin Med 1977; 90:* 955

5   Gray RW, Wilz DR, Caldas AE et al. *J Clin Endo Metab 1977; 45:* 299

6   Lemann J, Gray RW, Wilz DR et al. *Adv Exp Med Biol 1980; 128:* 427

7   Pak CYC, Ohata M, Lawrence EC et al. *J Clin Invest 1974; 54:* 387

8   Pabico RC, McKenna BA. *Kidney Int 1983; 23:* 131

9   Pabico RC, McKenna BA, Freeman RB. *Kidney Int 1975; 8:* 166

10   Walton RJ, Bijvoet ELM. *Lancet 1975; ii:* 309

Proc EDTA (1983) Vol 20

RELATIONSHIP BETWEEN SODIUM INTAKE, PROXIMAL TUBULAR FUNCTION AND CALCIUM EXCRETION IN NORMAL SUBJECTS AND IN IDIOPATHIC HYPERCALCIURIA

G Colussi, M Surian†, Maria Elisabetta De Ferrari, G Pontoriero, G Rombolà, B Brando, F Malberti†, P Cosci†, Adriana Aroldi*, Claudia Castelnovo*, L Minetti

Niguarda Ca' Granda Hospital, *Policlinico Hospital, Milan, and †Maggiore Hospital, Lodi, Italy

Summary

Proximal tubular function was studied with maximal water clearance studies in 15 controls (C), 22 Ca stone formers with idiopathic hypercalciuria (IH) and 10 normocalciuric Ca stone formers (NC). Distal delivery of glomerular filtrate (ClDD) and Na excretion were higher in IH and NC than in C; NaCl loading (6g/day) for seven days in C increased Na excretion and ClDD to similar levels as in IH and NC; the distribution of ClDD for any level of Na excretion was similar in C, NC and IH. NaCl loading in C slightly reduced renal phosphate threshold, which still remained higher than in IH on a free diet. It appears that reduced tubular reabsorption of glomerular filtrate in Ca stone formers is related to habitual high Na intake and is not peculiar to hypercalciuric patients. Habitual high Na intake is unlikely to be responsible for all the metabolic spectrum of idiopathic hypercalciuria.

Introduction

A renal proximal tubular defect, with reduced fractional reabsorption of sodium (Na) and of filtered fluid, has been suggested as a likely explanation for idiopathic hypercalciuria [1,2]; its physiopatholigical consequences would include reduced tubular reabsorption of phosphate (P) and hypophosphataemia, increased intestinal calcium (Ca) absorption and reduced distal tubule Ca reabsorption, resulting in hypercalciuria [2].

It has also been shown that, in hypercalciuric Ca stone formers, Ca excretion increases and plasma P concentrations fall when Na intake is increased [3]; according to these observations, it has been suggested that habitual high Na intake per se, might be an aetiological factor for idiopathic hypercalciuria [3].

We have evaluated the relationships between Na intake, proximal tubule Na reabsorption and Ca excretion in healthy people and in a group of Ca stone formers, as well as the changes in renal Na handling and Ca excretion after a chronic increase in Na intake.

Cases and methods

Fifteen healthy volunteers (C) (seven males and eight females, aged 24 to 48 years) and 32 idiopathic Ca stone formers (23 males and nine females, aged 18 to 50 years), were studied. Ten patients were normocalciuric (NC) (Ca excretion, UCaV, less than 320mg/day in males and less than 280mg/day in females, upper 95% values for healthy people, on a 1g Ca, unrestricted Na diet), 22 were hyper-calciuric (IH). After seven to 10 days of low Ca diet (approximately 400mg/day, achieved by avoiding dairy products) and unrestricted for Na, calorie and fluid intake, the patients and the controls underwent an ambulatory 24-hour urine collection for Ca, Na, P and creatinine determinations. The morning the collection ended, they came to the clinic for fasting blood and a maximum free water clearance study. Free water clearance studies were performed according to a standard protocol: the subjects remained supine throughout the study and got up only to void and drink; after drinking 20ml/kg body weight of distilled water in 20 to 30 minutes, they voided every 15 minutes and drank the same amount of distilled water; three to five collections with constant osmolality of less than 80mOsm/kg H_2O were obtained. Blood samples for Na, Cl, K, osmolality and creatinine were obtained at the time of the lowest urine osmolality. Eight C, seven IH and five NC repeated the same protocol seven days after the supplementation of their diet (kept constant for 400mg of Ca and unrestricted for Na intake) with 6g NaCl (as 1g tablets during the meals).

Plasma and urine osmolalities were measured using an Advanced Instruments 3D Osmometer; Ca by atomic absorption spectrophotometry; Na, Cl, K, P, creatinine by routine laboratory methods. Fractional delivery of filtered fluid to distal tubule was evaluated as 'chloride' term ($ClDD = C_{H_2O}/GFR + C_{Cl}/GFR$) a more accurate index of distal Na reabsorption [4].

Statistical analysis was performed by use of paired or unpaired Student's t test, as more appropriate.

Results

On low Ca, unrestricted Na diet IH had higher daily and fasting Ca excretion than C and NC (Table I), higher daily and fasting Na excretion, higher ClDD, and lower renal phosphate threshold (Tm_{PO_4}/GFR) than C; Na excretion, Tm_{PO_4}/GFR and ClDD were similar in IH and NC. Minimum urine osmolality was lower in IH (56.3 ± 10mOsm/kg H_2O) than in N (66.3 ± 11.9, $p<0.02$) and NC (65.3 ± 12.7, $p<0.05$), C_{H_2O}/GFR was lower in N ($9.3 \pm 3.6\%$) than in IH (13.6 ± 4.2, $p<0.005$) and NC (12 ± 2.9, $p<0.05$), fractional reabsorption of distal delivery ($C_{Cl}/C_{H_2O} + C_{Cl}$) was similar in N ($87.9 \pm 6.3\%$), IH (87.6 ± 4.9) and NC (85.1 ± 4.6). After NaCl supplementation, daily and fasting Na excretion rose in 8C to values as high as in IH on a free diet (Table II), ClDD rose accordingly to similar values, but Ca excretion remained unchanged and Tm_{PO_4}/GFR fell slightly but to still higher values than in IH. The results were similar if compared to all the group of IH. Almost all the plots of ClDD values related to daily Na excretion in IH and NC for which Na excretion was available fell within the 95 per cent confidence limits observed in C (Figure 1). There

456

TABLE I. Daily (UCaV and UNaV) and fasting (CaE and NaE) Ca and Na excretion, renal phosphate threshold (TmpO$_4$/GFR) and distal chloride delivery (CIDD) in normal subjects and Ca stone formers (number of cases in parentheses)

	UCaV mg/day	CaE mg/dl GFR	UNaV mEq/day	NaE mEq/L GFR	TmpO$_4$/GFR mg/dl GFR	CIDD %
C	132±47 (15)	0.03±0.03 (15)	150±51 (15)	1.07±0.87 (15)	3.8±0.6 (15)	10.6±4 (15)
IH	285±110[1] (22)	0.14±0.1[1] (22)	198±38[2] (10)	2.04±1.1[3] (22)	2.8±0.6[1] (22)	15.4±4.7[1] (22)
NC	153±63[4] (10)	0.08±0.05[5] [6] (10)	196±69 (8)	2.2±0.9[3] (10)	3.1±0.74[7] (10)	14.2±3.3[7] (10)

vs C, p<: [2]=0.05; [7]=0.02; [5]=0.01; [1]=0.001; [3]=0.005
vs IH, p<: [4]=0.001; [6]=0.05

TABLE II. Effects of 6g/day NaCl dietary supplementation in eight normal subjects (C) and seven idiopathic hypercalciuric patients (IH)

		UCaV mg/day	CaE mg/dl GFR	UNaV mEq/day	NaE mEq/L GFR	TmpO$_4$/GFR mg/dl GFR	CIDD %
C (n=8)	basal	135±55	0.03±0.02	135±35	0.73±0.6	3.99±0.5	9.6±2.8
	NaCl	146±76	0.04±0.03	230±46[1]	1.94±0.7[2]	3.62±0.7[2]	15.1±6.5[1]
	p<*	0.001	0.001	NS	NS	0.05	NS
IH (n=7)	basal	310±95[3]	0.17±0.12[6]	201±43[3]	2.66±1[3]	2.9 ±0.45[3]	16.8±4.4[3]
	NaCl	356±144	0.21±0.14	308±56[1]	3.78±1.24[4]	2.6 ±0.62	21.5±5.2[5]

Basal: free choice diet; NaCl: free choice diet + NaCl 6g/day
NaCl vs basal, p<: [2]=0.05; [5]=0.02; [4]=0.01; [1]=0.001
IH (basal) vs C (basal), p<: [6]=0.01; [3]=0.001
*: C(NaCl) vs IH (basal)

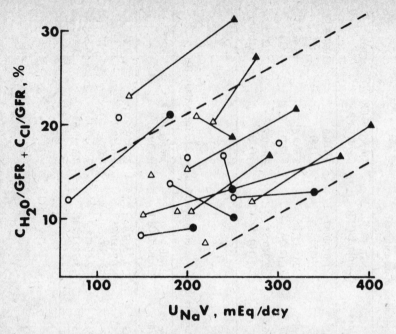

Figure 1. Relationship between 24-hour Na excretion and distal delivery of glomerular filtrate (C_{H_2O}/GFR + C_{Cl}/GFR). Dotted lines: 95 per cent confidence limits in controls (y=0.05 x 2.46, SEest=4.2, r=0.57, p<0.01). Open triangles: hypercalciuric patients, free diet; closed triangles: hypercalciuric patients, free diet + NaCl 6g; open circles: normocalciuric patients, free diet; closed circles: normocalciuric patients, free diet + NaCl 6g

were no significant correlations between Tm_{PO_4}/GFR vs ClDD and UNaV, and UCaV vs ClDD and UNaV, neither in C nor in the patients. UCaV did not change after NaCl supplementation in IH and slightly increased in five NC (from 178±70 to 205±41, p<0.05); in all the 12 Ca stone formers studied as a group UCaV increased from 238±125 to 293±141 (p<0.05).

Discussion

Our study confirms that IH have increased distal delivery of glomerular filtrate and, as a consequence, increased distal tubular reabsorption of Na and Cl while fractional reabsorption of distal delivery remains unchanged [2]. In our patients, the reduction in proximal tubular fluid reabsorption was correlated with Na intake: ClDD increased in C after NaCl loading to similar values as in IH, and was similarly increased in IH and in NC (who had as high Na excretion as IH) despite the absence of hypercalciuria in the latter. Thus, reduced proximal tubular Na reabsorption in Ca stone formers might not represent a tubular 'defect' but a physiological adaptation to habitual high Na intake. Higher than normal Na excretion in hypercalciuric patients was apparent also in the study of Lau et al [2].

Distal delivery of glomerular filtrate and Na excretion did not correlate with Tm_{PO_4}/GFR and Ca excretion neither in C nor in Ca stone formers; even though Tm_{PO_4}/GFR fell in C after NaCl loading, it still was higher than in IH on a free diet and was not accompanied by any change in Ca excretion; thus our study does not support the hypothesis that habitual high Na intake is responsible for all the metabolic spectrum of idiopathic hypercalciuria, as has been suggested [3]. Unlike in C, NaCl loading did slightly increase Ca excretion in all Ca stone formers; the increase might have been even greater if the patients had been on a higher Ca and/or lower Na diet. In conclusion, proximal tubular Na reabsorption in Ca stone formers is related to a habitual high Na intake, and is not peculiar to hypercalciuric patients; when Na intake is increased, Ca excretion may rise in Ca stone formers, but hypercalciuria does not appear in normocalciuric patients or in normal people. Thus idiopathic hypercalciuria does not seem to be strictly related to Na tubular handling.

Acknowledgments

We thank Mrs Paola Recino for her excellent technical assistance, and Mrs Ester Panagia for typing the manuscript.

References

1 Sutton RAL, Walker VR. *N Engl J Med 1980; 302:* 709
2 Lau YK, Wasserstein A, Westby R et al. *Min Electrolyte Metab 1982; 7:* 237
3 Muldowney FD, Freaney R, Maloney F. *Kidney Int 1982; 22:* 292
4 Danovitch GM. *Renal Physiol 1978; 1:* 56

Proc EDTA (1983) Vol 20

CALCIUM-LOADING TEST AND BONE DISEASE IN PATIENTS WITH UROLITHIASIS

B Lindergård, S Colleen, W Månsson, C Rademark, B Rogland

University Hospital, Lund, Sweden

Summary

A group of 121 patients with a history of multiple or complicated calcium urolithiasis were divided into three subgroups: normal, absorptive and renal/resorptive calciuria by means of a calcium-loading test. Patients with renal hypercalciuria had lower bone mineral content (BMC) than the other groups but did not differ in amount of bone or Tm_{PO_4}/GFR. The 24-hour urine calcium excretion was elevated in patients with renal and absorptive type of hypercalciuria but not in patients with normal calcium-loading test and there was no correlation to BMC. The c-AMP/creatinine seemed to discriminate patients with resorptive calciuria from patients with renal calciuria. It is suggested that only patients with renal hypercalciuria should be treated with calcium-retaining drugs such as thiazides.

Introduction

There are conflicting opinions in the literature regarding the value of differentiating hypercalciuria into subgroups [1, 2]. The present study attempts to clarify this subject and especially the relationship to bone metabolism in the subgroups.

Patients and methods

During 1977—1981, 121 patients with calcium urolithiasis were studied in our hospital. There were 34 women and 87 men, aged 20—60 years, with a serum creatinine less than 150μmol/L. Thirteen patients had multiple stones but had never been operated, whereas 108 patients had been operated for urolithiasis one or more times. Sixty patients had a family history of urolithiasis.

A calcium-loading test according to Pak [3] was performed in all.

During the following days, 2 x 24-hour urine collections were obtained for determination of calcium, phosphate and creatinine with the patients on a normal diet. The renal phosphate threshold was calculated as Tm_{PO_4}/GFR [4]. The bone mineral content (BMC) was measured on the distal forearm using a photon absorption technique [5]. The quantity of bone was estimated from the Barnett-Nordin [6] and the Exton-Smith [7] indices (D-d/D and D^2-d^2/D·L, where D = external diameter of bone, d = internal diamter, L = length of bone), both on X-ray pictures of 2nd metacarpal bones and on photon-absorption curves of radius and ulna of both arms. Cyclic AMP (cAMP) was determined with a protein binding assay and parathyroid hormone (PTH) with a radioimmunoassay with antiserum directed mainly against the C-terminal part of the hormone. The results of the urine analyses, the renal phosphate threshold and the photon absorption studies were compared with values in 114 normal controls, randomly chosen from the general population in our region. As Tm_{PO_4}/GFR and BMC were influenced by age we used the unit standard deviation, SD, for comparisons with the patients.

Results

The calcium-loading test separated the patients into three groups: those with normal calciuria (38%), with absorptive calciuria (25%) and with renal/resorptive calciuria (37%) (Figure 1). There were no clear differences in the urinary cAMP/creatinine ratio or serum PTH between the groups but the fasting urinary cAMP/creatinine (before calcium-loading) correlated positively with the fasting urinary calcium/creatinine ratio, signifying that patients with more severe renal calciuria were more parathyroid stimulated. Five patients with primary hyperparathyroidism were all in the renal/resorptive group of calciuria and the cAMP/creatinine, which was elevated or in the upper normal range before the load, was clearly elevated after the calcium load (Figure 1). The 24-hour urinary calcium/creatinine ratio was elevated in the absorptive and renal/resorptive group of patients but not in patients with normal calcium-loading test when compared to normal controls (Figure 2). The BMC was lower in patients with renal/resorptive calciuria compared to the other groups (Figure 3) and the BMC correlated negatively with the fasting urinary calcium/creatinine ratio (Figure 4). However, there were no deviations in BMC from normal controls, when all patients were taken together, and there was no correlation between the 24-hour urinary calcium and the BMC, nor within any separate group of calciuria.

The Tm_{PO_4}/GFR was not different from age-matched controls, and there was no difference between the groups. Only the five patients with hyperparathyroidism had lower values. Furthermore there was no correlation between Tm_{PO_4}/GFR and BMC or the parameters of bone quantity. The amount of bone evaluated as Exton-Smith index on the photon absorption curves was significantly lower in the total patient group than in the normal controls, but there were no differences between the separate groups of calciuria.

461

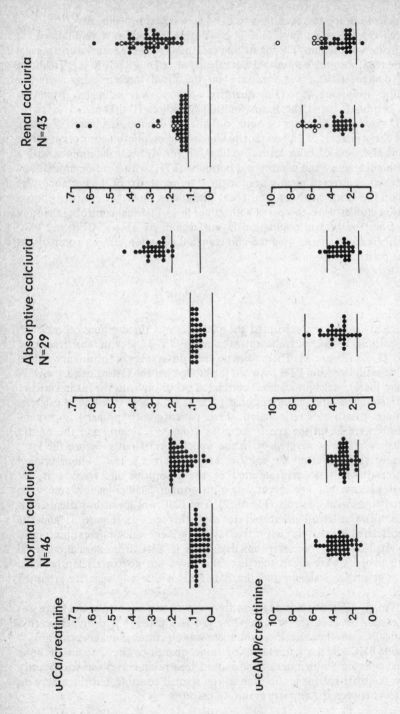

Figure 1. Groups of calciuria before and after calcium-loading test in 121 patients with calcium urolithiasis. Patients with primary hyperparathyroidism (resorptive) are denoted as open circles (o). Urinary calcium/creatinine is given in mg/mg and urinary cAMP/creatinine in μmol/gram creatinine. The horizontal lines indicate ± 2SD in normal controls

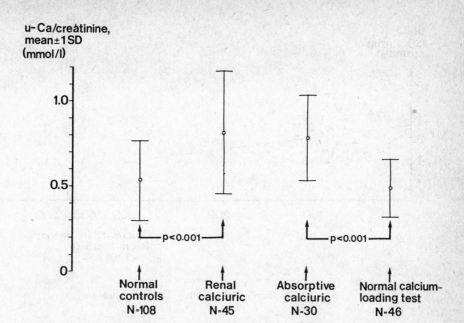

Figure 2. 24-hour urinary calcium/creatinine in normal controls and different groups of calciuria

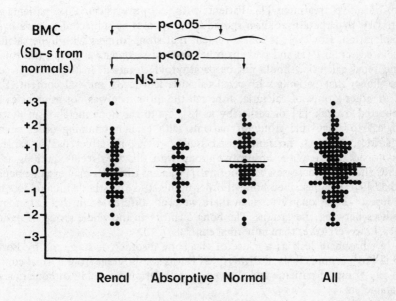

Figure 3. BMC in different groups of calciuria

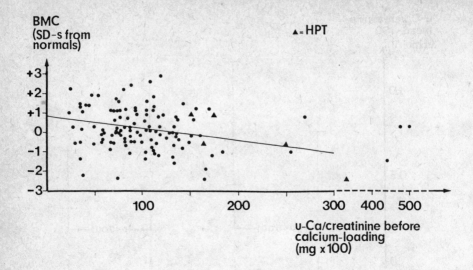

Figure 4. BMC in relation to fasting calcium/creatinine

Discussion

The main advantage of dividing patients with calcium urolithiasis into groups with absorptive, renal, resorptive and no hypercalciuria is to provide a basis for 'selective' treatment [1]. Patients with resorptive calciuria, i.e. patients with primary hyperparathyroidism should in most cases be subjected to parathyroid exploration. However, it is also evident that stone-formers with hypercalciuria, elevated serum PTH and perhaps other signs of secondary hyperparathyroidism and renal calciuria, should not be parathyroidectomised. In this study it could be shown that patients with renal calciuria had lower mineral content, BMC, than other groups of calciuria, although the difference was not as great as that reported by Pak [1] or earlier by us [8]. As to the bone metabolism it seems logical to treat this group of patients with calcium-retaining drugs such as thiazides, although no randomised study proving its effect has so far been published. To treat the absorptive group with thiazides seems dubious as the BMC then may increase above normal [1] and as thiazides may even be nephrotoxic [9]. The described bone disorder in this study is rather a mineral loss than a loss of bone quantity, since there were no differences in the Exton-Smith indices between the groups. The bone quantity in the whole group of patients was, however, lower than in normal controls.

A phosphate leak as a cause of the bone disorder, as suggested by Bordier et al [10], is unlikely as the Tm_{PO_4}/GFR was not different from normal controls in any group of patients and showed no correlation with BMC or bone quantity parameters.

References

1   Pak CYC, Nicar M, Northcutt C. *Contrib Nephrol 1982; 33:* 136
2   Peacock M. *Contrib Nephrol 1982; 33:* 152
3   Pak CYC, Kaplan R, Bone H et al. *N Engl J Med 1975; 292:* 497
4   Walton RJ, Bijvoet OLM. *Lancet 1975; ii:* 309
5   Lindergård B. *Scand J Urol Nephrol 1981; Suppl 59:* 1
6   Barnett E, Nordin BEC. *Clin Radiol 1960; 9:* 166
7   Exton-Smith AN, Millard PH, Payne PR, Wheeler EF. *Lancet 1969; ii:* 1154
8   Lindergård B. *Scand J Urol Nephrol 1980; Suppl 53:* 122
9   Harrington JT. *N Engl J Med 1983; 308:* 266
10 Bordier P, Ryckewart A, Gueris J, Rasmussen H. *Am J Med 1977; 63:* 398

MANAGEMENT OF INFECTED STONE DISEASE WITH HYDROXYUREA: A FIVE YEAR FOLLOW-UP

M J V Smith

Medical College of Virginia, Richmond, Virginia, USA

Summary

Hydroxyurea in a morning dose of 500mg along with Macrodantin, 100mg, has been used for more than five years as an adjunct to the management of retained struvite stones. Mild reversible toxicity occurs in 10 per cent. Urine sterility can be achieved in ninety per cent and no growth of the retained stone occurs.

Introduction

Hydroxyurea (HU) was suggested about six years ago as a useful adjunct in the management of retained struvite stones [1]. This work has been confirmed by at least two other authors [2,3].

It was distressing to hear that Martelli and his co-workers [3] found an increased incidence of toxic side effects with HU when compared to aceto-hydroxamic acid (AHA). The purpose of this report is to present the experience and results from more than five years of therapy with HU.

Material and methods

All patients who entered this study had a renal calculus that was radiopaque and which was presumed to be struvite. This presumption was based on the finding of residual stone after surgery for struvite stones or because of the characteristic appearance of the staghorn calculus associated with a urinary tract infection due to a urease-producing bacteria. All patients had consistently alkaline urine and all were infected with a proven urease-producing organism. No patient had an abnormal metabolic evaluation.

The experimental nature of the study was explained to all patients and an informed consent obtained. They were instructed how to record the pH of every voided urine using nitrazine paper. The patients were then given hydroxyurea, 500mg in the morning. No patient was given antibiotic therapy for the first three months of this study unless the clinical condition was such that this was essential.

All patients measured and recorded the pH of each voided urine for 24-hours once a week. They were seen at monthly intervals at the outset and this was stretched to three monthly intervals. The urine was usually cultured and a complete blood count and automated serum biochemical profile obtained which always included a blood sugar, creatinine, blood urea nitrogen, sodium, potassium, carbon dioxide, chloride, uric acid, calcium, phosphorus, total protein, albumin, cholesterol, total bilirubin, alkaline phosphatase, serum glutamic oxaloacetic transaminase, and lactic dehydrogenase.

A plain film was obtained at three monthly intervals which were eventually stretched to six monthly intervals. A 24-hour urine was also studied for calcium, phosphorus, magnesium, uric acid, oxalate and creatinine at regular intervals.

After three months, the patients were begun on nitrofurantoin (Macrodantin), 100mg in the morning.

Results

Our findings are reported in Tables I and II.

TABLE I. Hydroxyurea in 76 patients

	1 year	2 years	3 years	4 years	5 years
On Protocol:	48	40	34	27	21
Toxic:	9	0	0	0	0
Lost to follow-up:	7	6	3	2	1

NB: Approximately one-third dropout

TABLE II. Urine culture and stone

Years of entry:	1981 n = 8	1980 n = 6	1979 n = 7	1978 n = 6	1976 n = 21
Sterile:	7/8	6	6/7	5/6	19/21
Stone growth:	0	1	2	0	0
No change:	8	5	3	5	19
Decrease:	0	0	2	0	2

This Table represents studies on the patients during January — March 1983

In no patient was the feared complication of altered liver function, anaemia or leucopenia ever found. There were nine patients (12%) who experienced either myalgia, headache or nausea which occurred in the first six months of therapy.

Discussion

The problem with this work is that it has shown that it is safe to use low dosage of HU to decrease the pH of the urine, but no evidence is presented that this interferes with the struvite stone formation. Contemporary thoughts suggest that if the pH of the urine can be kept below pH6, then struvite should return into solution: i.e. the stone should dissolve. This has only occurred in four patients, but in only one has the stone completely disappeared.

Some of our earlier work has suggested that the formation of struvite stones was not only dependent upon the action of the bacteria urease in releasing excessive ammonium ions from urine but also, that the bacterial wall provided the matrix while the mitochondrial apatite provided the primordial cell of stone formation [4]. It is possible, thus, that the synergistic effect of HU and the antibiotic are in fact preventing bacterial growth and death. Thus, no further aggregation of stone growth occurs.

However, the dissolution of the stone rarely occurs because it is possible that the HU has no effect on urinary saturation in a similar way as AHA has no influence on the urinary saturation in spite of its good effect in long-term studies [5, 6]. This aspect was not studied for this report, but the data certainly will be reported in the future.

References

1 Smith MJV. *Urology 1978; 11:* 274
2 Carmignani G, Belgrano E, Puppo P et al. *Br J Urol 1980; 52:* 316
3 Martelli A, Bulli P, Cartecchia V. *Eur Urol 1981; 7:* 291
4 Keefe WE, Smith MJV. *Invest Urol 1977; 14:* 344
5 Burr RG, Nuseibeh I. *Br J Urol 1983; 55:* 162
6 Griffith DP, Moskowitz PA, Carlton CE. *J Urol 1976; 121:* 711

ACETOHYDROXAMATE IN STRUVITE STONES: IN VIVO STUDY

A Aroldi, G Graziani, C Castelnovo, G Colussi*,
M Surian*, A Mandressi†, E Mascheroni‡,
I Pazardjiklian‡, A Pagano‡, C Ponticelli

*Divisione di Nefrologia e Dialisi, *Ospedale Maggiore, Niguarda,
†Istituto di Urologia, and ‡Istituto di Igiene dell'Università di
Milano, Italy*

Summary

This report describes the results obtained with a combination of acetohydroxamic acid (AHA) and antibacterial agents in 13 patients with recurrent struvite stones complicated by refractory infections with urease-producing bacteria. Intravenous antibiotic pulses plus oral AHA achieved urine sterilisation in all. Then oral chemotherapy plus AHA was given for a mean period of 10.8 ± 5.4 months. In four patients, the urine remained sterile, but in all the patients urinary pH remained below 6.4 and urinary NH_4^+ below 40mg/dl. Despite the persistence of urea-splitting bacteria, the radiographic data showed an arrest of stone growth during the first year of treatment.

Introduction

Struvite stones grow rapidly during persistent urinary infection with urease-splitting bacteria. The enzyme urease splits urea to carbonic anhydride and ammonia (NH_4^+), which combines with magnesium and phosphates to rapidly precipitate as magnesium phosphate. For these reasons, this type of lithiasis must be treated very carefully. Until recently, no really effective therapy has been available. Following the introduction of the urease inhibitor, aceto-hydroxamic acid (AHA) which reduces ammonia production, therapeutic results have improved [1]. This report deals with the results obtained with a combination of AHA with antibacterial agents in 13 patients with recurrent struvite stones complicated by refractory urea-splitting infections.

Patients and methods

Intravenous (i.v.) pulses of antibiotics (AB) were administered to 13 patients with refractory urease-producing infections and struvite stones plus oral AHA (250mg x 4/day). The antibiotics administered were cefoxitime and tobramycin.

469

For five patients with mild renal failure, the doses were adjusted on the basis of the endogenous creatinine clearance. After five days all patients were given oral chemotherapy (pipemidic acid or trimethoprim) combined with AHA (250mg x 2, 3 or 4/day), which was continued for 6–15 months (mean 10.8 ± 5.4).

Urine cultures, total bacterial count (TBC) (col/ml), pH and NH_4^+ excretion, blood platelets, RBC, WBC, plasma creatinine, urea and aminotransferase were assessed every two weeks during the entire period.

Urine was collected under mineral oil, by spontaneous voiding, for the determination of pH (pH meter, Copenhagen) and NH_4^+ (mg/dl) (Fawcett and Scott's method) [2]. Urine samples for identification and counting of bacteria [3] were collected in a sterile container by spontaneous voiding. Abdominal X-rays were taken at the start of the therapy and every six months thereafter.

Persistent urinary sterilisation was defined as no bacteriuria for longer than six months.

Statistical analysis by Student t-test for paired data.

Results

Intravenous antibiotic pulses combined with oral AHA

Urine sterilisation and significant decreases in urinary pH and NH_4^+ were obtained in all patients after i.v. antibiotic pulses combined with oral AHA (Table I).

Oral chemotherapy combined with oral AHA

During treatment with oral chemotherapy and AHA, only four of 13 patients had persistently sterile urine. Transient sterilisation was obtained in four and in the other five patients, urinary infections recurred and persisted throughout treatment. In those patients, in whom bacterial growth persisted, the total bacterial counts, urine pH and NH_4^+ were lower than before treatment (Table I). In all patients urine pH remained below 6.4 and NH_4^+ below 40mg/dl (Table I). In the nine patients treated for 12 months, who served as their own controls, abdominal X-rays showed stabilisation of stone growth during therapy.

Red and white blood cells, plasma creatinine, urea and aminotransferase did not show any significant changes. A transient, dose-unrelated mild thrombocytopenia was observed in all patients after four to eight weeks of therapy, but the platelet counts returned to basal values without any discontinuation or decrease in drug dosage.

Side effects

1. Headaches were relatively common during the first days of treatment (77%), but disappeared spontaneously or responded to mild analgesics.
2. Four patients complained of a transient metallic taste.

470

TABLE I. TBC (col/ml) × 1000, urine pH and NH_4^+ (mg/dl) before and after the combination of oral AHA with five i.v. antibiotic (AB) pulses and during oral chemotherapy. All values are means ± SD and differ from values before AB + AHA, *p<0.001, †p<0.005, ‡p<0.01

	Before AB + AHA	After AB + AHA	During oral chemotherapy and AHA (500–1000mg/day)				
Months:			1	3	6	9	12
			Recurrent infection				
Number of patients	7	7	7	8	7	9	6
TBC	885 ± 220	0	385 ± 211	350 ± 141†	457 ± 310	657 ± 390	816 ± 240
pH	6.85 ± 0.34	5.68 ± 0.34†	6.12 ± 0.54	6.06 ± 0.70	6.01 ± 0.51	6.05 ± 0.45	5.95 ± 0.32‡
NH_4^+	79.8 ± 35.5	26.3 ± 12.6†	30.5 ± 9.88	28.0 ± 13.2‡	26.6 ± 11.5†	30.3 ± 9.12	30.0 ± 8.55‡
			Sterilised				
Number of patients	6	6	6	5	6	4	3
TBC	900 ± 160	0	0	0	0	0	0
pH	6.88 ± 0.46	5.64 ± 0.21†	5.90 ± 0.43‡	5.58 ± 0.31‡	5.42 ± 0.34*	6.02 ± 0.33‡	5.73 ± 0.30
NH_4^+	81.5 ± 36.1	28.5 ± 11.5†	28.3 ± 8.41‡	34.7 ± 8.40‡	31.8 ± 8.54‡	29.0 ± 12.5	25.9 ± 5.90

471

Discussion

AHA is known to be an irreversible, non-competitive, urease inhibitor [4]. The oral combination of AHA with i.v. antibiotic pulses sterilised the urine of all patients. During treatment with the oral AHA and chemotherapy combination there was prolonged bacterial eradication in only four. In the other nine patients only transitory urine sterilisation was obtained. Indeed, the presence of living bacteria on the surface of the stone makes permanent urinary tract sterilisation of these patients almost impossible. In spite of the recurrence of urease-producing infections and increased total bacterial count during treatment, urinary pH and NH_4^+ remained lower. It is interesting to note that all patients had been refractory to previous antibiotic treatment, while they had partial or total recoveries from infection during AHA administration.

Our results seem to suggest that concomitant chemotherapy and AHA treatment reduces the quantity of urease and blocks the urease that is produced. Moreover the lowering of urinary pH and NH_4^+ excretion should enhance the effects of the chemotherapy [5]. In conclusion, despite the persistence of urea-splitting bacterial strains, the combination of AHA and chemotherapy seems to arrest infection-induced calculogenesis in urine that has been rendered physiological by eradication of infection or inhibition of urease.

References

1 Griffith DP, Moskowitz PA, Feldman S. In Smith LN, ed. *Proc 4th Int Symposium on Urolithiasis Research.* New York: Plenum Press. 1981: 199–208
2 Fawcett JK, Scott JE. *J Clin Pathol 1960; 13:* 156
3 Pagano A, Russolo S, Paggi D. *Igiene Moderna 1981; 76:* 1245
4 Fishbein WN, Carbone PP, Hochstein HD. *Nature 1965; 208:* 46
5 Musher DM, Saenz C, Griffith DP. *Antimicrob Agents Chemother 1974; 5:* 106

Proc EDTA (1983) Vol 20

TREATMENT OF RENAL LITHIASIS ASSOCIATED WITH RENAL TUBULAR ACIDOSIS

C J Van Den Berg, T M Harrington, T W Bunch, A M Pierides

Mayo Clinic and Foundation, Rochester, MN, USA

Summary

In order to determine the incidence of renal lithiasis in patients with renal tubular acidosis and the effect of therapy on further stone formation, we reviewed the clinical and laboratory manifestations, X-ray findings, and treatment of 48 patients with renal tubular acidosis who were seen at the Mayo Clinic during the years 1970–1980. Thirty-four patients (70%) had radiological evidence of renal lithiasis which was the presenting symptom in 23 (48%) patients. In every instance the calculi were multiple and, with one exception, bilateral. While receiving therapy, 19 patients with renal lithiasis were followed for longer than one year with sequential uroradiographic studies. Fifteen of these patients were treated with oral base alone and thirteen had no evidence of new stone formation or continued growth of existing stones during therapy. The two patients with X-ray evidence of continued stone formation admitted to poor compliance. Four patients received initial treatment with an oral phosphorus supplement. Three of these four patients had radiographic evidence of continued renal stone formation during three, five and eight years of phosphate therapy. We conclude renal lithiasis is a frequent complication of renal tubular acidosis, and adequate base replacement is effective therapy to stop continued stone formation while oral phosphate therapy alone is often ineffective.

Introduction

Renal tubular acidosis is a clinical syndrome of hyperchloraemic metabolic acidosis resulting from renal tubular abnormalities while glomerular filtration rate is relatively well preserved [1]. Although patients with renal tubular acidosis may present with many different symptoms and physical findings, renal stone formation is a well-recognised manifestation of renal tubular acidosis and has been described [2, 3]. The precise documentation of this problem and especially the response of renal stone formation to appropriate treatment are less clear. We, therefore, characterised renal lithiasis seen in association with renal tubular

473

acidosis in regard to frequency, type, and response to treatment in 48 cases of renal tubular acidosis seen at the Mayo Clinic during a ten-year period.

Methods and materials

The clinical records of 48 patients with renal tubular acidosis seen at the Mayo Clinic between 1970 and 1980 were reviewed, and the clinical, laboratory, and therapeutic aspects of the case histories were examined. The diagnosis of renal tubular acidosis was based on the concurrence of a systemic acidosis (HCO_3 <20 mEq/L) with an inappropriately high urine pH (>5.5). In 23 patients the occurrence was spontaneous, 'complete renal tubular acidosis'. In 25 patients, systemic acidaemia was not present in a resting state, and the diagnosis, 'incomplete renal tubular acidosis' was confirmed by the above criteria present after challenge with oral ammonium chloride. In all patients, the presence or absence and the course of renal lithiasis were determined by excretory urography or a kidney-ureter-bladder radiographic study. Coincident disease was diagnosed by conventional criteria using the history, clinical examination, and laboratory procedures.

Results

General patient data, method of diagnosis, and the classification of renal tubular acidosis as to 'proximal' or 'distal' is shown in Table I. Of the 48 patients, 23 (48%) presented with complaints referrable to nephrolithiasis. Radiographic studies, however, revealed renal calculi in 34 of the 48 patients (70%). In every instance, the calculi were multiple and with one exception bilateral.

TABLE I. Renal tubular acidosis

48 patients	
Women 31	
Men 17	
Age range 10–71	
Diagnosis	
spontaneous	23
ammonium chloride load	25
Type of RTA	
proximal	4
distal	44

While receiving therapy, 19 patients with renal tubular acidosis and renal calculi were followed up for longer than one year with sequential kidney-ureter-bladder radiography or excretory urograms. The mean duration of follow-up was 55 months, median 48 months, and range 13–120 months. Fifteen of these 19 patients were treated with oral base (sodium bicarbonate or sodium and potassium citrate solutions) alone in amounts ranging from 60–120mEq daily. Thirteen of the 15 patients had metabolically inactive renal lithiasis during follow-up, that is they had no evidence of new stone formation or continued growth of an existing stone. Two of the 15 patients had X-ray evidence of continued stone formation. Both admitted to poor compliance. In one case oral base therapy was discontinued completely with stone growth documented over an 18-month period. With reinstitution of base therapy, the stone disease was metabolically inactive during the subsequent 44 months of therapy. In the second case, poor compliance was confirmed by persistently low urinary excretion of citrate. Four patients received initial treatment with oral phosphate supplement (1.6–2.4gm of phosphorus daily) as a neutral sodium and potassium salt. Three of these four patients had radiographic evidence of continued metabolically active renal lithiasis during three, five, and eight years of phosphate therapy.

Discussion

Although a rare cause of calcium renal lithiasis, accounting for less than one per cent of all patients who are calcium stone formers, type I renal tubular acidosis is frequently complicated by recurrent nephrolithiasis or nephrocalcinosis or both [1]. In our series, 34 of 48 patients had radiographic evidence of renal lithiasis which was often quite extensive consisting of multiple and bilateral calculi. In many instances there was extensive calcification within the renal parenchyma. Although we did not attempt to distinguish between nephro-calcinosis and extensive multiple small renal calculi, we were impressed with the obvious extensive renal calcification which complicates renal tubular acidosis, irrespective of whether the calcium was in the collecting system or in the renal parenchyma. The experience of other investigators [2] and our experience suggests that adequate oral base replacement is effective therapy for the pre-vention of calcium stone formation in patients with renal tubular acidosis. Three of four of our patients who received oral phosphorus supplements as the only treatment of renal tubular acidosis had continued metabolically active stone disease. While oral phosphate has been effective in the treatment of patients with metabolically active idiopathic renal lithiasis [3, 4], 2gm of phosphorus daily as a neutral salt does not supply adequate base to correct the metabolic abnormalities associated with renal tubular acidosis.

A number of metabolic abnormalities associated with renal tubular acidosis could predispose to calcium urolithiasis including an alkaline urine, hypercalciuria, and greatly decreased urinary excretion of citrate. While the propensity for formation of calcium phosphate crystals increases as the urine pH increases, the relatively alkaline urine pH in patients with renal tubular acidosis is more alkaline with appropriate base replacement. This occurs at the same time as stone formation ceases with adequate therapy, and it is hard to accept the premise that the relatively alkaline urine pH is a key factor for calcium stone formation in RTA. Hyper-calciuria was not a prominent feature of the initial laboratory investigation in our patients. In 29 patients whose initial investigation included a 24-hour urinary excretion of calcium, the mean value was 161mg with a range of 68–399. Normal values for urinary excretion of calcium in our patients on a diet of approximately 1gm of calcium daily are less than 275mg calcium per 24 hours.

With these findings it seems unlikely that hypercalciuria itself is a major risk factor for urolithiasis in our patients. In urine, citrate is a natural 'inhibitor' of the formation of calcium crystals. Citrate not only complexes with calcium reducing the activity of calcium ions but also may act in some independent fashion to inhibit crystal growth [5]. The urinary excretion of citrate is greatly decreased in patients with renal tubular acidosis and increases to normal values with adequate systemic base replacement [6]. In patients with renal tubular acidosis, the beneficial effect of systemic base replacement on the continued formation of calcium renal stones may be related to the increased urinary excretion of citrate. If decreased urinary excretion of citrate is a major risk factor for calcium stone formation in these patients, it provides a reliable marker to the adequacy of treatment, that is oral base therapy adequate to ensure increased urinary excretion of citrate to normal (400–600mg/24 hours).

References

1 Seldin DW, Wilson JD. In Stanbury JB, Wyngaarden JB, Fredrickson DS, eds. *Metabolic Basis of Inherited Disease.* New York: McGraw-Hill Book Co. 1966: 1230–1246
2 Gyory AZ, Edwards KDG. *Am J Med 1968; 45:* 43
3 Thomas WC Jr. *Trans Am Clin Climatol Assoc 1971; 83:* 113
4 Smith LH, Thomas WC Jr, Arnaud CD. In Cifuentes Delatte L, Rapado A, Hodgkinson A, eds. *Urinary Calculi: Recent Advances in Aetiology, Stone Structure and Treatment.* Basel: S Karger. 1973: 188–197
5 Smith LH, Meyer JL, McCall JT. In Cifuentes Delatte L, Rapado A, Hodgkinson A, eds. *Urinary Calculi: Recent Advances in Aetiology, Stone Structure and Treatment.* Basel: S Karger. 1973: 318–327
6 Morrissey JF, Ochoa M Jr, Lotspeich WD, Waterhouse C. *Ann Intern Med 1963; 58:* 159

DO THIAZIDES PREVENT RECURRENT IDIOPATHIC RENAL CALCIUM OXALATE STONES?

H Wolf, P Brocks, C Dahl

Hvidovre University Hospital, Hvidovre, Denmark

Summary

In a double-blind controlled clinical trial 62 patients with recurrent idiopathic renal calcium oxalate stone formation were allocated either to treatment with bendroflumethiazide, 2.5mg three times a day, or placebo. In each group the rate of stone formation during medication (average follow-up period 36 months) was compared with the rate of stone formation before medication (average control period 36 months). In both groups a similar striking fall in the rate of stone formation was found, indicating that thiazides in this study did not alter the spontaneous course of idiopathic renal calcium oxalate stone formation. It is doubtful whether life-long prophylaxis with thiazide is justified in patients with a moderate rate of stone formation.

Introduction

Thiazides are widely used in the prevention of recurrent renal calcium oxalate stones. This prophylaxis is based on the results from open clinical trials in which a beneficial effect on the prevention of recurrent renal calcium stones has been reported [1–4]. Such effect is in agreement with findings that thiazides reduce urinary excretion of calcium by about 50 per cent [5, 6] and reduces the stone forming potential in urine and abolishes the diurnal variation of the stone forming potential in urine [7]. However, although apparently very convincing, these studies were not double-blind controlled clinical trials.

This study is the first double-blind, controlled clinical study and preliminary results have already been reported [8].

Patients and methods

All patients with stones of the upper urinary tract referred to the department of urology were considered for this study. Eligible patients were aged 16–49, had passed or formed at least two stones in the preceding six years, were free from infection of the urinary tract, and had no well-defined metabolic causes of renal stone formation. The amount of calcium excreted in the urine was not used as a criterion of eligibility. The patients are treated with bendroflu-methiazide ('Centyl', Leo Pharmaceutical Products) 2.5mg three times daily or a placebo tablet three times daily for four years. Each patient gave informed consent in accordance with the Helsinki II declaration.

Registration of the rate of stone formation

Control period

The oldest radiograph taken within the preceding six years was obtained for investigation. Its date was taken as the start of the control period. Stones present at that time were not considered, whatever their fate. All stones formed de novo after that time, whether they had been passed, removed by surgery, or visualised by renal tomography at the start of medication (t_0), were counted and considered to have been formed during the control period. Episodes of renal colic alone were not considered indicative of new stone formation.

Treatment period

The patients were asked to collect all stones passed. Radiography including renal tomography was undertaken at t_0 and every 12 months for four years. Stones formed de novo during that period were again recorded.

For each group the number of patient years was obtained by summation of the years of observation. The stone-formation rate as expressed by the average number of stones formed per patient year was calculated by dividing the total number of stones formed by patient years.

Results

Random allocation to treatment or placebo has so far provided 33 patients in the thiazide group and 29 patients in the placebo group. All data on stone formation before and during medication with thiazide or placebo are presented in Table I. The rate of stone formation falls considerably in both groups – from 0.40 to 0.09 per patient year in the thiazide group and from 0.70 to 0.09 in the placebo group. The total of 16 stones formed in the two groups were in 13 different subjects. Thus during medication with thiazide or placebo no difference in the rate of stone formation could be seen. The expected number of stones with unchanged rate of stone formation is 36 in the thiazide-treated group and 61 in the placebo group. Thus, only 22 per cent of the expected number of stones were formed in the thiazide group and 13 per cent in the placebo group.

Discussion

This is to our knowledge the first controlled clinical trial of thiazide prophylaxis in idiopathic renal calcium stone formers. The reduction in the rate of stone

478

TABLE I. Stone formation before and during treatment with thiazide or placebo

Medication	Number of patients	Before treatment				During treatment			
		Average observation (years)	Patient years	Number of stones formed	Average number of stones/patient year	Average observation (years)	Patient years	Number of stones formed	Average number of stones/patient year
Thiazide	33	3.3	109	43	0.40	2.9	89	8	0.09
Placebo	29	3.0	87	61	0.70	3.0	87	8	0.09

formation observed by us during treatment with thiazide is in accordance with that seen in several open trials [1—4]. Yendt et al [3] found that the average number of stones formed per patient year fell from 0.57 to 0.03 in one group and from 1.1 to 0.53 in another. Backmann et al [2] reported a decrease from approximately 1.0 to about 0.16 per patient year. A similar sharp reduction was observed by Coe [4].

Of great surprise and interest, however, is our finding that the palcebo group showed a reduction in the rate of stone formation of the same magnitude as the thiazide group. It is hard to escape the conclusion that thiazide does not alter the spontaneous course of stone formation in idiopathic renal calcium stone formers.

The rate of stone formation in this series is moderate. We cannot be entirely sure that thiazide does not help patients with very aggressive stone formation. However, our data raise considerable doubt about the indication for life-long thiazide prophylaxis in the average renal calcium oxalate stone former. Others are encouraged to conduct similar controlled trials, and the results of one such trial have been reported [9], although the follow-up period of that study is limited.

Our study, however, stresses the importance of being cautious in instituting treatment of any kind to a large number of patients before substantial evidence of an effect is documented in controlled clinical trials.

References

1 Yendt ER, Cohanim M. *Kidney Int 1978; 13:* 397
2 Backmann U, Danielson BG, Johansson G et al. *Br J Urol 1979; 51:* 175
3 Yendt ER, Guay GF, Garcia DA. *Can Med Assoc J 1970; 102:* 614
4 Coe FL. *Ann Intern Med 1977; 97:* 404
5 Lamberg BA, Kuhlbäck B. *Scand J Clin Invest 1959; 11:* 351
6 Jørgensen FS. *Dan Med Bull 1976; 23:* 223
7 Brocks P, Christiansen C, Dirksen H et al. *Scand J Urol Nephrol.* In press
8 Brocks P, Dahl C, Wolf H et al. *Lancet 1981; ii:* 124
9 Scholz D, Schwille PO, Sigel A. *J Urol 1982; 128:* 903

PART XIV

GUEST LECTURES — HYPERTENSION

Chairmen: G Bianchi
N F Jones

Proc EDTA (1983) Vol 20

BODY SODIUM AND BLOOD PRESSURE: ABNORMAL AND DIFFERENT CORRELATIONS IN CONN'S SYNDROME, RENAL ARTERY STENOSIS AND ESSENTIAL HYPERTENSION

D L Davies, C Beretta-Piccoli, J J Brown, A M M Cumming, R Fraser, A Lasaridis, A F Lever, D McAreavey, J I S Robertson, P F Semple

Western Infirmary, Glasgow, United Kingdom

Introduction

The role of sodium in the pathogenesis of various forms of hypertension, and especially of essential hypertension, is of considerable interest. Currently, three main avenues are attracting attention. First, a variety of abnormalities affecting the transport of sodium and potassium across cell membranes have been described [1,2]. Professor Philip Meyer deals with some of these on page 489 of this volume. Second, it is suggested that the rise of arterial pressure with age in Western societies and thus the greater prevalence of hypertension results wholly or partly from increased dietary intake of sodium or decreased dietary intake of potassium or both [3]. Third, there is evidence that hypertension may result from a decreased ability of the kidney to excrete sodium at a given arterial pressure which then raises blood pressure to the point where sodium balance is restored. Conn's syndrome may be an example of this since the ability of the kidney to excrete sodium is reduced reversibly by excess corticosteroid [4]. The hypertension of chronic renal failure may be another instance where structural change within the kidney has a similar but irreversible effect.

In other hypertensive states there is sometimes sodium depletion. In unilateral renal artery stenosis sodium depletion may occur because blood pressure is raised by a mechanism which is not principally dependent on sodium retention. Sodium loss is then a consequence of the hypertension [5].

Thus, blood pressure may be controlled in part by a balance between the pressor effect of sodium retention and the natriuretic effect of increased blood pressure. In some hypertensive states blood pressure rises as a consequence of the first, in others sodium depletion is a consequence of the second.

Measurement of the body content of sodium is relevant to these mechanisms. In this paper we shall report such measurements in normal subjects and in patients with Conn's syndrome, unilateral renal artery stenosis and essential hypertension. Body sodium has been measured by neutron activation analysis which gives a value for total body sodium and by isotope dilution which estimates exchangeable sodium. Measurements made using both techniques on the same patient correlate well (r = 0.91, p <0.001). Details of the patients, of the techniques used for measuring body sodium and of other methods are given in papers on essential hypertension [6], Conn's syndrome [4] and renal artery stenosis [5].

Conn's syndrome

Exchangeable sodium was measured in 34 patients with untreated Conn's syndrome all having an aldosterone secreting adenoma. It was abnormally increased compared with measurements in 34 normal subjects matched for age and sex [4] and with 121 unmatched normal subjects (Table I). Total body sodium measured by activation analysis in 13 of these patients was increased to 128 ± 2.8 SEM per cent of predicted normal values. Exchangeable sodium (NaE) correlated positively and significantly with systolic and diastolic pressure in untreated patients (Table I). Treatment with spironolactone or surgical removal of the adrenal adenoma lowered blood pressure, restored a normal mean value for NaE and reduced to insignificance the correlation of NaE and blood pressure (Table I). Exchangeable sodium and blood pressure were not related in normal subjects (Table I).

TABLE I

| | Number | Mean NaE | Correlation Coefficient | | |
			NaE v SBP	NaE v DBP	Plasma K v DBP
Normal subjects	121	100.0	0.04	0.03	0.9
Untreated	34	116.7	0.64***	0.54***	−0.46**
Conn's syndrome					
Spironolactone	19	93.4	0.13	−0.06	−0.08
Post-surgical	23	98.0	0.09	0.01	0.31
Renal artery stenosis					
Untreated	25	96.1	−0.16	−0.54**	−0.34
Essential hypertension	91	99.1	0.44***	0.31*	−0.41***

Mean values of exchangeable sodium and coefficients of linear correlation for the exchangeable sodium (related to body surface area) and systolic blood pressure, for exchangeable sodium and diastolic blood pressure and plasma potassium and diastolic blood pressure. *p <0.05; **p <0.01; ***p <0.001

These results are compatible with a primary role for sodium retention in the hypertension of Conn's syndrome. Also suggesting this is the observation that mineralocorticoid hypertension in rats can be prevented if dietary sodium intake is reduced [7]. The mechanism by which sodium retention raises blood pressure is not so clear. Whole-body autoregulation is one possibility [8] but there is also the view that sodium retention stimulates release of a natriuretic agent with an inhibitory effect on sodium transport raising blood pressure by a direct action on vascular smooth muscle [9].

Renal artery stenosis

Exchangeable sodium was measured in 25 hypertensive patients with unilateral renal artery stenosis. With one exception all had a plasma urea concentration below 7mmol/L. Mean NaE for the group was close to normal (Table I), but the range of NaE was wider than normal. Six of the 25 had hyponatraemia at presentation with a plasma sodium concentration of 135mmol/L or less. Exchangeable sodium in these was much lower than in patients with normal plasma sodium. Plasma concentrations of angiotensin II and aldosterone were markedly increased in the hyponatraemic patients and hypokalaemia was present (Table II). For the group as a whole, NaE and diastolic blood pressure were inversely related (Table I).

TABLE II

	Unilateral Renal Artery Stenosis	
	I. Normal plasma sodium (n=19)	II. Hyponatraemia (n=6)
M/F	8/11	3/3
Age	40.8 ± 2.3	47.5 ± 6.9
BP: systolic mmHg	193.0 ± 5.0	219.0 ± 6.0*
diastolic mmHg	113.0 ± 3.0	133.0 ± 5.0**
Plasma concentrations of		
Na mMol/L	140.0 ± 0.7	129.0 ± 3.6***
K mMol/L	3.9 ± 0.1	2.9 ± 0.3***
Active Renin μU/ml	42.2 ± 22.6(n=11)	1648.0 ± 937.0(n=2)
Angiotensin II pg/ml	25.4 ± 4.3	309.2 ± 99.1***
Aldosterone pg/100ml	12.5 ± 1.8	38.3 ± 14.2**
Urea mMol/L	4.7 ± 1.1	4.2 ± 2.3
Creatinine clearance ml/min	104.0 ± 6.0	54.0 ± 7.0**
NaE% (BSA)	100.4 ± 1.8	85.6 ± 3.4***

Mean (± SEM) values for blood pressure, plasma concentrations of electrolytes, active renin, aldosterone and urea and creatinine clearance and exchangeable sodium (related to body surface area). Comparison by t-test is made of patients in groups I and II.
*$p<0.05$, **$p<0.01$, ***$p<0.001$

Twelve of the 25 patients had bilateral ureteric catheterisation which assesses separately the function of the two kidneys. Sodium excretion was invariably greater from the contralateral than from the kidney with the arterial stenosis and the rate of sodium excretion from this kidney (but not from the kidney with the arterial stenosis) correlated significantly both with NaE (r = -0.75, p <0.01) and with diastolic blood pressure at the time of catheterisation (r = +0.65, p <0.05).

This part of our study shows that sodium depletion occurs in some patients with unilateral renal artery stenosis which confirms earlier reports [10,11]. Sodium depletion is not an invariable finding however. Some of our patients had normal or slightly increased NaE and mean NaE for the larger group without hyponatraemia was 100.4 per cent of normal.

We also show that most of the sodium loss is from the relatively normal kidney and that the rate at which sodium is lost from this kidney relates to the deficit of body sodium and to arterial pressure. Sodium depletion and hyponatraemia were associated with secondary hyperaldosteronism (Table II). These findings are compatible with the view [11] that blood pressure is raised in unilateral renal artery stenosis by a mechanism not primarily involving sodium, that increased arterial pressure causes sodium loss from the contralateral kidney probably by pressure natriuresis. Secondary hyperaldosteronism is then a consequence of the sodium loss. If the increase of angiotensin II is sufficient to raise blood pressure further a vicious circle will develop with progressive sodium depletion stimulating renin and angiotensin II thereby raising blood pressure progressively.

Essential hypertension

Measurements of NaE were made in 91 patients with untreated essential hypertension [6]. Mean NaE for the group was close to 100 per cent of normal (Table I). However, there was also an abnormal relation of NaE with systolic and diastolic pressure in the essential hypertensives. No such relation was present in normal subjects. The relation was closest in men and in older patients with essential hypertension (r 0.64, p <0.001, for those of 49 years or more). There was no correlation of NaE and blood pressure in women or in younger patients (r -0.07 for patients under 35 years). Interestingly, mean NaE in young patients was subnormal [6]. As in Conn's syndrome there was a negative correlation of arterial pressure with plasma potassium concentration (Table I). This correlation was closer in young than in older patients [6].

Interpretation of these observations is less straightforward. Body sodium is abnormally related to arterial pressure in essential hypertension yet average body sodium is close to normal. This could mean that arterial pressure in patients with essential hypertension is abnormally responsive to changing body sodium, a given increase or decrease of body sodium producing a greater change of blood pressure in hypertensive than in normal subjects. Our data are compatible with a mechanism of this sort in older hypertensives but we see no evidence of it in young or female patients. We have discussed elsewhere [6] the possibility that the abnormal mechanism may develop in older patients as a consequence of hypertension of some other cause. Once developed it could perpetuate and exacerbate the hypertension.

The opposite correlation of body sodium and plasma potassium with arterial pressure and the significant correlation of arterial pressure with the ratio of plasma sodium and plasma potassium, and with the ratio of body sodium and body potassium [6] raises the possibility of abnormal corticosteroid secretion in essential hypertension. Against the idea is the normality of mean NaE and of mean exchangeable potassium [6]. However, some steroids may raise blood pressure without producing sodium retention. Measurements of corticosteroids in essential hypertension show only a minor abnormality in patients with essential hypertension [6].

Another possibility is that the relation of body sodium and blood pressure reflects an abnormality in the distribution of sodium between intracellular and extracellular compartments. There is the suggestion that an abnormality of this sort might result from an inhibitor of sodium transport causing hypertension by an action on vascular smooth muscle [1,2].

Our general conclusions from the comparison of body sodium in these three hypertensive states is that each shows a significant but different abnormality in the relation of body sodium and blood pressure. In Conn's syndrome the abnormality is to be expected from a knowledge of the action of mineralocorticoids in causing sodium retention; but there are doubts about the way in which sodium retention raises blood pressure [8]. In renal artery stenosis the correlation of body sodium and arterial pressure is the opposite of that in Conn's syndrome and while the explanation we have given for this may be correct there is no general agreement on why blood pressure rises in renal artery stenosis when body sodium is normal. In essential hypertension there is again an abnormality but it is not present in all groups of patients. Its significance is uncertain. It might relate to a mechanism causing hypertension, but it could be a consequence of increased blood pressure.

References

1   Blaustein MP. *Am J Physiol 1977; 232:* C165
2   DeWardener HW, MacGregor GA. *Kidney Int 1980; 18:* 1
3   Freis ED. *Circulation 1976; 53:* 589
4   Beretta-Piccoli C, Davies DL, Brown JJ et al. *J Hypertension 1983.* In press
5   McAreavey D, Brown JJ, Cumming AMM et al. *J Hypertension 1983.* In press
6   Beretta-Piccoli C, Davies DL, Boddy K et al. *Clin Sci 1982; 63:* 257
7   Green DM, Saunders FJ, Wahlgren N, Craig RL. *Am J Physiol 1952; 170:* 94
8   Schalekamp MADH, Wenting GJ, Man in 'T Veld AJ. *Clin Endocrinol Metab 1981; 10:* 397
9   Haddy F, Pamnani M, Clough D. *Clin Exp Hypertens 1978; 1:* 295
10 Barraclough MA. *Am J Med 1966; 40:* 265
11 Atkinson AB, Brown JJ, Davies DL et al. *Lancet 1979; ii:* 606

Open Discussion

JONES (Chairman) Can you detect any way in which the relationship between total exchangeable sodium and blood pressure in people who have had Conn's syndrome corrected by surgery, or other means, is different from normal?

LEVER Yes, only a minor difference, and it would please your co-chairman, because there is a correlation between that and urea. In other words it looks, if blood pressure is dependent on anything after you remove the Conn's tumour, it is a mild but significant correlation with urea. This suggests that renal function is now holding blood pressure up, when it does remain up, and this of course links with the idea that hypertension of any cause, when that cause is removed, can persist. The mechanism of the persistence some of us certainly believe might be related to the kidney.

BIANCHI (Chairman) I would like to take the opportunity of discussing the last slide in which you showed the sequence of causes and you pointed out the difficulty of dissecting primary cause from secondary. For this reason some years ago we did kidney transplantation in rats and we showed that hypertension could be transplanted with the kidney and this occurred also in the pre-hypertensive stage. I think that this could be taken as evidence that in the primary form the kidney is a leading abnormality to some extent at least in rats of the Milan strain and is causing all the other changes in natriuretic and other factors.

LEVER Well I think there is very strong evidence from you in your Milan strain and from the salt sensitive Dhal rat that this is true. There is less strong evidence in the other congenitally hypertensive animals that the hypertension is transplanted with the kidney. I think that this means that for your strain you have got the answer. However have you also got the answer in essential hypertension? I think that the evidence is quite good, from transplantation experiments in man, but it is not as good as it is in the rat. The rat data cannot be interpreted in any other way but the human data is less certain. You have got some nice pointers.

KERR (Newcastle upon Tyne) What do you think accounts for the persistence of salt sensitivity in the nephrectomised patient who was previously hypertensive? Certainly our experience is that such patients are much less sodium sensitive than they were before nephrectomy though they do remain salt sensitive, quite different from the relationship you showed for normal individuals. This applies whether their primary disease was glomerulonephritis, pyelonephritis or essential or malignant hypertension.

LEVER No, I don't know what the answer is, but it is true and indeed the referee of our recent Conn's syndrome paper which will appear shortly has made just the suggestion you have made. We should plot on our graphs for Conn's syndrome the regression for similar measurements in patients with bilateral nephrectomy. There is this sensitivity even after the kidneys have been removed, but it's a lot less. We should put the data that we have got and compare with that of the Conn's syndrome. It is an interesting thought, but I don't know the mechanism of the persisting sensitivity.

Proc EDTA (1983) Vol 20

ENDOGENOUS DIGITALIS-LIKE COMPOUND IN ESSENTIAL HYPERTENSION

Marie-Aude Devynck, Marie-Gabrielle Pernollet,
H De The, J B Rosenfeld, **P Meyer**

Hôpital Necker, Paris, France

Introduction

Gradients in concentrations of sodium (Na^+) and potassium (K^+) between intracellular and extracellular fluids stem essentially from the activity of the sodium pump. The sodium pump may be altered in certain pathological conditions, including essential hypertension [1–3], and may originate from either intrinsic cell membrane alterations or the action of circulating factor(s) or both. Endogenous pump inhibitors have recently been described in biological fluids [4–7] and in tissues [8–11]. These factors appear to be increased by sodium loading and volume expansion [12–14]. Several clinical and experimental investigations suggest that the reduction in sodium pump activity in primary hypertension may be secondary to an increased activity of such an inhibitor [13, 15]. The resulting increase in intracellular Na^+ may be of pathogenic significance.

The present study evaluates, by direct biochemical methods, the presence of Na^+ pump inhibitor(s) in plasma from hypertensive patients and the influence of antihypertensive therapy on these inhibitors.

Material and methods

Preparation of plasma extracts

Blood sampling and preparation of heat stable plasma extracts were performed as previously described [16]. The clear supernatants of boiled plasma were either tested immediately, frozen, lyophilised or not, and kept at $-80°C$ until analysis. Some plasma supernatants were subjected to the separation procedures previously reported [17]: briefly, a gel filtration where the inhibitory fraction was eluted just after the salt peak and anion exchange chromatography where the above fraction was resolved into three peaks. These three fractions, although not pure as shown by high pressure liquid chromatography on reverse phase, were characterised in terms of inhibition of ^{3}H-ouabain binding, Na^+,K^+-ATPase activity and ^{3}H-serotonin uptake by platelets.

^{3}H-ouabain binding to erythrocytes

Binding of ^{3}H-ouabain (17–32 Ci/mmol, Amersham) to erythrocytes was performed at equilibrium as described previously [16]. Number of pump units and affinity were calculated from Scatchard plots. The inhibition by plasma extracts was expressed as the decrease in apparent affinity given as per cent of the erythrocyte affinity in the absence of plasma.

Na^+,K^+-ATPase activity

The activity of the enzyme (EC 3.6.1.3., prepared from dog kidney, Sigma) was determined by hydrolysis of ^{32}P-ATP (Amersham, UK). At 80μl of the following medium: 100mM NaCl, 2.5mM EGTA, 4mM $MgCl_2$, 2mM ATP Na (Vanadate-free, Sigma), 160nCi ^{32}P-ATP and 80mM Tris-HCl buffered to 7.4, were added 10μl of plasma extracts corresponding to 190μl of boiled plasma supernate or ionic plasma-like solution and 10μl of enzyme suspension (3 x 10^{-3} unit). After 30 minutes of incubation at 37°C, the reaction was stopped by placing the tubes at 0°C and adding 100μl of 23% $HClO_4$. Liberated phosphates, separated from ATP adsorbed on acid-washed charcoal, were then counted.

Controls and patients

Seventy-one subjects on a free sodium diet were studied. Their blood pressure was recorded with a mercury manometer in the sitting position. They were divided into five groups as follows.

Group 1 comprises 21 normotensive healthy volunteers with no known family history of hypertension (13 males and 8 females, aged from 23 to 53 years, mean 32.1 ± 2.0); their mean blood pressure was 90.8 ± 1.9mmHg.

Group 2 included 21 normotensive healthy volunteers who had at least one parent with high blood pressure (13 males and 8 females, aged from 23 to 50 years, mean 34.4 ± 1.7); their mean blood pressure averaged 95.5 ± 2.0mmHg.

Group 3 comprises 21 hypertensive patients, untreated for at least two weeks (14 males and 7 females, aged from 22 to 71 years, mean 45.9 ± 3.2). Essential hypertension was diagnosed after careful clinical investigation. In all patients plasma Na^+ and K^+ were in the normal range.

Groups 4 and 5: Ten hypertensive patients were under antihypertensive therapy for at least three months. Five (2 males, three females, aged 40–84 years) were on thiazide diuretics (group 4), and their mean blood pressure was 123.8 ± 6.0 mmHg. Five (3 males and 2 females, aged 26–47 years) were on β-blocking agents (group 5); their mean blood pressure was 105.8 ± 5.3mmHg. None of the patients had significant change in plasma potassium.

Results

Inhibition of ^{3}H-ouabain binding and Na$^+$,K$^+$-ATPase activity

Plasma extracts from nearly half of the normotensive subjects, offspring of hypertensive parents, and of the essential hypertensive patients exerted a marked inhibitory effect on the two biochemical parameters used as tests of interaction with Na$^+$,K$^+$ pumps. A significant correlation ($r = 0.74$, $n = 44$) was obtained between the inhibition of ouabain binding to erythrocytes and that of ATP hydrolysis obtained in individual plasma extracts. As shown on Table I, average affinities for ouabain binding and Na$^+$,K$^+$-ATPase activities were significantly decreased by plasma extracts of hypertensives and normotensives with family history of hypertension when compared to normotensive controls.

Plasma from patients under thiazide therapy did not significantly inhibit ouabain binding, whereas plasma from patients receiving β-blockers inhibited ouabain binding to a greater degree when compared to that of untreated hypertensive patients (Table I).

TABLE I. Inhibition by plasma extracts of ^{3}H-ouabain binding, Na$^+$,K$^+$-ATPase activity and ^{3}H-serotonin uptake by platelets

	Number	^{3}H-ouabain binding[†]	Na$^+$,K$^+$-ATPase activity (%)	Platelet serotonin uptake
Boiled plasma supernatants				
Normotensives				
Without family history of hypertension	21−19	0.21 ± 0.4	2.6 ± 1.9	−
With family history of hypertension	21−13	0.67 ± 14*	13.8 ± 3.3*	−
Hypertensives				
Untreated	21−19	0.61 ± 0.15*	12.8 ± 3.3*	−
Treated with diuretics	5	0.29 ± 0.34	−	−
Treated with β-blockers	5	1.61 ± 0.42*	−	−
Low molecular weight anionic fractions[‡]				
1	3	0.33	4.3	1.3
2	3	0.66	2.6	1.7
3	3	0.52	6.5	2.0

† Inhibition expressed as indicated in 'Methods'
‡ Inhibition given as whole plasma equivalent concentration giving half maximal inhibition
* $p < 0.01$ by Student t-test when compared to normotensive controls

Three fractions, extracted from plasma by gel filtration and anion exchange chromatography also inhibited significantly ouabain binding and Na^+,K^+-dependent ATP hydrolysis (Table I). Their mean purification factors were estimated to reach 200, their inhibitory potency is given as the concentration of equivalent whole plasma giving half maximal inhibition, without taking into account possible losses during purification.

Discussion

A defect in transmembrane sodium transport, secondary to a plasmatic factor, has been suggested as a possible mechanism of essential hypertension. The hypothesis that a circulating inhibitor of the sodium pump exists in essential hypertensive patients has been examined by analysis of the effects of plasma on two specific features of the pump: sodium and potassium-dependent ATP hydrolysis and specific ouabain binding.

Several investigators had previously measured the changes induced by plasma and/or urine in transmembrane sodium and potassium fluxes, in intracellular sodium content, in the activity of glucose-6-phosphate dehydrogenase whose stimulation has been suggested to reflect inhibition of Na^+,K^+-ATPase [13], or recently in the activity of Na^+,K^+-ATPase itself [18]. The present method offers the following advantages: 1) it directly measures the activity of plasma inhibitor on its target enzyme, the Na^+,K^+-ATPase; 2) the simultaneous measurement of inhibition of ouabain binding on whole cells under conditions where an effect of plasma potassium is excluded establishes that this circulating compound either shares common structural determinants with the cardiotonic digitalis, or prevents ouabain binding by allosteric modification of the pump structure. It also confirms that the inhibition of the Na^+,K^+-ATPase activity is not due to circulating inhibitors such as vanadate or calcium ions which did not inhibit ouabain binding under our experimental conditions. Plasma values of this inhibitor were high in some essential hypertensives and in some normotensives born of hypertensive parents. This suggests that presence of the inhibitor is not secondary to high blood pressure and must either act in conjunction with other prohypertensive systems or induce long-term modifications before it raises blood pressure.

References

1   Wambach G, Helber A. *Clin Exp Hypertens 1981; 3(4):* 663
2   Postnov YV, Orlov SN, Shevchenko A, Adler AM. *Pflüger's Arch 1977; 371:* 263
3   Edmonson RPS, Thomas RD, Hilton PJ et al. *Lancet 1975; i:* 1003
4   Clarkson EM, Raw SM, De Wardener HE. *Kidney Int 1979; 16:* 710
5   Gruber KA, Whitaker JM, Buckalew Jr VM et al. *Nature 1980; 287:* 743
6   Licht A, Stein S, McGregor CW. *Kidney Int 1982; 21:* 339
7   Kramer HJ. *Klin Wochenschr 1981; 59:* 1225
8   Haupert GT, Sancho JM. *Proc Natl Acad Sci USA 1979; 76:* 4658
9   Fishman M. *Proc Natl Acad Sci USA 1979; 76:* 4661
10   Lichstein D, Samuelov S. *Proc Natl Acad Sci USA 1982; 79:* 1453
11   Raghavan SR, Gonick HC. *Proc Soc Exp Biol Med 1980; 164:* 101

12   Haddy FJ, Pamnani MB, Clough DL. *Life Sci 1979; 24:* 2105
13   De Wardener HE, Clarkson EM, Bitensky L et al. *Lancet 1981; i:* 411
14   Gonick HC, Kramer HJ, Paul W, Lu R. *Clin Sci Mol Med 1977; 53:* 329
15   Blaustein MP. *Am J Physiol 1977; 232:* C165
16   Devynck MA, Pernollet MG, Rosenfeld JB, Meyer P. *Br Med J 1983.* In press
17   Cloix JF, Miller ED, Pernollet MG et al. *C R Acad Sci (Paris) 1983; 296(III):* 213
18   Hamlyn JM, Ringel R, Shaeffer J et al. *Nature 1982; 300:* 650

Open Discussion

JONES (Chairman)   I imagine that most of the audience will be very familiar with your published work on the sodium potassium co-transport system and its defect in hypertension, and in the relatives of hypertensives. How do you see at present the relationship between the work you have described to us this morning and that particular transport system?

MEYER   There are two basic properties in hypertension which may occur in human beings and we have to define in what proportion of patients we see one phenomenon or the other. One phenomenon is the presence of a membrane alteration as shown in the rat which may affect the membrane in a different way according to genetic determination. The other possibility is that there are some circulating factor or factors which are capable of affecting the pump or another system. One has to define exactly what is the proportion of patients belonging to the first category and the patients belonging to the second category.

WOODS (Oman)   I have been following Dr Meyer's work about the effects of the various sodium transport problems in hypertension. If the normotensives with a family history have the same markers on the membrane, whether it be a membrane defect or whether it be a circulating inhibitor as our hypertensives have, what is the suggested mechanism by which over a 10—15 year period this defect contributes to hypertension?

MEYER   I don't know. The most likely explanation is that the progressive sodium retention in the cells leads to some changes which might increase the contractility of the arterial cells. It is possibly related to the action of sodium per se or change in the conformation and the sensitivity of contractile protein. Is it in relation to calcium influx, because in excitable cells there might be sodium calcium exchange? It will require some time to answer your question, possibly because it is quite difficult to study vascular and contractile cells. A great hope, I think, stems from study of platelets as they have contractile properties and that they are avid for calcium which might be estimated in those platelets. According to the work of Fritz Buhler there is a very good correlation between the amount of calcium which is within the platelets and the elevation of blood pressure.

PAPADIMITRIOU (Thessaloniki, Greece)   Are there any studies on sodium/ potassium transport via the red cell membrane concerning captopril administration? I am asking this because there are some recent reports concerning the direct effect of captopril on this transport system. This has been studied with propranolol a long time ago and it has been proven that there is massive efflux of potassium out of the cell. Are there any studies with captopril, concerning this effect?

MEYER No, I fully agree with the action of propranolol in vitro although this was tested at high doses. In vivo we have not made any systematic analysis of the variation of fluxes on isolated cells. With treatment, the only concern we have at the moment is to study the variation of the circulating inhibitor. Concerning your question on captopril I have no data, but in vivo I don't think it is of much importance. Again this has to be verified.

BERGSTRÖM (Stockholm) If you think that inhibition of the sodium pump is involved in the development of hypertension why are patients on chronic dialysis therapy not developing hypertension? We know that dialysis inhibits the pump and we know that you get an increase in intracellular sodium, so I think it's very puzzling why these patients do not develop hypertension.

MEYER Firstly I think we should remember a well established fact which is that in dogs or in humans having no renal function, the administration of ouabain or digitalin results in a marked, although transient, increase in blood pressure. In addition the administration of ouabain centrally administered in rats induces a rise in blood pressure both in the conscious and awake animal. Your question is somewhat similar to the one which was raised a few minutes ago. You are dealing with a phenomenon which is observed during a matter of months, or maybe years, but the time is something less important than the time which is necessary for high blood pressure to develop. This is one part of my answer, the second answer is that I do not think we should simplify something which is obviously very complicated. Hypertension is a polymorphic disease and it is possible that it represents several varieties of underlying diseases. The pump inhibitor may be involved but you have seen that it is increased in only half of the patients. There are other possibilities and your patients who do not develop hypertension may be lacking one of these other factors which have to be identified in the future.

BIANCHI (Chairman) It is important to recall here that the first idea that a natriuretic factor might have a role in essential hypertension stems from some data suggesting that there is a primary kidney defect in people with essential hypertension in that the kidney is unable to excrete sodium. This sodium retention is the first stimulus for the increase in natriuretic factors. Hypertension, according to this theory might be explained by both mechanisms, a defect in the kidney handling of sodium and a natriuretic factor that acts on the smooth muscle or at the sympathetic nerve terminal increasing blood pressure. Certainly it is really difficult to explain hypertension by the natriuretic factor alone, and I would be agreed with all of you that are rather doubtful about this as the only mechanism.

494

RITZ (Heidelberg) Dr Meyer, both you and other investigators of course use blood cells because of the ready availability and accessibility of this material. To what extent can this be extrapolated to resistant vessels? Recently work from Denmark* casts some doubt as to whether inhibition of the transport Na^+,K^+-ATPase in mesenteric arteries actually increases the contractile state of these resistance vessels.

MEYER Yes, a recent review by John Parker described extensively all similarities existing between the membranes of red blood cells and the membranes of other tissue investigated so far.†

*   Mulvaney MJ, Korsgaard N, Nyborg N, Nilsson H. *Clin Sci 1981; 61:* 615
†   Parker JC, Berkowitz LR. *Physiol Rev 1983; 63:* 261

Proc EDTA (1983) Vol 20

RENAL FUNCTION IN PREGNANT RATS WITH TWO-KIDNEY GOLDBLATT HYPERTENSION

A Dal Canton, M Sabbatini, C Esposito, M Altomonte, G Romano, F Uccello, G Conte, G Fuiano, D Russo, V E Andreucci

Second Faculty of Medicine, University of Naples, Naples, Italy

Summary

This study was carried out in female Wistar-Münich rats with two-kidney, one-clip hypertension, using clipped normotensive rats as controls. Metabolic studies were performed in the first two weeks of pregnancy, consisting of daily measurement of systolic blood pressure (BP) (tail-cuff), body weight (BW), and salt and water balance. At the end of metabolic studies, glomerular dynamics were studied in the unclipped kidney by micropuncture. During pregnancy, urinary output of Na^+ and water was greater in hypertensive than normotensive rats. The greater natriuresis accounted for a reduced Na^+ retention and a lower increase in maternal BW. Micropuncture studies showed an impaired renal autoregulation.

These results show that hypertension in pregnancy causes a salt-losing tendency, that may be secondary to incomplete renal autoregulation.

Introduction

Systemic hypertension alters renal sodium handling both in man [1] and in animals [2, 3]. This alteration may be manifest either as a greater natriuresis in hypertensives than in normotensives after saline loading ('exaggerated natriuresis'), or as a natriuretic response to a sudden change from normal to elevated blood pressure ('pressure natriuresis'). Both of these are short-term phenomena that are believed to be dependent upon acute modifications in intrarenal haemodynamics, secondary to transient insufficiency of renal autoregulation [1, 2].

Recently, we have shown a marked fall in afferent arteriole resistance in pregnant rats [4]. This renal vasodilatation might persistently blunt renal autoregulation in pregnancy, allowing for hypertension in this condition to result in a continued alteration in renal sodium handling. This study investigates the effects of hypertension on renal function in pregnant rats.

Methods

The studies were carried out in adult female Wistar-Münich rats, with glomeruli on the kidney surface, in which a silver clip (0.2mm i.d.) was placed on the right renal artery under light ether anaesthesia. After this manoeuvre, in 12 rats systolic blood pressure (measured daily by the tail-cuff method) rose over 150mmHg and remained elevated throughout the study. These were the hypertensive rats. In nine other rats, systolic blood pressure remained steadily normal ($\leqslant$130mmHg) despite insertion of the clip. These were the normotensive controls. All the rats were fed on a standard chow containing 0.12mmol Na^+/g and, after placing the clip, received hypotonic saline (70mmol NaCl/litre) to drink, instead of tap water. This policy of increasing Na^+ intake was necessary to avoid a return to normal blood pressure, which had occurred, in preliminary studies, in all of 10 rats with two-kidney, one clip hypertension receiving a normal Na^+ intake.

Metabolic studies

After placing the clip, all the rats were allowed to stabilise for three weeks, and then were mated over two days, the second of which was taken as day one of pregnancy. In the last three days before mating, and from the second to the fourteenth day of pregnancy, the rats were housed in individual metabolic cages. During metabolic housing, Na^+ and water balance, body weight, and systolic blood pressure (tail-cuff) were monitored daily. At the end of metabolic studies, five hypertensive rats and four normotensive rats were killed by decapitation and blood was collected in chilled EDTA containing vials for plasma renin (PRA) measurement (radioimmunoassay, Sorin, Saluggia, Italy). The other rats were used for micropuncture studies.

Micropuncture studies

Seven hypertensive rats and five normotensive rats were anaesthetised and the left (non-clipped) kidney was exposed for renal micropuncture, as previously described [5]. Micropuncture measurements included all parameters of glomerular dynamics. Technical details and methods of calculation have been thoroughly described in our previous papers [4, 6].

At the end of each study, the entire gravid uterus and its content was removed and weighed. The number of fetuses were registered.

Results

Metabolic studies

During pregnancy, mean systolic blood pressure ranged between 168 and 189 mmHg in hypertensive rats, and between 108 and 126mmHg in normotensive controls. Body weight was similar in hypertensive as in control rats before mating (185.3 ± 18.4g versus 179.5 ± 20.9g, NS), but rose less during pregnancy

500

TABLE I. Daily Na$^+$ intake and excretion in pregnant hypertensive (H) rats and normotensive (N) rats

	Before mating*						Days of pregnancy							
		2	3	4	5	6	7	8	9	10	11	12	13	14
							Sodium intake (mEq/day)							
H	3.17 ±1.06	6.57 ±3.79	6.32 ±2.69	6.67 ±4.25	6.01 ±2.97	6.09 ±2.37	5.72 ±2.23	5.63 ±1.77	6.71 ±2.63	5.98 ±1.58	6.56 ±2.25	6.62 ±2.25	6.01 ±2.51	6.76 ±3.19
N	3.36 ±0.99	3.15 ±1.08	3.52 ±1.10	3.48 ±1.37	3.85 ±0.84	3.44 ±0.92	3.38 ±0.82	3.85 ±0.85	3.88 ±0.89	4.20 ±0.67	4.26 ±0.89	4.06 ±0.60	3.71 ±1.43	3.49 ±1.69
p<	NS	0.05	0.01	0.05	0.05	0.01	0.01	0.05	0.01	0.01	0.01	0.05	0.05	0.05
							Sodium excretion (mEq/day)							
H	2.96 ±0.77	6.14 ±3.51	6.06 ±3.51	6.58 ±4.95	5.14 ±3.55	5.38 ±3.21	5.13 ±2.83	5.20 ±1.85	5.94 ±2.98	5.19 ±2.01	5.66 ±2.58	5.49 ±1.88	5.15 ±2.82	5.71 ±2.43
N	2.71 ±1.64	1.92 ±0.93	2.25 ±0.82	2.76 ±1.20	2.26 ±0.98	2.58 ±0.91	2.45 ±1.09	2.43 ±0.73	2.60 ±0.79	3.03 ±1.54	2.65 ±0.98	2.51 ±0.77	2.86 ±1.23	2.88 ±1.29
p<	NS	0.05	0.01	0.05	0.05	0.05	0.05	0.01	0.01	0.05	0.01	0.01	0.05	0.01

Values are means ± SD

* Mean of three days

TABLE II. Daily water intake and excretion in pregnant hypertensive (H) rats and normotensive (N) rats

	Before mating*						Days of pregnancy							
		2	3	4	5	6	7	8	9	10	11	12	13	14
Water intake (ml/day)														
H	30.9 ±5.8	68.9 ±55.5	67.3 ±42.8	75.3 ±59.9	61.3 ±38.4	63.8 ±34.9	56.3 ±33.0	57.3 ±28.1	70.2 ±42.6	60.0 ±20.8	65.6 ±32.0	60.5 ±30.0	57.2 ±28.5	69.2 ±36.0
N	26.9 ±10.7	28.1 ±8.0	28.7 ±10.6	30.0 ±10.6	31.5 ±9.6	29.9 ±8.5	30.4 ±9.2	33.9 ±20.2	29.2 ±7.9	34.7 ±9.7	36.9 ±14.6	32.2 ±9.0	36.4 ±11.3	36.4 ±14.1
$p<$	NS	NS	0.05	0.05	0.05	0.05	0.05	0.05	0.05	0.005	0.05	0.05	NS	0.05
Water excretion (ml/day)														
H	14.9 ±9.6	46.5 ±52.4	49.0 ±43.3	54.0 ±52.0	40.5 ±35.6	43.3 ±36.6	38.1 ±32.1	40.1 ±24.4	46.7 ±36.9	38.7 ±21.3	41.8 ±28.5	37.0 ±20.1	37.8 ±27.9	43.3 ±26.4
N	10.4 ±9.4	9.6 ±7.2	11.9 ±6.4	10.9 ±6.6	9.5 ±5.4	11.9 ±5.0	9.9 ±4.1	10.9 ±3.1	11.3 ±3.7	11.2 ±4.6	12.3 ±7.3	13.3 ±6.5	17.2 ±7.4	15.7 ±8.5
$p<$	NS	NS	0.05	0.05	0.05	0.05	0.05	0.005	0.05	0.005	0.01	0.005	0.05	0.01

Values are means ± SD

* Mean of three days

in hypertensive than in normotensive rats (fourteenth day; Δ BW 10.0 ± 20.9 versus 31.0 ± 16.0g, respectively, p<0.05). Mean daily values of Na^+ intake and Na^+ excretion in hypertensive and normotensive rats are shown in Table I. Both Na^+ intake and Na^+ excretion were similar in the two groups before mating. However, during pregnancy both Na^+ intake and Na^+ excretion were consistently greater in hypertensive than in normotensive rats. Cumulative daily Na^+ retention (daily Na^+ intake less daily Na^+ excretion) in days 2–14 of pregnancy averaged 1.22 ± 0.35mEq/day in normotensive rats, a value significantly greater than in hypertensive rats (0.69 ± 0.63mEq/day, p<0.01). Mean daily water intake and excretion in hypertensive and normotensive rats is shown in Table II. Both water intake and urinary water excretion were similar in the two groups, before mating. During pregnancy, however, water intake and water excretion were greater in hypertensive than in normotensive rats. In contrast with sodium, cumulative daily water retention (daily water intake less daily urinary water excretion) was not different in hypertensive and normotensive rats (20.9 ± 4.4 versus 20.3 ± 2.4ml/day, p>0.1).

Micropuncture studies

During micropuncture studies, mean blood pressure from femoral artery (systolic + 1/3 pulse pressure) averaged 131.8 ± 19.9mmHg in hypertensive rats versus 100.0 ± 8.9 in controls (p<0.01). Despite this increase in perfusion pressure, afferent arteriole resistance was only slightly, and not significantly, increased in hypertensive rats (2.8 ± 2.0 versus 2.0 ± 0.8 dyne/sec/cm^{-5}, p>0.1). Therefore, afferent arteriole plasma flow (AAPF) rose from 129.8 to 200.9nl/min. This rise of AAPF was not associated with any change in single nephron glomerular filtration rate (SNGFR) (35.4 ± 13.3 versus 35.4 ± 6.8nl/min), accounting for a lower single nephron filtration fraction in hypertensive rats (mean 0.22 versus 0.29).

The weight of conceptus averaged 11.2 ± 4.5g (with a mean number of 8.9 fetuses) in hypertensive rats, and 14.9 ± 2.8g (mean 10.2 fetuses) in normotensive rats, the difference being insignificant. PRA averaged 13.0 ± 5.6ng/ml/h in hypertensive rats and 14.9 ± 6.9ng/ml/h in normotensive rats (p>0.1).

Discussion

In this study, hypertensive rats excreted more Na^+ in urine than normotensive controls, and this natriuresis was associated with an increased Na^+ intake. A major conceptual problem with these results is whether Na^+ loss was the primary change in Na^+ handling, followed by enhanced Na^+ replacement, or vice versa. Theoretically, in fact, increased circulating angiotensin II in our hypertensive rats with two-kidney Goldblatt hypertension, might have been responsible for an increase in salt appetite [7], and thus for a primary increase in Na^+ introduction. In our study, however, PRA was similarly elevated in hypertensive and normotensive rats, excluding greater renin activity in the former as the cause of increased angiotensin II production. Admittedly, this does not exclude that either an increased angiotensin II sensitivity, or an angiotensin II independent

503

mechanism primarily increased salt appetite in hypertensive rats. The lower amount of Na^+ cumulated by hypertensive rats during pregnancy, however, strongly argues against this possibility. This reduced Na^+ retention, in fact, was not accounted for by a reduced need of Na^+ for producing the conceptus, since uterine weight was similar in normotensive and hypertensive rats, and, therefore, reflected in the latter an impaired accumulation of Na^+ in maternal body, most probably secondary to a renal salt-losing tendency. In hypertensive rats, the enhanced Na^+ excretion was associated with an increased urinary water output. This, however, did not result in a significant reduction of cumulative water retention. This result may reflect a greater ability of the kidney in pregnant rats to save water than Na^+, as shown by others [8]. Caution is necessary in drawing any conclusion, however, because in our, as well as in other studies [9], urinary water output amounted to about one-half of water intake, indicating an almost preponderant incalculable (extrarenal) than calculable (renal) water loss in the rat.

Micropuncture studies showed an almost unchanged afferent arteriole resistance, and a higher glomerular plasma flow, indicating impaired renal autoregulation in hypertensive rats. SNGFR was similar in hypertensive and normotensive rats and, therefore, single nephron filtration fraction (SNFF) was lower in the former. Defective renal autoregulation may be responsible for natriuresis by allowing transmission of a higher haemodynamic pressure within vasa recta and, therefore, reducing Na^+ reabsorption in Henle's loop [1]. The lower SNFF may contribute to the greater Na^+ excretion in hypertensive rats by reducing peritubular oncotic pressure and hence passive reabsorption in the proximal tubule [10].

References

1   Dal Canton A, Conte G, Fuiano G. *Nephron 1981; 27:* 123
2   Raeder M, Omvik JR, Kiil F. *Am J Physiol 1974; 226:* 989
3   Di Bona GF, Rios LL. *Am J Physiol 1978; 235:* 409
4   Dal Canton A, Conte G, Esposito C. *Kidney Int 1982; 22:* 608
5   Andreucci VE. *Manual of Renal Micropuncture.* Napoli: Idelson. 1980
6   Dal Canton A, Stanziale R, Corradi A. *Kidney Int 1977; 12:* 403
7   Buggy J, Fisher AE. *Nature 1974; 250:* 14
8   Lichton IJ. *Am J Physiol 1961; 201:* 765
9   Atherton JC, Dark JM, Garland HO. *J Physiol 1982; 330:* 81
10   Brenner BM, Falchuk K, Keimowitz R. *J Clin Invest 1969; 48:* 1519

Open Discussion

ALLISON (Glasgow)   I think you have a very interesting model but it's very difficult to disentangle the cause and effect, as in all models of hypertension. You've presented evidence about glomerular plasma flow which I accept, but you haven't told us anything about the tubular handling of sodium and water by your hypertensive pregnant rats. I am sure you must have this information. One can't make the conclusions you've made without telling us about the tubular handling of sodium and you must have measured it.

DAL CANTON Yes, I agree with you but other studies are necessary to study proximal and distal tubular absorption. Urinary excretion of potassium was more elevated in hypertensive than in normotensive rats and this may indicate that the distal delivery of sodium was increased. A reduced sodium reabsorption in proximal tubule is suggested also by the fact that in hypertensive rats single nephron filtration fraction was lower than in normotensive rats. In fact, glomerular plasma flow was increased, as you see, but single nephron GFR was unchanged and therefore a reduced peri-tubular oncotic pressure may be the cause of a reduced reabsorption of sodium in the proximal tubule.

ALLISON So single nephron glomerular filtration was not different?

DAL CANTON No, it was not different.

ALLISON So you must therefore assume that these rats did not reach filtration equilibrium because otherwise it would be dependent on glomerular plasma flow?

DAL CANTON Yes.

VAN YPERSELE (Brussels) If I understand you correctly you have hyper-perfusion of your glomeruli, analogous to that described by Brenner*. Did you check protein excretion in these rats and was it elevated?

DAL CANTON Yes, I checked it both as an absolute value and as a ratio between protein and creatinine excretion and it was not different from the protein excretion in normotensive rats.

ZOCCALI (Reggio, Italy) In your model you induced hypertension by clipping the renal artery and as Dr Lever has shown today in renal artery stenosis sodium balance can be negative. Do you think that the results that you have got are simply the effect of the renal artery stenosis or the renal artery stenosis plus pregnancy?

DAL CANTON I remind you that even the control rats had renal artery stenosis. The normotensive rats were rats that were clipped but remained normotensive. The difference should be related to hypertension not to clipping. However, it may be that Goldblatt hypertension per se increases sodium excretion but in our hypertensive rats this increase may be even more elevated.

LEVER (Chairman) Yes, it might have been quite interesting to add a second control group of non-pregnant rats since there are differences in GFR, renal plasma flow and sodium balance between the pregnant and the non-pregnant rat. They are all in the direction that you have shown comparing the hypertensive with the normotensive. In other words increased GFR, increased renal plasma flow and a tendency, particularly at the early stages of hypertension, of the pregnant rat to become salt deplete.

* Brenner BM, Meyer TW, Mostetter TM. *N Engl J Med 1982; 30:* 307

DAL CANTON We have studied this problem*. In normal pregnant rats GFR is increased as well as the glomerular plasma flow and the degree of this increase is similar to our normotensive rats.

LEVER So you have got that control group already?

DAL CANTON Yes.

BIANCHI (Italy) It is known that angiotensin may stimulate sodium appetite. You have shown that you have a decrease in total body sodium so it is important also to evaluate angiotensin II in these different experimental situations. Angiotensin II by itself can produce changes both in sodium intake and urinary sodium excretion. Did you measure angiotensin or renin?

DAL CANTON I expected you to ask this question Dr Bianchi. We have measured plasma renin activity in some hypertensive and normotensive rats and it was similar. This doesn't mean that angiotensin II values were similar. Another possibility is that sensitivity to angiotensin was different in hypertensive from normtensive rats. However, we are now planning to study a group of rats drinking saline and water and so to be able to see any difference in salt preference between hypertensive and normotensive rats.

LEVER Are they given a choice of sodium or water to drink?

DAL CANTON No.

LEVER Could I ask if your rats are Sprague-Dawley or Wistar?

DAL CANTON Wistar, only Wistar rats with glomeruli or the kidney surface to enable us to measure glomerular capillary pressure.

* Dal Canton A, Conte G, Esposito C et al. *Kidney Int 1982; 22:* 608

Proc EDTA (1983) Vol 20

ERYTHROCYTE SODIUM-POTASSIUM CO-TRANSPORT IN HYPERTENSION

D de Zeeuw, J F Jilderda, T Tepper

State University Hospital, Gronigen, The Netherlands

Summary

This paper reports on the measurement of sodium-potassium co-transport across red cell membranes in patients with hypertension and in normotensive volunteers. No differences were found in flux values between these two groups. Antihypertensive medication such as propranolol and enalapril (converting enzyme inhibitor) had no unequivocal effect on the measured cation transport. Individual diurnal and day-to-day variation of fluxes appear to be substantial. It is concluded that uniformity in the assay procedure may be of great importance before studying any difference in cation transport between various populations.

Introduction

The measurement of cation fluxes across cell membranes has become a very popular topic ever since the first data was published on a relation between defective fluxes and essential hypertension (EH). Apart from the scientific value of gathering more data to gain insight into the causes of hypertension, the individual flux values were thought to be of diagnostic importance in discriminating secondary and essential hypertension. The data however became more and more confusing since various investigators found different values for mean cation fluxes in controls as well as in hypertensive patients. Part of these discrepancies could be due to the various modifications that have been made with respect to the assay method. In addition various investigators measure different cation transport mechanisms and in different cells.

We have investigated some of the parameters that could possibly account for these discrepancies. Therefore the sodium-potassium co-transport was studied in patients with EH and in controls. In addition the effect of antihypertensive medication (converting enzyme inhibition vs propranolol) on the fluxes was analysed, and the confidence limits of the gathered sodium-potassium co-transport values were tested.

Patients and methods

Sodium-potassium co-transport was determined in 38 normotensive volunteers (21 ♂; 17 ♀) and in 33 patients with documented EH (17 ♂, 16 ♀). The mean age of both groups was 35 ± 12 yr (range 21 to 62 yr) and 47 ± 8 yr (range 24 to 63 yr), respectively. None of the patients were overweight. Antihypertensive medication had been withdrawn for at least one month before study. Blood pressure of all subjects was measured at 9.00 a.m. after 10 min of supine rest, and blood samples were drawn subsequently. Twenty-two patients were evaluated again after being on antihypertensive medication for at least 12 weeks. Half of the patients had taken propranolol (ranging from 40 to 120mg twice daily), whereas the other 11 had taken the converting enzyme inhibitor enalapril (5 to 20mg twice daily).

All blood samples (10ml mixed with 0.1ml 10 per cent EDTA) were processed within two hours of collection. Red cells were washed with saline thrice. Then they were incubated for 16 hours at 4°C under gentle rotation at eight per cent haematocrit in a medium containing (mmol/L): 50NaCl, 3KCl, 1EGTA, 200 cholinechloride, $1.25Na_3PO_4$, $1MgCl_2$, $1.25Na_2HPO_4$ and 0.01PCMBS (4°C; pH: 7.2). Thus cells were loaded with an equimolar amount of sodium and potassium (35mmol/L cells). Recovery of the red cells was achieved by one hour incubation (37°C) at a haematocrit of 10 per cent in a medium containing (mmol/L): 150NaCl, $1MgCl_2$, $5Na_2HPO_4$, 1EGTA, 4 cysteine, three inosine, 2 adenine and 10 glucose (37°C; pH: 7.2). After washing the cells five times, they were diluted to a haematocrit of six per cent with medium containing (mmol/L): $75MgCl_2$, 85 sucrose, five glucose, 0.1 ouabain, 10MOPS, one frusemide and Tris was added to reach pH 7.2 (37°C). Samples for measurement of sodium and potassium by Flamephotometry were taken at 0.5, 1, 1.5 and two hours after starting the incubation (37°C). Co-transport of sodium as well as potassium, was calculated from the difference between the slopes of the two linear regression lines that could be derived from the successive concentrations of each cation both when frusemide was absent and present in the incubation medium. All solutions used were freshly prepared on the day of measurement.

Results

Mean blood pressure in the control subjects was 122/74 ± 14/11mmHg. The hypertensive group had a mean blood pressure of 164/106 ± 17/8mmHg. Of the 22 hypertensives that were followed after medication the first 11 had mean blood pressures of 155/104 ± 10/5 before and 141/91 ± 15/9mmHg after propranolol, whereas the 11 patients on enalapril were 168/109 ± 17/8 and 138/92 ± 12/7 mmHg respectively.

Figure 1 shows the individual values of the sodium-potassium co-transport. There appears to be no difference between controls and hypertensives.

Antihypertensive treatment had no consistent effect on cation co-transport: in the propranolol group mean sodium flux (μmol/L/h) was 441 ± 201 before and 376 ± 188 after therapy, the median change being −5 per cent (range +6 to −64%). The enalapril group also failed to show a significant change: 346 ± 163

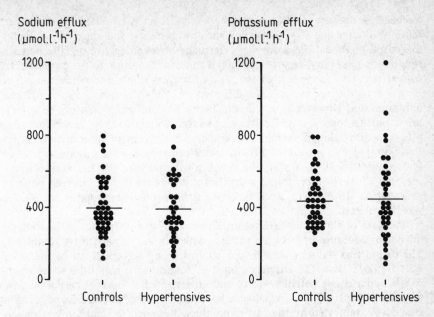

Figure 1.   Individual values of the sodium and potassium co-transport in normotensive
controls and patients with hypertension. The horizontal bars represent the mean values

before and 334 ± 144μmol/L/h after therapy, the median change was also −5 per cent with a range from +88 to −37 per cent. Potassium efflux measurements gave similar results including an even greater scatter in the percentage change.

To establish the confidence limits of this co-transport measurement the following tests were performed in six healthy normotensive volunteers: *Intra-assay* variation was measured as very low. Both for the sodium and potassium flux, the variation coefficient (VC) was less than three per cent in both the high and low range of cation fluxes. The VC within the cation fluxes of the same blood sample determined on two consecutive days was less than five per cent *(interassay)*. However when testing the *day-to-day* variation in the fluxes of an individual, the VC fluctuated from one to 37; in only two of the six subjects the VC of both sodium and potassium flux was less than seven per cent. In two of these volunteers co-transport was measured in blood samples taken at four different times in the day. Diurnal variation was six per cent in one subject and 22 per cent in the other. There was a tendency to lower fluxes towards the end of the day.

Discussion

A high systemic arterial blood pressure is a very common phenomenon in the western civilisation. The prevalence is estimated to be around 10–15 per cent. In 90 per cent of the subjects with high blood pressure no demonstrable cause will be found by means of the available diagnostic procedures. Thus, extensive

509

screening is needed to differentiate between EH and secondary hypertension. Since this screening has high costs and low benefits, and since the different diagnostic methods give a varying percentage of false negative or false positive results, the paper of Garay [1] promised an elegant solution to the problem. His data at that time, showed that the ratio of sodium efflux and potassium influx of the erythrocyte was able to differentiate 100 per cent between EH and normotension. However, since then a boom of conflicting data has been published on this topic. Some results point to the ouabain-sensitive cation flux [2], others to the sodium-potassium co-transport [3], or the lithium-sodium counter-transport [4] as a marker of EH. Whatever cell type or flux was studied, some investigators found no distinction between patients with EH and normotensive subjects, whereas others found a significant difference in flux between patients and controls. In the latter studies a considerable overlap between the two groups was still present.

The data of the present study furnish no proof of a difference in the sodium-potassium co-transport between patients with EH and normotensive volunteers. The cation flux values found in our control group agree with those found by others [5,6]. Thus, the difference must be found in the measured co-transport of the hypertensive patients. Garay and others [5] find a lower cation outflow whereas Adragna [7] reports a higher co-transport in the hypertensive population studied. As suggested by this last group these discrepancies could well be due to different sodium and potassium concentrations in the red cells used to assay the co-transport function. Apart from the method, it appears that other factors may well contribute to the differences such as: the selection of patients and control subjects, blood sampling, day-to-day variation, diurnal variations, dietary regimens, and medication. With respect to the selection of subjects it is difficult to assess any differences between the various studies. The previous antihypertensive medication and the time between withdrawal and assay might play a role. This was however, not confirmed by our data on the effects of propranolol and enalapril. We standardised blood sampling with respect to the position of the subject and the time of the day. The latter could be of importance since a diurnal variation in cation fluxes may well be present, according to our preliminary results. Furthermore, the substantial variation of the individual day-to-day flux values has to be taken into account in the evaluation of the flux differences between patients and controls. A dietary regimen such as a restricted sodium intake, which is often advised to a hypertensive patient, may interfere with the assay. In fact Edmondson [8] provided suggestive evidence for a positive correlation between plasma renin activity and (leucocyte) cation transport.

In conclusion, the results of the present study underline the need for a standardised experimental protocol when searching for differences in cation co-transport between hypertensives and controls. This was also suggested by Parker and Berkowitz in a recent review on this topic [9]. The observed individual diurnal and day-to-day variation of red cell cation transport may interfere with the assessment of a difference between groups of subjects. On the other hand, the observed variation might, after further study, lead to a better understanding of the factors that determine the activity of these transport mechanisms.

References

1   Garay RP, Meyer Ph. *Lancet 1979; i:* 349
2   Edmondson RPS, Thomas RD, Hilton PJ et al. *Lancet 1975; i:* 1003
3   Garay RP, Dagher G, Pernollet MG et al. *Nature 1980; 284:* 281
4   Canessa M, Adragna N, Solomon H et al. *N Engl J Med 1980; 302:* 772
5   Meyer Ph, Garay RP. *La Nouvell Presse Med 1982; 11:* 517
6   Swarts HGP, Bonting SL, Joep J et al. *Hypertension 1981; 6:* 641
7   Adragna N, Canessa M, Solomon H et al. *Hypertension 1982; 4:* 795
8   Edmondson RPS, MacGregor GA. *Br Med J 1981; 282:* 1267
9   Parker JC, Berkowitz LR. *Phys Reviews 1983; 63:* 285

Open Discussion

LEVER (Chairman)   It's my impression that what you have done now, and have still not completed, ought to have been done before anyone did any work whatsoever comparing normotensives and hypertensives. In other words there was no evidence on replicate variation, no studies of diurnal variation and no studies on the effects of previous drug treatment. The introduction of a new method without such ordinary regular checking of the method's validity before the first blast-off with normotensive and hypertensive data has to some extent obscured this potentially very important field. I think your paper is welcome and you are to be congratulated in producing, perhaps belatedly, things which ought to have been done a long time ago.

UNNAMED FROM HOLLAND   Did you check whether there is any relation between age and sodium efflux? If there is a relation between sodium efflux and age, the difference in age between the control group and the hypertensives may be critical.

de ZEEUW   Yes, you are quite right. We checked that, both in the normotensive population and also in the hypertensive subjects, and there is no correlation within the range of age that we have in our population, that is in people of approximately 20 to 60 years.

LEVER   How many patients did you put in that correlation?

de ZEEUW   There were 70 in both groups.

LEVER   The other possibility to consider, of course, is that it may not just be the age of the patient, it may be the age of the erythrocyte. A rapidly turning over population has a high proportion of young eager pumping erythrocytes which might have a rather different result than a population of rather subdued exhausted old erythrocytes. So survival of red cells may be important rather than any fundamental difference between cell transport in the two diseases.

de ZEEUW   I agree with you, I think that should also be checked but that doesn't explain that there is a diurnal variation.

LEVER Have all your hypertensives never been treated?

de ZEEUW Yes they were treated before but they were on at least four weeks of placebo therapy.

LEVER How do you know that hasn't affected them?

de ZEEUW This was in a multicentre study which we did with enalapril and so we had these regular checks every two weeks.

BIANCHI (Pisa) You put our group together with the people who found a lower co-transport, this is not correct because we observed that patients could have either a lower or higher co-transport compared to controls. The final results could well be that if you compare the averages of the controls and hypertensives you might come out with the similar values. Firstly can you give us some more detail about the technique you use? You mention that you overload the cells for 20 hours and then you measure the sodium efflux, but with what methods and what conditions?

de ZEEUW As you are probably aware if I gave a talk about the conditions in which I did the study I would be here for the next twenty minutes. I will suffice to say we use the same technique as Garay* described in his paper about measuring co-transport and we specially did this because the Paris group was one of the first groups to show this distinct difference between essential and secondary hypertension. We are well aware of the fact that after that a number of different techniques have been used, especially with respect to the loading of the erythrocytes for instance the group of Garraham and Rega† load their erythrocytes to about 60mmol internal sodium. This could well be the explanation for the fact that they find an increase instead of a decrease in sodium efflux.

BIANCHI Yes, I think this is very important for two reasons. First, are you sure that the variation during the day was mainly on sodium efflux while the potassium efflux was the same? By definition this is not co-transport but is something that selectively affects sodium but not potassium. The second point is you may have a 300 per cent change with menstrual cycle, and this should be taken into account in your interassay variations.

de ZEEUW I don't agree with you. I think that this even stresses the fact that measuring the co-transport in two populations without any restrictions is a bad thing to do. The six individuals, the normotensive volunteers, in which I measured the day-to-day variation in the urine were all male, in fact one of them was me.

SALTISSI (London) I wonder with the recognition of parathyroid hormone as a Na^+-K^+ ATPase inhibitor have you looked at the diurnal variation of Na^+-K^+

*Garay RP, Meyer Ph. *Lancet 1979; i:* 349
†Garraham P, Rega A. *J Physiol 1967; 193:* 459

512

co-transport in relation to parathyroid hormone or other diurnally varying hormones, particularly cortisol?

de ZEEUW We did not look at PTH but we did look at renin as was also published by Edmundson* and he found that renin was related to the ouabain sensitive sodium efflux. We measured renin in these subjects but we didn't find correlation with that.

* Edmundson RPS, MacGregor GA. *Br Med J 1981; 282:* 1267

Proc EDTA (1983) Vol 20

EFFECTS OF HAEMODIALYSIS ON ACTIVE AND INACTIVE RENIN IN NEPHRIC AND ANEPHRIC PATIENTS

F Vendemia, A Morganti*, A Scalia, C Sala*, L Turolo*, G D'Amico

*Ospedale S Carlo and Istituto Clinica Medica IV, Università di Milano, *Centro di Fisologia Clinica e Ipertensione, Ospedale Maggiore, Milano, Italy*

Summary

To investigate the origin, the mechanisms of regulation and the possible biological significance of inactive renin we examined the effects of haemodialysis on plasma active and inactive (cryoactivatable) renin in four anephric and in 10 nephric patients. Before haemodialysis inactive renin was similar in anephric and in the majority of nephric patients; this suggests that the source of the inactive enzyme is predominantly extrarenal. In response to haemodialysis active renin rose significantly in nephric patients whereas inactive renin showed minor and inconsistent increments in both groups. These results indicate that the response of the inactive enzyme to haemodialysis is less than that of its active counterpart and is unaffected by the presence of the kidneys. Therefore, it appears unlikely that inactive renin represents a circulating precursor of active renin.

Introduction

Plasma of man and of several animal species contains a renin-like enzyme whose ability to generate angiotensin can be revealed, in vitro, by several activating manipulations such as exposure to acid dialysis, low temperature or proteolytic enzymes [1,2]. The origin, the mechanisms of regulation and the biological significance of this so-called inactive renin are still undefined [3]. As to the site of origin, the observation that inactive renin is present also in plasma of anephric subjects [4] implies an extrarenal source of production. In animals renin-like enzymes have been identified in vascular tissue, uterus, brain and submaxillary glands; whether and to what extent these organs contribute to the maintenance of circulating inactive renin in man is unknown. As to the mechanisms of regulation it has been shown that during acute and chronic manoeuvres which affect the renin system, inactive renin may change in the same or opposite direction of active renin or remain unchanged [2]. Reciprocal changes of the two forms of the enzyme have been interpreted as the result of the possible conversion of one

514

into the other [5]; yet, clear evidence of such a transformation has not been demonstrated [3].

In the attempt to shed light on some of these issues, we examined whether and how haemodialysis, a well known stimulus for active renin, affects circulating inactive renin in nephric and anephric patients. The latter group are of particular interest as they lack the organ where part of the production and the conversion of inactive renin supposedly take place.

Methods

Fourteen ambulatory patients on chronic haemodialysis (EDTA stage 1–2) were studied; four of them had been bilaterally nephrectomised at least six years previously. None had previous kidney transplantation nor was on anti-hypertensive or steroid medication. Throughout the period of the study they were on their usual diet containing approximately 150mEq NaCl.

On the day of the study, after resting supine for one hour, the patients were weighed; thereafter three sphygmomanometric blood pressure and heart rate readings were recorded and blood samples for measurement of active and inactive renin, electrolytes and serum protein concentration were collected from the dialysis arterial line. A standardised haemodialysis was then initiated: filter $1m^2$, Q_B 320ml/min, ultrafiltration rate 500ml/hr, Q_D single pass 500ml/min, and dialysate Na^+ and K^+ concentrations 142 and 2mEq/L respectively. Dialysis proceeded for four hours with the patient remaining supine; during this time body weight, blood pressure and heart rate were recorded every 60 minutes. Immediately prior to the end of the procedure these variables were again recorded and blood samples were collected as before haemodialysis. For each patient these studies were repeated during three consecutive haemodialyses and the data obtained averaged.

Plasma renin activity was measured by radioimmunoassay according to Sealey et al [6]; in our laboratory the precision and the interassay reproducibility of this method are five per cent and 11 per cent respectively. To activate inactive renin one millilitre samples of plasma were incubated at $-5°C$ and pH 7.4 in a constant temperature shaking bath. After four days of exposure to cold samples were immediately processed. Plasma renin activity after cryo-activation (total renin) was measured by the same procedure as active renin; the precision and interassay variability for total renin is eight per cent and 12 per cent respectively. Inactive (cryoactivatable) renin is defined as the difference between total and active renin.

Statistical comparisons were made by Student's t test for paired and unpaired data, a value of p=0.05 being taken as the lowest level of significance. Correlation coefficients were calculated with the Pearson test.

Results

Table I summarises our results. Anephric patients were younger and had lower mean blood pressure than nephric patients (p<0.05 and 0.01 respectively); also, they had been on dialysis, on average, for a longer period of time.

TABLE I. Individual clinical and humoral data pre- and post-haemodialysis in nephric and anephric patients

Patients	Sex	Age (years)	Diagnosis	Duration haemodialysis (years)	MAP (mmHg)		Active renin (ng/ml/hr)		Inactive renin (ng/ml/hr)		ΔHR (b/min)	ΔWg (kg)	ΔK⁺ (mEq/L)
					Pre	Post	Pre	Post	Pre	Post			
Anephric													
ML	F	41	MHT	11	71	57	0.2	0.1	1.4	1.6	+ 7	-2.1	-4.1
CE	M	36	MHT	6	91	90	0.1	0.1	3.6	3.8	+ 8	-2.2	-1.8
MM	F	29	CGN	14	91	89	0.4	0.2	3.6	4.9	+ 7	-2.3	-2.4
RS	M	39	CGN	13	87	83	0.2	0.2	3.0	3.2	+10	-2.0	-1.5
X̄		36.2		11	85	80	0.2	0.2	2.9	3.4	+9.0	-2.2	-2.4
± SEM		±2.6		±1.8	±9	±15	±0.1	±0.1	±1.0	±1.4	±2.6	±0.1	±1.2
Nephric													
GG	F	69	PKD	10	119	124	0.1	0.1	1.2	1.4	+10	-1.3	-1.4
PA	M	54	PKD	7	94	89	0.7	1.2	1.2	1.2	- 2	-2.3	-1.4
MG	M	44	CGN	13	116	110	2.0	2.2	2.2	2.7	+ 8	-1.9	-2.7
VM	M	44	CGN	10	120	115	0.2	0.3	1.4	2.3	+10	-2.5	-1.3
GG	F	59	CPN	3	107	74	4.9	9.1	34.9	34.7	+ 3	-1.9	-1.0
MR	M	61	PKD	9	101	78	0.5	0.9	1.5	1.7	+28	-1.9	-1.9
RD	M	31	CGN	6	110	114	3.4	9.3	4.1	5.5	+ 3	-2.7	-2.5
VL	M	74	NAS	6	139	135	6.2	9.9	39.0	37.1	+14	-1.6	-1.8
GA	F	51	CGN	5	122	101	4.3	8.9	28.8	30.9	+10	-1.9	-1.5
GE	F	47	CGN	5	89	78	5.5	8.1	6.2	6.9	+ 8	-2.1	-1.7
X̄		53.4		7.4	112	102	2.8	5.0	12.0	12.4	+ 9	-2.0	-1.7
± SEM		±4.1		±1.0	±5	±1	±0.8	±1.4	±4.9	±4.8	±5.6	±0.1	±0.2

Abbreviations: MAP= mean arterial pressure; HR=heart rate; Wg=weight; K⁺=serum potassium; CGN=chronic glomerulonephritis; MHT=malignant hypertension; PKD=polycystic kidney disease; CPN=chronic pyelonephritis; NAS=nephroangiosclerosis

516

Before dialysis active renin varied, among nephric patients, from almost undetectable, comparable to those seen in the anephrics, to rather high values; these individual differences could be attributed to the duration and/or the nature of the underlying kidney disease. Inactive renin was higher in nephric patients, as a group, than in the anephrics; however, it is apparent that this difference was due to three subjects (GG, VL and GA) who had exceedingly high values. Since there were no obvious clinical reasons to explain this discrepancy these three patients have been restudied six months later and the data presented herein were confirmed. With the exclusion of these three subjects inactive renin was similar in the two groups (2.9 ± 1.0 vs 2.5 ± 0.7ng/ml/hr). There was a positive correlation between active and inactive renin ($r=0.77$, $p<0.01$) within the nephric patients.

Dialysis lowered blood pressure, body weight and serum potassium and increased heart rate almost to the same extent in the two groups; these changes were all significant ($p<0.05$ at least with the exception of those in blood pressure). Serum protein concentration rose by 11.8 per cent and by 16.4 per cent respectively in the anephric and nephric patients.

In response to these stimuli active renin remained, as expected, unchanged in the anephrics whereas increased in all but one of the nephrics; in these patients the mean percent increment in active renin, with respect to baseline values, was 68.5 per cent, the individual increments being correlated to pre-dialysis values ($r=0.78$, $p<0.01$) but not with the changes in weight, blood pressure, heart rate and potassium. In contrast, inactive renin had slight increments in the anephrics and was practically unchanged in the nephrics; even expressed as percent of baseline values the variations (+15% and +16% respectively) were lower ($p<0.05$ at least) than those of active renin in the nephric patients. It is of interest that inactive renin was practically unchanged also in those three subjects who had very high values before dialysis.

Discussion

Two relevant findings emerge from this study; first, cryoactivated renin was similar in anephric patients and in the majority of nephric patients. Since comparable concentrations of cryoactivated renin were found by ourselves and others in healthy subjects and in patients with essential hypertension and normal renal function [4,7], it appears that circulating inactive renin originates predominantly from extrarenal sources and that its secretion is not influenced by chronic renal failure 'per se'. Second, active renin clearly increased in response to haemodialysis in nephric patients whereas inactive renin was virtually unchanged in both groups of patients. Actually, in several subjects cryoactivated renin showed a tendency to increase; however, it must be appreciated that such minimal changes may well be due to the variability implicit in the method of measurement and/or to the haemodialysis induced haemoconcentration rather than to a real increase in secretion. Thus, the response, if any, of inactive renin to haemodialysis was smaller than that of its active counterpart and was unaffected by the presence of the kidneys, the organs where its conversion possibly occurs. Therefore, it seems unlikely that the inactive enzyme may represent a circulating precursor of the active form.

517

References

1 Overturf ML, Druilhet RE, Kirkendall WM. *Life Science 1979; 24:* 1913
2 Sealey JE, Atlas SA, Laragh JH. *Endocrinol Rev 1980; 1:* 365
3 Haber E, Carlson W. *Clin Exper Hypert 1982; A4(11–12):* 1995
4 Sealey JE, Moon C, Laragh JH, Atlas SA. *Circ Res 1977; 40 (Suppl I):* 41
5 Derkx FHM, Wenting GJ, Man In'T Veld AJ et al. *Clin Sci 1979; 56:* 115
6 Sealey JE, Laragh JH. *Cardiovasc Med 1977; 2:* 1079
7 Morganti A, Sala C, Turolo L, Zanchetti A. *Clin Exper Hypert 1982; A4(11–12):* 2403

Open Discussion

LEVER (Chairman) Why do you think inactive renin as a proportion of total renin is higher in the plasma of an anephric patient? The proportion of total renin which is inactive is much higher in anephrics and that is not entirely due to a decrease of active renin, it is an increase of inactive renin, why is that increase of inactive renin present?

MORGANTI (Milan) If I may answer, being a co-author with Dr Vendemia, your question about whether or not, in anephric patients, the levels of inactive renin are higher than in nephric patients, I must say that in our experience, as you have seen from our slide, inactive renin in anephric patients is not higher than in nephric patients.

KOKOT (Katowice, Poland) The reaction pattern of plasma renin activity to fluid loss in anephric patients is dependent upon the residual renal function. Could you tell us something about residual renal function of your nephric patients?

VENDEMIA These patients had all been on regular dialysis treatment for about 10 years, so that the kidney function was almost zero.

DAL CANTON (Naples) Since your patients had strikingly damaged kidneys, are the absolute values of inactive renin in your patients similar to those of patients with normal renal function?

VENDEMIA Yes, in another series of hypertensive and normotensive patients with normal renal function, the mean values were almost the same, about 2–3ng/ml/hr.

DRUKKER (Jerusalem, Israel) During dialysis some of your patients showed a rise in active plasma renin activity, especially those who had a high renin to start with. Now you showed, for the whole group, that heart rate went up and blood pressure fell. What happened in only those patients in whom renin increased, what happened to their blood pressure and heart rate?

VENDEMIA   In our patients the blood pressure during haemodialysis remained almost the same; there is a decrease but it was very small. In response to this small decrease in blood pressure we had a small increase in heart rate, regardless of the difference in renin. Perhaps this is because we had a high dialysate sodium and we standardised the ultrafiltration rate to 500ml per hour.

LEVER   I wonder if behind that last question lay the observation that over a long course of regular dialysis treatment, not just over the single act of dialysis, those patients in whom renin goes up tend to have a rise of blood pressure and develop the intractable hypertensive state?

VENDEMIA   No, all our patients were normotensive before and after dialysis.

Proc EDTA (1983) Vol 20

PLASMA RENIN ACTIVITY, BLOOD URIC ACID AND PLASMA VOLUME IN PREGNANCY-INDUCED HYPERTENSION

P Fievet, L Pleskov, I Desailly*, A Carayon†, J-F de Fremont,
B Coevoet, E Comoy‡, J E Demory§, P Verhoest§, J C Boulanger§,
A Fournier

Service de Néphrologie, CHU Amiens, *Laboratoire de Biochimie, CHU Amiens, †Laboratoire de Biochimie, CHU Pitié, Paris, ‡Laboratoire de Biochimie, Institut Gustave Roussy, Villejuif, and §Service de Gynécologie-Obstétrique, CHU Amiens, France

Summary

Plasma renin activity (PRA), plasma aldosterone (PA), blood uric acid (BUA), plasma concentrations of catecholamines (Pcat) and plasma volume (PV) were measured simultaneously in 24 patients with pregnancy-induced hypertension (PIH). This hypertensive group was divided into labile (LH) and persistent hypertension (PH) groups according to the response of their blood pressure to home bed rest. Compared to normal theoretical values, PV was decreased in both hypertensive groups (LH = -7%; PH = -14%). Compared to a control group (C) of 16 normotensive pregnant women, PRA was higher in LH and lower in PH whereas PA was lower in both hypertensive groups. BUA was higher than in C in both hypertensive groups. No difference in PCat was found between the three groups. In the PH group negative correlations were found between BUA and PRA, as well as between BUA and PV but no correlation between PRA and PV nor between Pcat and BUA were found.

In conclusion:

1. LH and PH are two pathophysiologically different entities in PIH.

2. In PH renin secretion is not appropriate to hypovolaemia and therefore not primarily involved in the pathogenesis of hypertension.

3. Hypovolaemia may play a role in the increase of BUA in PIH.

Introduction

Normal pregnancy is characterised by a plasma volume expansion and a stimulation of the renin-angiotensin-aldosterone system. During pregnancy-induced hypertension, plasma volume contraction has been demonstrated [1]. The results of studies on the renin-angiotensin-aldosterone system are controversial. Compared with normal pregnancy, some authors describe a stimulation of the system [2], others no difference [3], but the majority describe an inhibition [4]. There are few studies of plasma volume, blood uric acid and the renin-angiotensin-aldosterone system during pregnancy-induced hypertension. We report the results of such a study.

Patients and methods

Twenty-four hypertensive pregnant women have been studied and compared with 16 normotensive pregnant women. Hypertension was detected in the obstetric outpatient clinic by finding a blood pressure greater than 140/90mmHg, twice after 10 and 20 minutes sitting at rest. In the hypertensive group, hypertension was discovered after 20 weeks and all were normotensive before pregnancy and two months after delivery. The hypertensive women were studied in the nephrological outpatient clinic as soon as possible after the discovery of hypertension, according to the same protocol as the normotensive controls:

No patients had received drugs for at least one month;

All were ambulatory on a normal salt diet (confirmed by urinary sodium excretion and lack of weight loss since first examination for hypertension;

All arrived, fasting, between 8–10a.m., with a 24 hour urine collection and were weighed;

A venous catheter was inserted into an antecubital vein, the patient being in the supine position;

Blood pressure was measured after 30 minutes of rest in the lying position and then the blood samples were taken.

We distinguished two groups of hypertensive pregnant women according to the outcome of blood pressure after home bed rest has been prescribed:

1. The persistent hypertensive group consisted of 17 pregnant women who were found hypertensive not only in the obstetrical outpatient clinic but also, at least once, in the nephrological outpatient clinic.

2. The labile hypertensive group consisted of seven patients who were found hypertensive in the obstetrical outpatient clinic but who were not hypertensive in the nephrological outpatient clinic.

There is no difference between the persistent hypertensive group, the labile hypertensive group and the control group as regards age (respectively 27.2 ± 1, 25.4 ± 0.4, 28 ± 1 years), parity ratio (respectively 9/8, 3/4, 9/7 primigravida/multigravida), duration of pregnancy (respectively 31.5 ± 1.7, 31.2 ± 2.2, 31 ± 1.6 weeks), weight gain during pregnancy (respectively 12.5 ± 4.7, 9.4 ± 1.4, 10 ± 1.1kg) and natriuresis (respectively <12.2 ± 0.7, 10.2 ± 2.3, 13.3 ± 1.1, ratio of sodium excretion to creatinine excretion). The weight before pregnancy was significantly higher in the persistent hypertensive group than the control group (71.9 ± 3.7 versus 55.3 ± 2.4kg p<0.01). Mean arterial pressure is significantly higher at the first obstetrical examination in the persistent hypertension group and labile hypertensive group than in control group (respectively 116.1 ± 2.1, 111.6 ± 1.7 and 88 ± 3mm of Hg, p<0.01).

Methods

Blood samples handling

The blood samples for plasma renin activity (PRA) and aldosterone were taken into EDTA vacutainers put into ice and were centrifuged at 4°C within 30 minutes and then stored at −30°C, so that little cryoactivation could be expected. The samples for catecholamine measurement were taken into heparinised vacutainers and handled in the same way. The measurements were all made within three months so that deterioration of the samples was unlikely.

Analytical methods [6]

PRA was determined by the radioimmunoassay of angiotensin I; plasma aldosterone by radioimmunoassay; plasma catecholamines, epinephrine and norepinephrine by the radioenzymatic method of Da Prada; blood uric acid was measured by the method of Folin.

Plasma volume was determined by the Evan's Blue dilution method. Once the first blood sample was taken, 10cc of a solution containing 25mg of Evan's Blue was injected through the venous catheter. The patient was placed in left lateral lying position. Ten minutes later, a second blood sample was taken from the opposite arm. Concentration of Evan's Blue was determined by spectrophotometric method. The results have been expressed in percentage of normal theoretical values determined by Smith and Yarbrough [5], according to body surface and duration of pregnancy.

Statistical method

Comparisons of the groups were made using the Wilcoxon's test for non-paired data. Linear correlations were calculated with a small computer TI-55-II.

Results

The mean (± SEM) values of the various parameters observed in the three groups are summarised in Table I.

Plasma renin activity was significantly lower in the persistent hypertensive group than in control group and labile hypertensive group. Plasma renin activity was significantly higher in labile hypertensive group than in control group and persistent hypertensive group.

Plasma aldosterone values were significantly lower in the persistent hypertensive group and labile hypertensive group than in control groups (respectively 218 ± 52, 271 ± 58 and 533 ± 52pg/ml).

TABLE I. Biological data

Patients groups	Renin activity (ng/ml/h)	Plasma concentrations of				Uric acid (μmol/L)	Ratio Natriuresis/ Creatininuria (mmol/mmol)
		Aldosterone (pg/ml)	Epinephrine (pg/ml)	Norepinephrine (pg/ml)			
Non-pregnant control (NPC) (normal range)	0.7 – 3	120 – 180	10 – 100	100 – 350		180 – 420	
Pregnant control (PC) n = 16	6.7 ± 0.5	533 ± 52	56 ± 13	206 ± 32		240 ± 18	13.3 ± 1.1
Persistent hypertensive group (PH) n = 17	4.7 ± 0.3	218 ± 52	55.5 ± 11.3	292 ± 51		302 ± 16	12.2 ± 0.7
Labile hypertension group (LH) n = 7	12.2 ± 0.8	271 ± 58	83 ± 39.3	289 ± 57		298 ± 9	10.2 ± 2.3
Comparison significance							
PH vs PC	p<0.01	p<0.01	NS	NS		p<0.01	NS
LH vs PC	p<0.01	p<0.01	NS	NS		p<0.01	NS
PH vs LH	p<0.01	NS	NS	NS		NS	NS

523

There was no significant difference for plasma epinephrine and norepinephrine in the three groups.

Blood uric acid was significantly higher in the persistent hypertensive group and in labile hypertensive group than in control group (respectively 302 ± 16, 298 ± 9 and 240 ± 18μmol/L). There was no significant difference between the two hypertensive groups for their blood uric acid.

Plasma volume was decreased in the persistent hypertensive group and the labile hypertensive group (respectively –14.6 ± 3.2% and 7.2 ± 2.6%) compared to that of normal pregnancy. The difference between the two hypertensive groups however was not significant.

Linear correlation studies

There was a negative correlation between blood uric acid and plasma renin activity in the persistent hypertensive group (n = 17, r = 0.596, p<0.05), (Figure 1).

Plasma volume and blood uric acid were negatively correlated when all the hypertensive patients are considered (n = 22, r = 0.691, p<0.001) or when only the 17 patients with persistent hypertension are considered (n = 17, r = 0.695, p<0.01), (Figure 2).

There was no significant correlation between plasma renin activity and plasma volume.

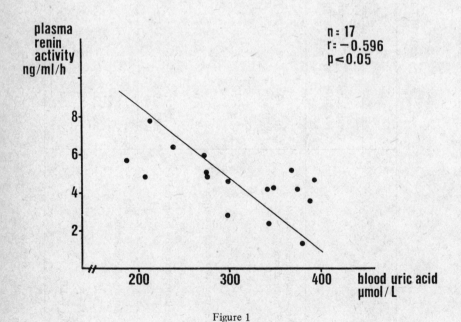

Figure 1

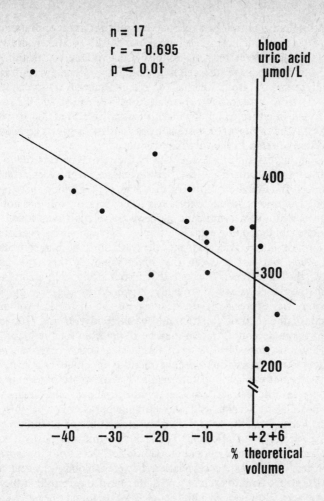

n = 17
r = − 0.695
p < 0.01

Figure 2

Discussion

Two kinds of pregnancy-induced hypertension were distinguished according to the response of blood pressure to home bed rest, the persistent hypertensive group and the labile hypertensive group. The persistent hypertensive group had a lower PRA than control patients whereas the labile hypertensive group had higher PRA than controls. These differences of PRA in the various hypertensive and control groups have already been found in a previous study [6], and cannot be explained by differences in clinical details, salt intake or plasma volume.

In both hypertensive groups, plasma volume has been found reduced compared to normal theoretical values, in agreement with the study of Gallery et al showing that plasma volume is contracted in hypertension induced by pregnancy [1]. In our study, this finding cannot be explained by salt restriction or diuretic therapy, since all patients had a normal salt intake and had not taken drugs for one month. In the labile hypertension group, plasma volume contraction is associated with a stimulation of the renin angiotensin system. In contrast, in the persistent hypertensive group, plasma volume contraction is associated with an inhibition of renin secretion. No correlation between PRA and plasma volume could be found in either group. The lack of negative correlation between PRA and volume in the group of persistent hypertension, suggests a maladaptation of the secretion of renin to the volaemic stimulus.

There is an increase in blood uric acid in the two hypertensive groups compared with control pregnant patients. Hypertensive pregnancies are associated with a reduced fractional excretion of uric acid [7] of which there is no good explanation. The role of lactate excess has been advocated but has not yet been proved. In our study, a significant negative correlation was found between plasma volume and blood uric acid. Beufils et al [7] found a correlation between the variations of blood uric acid and the variations of plasma volume in a sequential study but not between the direct values of these two parameters measured at the same time. The fact that in our study such a correlation was found with the direct values is probably explained by the way by which the plasma volume was expressed (the percentage of the theoretical volume) which is a function of the term of gestation and of the body surface. This correlation suggests that volume concentration may be responsible for the blood uric acid increase. However, since Beaufils et al found a reduction of plasma volume in intrauterine growth retardation without increase of blood uric acid, hypovolaemia per se cannot explain hyperuricaemia. The existence of a common factor which is able to reduce fractional excretion of uric acid and plasma volume is therefore postulated. Angiotensin and norepinephrine may be this common factor since Ferris et al [8] have shown that they both could induce a decrease of fractional excretion of uric acid. The lack of significant positive correlation between plasma norepinephrine and blood uric acid does not support the role of norepinephrine. The negative correlation between blood uric acid and PRA would at first glance tend to exclude a possible role of angiotensin in the elevation of blood uric acid. However, Symonds et al [9] have found a negative correlation between plasma renin activity and plasma concentrations of angiotensin II in pregnancy-induced hypertension, with higher concentrations of angiotensin II than in normotensive pregnant women, suggesting therefore a possible positive correlation of blood uric acid and angiotensin II. The discrepancy between high plasma concentrations of angiotensin II and low PRA may be explained by the release of angiotensin-like substance such as those reported to be released when uterine blood flow is reduced in pregnant dogs [10].

References

1 Gallery EDM, Hunyor SN, Gyory AZ. *Q J Med 1979; 192:* 593
2 Annat G, Raudrant D, Chappe J et al. *Obstet Gynecol 1978; 52:* 219
3 Gallery EDM, Stokes GS, Gyory AZ et al. *Clin Sci 1980; 59:* 49

4   Weir RJ, Doig A, Fraser R et al. In Lindheimer MD, Katz AJ, Zuspan FP, eds. *Hypertension in Pregnancy.* New York: John Wiley. 1976: 251–261
5   Smith RW, Yarbrough CJ. *Am J Obstet Gynecol 1967; 99:* 18
6   Fievet P, Coevoet B, Andrejak M et al. *Eur Heart J 1982; 3:* 33
7   Beaufils M, Uzan S, Don Simoni R et al. In Eisenbach GM, Brod J, eds. *Kidney and Pregnancy.* Basel: Karger. 1980: 132–136
8   Ferris TF, Gorden P. *Am J Med 1968; 44:* 359
9   Symonds EM, Broughton Pipkin F, Craven DJ. *Br J Obstet Gynecol 1975; 82:* 643
10 Bell C. *Am J Obstet Gynecol 1973; 117:* 1088

Open Discussion

MANN (Heidelberg) Plasma volume was not measured in controls, but derived from data on a different population, which may slightly invalidate the findings.

FOURNIER We did not measure plasma volumes in controls because of ethical difficulties so we used the published data of Yarbrough*.

MANN Were these also derived from the Evans blue dilution technique?

FOURNIER Yes, of course we used data derived from the same technique as that used in our study.

DAL CANTON (Naples) I would like to emphasise that your results in women are in full agreement with our results in rats. You have found hypovolaemia and this may well have been caused by a greater natriuresis until a new steady state had been obtained. You would not see this because your women were in a steady state and they had a similar sodium excretion as normotensive patients. In your opinion is this hypovolaemia related to the higher incidence of toxaemia induced by hypertension in pregnancy?

FOURNIER You're asking me if the hypovolaemia is just a consequence of the increase in blood pressure?

DAL CANTON Yes, I mean the hypovolaemia may be a cause of toxaemia.

FOURNIER Well it's difficult to say from my data as we have no sequential data up to now. You may think that hypovolaemia, by stimulating some vaso-constricting factors, may induce the hypertension with hypovolaemia, but I have no data on that.

LEVER (Chairman) Are you asking whether there are not two different forms of hypertension but one which may be the precursor of the other, is that what you are saying?

* Smith RW, Yarbrough CJ. *Am J Obstet Gynecol 1967; 99:* 18

527

DAL CANTON No, in my opinion there might be this sequence of events; greater natriuresis in essential hypertensive women with hypovolaemia lowering uterine perfusion, producing uterine ischaemia and consequently toxaemia.

KLEINKNECHT (Paris) According to your results and data in the literature, do you recommend volume expansion in hypertensive pregnant women, and if so what will be the expected benefit especially for the fetus?

FOURNIER That's a very difficult question to give a good practical answer, because we do not have the data. I think the first thing to do would be to cautiously expand as much as possible the blood volume. In a situation where the vessels are vasoconstricted you may induce pulmonary oedema when you induce plasma expansion. In our experience this has been done, not by us but in other obstetrical clinics and we have had three cases of toxaemia with convulsion and two with pulmonary oedema and when we made a haemodynamic study we had an increase in pulmonary artery wedge pressure. I would caution about the use of plasma expansion in women with hypertension.

BIANCHI (Pisa) We have seen recently a positive correlation between serum uric acid and sodium lithium counter transport. As you know, serum uric acid is reabsorbed mainly in proximal tubules by a mechanism that is essentially similar to this type of counter transport mechanism. A suggestion that might explain your data could be that there is an increase in sodium excretion because of a defect in autoregulation and then a secondary increase in proximal tubular reabsorption in an attempt to counteract this effect, without succeeding because the final result is decrease in plasma volume. This increase in proximal tubular absorption per se may lead to an increase in serum uric acid. In this way you may explain both the negative correlation between the serum uric acid and plasma volume and the data relating to serum uric acid and proximal tubular reabsorption. It is just a suggestion.

DORHOUT MEES (Utrecht, The Netherlands) There was a striking discrepancy between your aldosterone and plasma renin. Could that be related to a decrease in progesterone which is known to have an anti-aldosterone action?

FOURNIER Yes, we have measured progesterone but there was no signficiant difference in the group.

PEDERSEN (Åarhus, Denmark) Do you think there is a problem in using plasma renin activity in evaluating the renin aldosterone system? I think there is a problem because the renin substrate is increased during pregnancy and your method is dependent on the substrate concentration. I think it would have been better to use plasma renin concentration or plasma angiotensin II for evaluating the system.

FOURNIER I think there has been a study which showed that the increase in substrate was the same in the control and in hypertensive patients, we have not measured substrate.

EL MATRI (Tunis, Tunisia) Please can you give further information about your cases? Were they only pregnancy-induced hypertension or hypertension with underlying glomerulonephritis?

FOURNIER None had proteinuria two months after delivery and only three of the 24 had proteinuria. The patients had pregnancy-induced hypertension.

EL MATRI In your cases you had low renin, had they been treated with beta-blockers?

FOURNIER No, they were all without treatment when we measured these parameters. They had never been treated.

EL MATRI In that case do you advise not treating patients with low plasma renin by beta-blockers?

FOURNIER The point is that beta-blockers act on hypertension not only by decreasing plasma renin. There is clinical data from an English group showing that atenolol, and also data from Glasgow with labetalol, showing that it is good for the pregnant woman and the fetus.

SEVERE SIDE-EFFECTS OF CAPTOPRIL IN ADVANCED CHRONIC KIDNEY INSUFFICIENCY

V Beroniade

Faculté de Médecine Université de Montréal et Hôtel-Dieu de Montréal, Québec, Canada

Summary

Using equal or lower than manufacturer's recommended doses of Captopril in 10 hypertensive patients with creatinine clearance less than 30ml/min severe side-effects were observed in four cases. The adverse reactions continued after stopping the drug. One case developed symptomatic thrombocytopenia; one other, a lethal infected exfoliative dermatitis and an irreversible deterioration of her renal function. The other two cases demonstrated severe aggravation of their CRF, one requiring dialysis. The protective effect of dialysis against these side-effects is obvious in this series and dialysis may also accelerate the resolution of the complications. Suggestions for the management of this kind of patient with Captopril are made.

Introduction

Captropril (Capoten®, Squibb) is the only orally effective converting enzyme inhibitor available on the North American market and has proved an extremely potent antihypertensive drug, succeeding in controlling resistant hypertension, especially those types mediated by the renin-angiotensin system [1]. It is mainly eliminated by the kidney with an elimination rate constant which closely parallels the endogenous creatinine clearance (C_{cr}) [2]. Guidelines for adjusting the dose interval in patients with chronic renal failure (CRF) have been suggested [1]. Theoretically, similar plasma concentrations can be obtained by proportionately decreasing the individual Captopril dose [2].

A rather high incidence of troublesome, or even serious side-effects have been associated with Captopril. There is a general impression [see 1, pages 438—439] that the incidence of adverse effects is significantly lower if patients with renal dysfunction are excluded from statistical studies.

The present paper confirms the impression that advanced CRF patients are particularly prone to develop severe side-effects to Captopril and discusses the alterations of dosage in this category of patients.

Material and methods

Ten patients with advanced CRF ($C_{cr} \leqslant 30ml/min$) of different causes have been treated with Captopril in the last year. Two of them were on chronic haemodialysis when Captopril was started: a third patient was on acute peritoneal dialysis for a probable acute interstitial nephritis, presumably secondary to chlorthalidone.

The dosage of Captopril varied between 12.5mg every 48 hours to 25mg b.d., with the exception of one patient who required a dose of 50mg t.i.d. for good hypertension control. In half the cases, including the three being dialysed, all other antihypertensive drugs could be stopped, either before or immediately following the introduction of Captopril.

In the remaining five patients, three also received adjusted doses of frusemide, while the other two needed in addition a beta-blocker or clonidine. During the admission period, the blood pressure was measured regularly in supine and upright positions every half-hour for the first interval of two hours following the administration of Captopril, and subsequently every two hours. Plasma creatinine (P_{cr}), urea, Na, K, liver function tests, Hb, white cell count and urinalysis were checked at least every other day.

During the initial outpatient period the same tests were performed at ten day intervals for one month and then at longer intervals, depending on the degree of blood pressure control on each patient.

TABLE I. Description of cases which presented major side-effects

Patient number	Age	Sex	Diagnostic
1	46	M	Repeated acute pulmonary oedema. Severe, resistant, renovascular hypertension (frusemide, minoxidil, clonidine, metoprolol, hydralazine, methyldopa). CRF ($P_{cr} = 360\mu mol/ml$, $C_{cr} = 10.3ml/min$). Nephrotic syndrome of unknown aetiology (proteinuria = 1.5–2.7g/day). Complex haematological disorder: haemolytic anaemia, thrombocytopenia (80–94,000/μl), circulating anticoagulant, Raynaud syndrome. Autopsy (five months later): bilateral renal artery stenosis, nephrosclerosis. No aetiology found for the nephrotic syndrome and the haematological disorder.
2	69	F	Acute pulmonary oedema. Severe, resistant hypertension (pindolol, chlorthalidone, nipride, frusemide, clonidine methyldopa). CRF ($P_{cr} = 202\mu mol/ml$, $C_{cr} = 29ml/min$) with recent acute exacerbation, necessitating peritoneal dialysis (probably acute interstitial nephritis). Autopsy (80 days later): nephrosclerosis, no renal artery stenosis.
3	26	F	Acute pulmonary oedema. CRF ($P_{cr} = 325\mu mol/ml$, $C_{cr} = 14.8ml/min$). Severe, resistant hypertension (frusemide, hydralazine, clonidine). Severe congenital immunodeficiency syndrome (2.5% gamma globulin, 3600 leucocytes/μl. Autopsy (10 months later): no renal artery stenosis.
4	71	F	Acute pulmonary oedema. Severe, resistant hypertension (frusemide, nipride). CRF ($P_{cr} = 228\mu mol/ml$, $C_{cr} = 23.9ml/min$). Chronic pyelonephritis.

TABLE II. Major side effects of Captopril in four advanced CRF patients

Patient No.	P_{cr} (μmol/ml) C_{cr} (ml/min)	C dosage	SIDE-EFFECTS Type	Day of: appearance max. intensity	Duration (days)	Duration of control of BP (days after stopping Captopril)	Initial evolution of C_{cr} (under Captopril treatment)
1.	413.6 9.0	12.5mg every 48 hr for 9 days	Thrombocytopenia with epistaxis: Leucopenia: Proteinuria:	9 (29000/μl) 11 (23000/μl) 9 (4200/μl) 11 (3200/μl) 4 (9.1g/24hr)	5 5 22 (4.2g)	10	Increasing progressively: 12ml/min at 4th day
2.	536.8 11.0	12.5mg b.d. x 3d 25mg b.d. x 49d 12.5mg b.d. x 9d	Rash: exfoliative dermatitis: Eosinophilia: Acute renal failure with final oligoanuria:	34 47 55–61 61 (2530/μl) 58	at exitus at exitus 13 at exitus	21	Very variable for the first 58d, but lower than pre-treatment values
3.	440.0 10.9	12.5mg b.d. x 10d	Acute renal failure with oligoanuria	6	10*	12	Increasing progressively the first 5 days (up to 13.7ml/min), then suddenly deteriorating
4.	228.0 23.9	25mg b.d. x 1d 25mg t.d.s. x 3d 50mg t.d.s. x 2d	Acute renal failure with oligoanuria: Rash: Eosinophilia:	4 4 11 (600/μl) 16 (1920/μl)	12† 11 20	21	Continuously deteriorating (first measured on the 4th day of treatment)

* Pc = 996μmol/ml, the 10th day. Ten days later 633μmol/ml, but 2 days after 472μmol/ml.

† three days later, Pcr = 281μmol/ml, but 4 months later 211μmol/ml. Two haemodialyses were required: on the 9th and the 11th day after stopping Captopril

Results

Six patients did not show any adverse effects which could be associated with Captopril, except for a significant increase of plasma K (from 3.7 ± 0.3 to 4.6 ± 0.6mEq/L). Both haemodialysis patients were in this group.

The four other patients had severe adverse effects most probably related to Captopril. All are described in some detail in Tables I and II.

Discussion

Despite the use of well-adjusted Captopril dosage [1, 3], the incidence and severity of side-effects were rather high in this series: oligoanuria was present in three (requiring dialysis in two), rashes in two (with one case evolving into a severe lethal exfoliative dermatitis), mild leucopenia in two with severe symptomatic thrombocytopenia in one case and possible exacerbation of pre-existing protein-uria in one of the cases. This observation is notably in contrast with the good tolerance of full Captopril dosage in patients with equivalent or more advanced CRF (see 1, Table I). Also it contrasts with the results of one other study [4], where major side-effects were observed only in patients with advanced CRF treated with a full dose of Captopril. .

We are not aware of any other report of symptomatic thrombocytopenia (blood pressure in our patient was normal on the day of the epistaxis). Thrombo-cytopenia was encountered only in 11 of 6000 cases [5]. It is worth mentioning that this patient's platelet count was abnormally low even before Captopril and he had a rather complex haematological disorder.

Surprisingly, another patient suffering from a congenital immunodeficiency syndrome with leucopenia did not develop thrombocytopenia. In her, only a slight decrease was noted in the leucocyte count.

Exfoliative dermatitis as a side-effect of Captopril has only been reported once previously [6]. The significantly increased proteinuria appeared too early (in this one case of nephrotic syndrome of undetermined aetiology) to be attributed to Captopril. The frequent deterioration of renal function is too severe to be attributed simply to blood pressure reduction. In the medical literature such severe renal deterioration is considered specific for cases of bilateral renal artery stenosis [7]. In our study, however, the only case presenting with this condition (case 1) showed progressive improvement in kidney function during Captopril administration. In another patient (case 3), a similar improvement was observed in the first five days of treatment, preceding a subsequent severe deterioration. In fact, most of the published experimental and clinical studies found an increase of renal plasma flow and glomerular filtration rate, even in acute renal failure experiments [see 1, page 422]. Most probably the severe deterioration of renal function observed in this series (two of three patients needing dialysis) had an organic basis, either a nephrotoxic or an allergic one. The association of signifi-cant eosinophilia in two cases favours the latter aetiology, even though no eosinophils were found in the urine. Perhaps the third case, whose eosinophil count increased from $36/\mu l$ to $189/\mu l$, was not able to produce an absolute eosinophilia due to her congenital immunologic disease.

The fact of a delay in blood pressure increase after the side-effects resolved (suggesting that enough Captopril persisted in the circulation) seems to us against the hypothesis that an elevated plasma kinin concentration [see 3, page 33] is responsible for some side-effects (rashes).

The resolution of some side-effects of Captopril in spite of continuation of the treatment, as well as the protective effect of dialysis, are against an allergic mechanism, whereas the coincidence between dialysis and restoration of renal function of case 4 favours a nephrotoxic mechanism.

We have already concluded [8] that in CRF patients Captopril should be started at the lowest possible dose (12.5mg) and, if it proves effective, should not be repeated before a significant increase in blood pressure occurs. The interval for the administration of Captopril can be clearly determined in this manner. Once the dose and interval are established, loss of blood pressure control means, in most of the cases, an unrecognised salt and water retention. The addition or increase in dosage of a diuretic will re-establish the effectiveness of the given dose of Captopril.

Recent studies [9] showed almost a similar effectiveness of a dose of 150mg t.d.s. and of 25mg t.d.s. of Captopril in resistant hypertension associated with CRF, even if the same doses of diuretic are maintained. This means higher dosage adds mostly toxic effects with very little benefit on blood pressure control.

Considering the present experience, we are in favour of adding another anti-hypertensive drug to the combination of diuretic and Captopril rather than increasing the dose above 25mg b.d. in patients with C_{cr} less than 30ml/min, or 12.5mg b.d. in patients with C_{cr} less than 10ml/min.

The dialysance of Captopril, evaluated at 65 per cent of C_{cr} [10], could be a good means for rapidly correcting its side-effects after stopping the drug. Despite the high dialysance of Captopril we did not have to add the equivalent of 50 per cent of the regular dose after each dialysis, as recommended by others [see 3, page 35], probably because ultrafiltration rendered our patients more sensitive to Captopril. This suggests that smaller doses may be effective in well dehydrated patients.

Conclusions

1. Even the present recommended dose of Captopril in CRF patients can produce a high incidence of major side-effects.

2. For this reason the lowest possible dose should be tried initially and, if effective, should not be repeated until a significant increase in blood pressure occurs.

3. If not effective, the dose can be increased, but not above a 'reasonable' amount. There is the possibility that unresponsiveness to rather large doses of Captopril may be due to insufficient dehydration.

4. In any event, before the pharmacodynamics and the pharmacokinetics of Captopril in CRF are better known, it seems preferable to add to the combination of diuretic and Captopril another antihypertensive drug, rather than increasing the dose of Captopril.

References

1   Heel RC, Brogden RN, Speight IM et al. *Drugs 1980; 20:* 409
2   Rommel AJ, Pierides AM, Heald A. *Clin Pharmacol Ther 1980; 27:* 282
3   Romankiewicz JA, Brogden RN, Heel RC et al. *Drugs 1983; 25:* 6
4   Isles CG, Hodsman GP, Robertson JIS. *Lancet 1983; i:* 355
5   Cooper RA. *Arch Intern Med 1983; 143:* 659
6   Solinger AM. *Cutis 1982; 29:* 473
7   Hricick DE, Browning PJ, Kopelman R et al. *N Engl J Med 1983; 308:* 373
8   Beroniade V. In Genest J, Kuchel O, Hamet P, eds. *Hypertension 2nd Edition.* New York: McGraw Hill. In press
9   Smith SJ, Markanu ND, MacGregor GA. *Lancet 1982; ii:* 1460
10   Hirakata H, Onoyama K, Iseki K et al. *Clin Nephrol 1981; 16:* 321

Open Discussion

MANN (Heidelberg) Regarding the first case with haemolytic anaemia, increased creatinine, severe hypertension and thrombocytopenia did you consider a diagnosis of haemolytic uraemic syndrome?

BERONIADE The case was well studied during the episode and five months after the thrombocytopenia she died and we had an autopsy. We did not find any aetiology either for the nephrotic syndrome or the haematological problem. It was certainly not a case of haemolytic uraemic syndrome.

ANDREUCCI (Naples) I am afraid that you don't have renal biopsies on these patients.

BERONIADE But we have, some months later, autopsies in three of the patients.

ANDREUCCI And what did you find?

BERONIADE As I told you, the first patient died five months after, and this was the only one in whom we confirm a bilateral stenosis of the renal artery. The second one was exfoliative dermatitis which infected the skin.

ANDREUCCI What was the renal histology?

BERONIADE Only nephrosclerosis in the second case, and in the third the autopsy took place six months later and there was diabetic nephropathy.

ANDREUCCI You know that there are two kinds of acute renal failure after Captopril. One is acute interstitial nephritis of the immunological type; this can happen with many drugs and it has been described after Captopril*. The other type has been reported in patients with one functioning kidney and renal

* Farrow PR, Wilkinson R. *Br Med J 1979; 1:* 1680

535

artery stenosis and in patients with bilateral renal artery stenosis. Two articles have appeared recently in the *New England Journal of Medicine**. It was considered as a functional renal failure and attributed to inhibition of angiotensin-induced vasoconstriction of the efferent glomerular arteriole. While I agree on the functional type of acute renal failure I disagree on the suggested mechanism because we have proven that angiotensin II exerts its vasoconstrictive effect only on the afferent arteriole. I personally think that the functional renal failure occurring after Captopril administration is due to salt depletion because Captopril is usually given with diuretics. Captopril itself may cause natriuresis since it stimulates prostaglandin release and prostglandins are known to cause salt excretion. As a matter of fact the effect of Captopril on blood pressure is immediate whereas the decrease in renal function occurs later after many days and it returns to normal as soon as Captopril administration is discontinued. We have observed this in a young transplant patient with renal artery stenosis; acute renal failure occurred on two occasions both times after several days of Captopril therapy and in both occasions it was reversed by discontinuation of Captopril.

BERONIADE I know very well your quoted article about the renal function disturbances in patients with bilateral renal artery stenosis treated with Captopril, but as was presented in the paper the only case who has this condition in our series did not have any trouble with his kidney function. Secondly I don't think that the deterioration of kidney function was only on a 'functional' or a pre-renal basis because as you could see in the last case acute renal failure lasted for 14 days and needed two haemodialyses before renal function started again. So I think the renal insufficiency has an organic basis, but of course I cannot say whether the lesion was an acute interstitial nephritis or an acute tubular necrosis.

MORGANTI (Milan) I understand that in some of your patients blood pressure remained low or returned to normal after stopping the drug for several days, in one case 21 days. Now did you try to evaluate, during this period, whether the classical mechanism responsible for the blood pressure is still active, I mean the blockade of angiotensin II by measuring, for instance, plasma renin activity?

BERONIADE In two cases we measured the plasma renin activity. In one case about six days and in the other case about 10 days after stopping the drug. The blood pressure was at that time under control and the renin was very high.

MORGANTI So there was still active blockade of angiotensin?

BERONIADE Yes. I think we can say that.

EL MATRI (Tunis, Tunisia) In our experience we have observed four cases of leucopenia in renal insufficiency patients. One case was pancytopenic but in the three others we observed an increase of white blood count one or two days after

---

*   Hricik DE, Browning PJ, Kopelman R et al. *N Engl J Med 1983; 308:* 373
     Curtis JJ, Luke RG, Whelchel JD et al. *N Engl J Med 1983; 308:* 377

discontinuing treatment. In these patients, who again developed leucopenia on Captopril, we continued the treatment on a dose of 50—100mg daily and observed a quick return to normal of the white blood count. We think they were not cases of haematological toxicity but a new distribution of white blood cells by some effect of Captopril. Have you observed such a phenomenon?

LEVER (Chairman) Our own experience is of 100 normal patients treated with Captopril. I think it was a shame that this otherwise very good drug was introduced at far too high a dose. Initially we gave our patients 450mg daily and all the serious side effects that we have seen, and there were seven in 100, were in the patients with mildly impaired or seriously impaired renal function and getting this higher dose. I think the real message about Captopril is that it is good provided you don't give it in too large a dose, it's effective in a low dose, and watch particularly in patients who have renal failure because that's where the trouble lies.

BERONIADE Yes that was my message.

Proc EDTA (1983) Vol 20

RESTENOSIS OF THE RENAL ARTERY AFTER PERCUTANEOUS TRANSLUMINAL RENAL ANGIOPLASTY: AN INEVITABLE OUTCOME?

K J Kuiper, P E de Jong, D de Zeeuw, K H Schuur, G K van der Hem

State University Hospital, Groningen, The Netherlands

Summary

We performed follow-up studies in 26 patients four to 36 months after percutaneous transluminal renal angioplasty. Restenosis was found in 47 per cent of the patients who had an atherosclerotic type of stenosis and in 14 per cent of the patients with fibromuscular dysplasia. We could not detect any significant differences between the atherosclerotic patients who did develop restenosis and those who did not. In fact, the presence of generalised atherosclerosis, the severity of the stenosis and the initial success of the dilatation were similar in the two groups. It thus cannot be predicted which patients will develop restenosis.

Introduction

Since its introduction in 1978, percutaneous transluminal renal angioplasty (PTRA) has received an increasing popularity as a treatment of renal artery stenosis [1–3]. The obvious reason is the relative simplicity of the procedure compared to surgical intervention. Moreover, the initial results were promising. Blood pressure (BP) appears to improve in about 80–90 per cent of all patients after dilatation, whereas complications vary from 5–10 per cent [1–3].

The first long-term results however, are not too encouraging. Follow-up studies show that restenosis develops frequently in patients with atherosclerotic (AS) lesions of the renal artery [4,5]. Grim et al even found restenosis to occur in 100 per cent of AS patients [5]. In contrast, PTRA appears to have a more permanent dilating effect on a fibromuscular dysplasia (FMD) type of stenosis. It is of great interest to know whether characteristics other than the type of stenosis will predict re-occurrence of the dilated stenosis.

Therefore we present follow-up data on 26 patients in whom PTRA was performed. In particular we studied the clinical and angiographic indices that could possibly predict the long-term success of therapy.

Patients and methods

From January 1980 to May 1982 PTRA was performed in 44 consecutive hypertensive patients with renal artery stenosis. Dilatation was carried out with the aid of a Grüntzig double lumen balloon catheter. Angiography was performed prior to and directly after the dilatation. All patients received acetylsalicylic acid 500mg every other day three days before and for at least six months after PTRA. Calcium heparin 5000U was given subcutaneously twice daily for one week starting the day before dilatation. Screening of the patients before PTRA focused on the symptoms of generalised atherosclerosis and cardiovascular disease.

The angiograms made prior to PTRA were shown to five independent observers. They were unanimous in their diagnosis of the type of stenosis (AS or FMD) in 42 out of the 44 patients. In nine out of these patients the procedure could not be carried out because the balloon catheter could not be introduced through the stenosis. In two of these nine patients the renal artery occluded due to the procedure and in one patient subintimal passage of the catheter occurred. These nine patients were either operated or treated with antihypertensive medication.

In the remaining 33 patients the angiogram performed after PTRA showed a successful dilatation of the renal artery. Twenty-four of these 33 patients had AS-stenosis (15 male and 9 female) and nine subjects had a FMD-type of stenosis (all female). In the AS-group the stenosis was localised unilaterally in 10 patients, bilaterally in five (also dilated bilaterally) and in nine patients there was a unilateral stenosis with an occlusion of the contralateral artery. In the FMD-group eight patients had a unilateral stenosis and the other one showed a bilateral localisation of the FMD-lesion (dilated at both sides). At least four months after the dilatation patients were asked to co-operate in a study to evaluate the frequency of restenosis. Informed consent was obtained from 26 out of the 33 patients (19 with AS and 7 with FMD). In these patients angiography was performed after 12 months (median, range 4–36) in the AS-group and after 15 months (median, range 6–34) in the FMD-group.

The angiograms done prior to PTRA, directly after the procedure and at follow-up were compared with respect to the minimal diameter of the stenosis and the degree of the stenosis, expressed as a percentage (diameter of the artery at the site of the stenosis divided by the diameter of the artery proximal to the stenosis x 100) Also the size of the kidney measured by perimeter as kidney surface area was studied.

The effect of PTRA on BP was scored to be beneficial when antihypertensive medication could be diminished or stopped with a diastolic BP stabilised below 95mmHg.

Statistical analysis was performed using Wilcoxon two sample test and Wilcoxon test for paired data.

Results

The initial BP effect after PTRA was beneficial in 19 out of the 33 patients (58%) in whom the procedure was technically successful. Considering only

539

the patients with unilateral stenosis (n=18) and those with a bilaterally treated stenosis (n=6), BP improved in 75 per cent (67 per cent of the AS-group and 89 per cent of the FMD-group). Follow-up angiography was performed in 19 AS-patients and in seven FMD-patients.

Follow-up in patients with AS-lesions (n=19)

In this group the initial stenosis was localised unilaterally in seven subjects and bilaterally in five; in the other seven subjects a unilateral stenosis with a contra-lateral occluded artery was present.

Restenosis was found in nine out of the 19 AS-patients (47%). In the other 10 AS-patients (53%) the renal artery was patent. The group with restenosis was not significantly different from the group without restenosis with respect to the time between PTRA and follow-up angiography (11 months, range 4–34, in the restenosis group compared to 24 months, range 7–36, in the non-restenosis group), age (55 years, range 44–66, compared to 51 years, range 41–58, respectively) or duration of hypertension (5 years, range 1–19, versus 1.5 years, range 1–13). In both the restenosis group and the non-restenosis group five patients with a history of generalised atherosclerosis (angina pectoris, myocardial infarction, cerebrovascular or peripheral vascular disease) were present. Also in both groups six patients had evidence of bilateral stenosis or unilateral stenosis with contralateral occlusion. There was a slight although not significant preponderance of male subjects in the restenosis group (7 out of 9 patients) compared to five out of 10 patients in the group without restenosis. When evaluating the initial BP effect in the patients with unilateral stenosis or a bilaterally treated stenosis in our AS follow-up group (n=12), BP had improved in four out of the six patients (67%) who developed a restenosis and in five out of six patients (83%) who showed a patent artery at follow-up. Of the four patients in the restenosis group who had a good initial effect on BP two patients had developed hyper-tension again at the time of the follow-up studies. Thus, in two patients a restenosis appeared without recurrence of hypertension. None of the subjects in the group without restenosis who had a good initial effect on BP had developed hypertension again at follow-up.

The angiographic data of the patients in both the stenosis and the non-stenosis group are given in Table I. There was no significant difference between the two groups with respect to the characteristics of the stenosis prior to PTRA. Also the success of dilatation was not different between the two groups: 54 per cent stenosis before and 17 per cent after PTRA in the restenosis group compared to 61 per cent stenosis before and 29 per cent after PTRA in the non-restenosis group. In some patients who had developed restenosis the artery was even more stenotic at follow-up compared to the situation prior to the dilatation. None of these patients had a complete obstruction of the renal artery. On the other hand in some of the patients who had no restenosis the visible effect of the dilatation had even improved on the control angiogram compared to the situation directly after PTRA; this difference was not significant for the total group.

TABLE I. Angiographic data of the renal artery stenosis in patients with restenosis and in patients without restenosis on follow-up angiography. Median and range are given

	Restenosis			No Restenosis		
	pre-PTRA	post-PTRA	follow-up	pre-PTRA	post-PTRA	follow-up
Minimum diameter	2	4	2	2	5	5
(mm)	(1–4)	(2–6)	(1–5)	(1–6)	(3–6)	(3–6)
Degree of stenosis	54	17	64	61	29	20
(%)	(30–86)	(0–64)	(28–86)	(11–86)	(0–48)	(0–50)
Kidney surface area	53	55	53	58	58	61
(cm²)	(38–75)	(38–74)	(39–71)	(31–92)	(32–93)	(38–83)

Follow-up in the FMD-group (n=7)

In this group restenosis was observed in only one patient (14%). This patient had hypertension again at the time of follow-up angiography. In the other six patients hypertension had not recurred.

Discussion

Recurrence of stenosis after PTRA was found in 47 per cent of the patients with an atherosclerotic type of stenosis and in 14 per cent of the patients with FMD. This confirms earlier studies that restenosis seldom occurs in patients with FMD whereas it is rather frequent in AS-lesions [4,5]. It is important to stress however that we, in contrast to the studies of Grim et al [5], found at least half of the patients with an AS-stenosis to have no recurrence of the stenosis after a follow-up of approximately two years.

We could not demonstrate significant differences between the group with restenosis and the group who had a patent renal artery at follow-up. One could expect patients with generalised atherosclerotic disease to be more prone to recurrence of the stenosis. However, also in the group without restenosis half of the patients had widespread systemic atherosclerosis as shown by a positive history of cardiovascular disease and/or by the presence of bilateral renal vascular pathology. One could also suggest that patients with a more severe stenosis or patients in which the dilatation was not so successful should more often develop restenosis. This could be estimated from the PRA-ratio prior to PTRA, from the effect of the procedure on the renal artery diameter at the post PTRA angiography and from the effect on BP. Also with respect to these parameters we could not detect any differences between the two groups. Information on PRA-ratio is not included. The data are not conclusive since there were only three and four patients with a unilateral stenosis in the restenosis and non-restenosis group, respectively.

When discussing the occurrence of restenosis after PTRA, one should realise that atherosclerosis of the renal artery in itself without any intervention can also be progressive and can finally lead to occlusion of the artery [6,7]. In some of our patients with restenosis the stenosis indeed was more severe at follow-up. None had complete occlusion of the artery at that time. Redilatation was possible in some although not all patients. In others surgical intervention was chosen.

Two subjects in the AS-group in whom BP initially had improved after PTRA, had developed hypertension again. They indeed showed a restenosis at the follow-up angiography. The one FMD patient who had hypertension again also had a restenosis, suggesting that angiography should be repeated in patients in whom BP after an initial improvement deteriorates again. On the other hand two patients out of the restenosis group had no increase of BP at the time restenosis was documented.

In some of the patients who showed a patent renal artery at follow-up, the result of dilatation had even improved compared to the direct post PTRA angiography. This shows that the ultimate success of the procedure cannot be predicted from the angiography made directly after dilatation.

We conclude restenosis occurs in about half of the patients with an AS lesion. We cannot give however, any parameter that predicts which patient will develop restenosis and which patient will not. Since at least half of the patients, including some with generalised atherosclerosis and some with severe stenosis, do not develop restenosis we suggest PTRA as a first choice of treatment of atherosclerotic renal artery stenosis. Close follow-up is warranted and in a situation of restenosis surgical intervention should be considered.

Acknowledgments

We are grateful to Dr AJM Donker for reviewing the angiograms.

References

1   Grüntzig A, Kuhlmann U, Vetter W et al. *Lancet 1978; i:* 801
2   Mahler F, Krneta A, Haertel M. *Ann Int Med 1979; 90:* 56
3   Medias NE, Ball JT, Millan VG. *Am J Med 1981; 76:* 1078
4   Kuhlmann U, Vetter W, Furrer J et al. *Ann Int Med 1980; 92:* 1
5   Grim CE, Luft FC, Yune HJ et al. *Proc 8th Int Congr Nephrol Athens 1981;* 1154
6   Wollenweber J, Sheps SG, Davis GD. *Am J Cardiol 1968; 21:* 60
7   Meaney TF, Dustan HP, McCormack LJ. *Radiology 1968; 91:* 887

Open Discussion

KLEINKNECHT (Paris) In your study angioplasty was performed successfully. Have you any patients with renal artery stenosis in whom you had immediate side effects such as arterial rupture?

de JONG Indeed we had. I showed you that we had 35 subjects with successfully performed angioplasty. In 44 subjects we tried to perform angioplasty and in nine patients we were not able to get good results. In these subjects it was due to the fact that, in some, the curve of the renal artery to the aorta could not be passed by the Grüntzig catheter and in two patients the renal artery was completely occluded by the manipulation of the guide wire through the stenosis. Moreover we had two patients with segmental infarction during the procedure, so four of the 44 patients had a rather severe complication.

LEVER (Chairman) Did you have to operate on those four?

de JONG We operated later on, not immediately after the procedure.

LEVER And you're still happy to recommend this as a first line treatment, with reconstructive surgery or nephrectomy if it fails?

de JONG I believe this is the treatment of first choice. I have to add that we believe that it is a treatment that should be performed in experienced centres. Therefore it is probably better not to state that it's the first line treatment for renal hypertension.

LEVER Have you any evidence that your first patients did worse than those treated subsequently? Have you got better as you got more experience?

de JONG No, that was not the situation.

DAL CANTON (Naples, Italy) We have also had some experience with percutaneous angioplasty, some of which will be presented this afternoon, our results were not so negative as yours. In our 10 patients four of which were atherosclerotic, the overall success rate at a mean follow-up of 17.5 months was 90 per cent. There were no apparent recurrences of stenosis as judged by the results of hypertension. We had three repeat angiographies at three to five months after the first dilatation. These angiographies were performed in one case because of a very narrow stenosis and in two cases because of difficulty in controlling hypertension. Despite these negative results of hypertension the dilatation was still permanent.

de JONG Am I correct in thinking that most of your patients were patients with fibromuscular dysplasia?

DAL CANTON Six of 10.

de JONG I agree fully that in those patients the results are indeed better. It is not a conclusion of my paper that we are not positive about the angioplasty in patients with an atherosclerotic type of stenosis. The results on blood pressure in those patients are not as good as patients having muscular dysplasia. We had a lot of patients with bilateral pathology and also a number of patients, in the series of 35 there were nine, with a unilateral stenosis and a contralateral occlusion. In those patients we cannot expect blood pressure to improve much. In these patients the contralateral kidney was operated on later on.

LEVER The issue really is whether everybody finds fibromuscular hyperplasia responding better than atheromatous stenosis, whether with surgery or balloon catheterisation. The issue really is whether balloon catheterisation for fibromuscular hyperplasia is better than surgery and similarly for atherosclerosis.

SCHREIBER (Cleveland, USA) Our experience with PTA is not encouraging, especially in individuals with extra renal atherosclerosis with significant peripheral vascular disease and cerebral vascular disease. We approach these patients surgically as opposed to doing angioplasty, both because of the high complication rate as well as the increased incidence of restenosis when these individuals were re-angiogrammed at a later date. The Chairman's point about medial hyperplasia or fibrous dysplasia may be a very good one and there has not been a collaborative study looking at this very question. In the patients with fibrous disease there may be less complications as well as a greater incidence of success. Two important points need to be brought out. The first is that with different centres the technique of doing PTA differs. There may need to be some standardisation of the technique as well as the development of expertise in this area. The second point is in animal models it has been shown that following damage to the intima or endothelial surface it may result in an increased predisposition to develop progressive atherosclerosis if blood pressure in fact is not controlled. In those individuals who have extra renal atherosclerosis the mechanism of hypertension is multifactorial, and still needs medication and close follow-up. I think if you angioplasty an individual with extra renal atherosclerosis then you need to be very compulsive about controlling hypertension because theoretically the rate of restenosis in those individuals may be very high if the blood pressure remains high.

MORGANTI (Milan, Italy) After successful dilatation how long does it take for blood pressure to return to normal?

de JONG That is a difficult question. We have observed in about the first 10 or 15 patients which we dilated that immediately after the procedure a rather sharp fall in blood pressure occurs at least in the first four hours after the procedure. Later on we stopped or diminished the antihypertensive medication used by these patients before the procedure and this last group of patients mostly were dilated without any medication at all. In that situation we observed that the fall in blood pressure in the first hours after the procedure was not as marked as in the group which had concomitant antihypertensive medication. In another group of patients the blood pressure decline was observed in the first few days after the procedure.

544

DAVID (Brazil) Do you have any experience about restenosis after percutaneous angioplasty in kidney transplant?

de JONG No, we have not done that.

Proc EDTA (1983) Vol 20

CHEMICAL RENAL MEDULLECTOMY AND EXPERIMENTAL HYPERTENSION

G I Russell, R F Bing*, D Taverner*, J D Swales*, H Thurston*

*Leicester General Hospital, and *Department of Medicine, University of Leicester, United Kingdom*

Summary

The possible vasodepressor role of the renal medulla was studied by chemical medullectomy (i.v. bromoethylamine hydrobromide) in rats. A significant increase in blood pressure (BP) was observed 10 weeks after injection which related to the increase in urinary volume and decrease in urinary prostaglandin E_2 (PGE_2) in medullectomised rats, but not to plasma renin concentration (PRC). Creatinine clearance was unchanged. The differences between control and medullary damaged rats were maintained over a wide range of sodium intakes although the patterns of response were similar in the two groups. The increase in BP observed following renal medullectomy is likely to be secondary to a reduction in interstitial cell function.

Introduction

Studies have indicated that the renal medulla may have an antihypertensive role in rats with experimental hypertension [1, 2]. Vasodepressor properties of the renal medulla appear to originate in the renal medullary interstitial cells which contain prostaglandins, particularly E_2 [3], and antihypertensive lipids [1].

Bromoethylamine hydrobromide selectively ablates the renal medulla [4] and it has been reported that this compound exacerbates experimental renovascular hypertension [5] and reduces the fall in blood pressure after unclipping in two-kidney one clip hypertension in the rat [2].

Accordingly, we have studied the effects of chemical renal medullectomy produced with bromoethylamine, on blood pressure, urinary prostaglandin E_2 (PGE_2) and plasma renin concentration (PRC) in normal rats, together with the effects of altering sodium intake in these animals.

Methods

White female Wistar rats were used and maintained on standard rat chow except where stated. Chemical renal medullectomy was performed by a single intravenous injection of bromoethylamine hydrobromide (200mg/kg BW, Sigma, UK) in saline. Control rats were injected with an equivalent volume of 0.9 per cent saline alone. All animals were housed individually throughout the study. Two separate groups of rats were studied.

a) Acute effect of renal medullary damage on sodium balance

Rats were housed in metabolic cages and after a two day run-in period were either injected with bromoethylamine or saline and balances continued for seven days. PRC was measured before and after injection. Cumulative sodium balance was calculated as previously described [6]. Direct blood pressure (BP) was measured within one week of completion of the balances [2].

b) Responses to changes in sodium intake in rats with established renal medullary damage

Rats injected with bromoethylamine or saline alone two weeks previously were allocated randomly to either normal, low sodium (edosol and deionised water) or high salt (standard diet and one per cent saline to drink) diet for a period of two weeks. Dietary regimes were then changed so that all rats received the three diets in rotation, each for a two-week period. At the end of each dietary period a 24-hour urine sample was collected. This was cooled immediately and stored at $-70°C$ and used for the estimation of volume, sodium content, PGE_2 [7] and creatinine excretion. At the same time a plasma sample was taken for PRC and creatinine estimation [2]. At the end of this study rats were returned to a normal diet and two weeks later direct blood pressure measured [2].

Statistical analysis

Results are expressed as mean ± SEM. Comparisons between and within groups were by unpaired and paired Student t-test respectively. PRC was logarithmically transformed before analysis.

Results

a) Acute effect of renal medullary damage on sodium balance (Table I)

TABLE I. Urine volume, weight and cumulative seven day sodium balance in chemically medullectomised and control rats (mean ± SEM)

	Bromoethylamine (n = 13)			Control group (n = 8)		
	−1	days	7	−1	days	7
U volume (ml)	12.2 ± 1.7		24.9 ± 2.4*	9.3 ± 3.0		11.8 ± 2.5
Body weight (g)	183 ± 5		174 ± 5*	188 ± 2		189 ± 3
Cumulative sodium balance (mmol)	+0.07 ± 0.07		−0.06 ± 0.41	+0.10 ± 0.11		+0.30 ± 0.30

* Difference from value on day −1, p<0.05

547

In all 13 rats that received bromoethylamine there was an immediate diuresis. Urine volume increased to over 20ml/day in the first 24 hours following the injection. During the next six days urine volume remained elevated and was significantly greater than baseline volume on day 7 ($p < 0.01$). Urine volume was unchanged in the control group.

Sodium balance became negative in the 24 hours following bromoethylamine (-0.65 ± 0.12mmol/day) but corrected over the next six days, so that the cumulative sodium balance for the seven days after injection was -0.12 ± 0.4 mmol. In contrast, the control group retained sodium for the first four days after injection but by day seven cumulative sodium balance ($+0.2 \pm 0.24$mmol) was not significantly different from baseline or from the bromoethylamine group ($p > 0.5$). At seven days the bromoethylamine group had a significant fall in body weight ($p < 0.01$, Table I) and PRC was slightly higher (167 ± 29ng AI/ml/hr) than in the control group (121 ± 41, $p > 0.1$).

b) *Responses to changes in sodium intake in rats with established medullary damage (Figure 1)*

i) *Normal diet:* Urine volume was increased ($p < 0.01$) and daily excretion was higher ($p < 0.05$), whereas urinary PGE_2 was significantly reduced ($p < 0.01$) in medullectomised rats compared to controls. PRC, plasma osmolality and body weight were not significantly different. Serum creatinine was the same in both groups (medullectomised = 60 ± 2, control = $55 \pm 2\mu$mol/L) with creatinine clearance slightly higher in the medullectomised group (0.9 ± 0.05 vs 0.8 ± 0.07 ml/min).

ii) *High salt:* Urine volume increased significantly in both groups after two weeks although the difference between the two groups was maintained. Urine sodium excretion rose in both groups but the increase was significantly greater in the medullectomised group ($p < 0.01$). Urinary PGE_2 increased on a high salt intake in proportion to the baseline value, thus maintaining the difference between the two groups. PRC fell but this was only significant for the medullectomised group. Body weight increased significantly in the latter.

iii) *Low salt:* Urine sodium was reduced to very low levels and PRC was elevated to a similar degree in both groups. Urine volume in the medullectomised group was similar to that when on a normal diet but was higher in the control group. Urinary PGE_2 was similar to that on a normal diet in both groups.

Direct blood pressure

When measured on day 14 after injection in rats in study (a), BP was higher in medullectomised animals compared to controls (130 ± 3.6mmHg, vs 123 ± 4.2, $p > 0.1$). On week 10 after injection this increase in BP was significant: study (b) (136 ± 3.3 vs 118 ± 4.5mmHg, $p < 0.01$). At 10 weeks there was a positive correlation between direct BP and daily urine volume ($r = 0.6$, $p < 0.01$) and a negative correlation with urinary PGE_2 ($r = -0.43$, $p < 0.05$), but no significant correlation with PRC ($r = 0.01$).

548

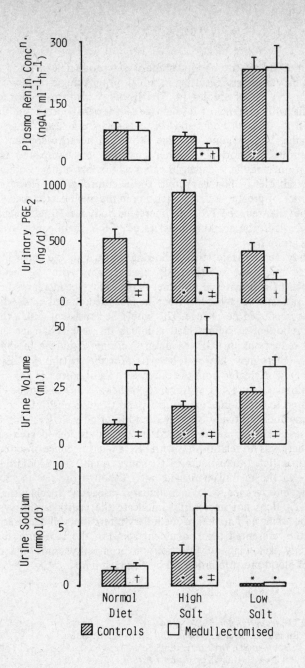

Figure 1. Daily urine volume, sodium and PGE_2 excretion and PRC in control (hatched columns, n = 10) and renal medullary damaged rats (open columns, n = 13) on normal, high salt and low salt diets. (Mean ± SEM, *$p < 0.05$ for differences within each group, †$p < 0.05$ and ‡$p < 0.01$ for differences between control and medullectomised rats)

Discussion

A single injection of bromoethylamine is a reproducible method of inducing renal medullary necrosis, resulting in a high urine volume of low osmolality as seen in this and earlier studies [4, 5]. Histology confirmed destruction of the renal papilla with minimal or no damage to the renal cortex and urine volume increased in the first 24 hours and this persisted for at least 10 weeks. Despite the continuing high volume of urine the initial negative sodium balance was rapidly returned to normal. Further evidence for unimpaired renal sodium conservation in medullary damaged rats was the low urinary sodium excretion on the low salt diet, which was similar to the control group. However, there was some evidence of greater sodium retention in the medullectomised group on the high salt diet, i.e. reduced PRC and increased body weight, although the administration of salt in the drinking water resulted in a significantly greater sodium load in this group.

This study demonstrates that following damage to the renal medulla there is a marked reduction in urinary PGE_2 consistent with the medulla being a major source of this material in urine. A high salt diet increased urinary PGE_2 in normal rats and to a lesser extent in medullectomised rats, whereas a low sodium diet produced no change. This would be consistent with a role for PGE_2 in the excretion of a sodium load although in medulla-damaged rats, despite substantial reductions in PGE_2, sodium excretion could be modulated within wide limits. There may, however, be a role for the remaining PGE_2 production which probably originates from the outer medulla or cortex [8].

Direct blood pressure was significantly higher at 10 weeks in medullectomised rats compared to saline injected controls and this was positively correlated with urine volume and negatively correlated within urinary PGE_2. This suggests that the increase in blood pressure could be related to the degree of medullary damage. There was no relationship with PRC and no evidence of sodium retention on the normal diet. Interestingly PRC changes on different sodium intakes were appropriate in the medulla-damaged rats. Although the rise in blood pressure may follow interference with a medullary vasoactive mechanism, the fall in urinary PGE_2 does not necessarily implicate the prostaglandin system as this may only be acting as a marker of medullary interstitial cell damage.

The results presented here document some of the biochemical sequelae of medullectomy following an injection of bromoethylamine and confirm the elevation of blood pressure produced by this technique.

References

1 Muirhead EE. *Hypertension 1980; 2:* 444
2 Bing RF, Russell GI, Swales JD et al. *Clin Sci 1981; 61:* 335s
3 Anggard E, Bohman SO, Griffin JE et al. *Acta Physiol Scand 1972; 84:* 231
4 Murray G, Wyllie RG, Hill GS et al. *Am J Pathol 1972; 67:* 285
5 Heptinstall RH, Salyer DC, Salyer WR. *Am J Path 1975; 78:* 297
6 Thurston H, Bing RF, Swales JD. *Hypertension 1980; 2:* 256
7 Auletta FJ, Zusman RM, Caldwell BV. *Clin Chem 1974; 20:* 1580
8 Dunn MJ, Hood VL. *Am J Physiol 1977; 233:* F169

Proc EDTA (1983) Vol 20

EPIDEMIOLOGY OF HYPERTENSION IN CHILDREN

A Papa, A Dal Canton, A Capuano, G Conte, L D'Avanzo, F D'Anna,
N Lavecchia, V E Andreucci

Second Faculty of Medicine, University of Naples, Italy

Summary

In 1979–80, a cross-sectional study was carried out in 7118 Neapolitan school
children aged 10–15 years. In 1980–81 and 1981–82 a longitudinal study was
performed in a group of children with blood pressure above the mean + 1SD
(in age and sex related peers) and in a group with blood pressure <mean + 1SD.
In the whole population blood pressure increased with age from 10 to 14 years.
The major determinant of blood pressure was body weight, followed by heart
rate. Three hundred and ninety-eight children (5.6%) were hypertensive having
blood pressure >mean + 2SD. In children followed longitudinally, blood pressure
was very labile; only 13 per cent of those originally having blood pressure mean
+ 1SD, in fact, remained in the same category. All of these, however, had blood
pressure >mean + 2SD throughout the study.

Introduction

In the last decade, the increasing awareness that essential hypertension in adults
may be preceded by a borderline elevation of blood pressure (BP) in childhood,
has increased the need for exactly defining the limits of normal BP in children.
To determine these limits, several epidemiological studies have been performed,
mainly on groups of North American children [1–3]. From these studies,
regional differences in the frequency distribution of BP have clearly emerged,
dependent on both ethnic and environmental factors. It has become evident,
therefore, that the limits of normal BP in a given child population can only be
determined by obtaining the frequency distribution of BP in that same population.

This paper reports on an epidemiological study performed on a population of
South European students, in Naples. In the school year 1979–80, a cross-sectional
study was carried out to determine the frequency distribution of BP in our
population. In the two successive years a longitudinal study was performed,
to define the BP in our children which predicts persistent hypertension.

Methods

Cross-sectional study

In the school year 1979–80, 7118 students, aged 10–15 years, attending the Public School in Naples (grades 7–10), were examined in their schools personally by the authors. Blood pressure was measured in a seated position by auscultation and mercury manometers. Cuffs were used covering at least two-thirds and encompassing the circumference of the upper arm. Three pressure readings were recorded, i.e. at the point of appearance (systolic blood pressure, SBP), at the point of muffling (intermediate diastolic blood pressure, IBP) and at the point of disappearance (diastolic blood pressure, DBP) of Korotkoff sounds. Readings were taken to the closest 2mmHg. The height was measured and the weight recorded with the subjects clothed and shoeless. Finally, heart rate was recorded and the date of menarche was noted in girls.

In children whose SBP or IBP or DBP values were higher than 135 or 90 or 85mmHg, respectively, a second blood pressure measurement was obtained after resting quietly for at least 30 minutes. Children whose SBP or IBP or DBP remained elevated were invited to hospital within the next week and their blood pressure taken again.

Longitudinal study

In the school year 1980–81, 72 children were randomly selected from those having in the 1979–80 study a BP greater than the mean + 1SD (in their age and sex matched peers), and 60 children were selected from those having a BP <mean + 1SD. All these children were called to hospital where BP, body weight, heart rate and height were recorded, and Fractional Sodium Excretion (FE_{Na}) calculated, using a spontaneous urine collection and a simultaneous blood sample for measurement of urine and plasma Na^+ and creatinine concentrations.

In the school year 1981–82, the same children were called to another visit, at which the same measurements as in 1980–81 were performed. In addition, plasma renin activity was measured by radioimmunoassay (Sorin Biomedica, Saluggia, Milan) both in the standing position, and after one hour of supine rest in bed.

Statistical methods

Statistical analysis including simple statistics, analysis of variance, simple correlation coefficients, the unpaired t test, and multiple regression analysis, was performed by IBM computer (SPSS batch system).

Results

Cross sectional study

The mean values of blood pressures in the various age and sex divided cohorts are shown in Table I. Blood pressures rose with age from 10 to 14 years and

TABLE I. Mean blood pressure in school children in Naples

Age (years)	MALES				FEMALES			
	SBP	IBP mmHg	DBP	N	SBP	IBP mmHg	DBP	N
10	110.4 ±13.4	70.7 9.6	65.6 9.6	253	111.4 ±13.5	71.3 10.0	65.8 10.6	218
11	112.9 ±13.2	72.8 10.4	67.5 10.4	1032	113.9 ±13.2	73.1 9.7	68.1 9.9	922
12	114.5 ±13.1	72.8 10.4	67.1 10.7	1237	117.2** ±13.5	74.9** 9.8	69.7** 10.0	1021
13	118.4 ±13.2	74.1 10.0	68.2 10.2	830	119.8* ±13.7	76.9** 10.1	71.6** 10.6	850
14	121.0 ±14.1	74.3 10.7	68.8 10.9	348	121.5 ±12.5	78.6** 11.3	73.6** 11.4	225
15	120.6 ±12.2	74.0 11.2	69.2 11.5	110	118.0 ±12.9	75.6 10.7	70.4 11.6	69

* p<0.05
** p<0.001
N = number of children
Values are mean ± SD

apparently decreased a little at 15 years. Systolic blood pressure was significantly higher in females than in males aged 12 and 13 years, and both diastolic blood pressures were significantly more elevated in females aged 12, 13 and 14 years. Blood pressures were significantly higher post-menarche than pre-menarche in females aged 10–13 years. In the whole population a significant linear relation occurred between blood pressures and body weight (BW), height (H), heart rate (HR) and Ponderal Index (PI) (Table II). In addition, children with SBP, IBP or DBP values greater than the mean + 1SD had a greater BW (49.0 ± 25.1 vs 44.1 ± 8.4kg, p<0.0001) and HR (90.7 ± 25.1 vs 85.9 ± 16.7 beats/min, p<0.0001), and a lower Ponderal Index (42.3 ± 8.4 vs 43.1 ± 8.4cm/$^3\sqrt{kg}$, p<0.0001) than their peers with blood pressures lower than the mean + 1SD. Stepwise multiple

TABLE II. Relationship between SBP, IBP and DBP with HR, BW and Ponderal Index

	HR	BW	PI
SBP	x 0.23 + 96*	x 0.571 + 90*	−x 1.24 + 90**
IBP	x 0.10 + 65*	x 0.025 + 63**	−x 0.877 + 114*
DBP	x 0.083 + 62*	x 0.125 + 58*	−x 0.795 + 103*

* p<0.01
** p<0.001

regression analysis was performed with SBP, IBP or DBP as dependent variables, and BW, HR, Age, and H as independent variables. In the whole population, the independent variables altogether accounted for 10.4 per cent of variance of SBP, 7.2 per cent of variance of IBP, and 5.6 per cent of that of DBP. The major determinant of variability of SBP was body weight (8.2%), followed by heart rate (2.1%). Similarly, body weight accounted for the greatest portion of explained variance of IBP and DBP (5.4% and 4.7%, respectively). Multiple regression analysis in age-cohorts showed that body weight was the major determinant of SBP in all age groups, and of IBP and DBP in children aged 10 to 14 years. In the 15 year group, instead, heart rate was the major determinant of IBP and DBP. Table III shows the incidence of hypertension with three

TABLE III. Incidence of hypertension with different selection criteria

	MALES		FEMALES		TOTAL	
	No.	%	No.	%	No.	%
SBP ≥135mmHg	266	7.0	312	9.4	578	8.1
IBP ≥ 90mmHg	237	6.2	281	8.5	518	7.3
DBP ≥ 85mmHg	166	4.3	219	6.6	385	5.4
SBP ≥135 and/or IBP ≥ 90 and/or DBP ≥ 85mmHg	356	9.3	401	12.1	757	10.6
SBP ≥140mmHg	175	4.6	212	6.4	387	5.4
DBP ≥ 90mmHg	90	2.4	114	3.4	204	2.9
SBP ≥140mmHg and/or DBP ≥ 90mmHg	197	5.2	243	7.3	440	6.2
SBP ≥ mean + 2SD	100	2.6	105	3.2	205	2.9
IBP ≥ mean + 2SD	49	1.3	55	1.7	104	1.5
DBP ≥ mean + 2SD	27	0.7	62	1.9	89	1.2
SBP and/or IBP and/or DBP ≥ mean + 2SD					398	5.6

different selection criteria. Systolic hypertension, defined as a SBP ≥135mmHg occurred in seven per cent of males, and in 9.4 per cent of females. A SBP ≥140 mmHg occurred in 4.6 per cent of males and 6.4 per cent of females. The incidence of systolic hypertension was further reduced to 2.6 per cent of males and 3.2 per cent of females when a SBP ≥ mean + 2SD was the selection criterion. In males aged 12−15 years, and in females aged 11−15 years, SBP + 2SD was greater than 140mmHg. Diastolic hypertension, defined as a DBP ≥85mmHg occurred in 4.3 per cent of males and 6.6 per cent of females. A DBP ≥90mmHg occurred in 2.4 per cent of males and 3.4 per cent of females. Finally, 0.7 per cent of males and 1.9 per cent of females had a DBP ≥ mean + 2SD.

In children with SBP $\geq$ 135 and/or IBP $\geq$ 90 and/or DBP $\geq$ 85mmHg a new measurement after 30 minutes supine rest confirmed hypertension in 67 per cent (n = 512). Three hundred and ninety-six out of these 512 came to the hospital one week later, and hypertension was confirmed in 66 per cent (n = 261).

Longitudinal study

In 1981, only 35 per cent of children who had a systolic and/or diastolic BP $>$ mean + 1 SD in 1979–80 were unchanged. In addition, 26 per cent of children with previous BP $<$ mean + 1 SD, had now BP $>$ mean + 1 SD. In this latter group, the changes to a more elevated BP was associated with a significant decrease of Ponderal Index (43.3 to 42.8cm/$^3\sqrt{kg}$, p<0.05). In 1982 the number of children with BP persistently $>$ mean + 1 SD was further reduced to 13 per cent (n = 8). In these eight children the BP had been greater than the mean + 2 SD throughout the study.

FE_{Na} and PRA values were similar in normotensive and hypertensive children.

Discussion

This is the first study defining the mean values and the frequency distribution of blood pressure in a large Mediterranean childhood community. In contrast with other populations of the same age both in Europe and in North America [1–5], in our population BP was more frequently elevated in females than in males. Whether this difference is due to an earlier menarche in our girls is a possibility that requires appropriate investigation.

In our population, the major determinant of variability of BP was body weight. Thus, the finding of a significantly lower Ponderal Index in children with BP greater than the mean + 1 SD, and the significant decrease in Ponderal Index associated with a change from a lower to a higher BP rank in a group of children followed longitudinally, support the possibility that obesity favours hypertension in the young [6].

Heart rate was another significant determinant of BP in all age-groups, and the major determinant of diastolic blood pressure at 15 years, suggesting that an increased cardiac activity may be associated with a tendency toward diastolic hypertension.

Our study confirms that hypertension occurs in the young. A major conceptual and practical problem, however, is to establish the limits for normal blood pressure in childhood. Ideally, these limits should be defined for any given population taking into account the frequency distribution of BP in that population. Our study suggests that a BP greater than the mean (in age and sex related peers) + 2 SD is predictive of a persistent hypertension and, therefore, can be used to select those children that are already hypertensive. With this criterion, the incidence of hypertension in our population was of 5.6 per cent. Clearly, this selection criterion will not include all children at risk for future essential hypertension. Other, less restrictive criteria, such as a BP greater than the mean + 1 SD are to be used for this purpose. The great lability of BP in children, however, indicates that only longitudinal studies by which children are followed to adulthood will perhaps establish the limits of BP in childhood predictive of hypertension in adulthood.

References

1   Rames RK, Clarke WR, Connor WE et al. *Pediatrics 1978; 61:* 245
2   Gutgesell M, Terrel G, Labarthe D. *Hypertension 1981; 3:* 39
3   Cornoni-Huntley J, Harlan WR, Leaverton PE. *Hypertension 1979; 1:* 566
4   Morrison JA, Khoury P, Kelly K et al. *Am J Epidemiol 1980; 111:* 156
5   Aullen JP. *Nouv Presse Med 1978; 7:* 1171
6   Lauer RM, Connor WE, Leaverton PE et al. *J Pediatrics 1975; 86:* 697

Proc EDTA (1983) Vol 20

INFLUENCE OF HEAD-OUT WATER IMMERSION ON PLASMA RENIN ACTIVITY, ALDOSTERONE, VASOPRESSIN AND BLOOD PRESSURE IN LATE PREGNANCY TOXAEMIA

F Kokot, J Ulman, A Cekański

Silesian School of Medicine, Katowice, Poland

Summary

In 39 healthy pregnant women and 45 women with mild or moderate late pregnancy toxaemia (LPT) the influence of head-out water immersion on blood pressure, the renin-aldosterone system, vasopressin and plasma osmolality was examined. Water immersion induced a prompt and marked fall in systolic and diastolic blood pressure, which was significantly higher in LPT women. Simultaneously a significant decrease of plasma renin activity, aldosterone and vasopressin was noted both in healthy and toxaemic pregnant women. In contrast to healthy pregnant women in LPT haemodilution was not observed in the early phase of water immersion.

Introduction

Late pregnancy toxaemia (LPT) is characterised by high maternal and fetal morbidity and mortality. Hypertension, oedema and proteinuria appearing in the last trimester of pregnancy are the main symptoms of LPT. Excessive fluid shift from the vascular bed into the interstitial fluid space (clinically visualised by oedema) may be involved in the pathogenesis of pregnancy induced hypertension (PIH) by triggering mechanisms which are counteracting intravascular fluid loss. The present work aimed: 1) to prove this hypothesis, and 2) to clarify the importance of the renin-angiotensin-aldosterone system (RAAS) and vasopressin (AVP) in the pathogenesis of PIH.

Material and methods

Two groups of pregnant women were examined: the first consisted of 39 healthy subjects some days before the calculated term of delivery, with a mean age of 24.6 ± 0.6 years (mean ± SEM). The second comprised 45 women with signs of mild or moderate LPT at the 29–42 week of gestation. The mean age of this group was 27.1 ± 0.82 years. Two to three hours after breakfast all women were immersed to the neck in a bath filled with tap water at 35–36°C. The women remained in this bath in a semireclining position. At 3, 30 and 60 minutes after water immersion blood pressure measurements and pulse rate counts were performed and antecubital venous blood samples were withdrawn for the estimation of plasma renin activity (PRA), plasma aldosterone (ALD), vasopressin (AVP) and plasma osmolality. No food was served during water immersion. PRA, ALD and AVP were assayed by radioimmunoassay [1], plasma osmolality by a digital micro-osmometer (Roebling). Statistical evaluation of the results were performed by the Student t test.

TABLE I. Systolic (SBP) and diastolic (DBP) blood pressure, plasma renin activity (PRA), plasma aldosterone (ALD), vasopressin (AVP) and osmolality and pulse rate in normal pregnancy (NP) and pregnant women with late pregnancy toxaemia (LPT). Means ± SEM. The degree of statistical significance concerns the difference between 0 min and 30 or 60 min values

	Minutes	Normal pregnancy (NP)	LPT women (LPT)	Statistical significance of NP–LPT
SBP mmHg	0	117.82 ± 1.84	146.33 ± 3.05	p < 0.001
	30	109.1 ± 1.68	131.11 ± 2.30	p < 0.001
	60	105.51 ± 1.71	127.55 ± 2.29	p < 0.001
DBP mmHg	0	72.94 ± 1.61	93.77 ± 1.38	p < 0.001
	30	67.05 ± 1.48	81.44 ± 2.03	p < 0.001
	60	64.74 ± 1.79	80.44 ± 1.86	p < 0.001
PRA ng/ml/hr	0	14.2 ± 1.91	15.75 ± 2.39	NS
	30	10.0 ± 1.57	8.62 ± 1.19	NS
	60	5.8 ± 0.88	5.34 ± 0.63	NS
ALD ng %	0	43.8 ± 5.78	35.31 ± 3.61	NS
	30	34.1 ± 2.40	29.10 ± 3.14	NS
	60	26.2 ± 1.18	23.29 ± 2.60	NS
AVP pg/ml	0	4.2 ± 0.84	3.18 ± 0.35	NS
	30	2.7 ± 0.83	2.08 ± 0.27	NS
	60	1.6 ± 0.21	1.45 ± 0.20	NS
Osmolality mmol/kg/H_2O	0	287.2 ± 1.04	281.0 ± 1.72	p < 0.02
	30	284.1 ± 1.29	282.2 ± 1.56	NS
	60	282.9 ± 0.41	280.2 ± 1.56	NS
Pulse rate/min	0	76 ± 2.65	72 ± 1.87	NS
	30	71 ± 2.08	65 ± 2.08	p < 0.05
	60	68 ± 1.94	64.8 ± 1.83	NS

NS = not significant

558

Results

Blood pressure

Water immersion was followed by a significant drop in systolic and diastolic blood pressure both in healthy pregnant and LPT women (Table I). Thirty minutes after water immersion the absolute decrease in systolic and diastolic blood pressure in LPT women was nearly twice that of normal pregnant women.

Plasma renin activity and plasma aldosterone

After water immersion a significant fall of PRA and ALD was noted, which was very similar both in healthy and pre-eclamptic pregnant women (Table I). After 60 minutes of water immersion PRA fell to 39 per cent of the basal value in normal pregnant women and to 30 per cent in LPT. The respective values for plasma aldosterone were 60 per cent and 66 per cent and did not differ significantly between each group.

Plasma vasopressin (AVP)

Basal plasma AVP in LPT women was lower (although statistically insignificant) than in normal pregnant women. After water immersion a significant decrease of AVP was observed both in healthy and LPT women. The magnitude of this decrease was similar in both groups of pregnant women.

Plasma osmolality

Basal plasma osmolality was significantly higher in normal pregnant women than in LPT ($p < 0.02$). In contrast to normal pregnant women in LPT water immersion was not accompanied by a significant decrease in plasma osmolality.

Pulse rate

In both groups of pregnant women similar basal values of pulse rate were observed which decreased significantly after water immersion.

No significant correlation was found between blood pressure changes and the behaviour of PRA, ALD, AVP and osmolality during water immersion both in healthy pregnant and pre-eclamptic women.

Discussion

From the results obtained in this study it follows clearly that water immersion of healthy pregnant and LPT women is followed by a significant fall both of systolic and diastolic blood pressure, and suppression of the renin-aldosterone system and vasopressin. In addition in healthy pregnant women a significant decline in plasma osmolality was observed. This decline was absent in LPT women. The following two questions arise: 1) how can the stated hormonal changes be explained? and 2) do LPT women differ from healthy pregnant women in the endocrine reaction pattern induced by water immersion?

It has been known for several years that water immersion to the neck produces a redistribution of plasma volume with a relative increase in intrathoracic volume [2] and an increase in plasma volume caused by a fluid shift from the extracellular or/and intracellular fluid space [3, 4].

Since both the renin-aldosterone system and antidiuretic hormone are controlled by similar 'volume' receptors [5] suppression of these hormones during water immersion may be anticipated. In fact several investigators have observed a significant suppression of the renin-aldosterone system during water immersion [2, 3]. In healthy subjects water immersion was also accompanied by a significant fall in plasma AVP [3]. In our present study the endocrine responses in pregnant women were comparable to those reported in the literature for healthy non-pregnant subjects. Thus it seems that in healthy pregnant and LPT women both the renin-aldosterone system and AVP secretion are controlled by similar volume receptors as in non-pregnant subjects. From the results of our study it also follows that water immersion-induced endocrine alterations in LPT women do not differ significantly from those reported in healthy pregnant subjects.

Despite similar water immersion-induced endocrine responses the two groups of pregnant women showed different responses in plasma osmolality. In normal pregnant women water immersion was accompanied by a significant fall in plasma osmolality while in contrast in LPT women the fall was only slight and statistically not significant. From these results it follows that in healthy pregnant women, as in non-pregnant healthy subjects [3, 4], water immersion is followed by haemodilution. The fall in plasma osmolality suggests a shift of hypotonic fluid to the intravascular fluid space [4]. The exact mechanism of water immersion-induced hypotonicity remains to be elucidated.

Our results revealed the presence of abnormal fluid metabolism in LPT women which was characterised by the absence of haemodilution in the early phase of water immersion. The observed altered water-electrolyte metabolism could be caused by an abnormal permeability of the capillary or venular walls in LPT.

As already shown in this study no significant correlation was found between blood pressure changes and endocrine reaction patterns induced by water immersion. This seems to indicate, that factors other than the renin-aldosterone system and AVP are also involved in the pathogenesis of pregnancy-induced hypertension.

Whether water immersion could be used as a safe and innocuous tool to treat LPT women remains to be further investigated.

Conclusions

1. Both healthy pregnant and LPT women are characterised by a 'physiological' endocrine reaction pattern induced by water immersion.

2. Factors other than the renin-aldosterone system and vasopressin seem to be involved in the pathogenesis of hypertension in LPT women.

3. Women with LPT are characterised by an absence of haemodilution in the early phase of water immersion.

560

References

1. Kokot F, Stupnicki R. *Metody Radioimmunologiczne i Radiokompetycyjne Stosowane w Klinice.* Warsaw: State Publisher of Medical Books. 1979: 128, 212, 260
2. Epstein M. *Circ Res 1976; 39:* 619
3. Greenleaf JE, Shvartz F, Keil LC. *Aviat Space Environ Med 1981; 52:* 320
4. Khosla SS, DuBois AB. *J Appl Physiol 1979; 46:* 703
5. Bonjour JP, Malvin RL. *Am J Physiol 1970; 218:* 1555

SPECIFIC ANGIOTENSIN BINDING TO HUMAN BLOOD CELLS

J F E Mann, Jeanne M Sis, E Ritz

Medizinische Klinik, Universität Heidelberg, Heidelberg, FRG

Introduction

Angiotensin II, the effector peptide of the renin-angiotensin-system, acts on its target cells by specific, cell-surface receptors. The binding characteristics and functional changes have been well characterised in several organs of various animal species [1–3]. For obvious reasons, specific binding of angiotensin to human organs cannot readily be studied. Only blood cells can be used for controlled and repeated studies. We therefore investigated whether angiotensin binds specifically to human blood cells. Such binding sites could serve as indicators for physiologically more relevant receptors, for example on adrenal cells.

Materials and methods

Studies with platelets

Blood was obtained from healthy volunteers, anticoagulated with sodium-citrate, and centrifuged at 200g for 10 minutes. Platelet rich plasma was separated, washed twice with 10 volumes of Hank's buffer containing 5mM ethylenediamine-tetra-acetate (EDTA), 1mM di-isopropylfluorophosphate (DFP), 0.2 per cent bovine serum albumin (BSA) (pH 7.4, 'assay-buffer'), and the pellet was resuspended in the assay buffer to a concentration of 10^6 cells/μl. The final incubation volume was 100μl. ^{125}I-angiotensin II was incubated with the platelets at 37°C. To determine non-specific binding, unlabelled (Ile^5)-angiotensin II (10^5M) was added. The incubation was stopped by adding 2ml of chilled saline. Bound from free hormone was separated by centrifugation at 4°C, and radioactivity in the pellet measured in a gamma-well-counter.

Studies with mononuclear leucocytes

Blood from healthy volunteers, anticoagulated with sodium-citrate, was centrifuged at 200g for 10 minutes. Platelet-rich plasma was discarded and replaced by an equal volume of sodium phosphate buffer (0.1M, pH 7.4). Mononuclear leucocytes were then prepared by centrifugation through a ficoll-isopaque density gradient. Cells were then further processed as described for the platelets. Final incubation volume was 100–200μl for 10^4 cells/μl.

Results

Studies with platelets

When platelets were incubated with ^{125}I-angiotensin II (0.05nM) at 37°C for three hours in the presence of 1mM DFP, thin-layer chromatography showed no evidence of peptide degradation. However, with various other proteinase-inhibitors (e.g. phenylmethysulfuronyl-fluoride, dithiothreitol), the octapeptide was degraded. Platelets showed a time-dependent uptake of ^{125}I-angiotensin II which was suppressed by greater than 90 per cent unlabelled angiotensin II (Figure 1). At 22°C, binding of ^{125}I-angiotensin II was slower and did not reach a plateau within three hours. With increasing concentrations of ^{125}I-angiotensin II, binding was saturable and reached a plateau between 0.2 and 0.4nM ^{125}I-angiotensin II. Scatchard plots were calculated from incubations with increasing concentrations of ^{125}I-angiotensin II in several volunteers. Some variation was observed for the calculated maximum number of binding sites, but not for

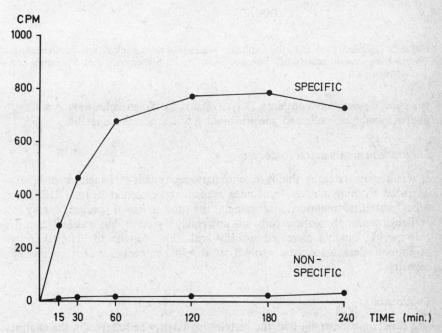

Figure 1. Time course of ^{125}I-angiotensin II binding to human platelets. For details see text

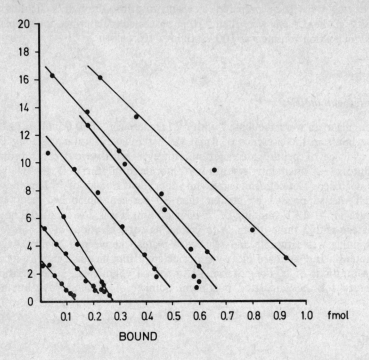

B/F x 100

Figure 2. Scatchard plots from incubations of platelets of several volunteers with increasing, saturating concentrations of ^{125}I-angiotensin II. Each regression line represents one individual

apparent dissociation constants (K_D) (Figure 2). When cells were lysed and plasma membranes collected, specific binding was almost undetectable.

Studies with mononuclear leucocytes

It was demonstrated by thin-layer chromatography that ^{125}I-angiotensin II was degraded by mononuclear leucocytes even in the presence of 1mM DFP and other proteinase-inhibitors. Accordingly, the time course of specific binding of ^{125}I-angiotensin II to these cells did not reach a plateua, but was bell-shaped. Non-specific binding increased steadily with time. Similar to platelets, lysis of mononuclear leucocytes resulted in a >90 per cent decrease in binding capacity.

Comments

Our results demonstrate, that the platelet model may be suitable for the clinical study of human angiotensin receptors. This is in accordance with one study [4], but is contradictory to another [5] on stable binding of angiotensin II to mononuclear leucocytes but not to platelets. In conjunction with the wealth of data on angiotensin receptors in animals, further studies with the platelet receptor should delineate angiotensin receptor regulation in man.

References

1 Catt KJ, Harwood JP, Aguilera G, Dufau ML. *Nature 1979; 280:* 109
2 Gunther St, Gimbrone MA, Wayne Alexander R. *Circ Res 1980; 47:* 278
3 Mann JFE, Schiller PW, Schiffrin EL et al. *Am J Physiol 1981; 241:* R124
4 Moore TJ, Williams GH. *Circ Res 1982; 51:* 314
5 Shimada K, Yazaki Y. *J Biochem 1978; 84:* 1013

PRORENIN AND BETA-BLOCKADE IN HYPERTENSION

F McKenna, A M Davison

St James's University Hospital, Leeds, United Kingdom

Summary

The role of prorenin in relation to beta-blockade has received little attention. We have studied both active renin and prorenin before and during treatment of hypertension with either nadolol or metoprolol in 44 patients. The ratio of active renin to prorenin before treatment was the best predictor of response; the fall in active renin with treatment did not correlate with the fall in blood pressure, whereas prorenin showed an inverse correlation. We suggest that plasma prorenin is an important indicator of the renin status in hypertensive patients.

Introduction

The significance of plasma renin as a predictor of efficacy of beta-blockade in the treatment of hypertension is controversial. Buhler et al demonstrated a close correlation between pre-treatment renin and response to treatment with propranolol [1], but the majority of subsequent studies have failed to repeat their findings [2]. The reasons for this are unclear, although in some studies this can be explained by the inadvertent assay of a combination of both inactive (prorenin) and active renin, the prorenin masking the values of active renin [3].

Prorenin itself has received little attention other than to be recognised as a hazard in renin assay methodology; its physiological role remains unknown. The importance of cardioselectivity of beta-blockers on the secretion of active renin has been studied but this has not been evaluated with respect to prorenin. We therefore examined a selective (metoprolol) and non-selective (nadolol) beta-blocker to compare the effect of these drugs in the treatment of hypertension and to correlate their hypotensive effect with both active renin and prorenin.

566

Methods

Patients

Forty-eight patients aged 21—65 years with essential (38 patients) or renal (10 patients) hypertension attending a hypertension outpatient clinic were studied. Exclusion criteria were the presence of heart disease, asthma, diabetes mellitus, previous stroke, liver disease or renal failure (serum creatinine >150 μmol/L). All patients gave their informed consent.

Trial design

The trial was of a double-blind placebo run-in design, comparing once daily doses of nadolol with metoprolol. Previous anti-hypertensive therapy (including diuretics) was stopped prior to entry. Following a four week period of control observations on placebo, patients were randomly allocated to receive (double-blind) either nadolol 80mg or metoprolol 100mg tablets. Visits were at -4, -2, 0, 2, 6, 10, 14 and 18 weeks. Initial dose of active drug was one tablet daily commencing at week 0. Dosage was thereafter increased at each visit until either erect diastolic blood pressure was less than 90mmHg or to a maximum of four tablets daily. Patients were seen 24 hours after taking their last tablet; blood pressure and heart rate were recorded after five minutes recumbency, after standing for one minute, and during, at the end of and two minutes after a five minute exercise on a static bicycle ergometer with a 70 watt load. Blood pressure was measured indirectly using a mercury manometer; the diastolic blood pressure was taken as Korotkov phase IV. Each blood pressure recording was the mean of three readings. Patients were requested to maintain their usual dietary sodium intake throughout the study.

Samples for renin and biochemistry were taken after five minutes recumbency, at 0 and 18 weeks. Blood for renin was collected into EDTA tubes on ice and then centrifuged at 4°C, the plasma being stored at -20°C until analysis. Active renin was measured by radioimmunoassay of angiotensin I generated at 37°C for one hour in pH 5.3 buffer [4]. Total renin was estimated by exposing the serum to trypsin (1mg per ml) with angiotensin I generation as above. Prorenin was calculated as total renin minus active renin.

Statistical analysis

Differences between the groups were analysed by Student's t-test; correlation between blood pressure and renin was by Pearson correlation coefficients and verified by Kendal rank correlation.

Results

Forty-four patients (35 essential hypertension, 9 renal hypertension) completed the study, 22 patients on each drug. Four patients were withdrawn; one for non-compliance, one for bronchospasm (on nadolol), one for fluid retention (on placebo) and one for an unacceptable increase in blood pressure whilst on placebo.

TABLE I. Blood pressure and heart rate before and after beta-blockade

	Week	SUPINE			ERECT			MID EXERCISE			END EXERCISE			POST EXERCISE		
		Systolic blood pressure mmHg	Diastolic blood pressure mmHg	Pulse rate (beats/ min)	Systolic blood pressure mmHg	Diastolic blood pressure mmHg	Pulse rate (beats/ min)	Systolic blood pressure mmHg	Diastolic blood pressure mmHg	Pulse rate (beats/ min)	Systolic blood pressure mmHg	Diastolic blood pressure mmHg	Pulse rate (beats/ min)	Systolic blood pressure mmHg	Diastolic blood pressure mmHg	Pulse rate (beats/ min)
Nadolol	0	165.4	100.0	86.6	161.9	102.9	90.8	198.0	109.8	131.9	193.6	102.1	132.1	158.5	102.9	98.2
	18	152.6	88.7	59.3	148.0*	92.2	62.3	174.7	97.2	127.2	171.3	90.4	101.0	145.6	90.6	65.7
Metoprolol	0	161.9	100.9	82.9	162.6	106.0	89.3	204.5	112.4	99.7	195.5	100.7	128.9	164.9	105.6	95.2
	18	145.3	88.7	73.9	148.6	95.7	78.4	180.5	98.7	117.1	177.9	89.9	120.0	146.1	92.3	80.8

Differences between blood pressure at week 0 and week 18, $p < 0.001$ except * where $p < 0.05$

Effects on blood pressure and heart rate (Table I)

Blood pressure was reduced equally by both drugs before, during and after exercise. Both drugs reduced heart rate, the effect of nadolol being greater than that of metoprolol. After 18 weeks' treatment the mean daily dose of metoprolol was 291mg/day and of nadolol was 189mg/day.

Effects on plasma renin

There was no difference between the two groups in the pre-treatment values of either active renin, prorenin or total renin. There was a slight rise in total renin with treatment (14.5–16.0ng/ml/hour) although this failed to reach significance. Active renin decreased with treatments (2.6–1.7ng/ml/hour $p<0.001$) and prorenin increased significantly (11.8–14.3ng/ml/hour $p<0.02$).

Correlation between fall in blood pressure and pre-treatment renin

There was a direct correlation in all patients between the pre-treatment active renin and the fall in systolic ($p<0.02$, $r = 0.37$) and diastolic ($p<0.02$, $r = 0.36$) pressure whilst standing, and with the diastolic pressure after exercise ($p<0.05$, $r = 0.35$). There was a similar correlation with diastolic pressure with nadolol ($p<0.02$, $r = 0.53$) but not with metoprolol.

There was an inverse correlation between pre-treatment prorenin and the fall in supine diastolic pressure in all patients ($p<0.05$, $r = -0.33$). There was a significant inverse correlation with diastolic pressure whilst supine ($p<0.002$, $r = -0.62$), erect ($p<0.05$, $r = -0.43$) and after exercise ($p<0.02$, $r = -0.55$) with metoprolol, but a lack of correlation with nadolol.

There was a positive correlation between the ratio of active to prorenin before treatments and the fall in systolic ($p<0.01$, $r = 0.40$) and diastolic ($p<0.005$, $r = 0.42$) pressure whilst standing, and the systolic ($p<0.005$, $r = 0.45$) and diastolic ($p<0.025$, $r = 0.37$) pressure after exercise, without any difference between either drugs.

Relation between fall in blood pressure and changes in renin

There was no correlation between the fall in blood pressure and the fall in active renin when the groups were assessed either separately or together.

There was an inverse correlation between the increase in prorenin and the fall in systolic ($p<0.05$, $r = -0.36$) and diastolic ($p<0.05$, $r = -0.34$) pressure whilst standing and with the diastolic pressure after exercise ($p<0.005$, $r = -0.49$), without any difference between the two groups.

There was a positive correlation between the change in ratio of active to prorenin and the fall in systolic ($p<0.02$, $r = 0.39$) and diastolic ($p<0.05$, $r = 0.32$) pressure whilst standing and the diastolic pressure after exercise ($p<0.02$, $r = 0.42$). There was a significant correlation in the nadolol group with the fall in systolic pressure after exercise ($p<0.02$, $r = 0.55$).

There was a within-patient correlation between active renin and prorenin prior to beta-blockade (p<0.025, r = 0.34); the correlation was stronger after treatment (p<0.001, r = 0.55).

Discussion

The presence of a circulating inactive precursor of renin, so-called prorenin, has been the subject of recent review [5]. Its response to both physiological stimuli and drugs differs from active renin [6], and as prorenin constitutes the majority of circulating renin the inadvertent assay of total renin (active + prorenin) may mask any correlation between the hypotensive effect of beta-blockade and renin. This may explain the failure of some studies to find such a correlation, but negative results in others which have measured active rather than total renin are more difficult to explain.

The role of prorenin as a predictor of reponse to beta-blockade has not previously been evaluated, although Atlas et al [7] have demonstrated an inverse correlation between an increase in prorenin and the fall in systolic pressure during treatment with propranolol. It is likely however, that in their studies the value of prorenin was underestimated as they used a cryo-activation procedure which we believe to be less efficient than the use of a proteolytic enzyme such as trypsin.

We have demonstrated a correlation between the reduction in blood pressure to beta-blockade and both the pre-treatment active renin and its ratio with prorenin. In addition we have demonstrated some correlation with pre-treatment prorenin. The effect of beta-blockade was correlated both with the rise in prorenin and the change in ratio of active to prorenin, but not with the fall in active renin alone. This suggests that prorenin may be a better indicator of renin status than active renin which is more sensitive to variation from posture and salt intake. Also, because the fraction of prorenin is much greater than active renin, only a small proportion of prorenin needs to be cryo-activated (e.g. during collection and storage of samples) to significantly alter the assay value of active renin. These results demonstrate the importance of estimating both active renin and prorenin in order to recognise important correlates with treatment.

We found little difference between the selective and non-selective beta-blocker except on the correlation between their hypotensive effect and the pre-treatment values of renin, which is difficult to explain. Some debate has centred on the relevance of cardioselectivity to the effect of beta-blockers on renin secretion [8]. We did not demonstrate a difference between the two drugs on either the fall in active renin or the rise in prorenin with treatment.

These findings strongly support the concept that not only is the renin status of hypertensive patients relevant in their response to beta-blockade but suggest that the mode of action of the drugs may be related to the renin-angiotensin system. The best responders to beta-blockade were patients with a high ratio of active renin to prorenin, i.e. a high active renin and low prorenin. We would like to postulate that the in vivo activation of prorenin to active renin in such patients is accelerated and that beta-blockade reduces activation of prorenin and tends to return the system to normal. Observation of a stronger correlation between active and prorenin within patients after treatment also supports this.

We conclude from the results of this study that plasma renin is an important indicator of the response to treatment of hypertension with beta-blockers. It is necessary to measure both active renin and prorenin as the ratio between the two offers the best indicator of response. We suggest that this study helps to explain some of the current controversy.

Acknowledgments

We would like to thank E R Squibb & Company Limited for their financial support for this study. We also thank Dr K MacRae, Senior Lecturer in Statistics, Charing Cross Hospital Medical School, for undertaking the statistical analyses and The Yorkshire Kidney Research Fund for the use of their research laboratory.

References

1 Buhler FR, Laragh JH, Baer L et al. *N Engl J Med 1972; 287:* 1209
2 Prichard BNC. *Br J Clin Pharmacol 1978; 5:* 379
3 Amery A, Lijnen P, Fagard R, Reybrouck T. *Lancet 1976; ii:* 849
4 Haber E, Koeruer T, Page LB et al. *J Clin Endocrinol Metab 1969; 29:* 1349
5 Sealey JE, Atlas SA, Laragh JH. *Clin Sci 1982; 63:* 133s
6 Derkx FHM, Gool JMG, Wenting GJ et al. *Lancet 1976; ii:* 496
7 Atlas SA, Sealey JE, Laragh JH, Moon C. *Lancet 1977; ii:* 785
8 Weber MA, Stokes GS, Gain JM. *J Clin Invest 1974; 54:* 1413

INCREASE IN SERUM POTASSIUM CAUSED BY BETA-2 ADRENERGIC BLOCKADE IN TERMINAL RENAL FAILURE: ABSENCE OF MEDIATION BY INSULIN OR ALDOSTERONE

P Arrizabalaga, J Montoliu, A Martinez Vea,
L Andreu, J López Pedret, L Revert

Hospital Clinic, University of Barcelona, Spain

Summary

To test the hypothesis that beta-blockade might impair potassium (K) tolerance in terminal renal failure we gave propranolol, and then atenolol, to a group of 12 clinically stable non-diabetic patients on chronic haemodialysis and on a constant diet containing approximately 50mEq of K/day.

Propranolol, 60 to 80mg/day for 10 days induced a significant increase in predialysis serum K from 5.1 ± 0.1 to 5.8 ± 0.2mEq/L ($p < 0.005$). Atenolol (50mg/day for 10 days) in the same group of patients did not produce a significant change in predialysis serum K (5.5 ± 0.2 vs 5.2 ± 0.2mEq/L). Both propranolol and atenolol decreased heart rate but neither drug induced significant changes in plasma aldosterone, arterial pH, serum insulin or blood glucose. Thus in haemodialysis patients, beta-2 adrenergic blockade by propranolol is associated with a significant increase in serum K not mediated by pH, aldosterone or insulin, and probably due to inhibition of intracellular K uptake. Selective beta-1 adrenergic blockade by atenolol at low doses does not change serum K, and therefore, if indicated, cardioselective beta-blockers might be preferable to non-selective drugs in haemodialysis patients.

Introduction

The balance between intracellular and extracellular potassium (K) content is influenced by pH, plasma bicarbonate, aldosterone and insulin [1]. In addition, beta-adrenergic stimulation has been recently shown to induce intracellular K uptake in normal subjects [2, 3] through a mechanism involving stimulation of the beta-2 adrenoreceptor [4] and independent from insulin or aldosterone changes [3].

In approximately half of uraemic patients, we have noted that an epinephrine infusion lowers serum K. This effect is not mediated by changes in arterial pH, serum insulin or aldosterone and the simultaneous administration of propranolol blocks the effect of epinephrine on serum K [5]. Accordingly, beta-blockade might be expected to impair K tolerance in renal failure. To test this hypothesis we gave propranolol and then atenolol to a group of haemodialysis patients to determine if these drugs could modify the equilibrium between intracellular and extracellular K.

Methods

After informed consent, 12 essentially anuric, non-diabetic and clinically stable haemodialysis patients were selected to participate in the study. There were six males and six females, aged 35 to 71 years (mean 54 years). Time on dialysis ranged from 6 to 108 months (mean 66 months). All patients were normotensive or had occasional and slight volume-dependent hypertension. Throughout the study the patients were maintained on their usual diet, containing approximately 50mEq of K/day. No clinical incidences that could result in hypercatabolism occurred during the study period. No patient was taking medication other than aluminium hydroxide and/or iron. Atrioventricular block or clinically evident liver disease was absent in every case.

Propranolol was administered for 10 days; 60mg/day in three divided doses to patients with dry weights up to 60kg, patients over 60kg received 80mg of propranolol/day in two divided doses.

Immediately before and after the period of drug administration, the following pre-haemodialysis values were measured: blood pressure, heart rate, arterial pH, blood glucose, and serum K by standard techniques, and serum insulin and aldosterone by radioimmunoassay.

After completion of the propranolol trial there was a two week period without beta-blocking medication followed by a second phase using the cardioselective beta-1 blocker atenolol in a single daily dose of 50mg for 10 days. The dose was kept intentionally low to avoid losing cardioselectivity. The same procedures and laboratory determinations carried out during the propranolol trial were employed during atenolol administration.

Patient compliance was ensured by tablet counts and by monitoring heart rate.

Results

Two patients were withdrawn from the study, one for non-compliance and one for intolerance to medication (hypotension during dialysis) in the other patient.

In the remaining 10 patients, propranolol induced a significant increase in serum K, from 5.1 ± 0.1mEq/L ($\pm$ = SEM) to 5.8 ± 0.2mEq/L ($p < 0.005$). In this group of patients, a control serum K measured three months prior to the initiation of the study, was essentially equal to that obtained immediately before the initiation of propranolol (Figure 1).

Two additional patients denied permission for continuation of the study with atenolol. In the remaining eight patients from the original group, atenolol did not produce a significant change in predialysis serum K, which in fact decreased slightly, from 5.5 ± 0.2 to 5.2 ± 0.2mEq/L, p = NS (Figure 1).

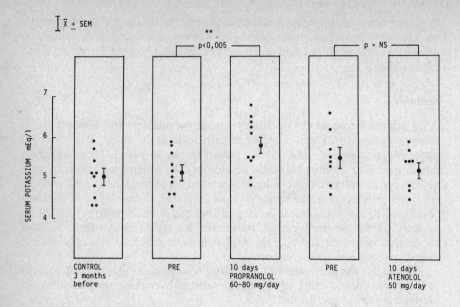

Figure 1. Changes in serum K induced by propranolol and atenolol in haemodialysis patients

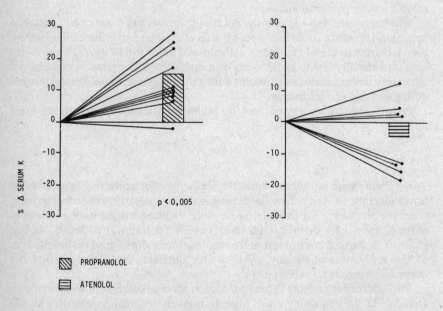

Figure 2. Percent change in serum K in relation to basal values after administration of propranolol or atenolol. Bars for each drug indicate mean magnitude of percentual change

In relative terms, propranolol induced a 14 ± 3 per cent increase in serum K in relation to basal values, whereas atenolol actually favoured a small decrement (−4 ± 4%) (Figure 2). The comparison in the difference in the percentual changes in serum K observed with the two drugs was statistically significant (p<0.005).

Both propranolol and atenolol decreased heart rate (72 ± 2 to 66 ± 2 and 76 ± 3 to 62 ± 3 beats per minute respectively, p<0.02 for both). As shown in Table I, neither propranolol nor atenolol induced significant changes in pre-dialysis plasma aldosterone, arterial pH, serum insulin or blood glucose.

TABLE I. Values of various measurements before and 10 days after propranolol or atenolol

	Heart rate beats/min	Mean arterial blood pressure mmHg	Renin activity ng ml^{-1}h^{-1}	Plasma aldosterone ng/dl	Serum glucose mg/dl	Serum insulin mU/ml	Arterial pH
			PROPRANOLOL				
Pre	72±2	108± 8	1.19±0.7	57 ±11	90.4±5	31.6±6	7.34±0.01
At 10 days	66±2	108± 8	0.26±0.1	51 ±10.7	93.3±3.5	29.6±3.5	7.34±0.01
p	<0.02*	NS	NS	NS	NS	NS	NS
			ATENOLOL				
Pre	76±3	107± 8	1.13±0.5	63.7±14	94.5±3.7	23.6±2.7	7.34±0.01
At 10 days	62±3	107±13	0.68±0.4	44.6±18	88 ±3.3	18 ±1.7	7.35±0.01
p	<0.02*	NS	NS	NS	NS	NS	NS

* In relation to initial values

Discussion

The results obtained in this study indicate that the use of propranolol in haemo-dialysis patients is associated with a significant rise in serum K. Since there were no simultaneous changes in arterial pH, blood glucose, serum insulin or plasma aldosterone, it must be deduced that the increase in serum K seen with propranolol was not mediated by any of these factors and was probably due to inhibition of beta adrenergic facilitation of intracellular K uptake. Furthermore, this effect seems to be due to specific blockade of a beta-2 adrenergic receptor, because the administration in the same group of patients of the cardioselective beta-1 blocker atenolol at low doses failed to produce any significant change in serum K or in the other parameters measured, with the exception of heart rate. In addition the existence in our patients of end-stage renal failure with negligible residual urine output makes it highly unlikely that variations in the urinary excretion of K could have accounted for the decrease in serum K. It could be argued that whereas propranolol and atenolol are supposed to have similar beta-blocking

575

potency, as measured by their inhibition of isoproterenol-induced tachycardia [6], some of our patients received atenolol doses that were slightly lower than those used for propranolol. However, whereas propranolol is metabolised mainly by the liver, atenolol has a predominant renal route of excretion and small doses can accumulate in patients with renal failure [7]. We have observed severe hypotension caused by a single 100mg dose of atenolol [8], and indeed in this study, the reduction in heart rate was more pronounced with atenolol than with propranolol. Therefore we believe that the disparity between atenolol and propranolol with respect to their action on serum K in this group of patients cannot be explained by dose differences, which were minimal.

An increase in serum K has been observed in normal subjects during propranolol treatment [9]. Recently, this increase has been shown to be unrelated to the renin-angiotensin-aldosterone system [10], thus lending further support to our hypothesis of a mechanism based on blockade of the normal beta-2 adrenergic facilitation of intracellular K uptake. Nevertheless it should be noted that while the increase in serum K with the use of propranolol in normal subjects is small and clinically insignificant [9, 10], patients with renal failure are obviously at an increased risk of hyperkalaemia from beta-blockade.

Beta-blockers are commonly employed in patients with chronic renal failure, for the treatment of hypertension or ischaemic heart disease. The results of this study favour the view that propranolol should be used with caution in this group of patients because it can accentuate their spontaneous tendency to hyperkalaemia. When indicated, and since they do not seem to adversely influence serum K, cardioselective beta-blockers at low doses are therefore preferable to non-selective drugs.

Acknowledgments

The authors thank Dr A Botey for helpful suggestions and advice, the staff of the Hormonal Laboratory for their co-operation and Ms Isabel Roselló for help in the preparation of this manuscript.

References

1   Sterns RH, Cox M, Feig PU Singler I. *Medicine (Baltimore) 1980; 60:* 330
2   Rosa RM, Silva PS, Young JB et al. *N Engl J Med 1980; 302:* 431
3   De Fronzo RA, Bia M, Birkhead G. *Kidney Int 1981; 20:* 83
4   Tyler K, De Fronzo R, Bia M. *Kidney Int 1982; 21:* 159 (abstract)
5   Martinez Vea A, Montoliu J, Andreu L et al. *Proc EDTA 1982; 19:* 756
6   McDevitt DG. *Br J Clin Pharmacol 1977; 4:* 413
7   McAinsh J, Holmes BF, Smith S et al. *Clin Pharmacol Ther 1980; 28:* 302
8   Montoliu J, Botey A, Darnell A, Revert L. *Med Clin (Barc) 1981; 76:* 365
9   Buhler FR, Burkart E, Lutold BE et al. *Am J Cardiol 1975; 36:* 653
10   Traub YM, Rabinov M, Rosenfeld JB, Treuherr S. *Clin Pharmacol Ther 1980; 28:* 765

EFFECTS OF ENALAPRIL ON BLOOD PRESSURE AND RENAL HAEMODYNAMICS IN ESSENTIAL HYPERTENSION

G J Navis, P E de Jong, A J M Donker, D de Zeeuw

State University Hospital, Gronigen, The Netherlands

Summary

The effects of enalapril were assessed in a double-blind study versus propranolol. Twenty-two patients with essential hypertension were titrated with either enalapril (5, 10 and 20mg twice daily) or propranolol (40, 80 and 120mg twice daily). With propranolol blood pressure decreased from 154/101 ± 4/1 to 146/98 ± 5/2mmHg (mean ± SEM); with enalapril it decreased from 151/103 ± 3/1 to 134/92 ± 4/2mmHg, both after 12 weeks of therapy. Effective renal plasma flow remained unchanged in the propranolol group whereas it increased from 413 ± 19 to 445 ± 27ml/min ($p < 0.05$) with enalapril. Glomerular filtration rate remained unchanged at either medication. Enalapril is an effective anti-hypertensive agent with a favourable effect on renal haemodynamics.

Introduction

Angiotensin converting enzyme (ACE) inhibitors are potent anti-hypertensive agents in essential as well as renal hypertension. The effect of these drugs on renal haemodynamics is of interest as their predominant mode of action is thought to be blockade of the renin-angiotensin-aldosterone system [1]. Captopril was found to increase renal plasma flow in essential hypertension (EH) in spite of a concomitant fall in blood pressure (BP) [2]. Recently a series of new ACE-inhibitors not containing an SH-group like captopril have been developed [3]. The absence of the SH-group could be of value as this mercapto group is suspected of playing a key role in the pathogenesis of several side effects of captopril [4], especially with high doses, and in certain high-risk patients. We investigated the renal and systemic effects of one of these new agents, enalapril (MK 421), in uncomplicated mild to moderate EH in a double-blind study with propranolol.

Patients and methods

Twenty-two patients with a mild to moderate EH defined as a supine diastolic BP of 95–115mmHg after at least four weeks of placebo therapy were studied.

All had normal renal and hepatic function and all had stopped previous anti-hypertensive medication. They visited the outpatient clinic twice weekly for four months. They were instructed to adhere to a diet containing 100mmol of sodium and 100mmol of potassium daily. BP was measured after 10 minutes of supine rest with a standard mercury sphygmomanometer; the average of three sequential readings was recorded.

Diastolic BP was taken at the disappearance of the audible pulse beat (Korotkoff V). Twenty-four hour urine was collected the day preceding each visit for determination of urine volume, sodium excretion and creatinine excretion. After stabilisation of BP on placebo the patients were randomised to receive either enalapril (5mg twice daily) or propranolol (40mg twice daily). The dosage was increased after four and eight weeks of therapy to 10 and 20mg enalapril twice daily and to 80 and 120mg propranolol twice daily, respectively, if the diastolic BP did not fall below 90mmHg. Renal function studies were performed before starting active therapy, on the lowest dose of either medication (after 4 weeks) and on the highest dose of either medication (after 12 weeks). Effective renal plasma flow (ERPF) and glomerular filtration rate (GFR) were measured simultaneously using a constant infusion of ^{131}I-Hippuran and ^{125}I-iothalamate, respectively [5]. Results are expressed as values per 1.73m^2 body surface area. During a further period of 12 weeks, hydrochloro-thiazide was added in either group if inadequate BP control had been achieved on propranolol or enalapril alone.

The Wilcoxon two-sample test and the Wilcoxon test for paired data were used for statistical analysis.

Results

Both patient groups were similar with respect to their mean age, sex-ratio, Quetelet-index, duration of the hypertension and initial BP. In the propranolol group only three of 11 patients achieved the criterion for satisfactory BP control (diastolic BP < 90mmHg). Supine BP decreased from 154/101 ± 4/1mmHg (mean ± SEM) on placebo to 148/94 ± 5/3 and 146/98 ± 5/2mmHg after four and 12 weeks, respectively. After 12 weeks the dose was 40mg b.d. in two patients, 80mg b.d. in three patients and 120mg b.d. in six patients. Thus, in eight of these 11 patients diastolic BP remained ≥ 90mmHg and additional therapy was needed. In the enalapril group five of 11 patients achieved BP control with enalapril only. BP decreased from 151/103 ± 3/1mmHg on placebo to 140/93 ± 5/2 and 134/92 ± 4/2mmHg after four and 12 weeks, respectively. The dose after 12 weeks was 5mg b.d. in two patients, 10mg b.d. in three patients and 20mg b.d. in six patients. The latter patients needed additional therapy.

Heart rate decreased from 70 ± 3 (mean ± SEM) to 63 ± 3 (p < 0.01) and 62 ± 2 beats per minute (p < 0.01) after four and 12 weeks in the propranolol group. In the enalapril group heart rate did not change (67 ± 3 versus 68 ± 3 and 67 ±3, respectively). Body weight did not change in the propranolol group (75.5 ± 5.0kg (mean ± SEM) versus 75 ± 4.1 (ns) and 74.6 ± 5.0kg (ns) after 4 and 12 weeks); in the enalapril group however, body weight decreased from

77.8 ± 4.1kg to 77.3 ± 6.9 (ns) and 75.9 ± 4.1kg (p < 0.01), respectively. No significant differences in 24-hour sodium excretion were found between the propranolol group and the enalapril group, neither on placebo nor during active therapy. Sodium excretion also did not change during the treatment period in either of the groups. In the propranolol group sodium excretion was 121 ± 11mmol/24 h (mean ± SEM), 131 ± 18 (ns) and 141 ± 17mmol/24 h (ns) at 0, 4 and 12 weeks, respectively; in the enalapril group sodium excretion was 136 ± 21, 121 ± 21 (ns) and 119 ± 14mmol/24 h (ns), respectively.

In the propranolol group ERPF did not change (423 ± 24ml/min (mean ± SEM) on placebo versus 418 ± 27ml/min (ns) after four weeks treatment with 40mg twice daily and 418 ± 30ml/min (ns) after 12 weeks of treatment (Figure 1). GFR did not change either: 105 ± 4ml/min versus 104 ± 5 (ns) and 105 ± 5ml/min (ns) after four and 12 weeks. As a consequence filtration fraction (FF) remained unchanged: 0.25 ± 0.01 (mean ± SEM) versus 0.25 ± 0.01 (ns) and 0.26 ± 0.01 (ns). In the enalapril group however, ERPF increased from 413 ± 19ml/min to 431 ± 22ml/min (ns) after four weeks of treatment with

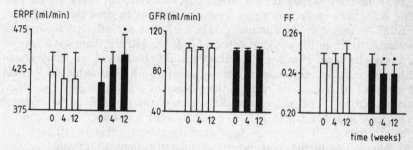

Figure 1. Effects of titration with propranolol (open bars) and enalapril (closed bars) on effective renal plasma flow, glomerular filtration rate and filtration fraction. Results are shown as mean ± SEM : p < 0.05 for differences with values at week 0

5mg twice daily, and to 445 ± 27ml/min (p < 0.05) after 12 weeks of treatment. GFR did not change: 102 ± 3ml/min on placebo versus 102 ± 3 (ns) and 103 ± 3ml/min (ns) after four weeks and 12 weeks, respectively. FF decreased from 0.25 ± 0.01 to 0.24 ± 0.01 (p < 0.05) and 0.24 ± 0.01 (p < 0.05) after four and 12 weeks therapy.

During the extension period hydrochlorothiazide was added to the medication in eight patients receiving propranolol, resulting in a further fall in BP from 146/98 ± 5/2 to 132/88 ± 3/2mmHg (mean ± SEM of 11 patients) after another 12 weeks. In the enalapril group hydrochlorothiazide was added in six patients and resulted in a further fall in BP from 134/92 ± 4/2 to 120/82 ± 6/2mmHg (mean ± SEM of 11 patients).

Minor side effects were observed in the propranolol group in two patients (stuffy nose, cold hands and feet). On careful screening of physical (particularly with respect to rash, fever, arthralgia and ageusia), immunological (anti-nuclear antibodies), haematological (w.b.c, oesinophils, differential count) and biochemical (electrolytes, transaminases, urinary protein) parameters, no side effects were observed that could be attributed to the use of enalapril.

Discussion

Enalapril appears an effective anti-hypertensive drug. A fall in BP, with a mean decrease of diastolic BP of 12 per cent, occurred in all patients and five out of 11 patients achieved normotension without additional therapy. It can be argued that these results are not impressive, more than half of the patients requiring additional therapy. However, BP decrease with enalapril was greater than with propranolol, though not statistically significant. Furthermore, in our study salt intake, though limited, was not restricted rigorously. From the experience with other ACE-inhibitors it can be expected that a more rigid dietary regimen could augment the hypotensive effect of enalapril [6].

The reduction of body weight observed in the enalapril group is of interest. The mechanism of this weight reduction could not be assessed with certainty as calorie intake was not standardised. However, the difference between the groups suggests the weight reduction in the enalapril group to be due to an intrinsic characteristic of enalapril. A natriuretic effect could well account for a decrease in body weight of this magnitude, however, our study design with urine collections every two weeks does not allow us to draw this conclusion.

ERPF increased in the enalapril group, GFR was not affected whereas BP decreased. A fall in BP would be expected to lower ERPF if there was unaltered renal vascular tone. However, the decrease in BP obtained in our study is well within the range of renal auto-regulation, therefore ERPF as well as GFR could be expected to remain unaltered in the absence of a direct effect on the renal vascular bed [7]. The increase in ERPF with unaltered GFR in the enalapril group, resulting in a fall in FF, is consistent with a vasodilator effect on the efferent arteriole. It should be kept in mind however, that redistribution of renal blood flow to the more superficial cortical nephrons that could account for the same net effect [8], is by no means excluded. Since GFR is determined by both MAP and ERPF [7], and since we found an inverse change in MAP and ERPF with a constant GFR in the enalapril group, we evaluated whether the individual changes in GFR correlated with the changes in the product of MAP and ERPF. This correlation was not statistically significant after four and 12 weeks of therapy. However, the strong correlation that has been found between the absolute values of GFR and the product of MAP and ERPF, leads us to suggest the maintained GFR to be determined by the inverse changes in MAP and ERPF.

A similar effect on renal haemodynamics in EH has been observed with other ACE-inhibitors [3]. The increase in ERPF with decreased FF has been considered a partial reversal of the abnormalities in renal haemodynamics characteristic of established EH [9]. It seems logical to consider the correction of target organ abnormalities as a beneficial feature of certain forms of anti-hypertensive treatment as compared to other forms. However, whether additional protection against final renal damage is really provided, has to be investigated in long-term studies.

Enalapril was tolerated well in our study and most patients reported feeling better on this treatment that on their previous medication. With respect to the safety of the drug no definite conclusions can be drawn, as doses used were low and patients from high-risk groups (impaired renal function and/or auto-immune disease) were excluded. A feeling of well-being of the patient is known to improve patient's compliance, especially in asymptomatic hypertensives. From this point of view enalapril deserves consideration as a drug to be used in the first line of treatment. However, in considering a drug for maintenance therapy of hypertension the ultimate criterion should be a decrease in morbidity and mortality [10]. In this respect the frequent need of additional therapy such as diuretics, that could induce unfavourable metabolic changes, should be taken into account.

In summary, enalapril appears to be an effective anti-hypertensive drug with a beneficial effect on renal haemodynamics. The long-term effects on morbidity and mortality however remain to be investigated.

Acknowledgments

We would like to thank Mrs A Drent-Bremer and Mrs PT Hesling-Kuiper for their assistance in performing the renal function studies and patient administration. Furthermore, we would like to acknowledge the support of the hypertension outpatient clinic (head: Mr BS ten Berge MD).

This work was supported by a grant of Merck, Sharp and Dohme RL. Drugs were supplied by MSD.

Renal function studies were performed by a grant (C9VI) of the Dutch Kidney Foundation (Nier Stichting Nederland).

References

1　Brunner HR, Waeber B, Turini GA et al. In Laragh JH, Bühler FR, Seldin DW, eds. *Frontiers in Hypertension Research.* New York, Heidelberg, Berlin: Springer-Verlag. 1981: 503–516
2　Zimmerman BG, Wong PC. In Horovitz ZP, ed. *Angiotensin Converting Enzyme Inhibitors.* Baltimore, Münich: Urban and Schwarzenberg. 1981: 239–253
3　Patchett AA, Harris E, Tristam EW et al. *Nature 1980; 288:* 280
4　Hoorntje SJ, Kallenberg CGM, Weening JJ et al. *Lancet 1980; i:* 1212
5　Donker AJM, van der Hem GK, Sluiter WJ, Beekhuis H. *Neth J Med 1977; 20:* 97
6　Atkinson AB, Brown JJ, Lever AF et al. *Lancet 1980; ii:* 105
7　Reubi FC. *Europ J Clin Pharmacol 1978; 13:* 185
8　Bailie MD, Barbour JA. *Am J Physiol 1975; 228:* 850
9　Hollenberg NK. In Laragh JH, Bühler FR, Seldin DW, eds. *Frontiers in Hypertension Research.* New York, Heidelberg, Berlin: Springer-Verlag. 1981: 143–147
10　Dollery CT. *Clin Sci 1981; 61:* 413,S420

Proc EDTA (1983) Vol 20

PERCUTANEOUS ANGIOPLASTY FOR TREATMENT OF RENOVASCULAR HYPERTENSION

A Dal Canton, D Russo, V Iaccarino, A Caputo, F D'Anna,
V E Andreucci

Second Faculty of Medicine, University of Naples, Italy

Summary

In this study, 10 patients with renovascular hypertension were treated with percutaneous transluminal angioplasty (PTA). The obstructive lesion was atherosclerotic in four cases, fibrodysplastic in five, and mixed in one. Stenosis was bilateral in two patients. Before PTA, all patients had sustained hypertension, in nine despite medication. Immediately after PTA, hypertension was cured (BP≤ 140/90mmHg without medication) in six patients, and improved (either a BP≤ 140/90 or a decrease in diastolic BP>15mmHg, with equal or less medication) in three patients. The one failure occurred in the only patient in which PTA did not achieve a complete dilatation of the stenosed artery. The overall success rate was 90 per cent after a mean follow-up of 17.5 months.

Introduction

Percutaneous transluminal angioplasty, originally developed by Dotter and Judkins [1], and since refined by Grüntzig and Kempe [2], has been recently used to treat renal artery stenosis, with encouraging results [3–5]. We report here our experience with PTA in 10 patients with renovascular hypertension.

Patients and methods

The study was performed in 10 patients who gave informed consent to the angioplastic procedure. Clinical data on these patients are given in Table I. Eight were males, and two females. Age ranged from 19 to 57 years, and the duration of hypertension varied from seven months to 19 years. All patients had normal renal function (serum creatinine < 1.5mg/100ml). Nine patients were on hypertensive medication, but all with unsatisfactory results. In all patients, renovascular disease was documented by angiography. A bilateral stenosis was shown in two cases (No 7 and No 8). The obstructive lesion was of atherosclerotic

TABLE I. Clinical data in 10 patients with renovascular hypertension before treatment with angioplasty

Case	Age Sex†	Blood Pressure mmHg	Duration of hypertension	Medication	Site and type+ of renal artery stenosis	Renal vein Renin ratio*
1	19 yr F	160/120	12 months	Propranolol Clonidine Chlorothiazide Amiloride	Left, Fi	1.47
2	23 yr M	170/110	16 months	Atenolol Chlorothiazide Amiloride	Right, Fi	1.1
3	30 yr M	210/110	3 years	Labetalol Hydralazine	Left, Fi	1.6
4	45 yr M	145/105	7 months	Atenolol Chlorothiazide Amiloride	Left, A	Not performed
5	57 yr M	200/120	5 years	Spironolactone Hydralazine Atenolol	Right, A	7.0
6	37 yr M	200/120	4 years	Atenolol Captopril Hydralazine	Left, Polar A	1.5
7	24 yr F	190/120	4 years	Atenolol Hydralazine	Bilateral, Fi	1.2
8	40 yr F	250/140	16 years	Frusemide Acebutolol Hydralazine	Bilateral Right, Fi Left, A	1.7
9	29 yr M	200/120	2 years		Right, Fi	2.8
10	53 yr M	200/130	19 years	Atenolol Methyldopa Hydralazine	Left, A	1.1

† M = Male; F = Female. +A = Atherosclerotic; Fi = Fibrodysplastic
* = Stenotic vs non stenotic side. In patients with bilateral stenoses, the ratio is between the more obstructed and the less obstructed side

type in four cases, of fibrodysplastic type in five, and mixed in one case (No 8, with a fibrodysplastic stenosis on the left side and an atherosclerotic one on the right side). Renal vein renin ratio was obtained in nine patients, and indicated lateralisation (ratio ⩾1.5) in five, including patient No 8 with bilateral stenoses. The ratio, instead, was clearly negative in the other patient with bilateral lesions (No 7), and in patients No 2 and 10; in patient No 1 a borderline value of 1.47 was obtained. In all patients, PTA was performed by means of a Grüntzig balloon catheter of appropriate size (5 to 7 F) introduced over a guide wire to the stenotic artery. The balloon was inflated for 10 to 15 seconds at a pressure of four to six atmospheres, and this manoeuvre was usually repeated two to three times. A control angiogram was obtained in all patients one hour following PTA. In patient Nos 1, 2, 3 and 10 repeat angiography was carried out one week to five months after PTA. In all patients, a complete clinical examination was performed at monthly intervals after PTA. Hypertension was considered as cured when blood pressure was ≤ 140/90mmHg without any medication, and improved when blood pressure was ≤ 140/90mmHg, or the diastolic blood pressure was reduced by at least 15mmHg, with the same or less anti-hypertensive medication than before angioplasty.

No anticoagulant therapy was administered, either during or following PTA.

Results

Complete dilatation of renal artery stenosis (bilateral in patient Nos 7 and 8) was documented one hour after PTA in all patients, except No 9. Even in this patient, however, the degree of stenosis was markedly reduced from 80 to 20 per cent of the luminal diameter. A repeat angiography was carried out in patient Nos 1, 2, 3 and 10. In patient No 1, the repeat examination was performed as early as one week after PTA, because hypertension had been unmodified by the procedure; a partial recurrence of the obstructive lesion was observed, and the stenosis was successfully redilated. An original stenosis greater than 80 per cent was the reason for confirming the effects of PTA after three and five months, respectively, in patient Nos 2 and 3, in both a complete dilatation was documented. In patient No 10, angiography was repeated after PTA because continued medication, with troublesome side effects, was still needed to treat hypertension. However in this patient, complete correction of the stenosis was confirmed.

The effects of PTA on blood pressure are summarised in Table II. One week after PTA, hypertension was cured in six patients (4 fibrodysplastic, 1 atherosclerotic, and 1 mixed), and was improved in three patients (all atherosclerotic). PTA was considered unsuccessful in patient No 9 (fibrodysplastic), because in this patient a reduction in blood pressure occurred only after medication with captopril was introduced. It is of interest that this unique failure occurred in only the one patient in whom an incomplete dilatation of renal artery stenosis was achieved.

Patients were followed up for five to 25 months (mean 17.5 months). At the most recent follow-up, three patients were cured (2 fibrodysplastic and 1 atherosclerotic), after a time interval from PTA of at least two years. Six patients were improved, three of which had normal blood pressure with much less medication than before PTA. In the combined cured and improved group, mean reduction in systolic blood pressure was of 51.7mmHg, and in diastolic blood pressure of 36.1mmHg. All of the four patients with a significant renal vein renin ratio in which a complete renal artery dilatation was obtained were either cured or improved. Renin ratio was positive also in patient No 9, in whom hypertension was not improved by PTA; however, no conclusion on the predictive value of renin ratio can be drawn from this result, since in patient No 9 the dilatation of renal artery stenosis was incomplete. Cure or improvement,

TABLE II. Effects of percutaneous transluminal dilatation on blood pressure in patients with renovascular hypertension

| Case | 1 week after angioplasty | | Most recent follow-up | | |
	Blood Pressure mmHg	Medication	Blood Pressure mmHg	Medication	Time since angioplasty
1*	130/90	–	140/90	Chlorothiazide	20 months
2	130/80	–	130/70	–	25 months
3	140/90	–	130/80	Atenolol	16 months
4	120/80	–	130/80	–	24 months
5	180/80	–	160/80	–	18 months
6	150/90	Captopril Hydralazine Atenolol	150/90	Captopril Hydralazine Atenolol	22 months
7	130/80	–	140/90	–	24 months
8	140/90	–	130/90	Atenolol	8 months
9	160/110	Captopril	150/80	Captopril	5 months
10	160/90	Hydralazine Atenolol Methyldopa	150/80	Hydralazine Atenolol Methyldopa	13 months

* In this case, data after the second PTA are reported

however, also occurred in four patients with negative ratios.

No major complication occurred in our patients following PTA. Transient hypotension occurred in most immediately after the procedure, which was easily treated by saline infusion. In two patients an inguinal haematoma was caused by femoral vein catheterisation, this healed by spontaneous reabsorption. In all patients, renal function remained normal at the last follow-up.

Discussion

Our results show that PTA can successfully dilate renal artery stenoses, both of fibrodysplastic and of atherosclerotic type. Eleven of the 12 stenoses in our 10 patients appeared completely dilated immediately after PTA, and even in the only case in which dilatation was incomplete (No 9), a marked reduction of the degree of stenosis was achieved.

The correction of renal artery stenoses was followed within one week by a return to normal blood pressure in five patients, improvement in three, and persistence of similar hypertension in only two cases. In one of these two cases, the stenosis had partially recurred, and normal blood pressure was achieved immediately after redilatation. The other case was that (No 9) with incomplete dilatation refused a further angioplastic procedure, was treated with captopril, and was considered a failure. A greater than 90 per cent short-term success rate was therefore obtained with PTA.

A major concern with relying on PTA for treatment of renovascular hypertension, however, is that its long-term efficacy has not yet been established [6]. In our patients, a repeat angiography was not performed routinely. In three cases, however, complete correction of the stenosis was confirmed angiographically three to five months after PTA. Further information on the duration of the effects of PTA was given by follow-up studies. Three patients, were still cured after two years. In another three, blood pressure was normal after eight to 20 months, with much less medication than before PTA. Finally, in three patients hypertension was improved, even if not normal, after 13—22 months. The overall success rate, therefore, was 90 per cent at a mean time of 17.5 months after angioplasty. These results clearly show that PTA is an effective treatment of renovascular hypertension even in the long-term, and strongly suggests that the sustained anti-hypertensive effect of PTA was associated with a persistent dilatation of the renal artery stenoses.

Admittedly, only prospective, randomised trials can definitely establish the value of PTA compared to traditional treatment of renovascular hypertension. Our results, however, seem to compare favourably with those reported by others for surgical treatment. A Co-operative Study on Renovascular Hypertension, involving 15 centres in the United States, in fact, reported an overall 50 per cent success rate; 35 per cent of successful cases, however, required nephrectomy, and the overall surgical mortality rate was of 6.8 per cent [7]. Better results were obtained by Lankford et al, who reported a 90 per cent cured-improved rate, and a five per cent postoperative mortality (8). Nephrectomy, however, was carried out in 24 per cent of patients treated by these authors, even though they emphasised their desire to preserve renal mass.

Finally, in our study, while confirming the predictive value of a renal vein renin ratio of 1.5, there was an exceptional rate (100%) of false negative ratios. These results further stress the value of a simple non surgical procedure, such as PTA, in an attempt at treatment of renovascular disease even in the absence of a clear prognostic indication.

References

1   Dotter CT, Judkins MP. *Circulation 1964; 30:* 654
2   Grüntzig A, Kempe DA. *Am J Roentgenol 1974; 132:* 547
3   Grüntzig A, Vetter W, Meier B et al. *Lancet 1978; i:* 801
4   Tegtmayer CJ, Teates CD, Crigler N et al. *Radiology 1981; 140:* 323
5   Tegtmayer CJ. *Arch Int Med 1982; 12:* 1085
6   Editorial. *Ann Intern Med 1980; 92:* 117
7   Foster JH, Maxwell MH, Franklin SS et al. *JAMA 1975; 231:* 1043
8   Lankfort NS, Donohue JP, Grim CE et al. *J Urol 1979; 122:* 439

Proc EDTA (1983) Vol 20

RENAL REVASCULARISATION IN 36 PATIENTS WITH CHRONIC TOTAL OCCLUSION OF THE RENAL ARTERY

G Dostal, J J Heihoff, H D Jakubowski, F W Eigler

University Clinic, Essen, FRG

Summary

From 1972 to 1982 36 patients with totally occluded renal arteries were operated on. Contralateral stenosis existed in 11 patients, in five of whom a bilateral operative procedure and in three of whom an additional intraluminal dilatation was performed. A revascularisation of the occluded artery was performed in 33 and a primary nephrectomy in three patients. Hospital mortality was 14 per cent, the causes of death being cardiac or cerebral complications. In spite of cure or improvement of hypertension in 75 per cent of all patients and improvement or stabilisation of pre-operative azotaemia in 11 patients, the significant postoperative mortality indicates the difficult problem of proper selection of patients for operation.

Introduction

The indications for revascularisation of chronic total renal artery occlusion are controversial. It is well known that gradual complete renal artery occlusion can occur with maintenance of renal viability from a collateral arterial supply [1–4]. However, there is doubt whether a patient with a totally occluded renal artery should undergo reconstruction, especially when the kidney supplied by the occluded artery is not functioning properly. The purpose of this study was to determine the long-term results of surgical treatment of the totally occluded renal artery in a review of 36 patients.

Patients and methods

From 1972 to 1982 36 patients underwent operation for chronic total occlusion of a renal artery. There were 21 men and 15 women ranging in age from 27 to 63 years, mean 47.4 years. Patients with acute thromboses and those whose occlusions were caused by emboli or trauma were not included in this review. Functionally important stenotic disease of the contralateral renal artery was present in 11 patients. No patient had bilateral renal artery occlusions. Occlusions occurred on the left in 19 and on the right in 17 patients. Impaired renal function, evident by a serum creatinine greater than 1.5/dl, was documented in 17 patients (range 1.5 to 7.9, mean 3.0mg/dl).

Arteriographic studies were performed in all 36 patients. Functional tests, especially renal vein renin assay or Saralasin test, were not considered necessary and were conducted only occasionally.

Reconstruction of the totally occluded renal artery was performed in 33 of the 36 patients: 11 underwent thromboendarterectomy; seven thromboendarterectomy and patch graft; 10 aorto-renal reimplantation and five aorto-renal bypass. In addition five patients underwent contralateral reconstructive procedures during the operation. Three patients were treated by primary nephrectomy. Percutaneous intraluminal dilatation was performed in another three patients with additional contralateral stenosis. In three patients additional vascular procedures were performed at the same time.

Thirty-one surviving patients were followed up at intervals ranging from 11 to 131 months (mean interval 43.3 months), six being lost to follow-up at different times postoperatively. At follow-up blood pressure was determined, and the functional status of the kidney was evaluated by determination of serum creatinine. Aortography was used only in six patients.

Results

Mortality

There were five perioperative deaths, resulting in an overall mortality rate of 13.9 per cent. These deaths followed myocardial infarction at the day of operation and six days postoperatively in two patients, myocardial failure two and seven days postoperatively in two patients and a cerebrovascular accident four days postoperatively in one patient.

There were three late deaths 7.5 to 114 months postoperatively. In one case the patient died of myocardial infarction 7.5 months after bilateral revascularisation of the renal arteries during revascularisation for an acute iliac artery occlusion. The second patient died of myocardial failure 30 months after revascularisation of the occluded artery of a solitary kidney during hospitalisation because of an ascending thrombosis of the aorta including the left reconstructed artery. The third patient died of lung carcinoma 114 months after reconstruction of the renal artery.

Complications

Thrombosis of the revascularised occluded renal artery occurred between the day of operation and the 27th postoperative day in six patients. A thrombectomy was performed in two patients. In three patients the thrombosis caused a secondary nephrectomy. In one of the thrombectomised patients a re-thrombosis was found six weeks later without further consequences. One kidney had to be removed on the fourth postoperative day due to intraparenchymal haemorrhage with massive haematuria. Thus altogether six kidneys were lost following reconstruction, resulting in a total operative failure rate of 18.2 per cent, if lethal events are excluded. Taking into account only the 31 surviving patients and including three primary nephrectomies long-lasting revascularisation was achieved in 23 patients or 64 per cent.

Postoperative blood pressure

Blood pressure responses have been defined in an earlier article from this institution [5]. According to this classification eight patients were cured, 19 patients improved and four were failures (Table I). That means a success rate of 87 per cent considering the 31 surviving patients, which is reduced to 75 per cent if all 36 patients are taken into consideration.

TABLE I. Response of blood pressure in correlation to operative method performed

Operative procedure	n	Blood pressure cured	improved	failure	death
Thromboendarterectomy with or without patch	16	3	8	3	2
Aortorenal reimplantation	10	3	6		1
Aortorenal bypass	3		1	1	1
Primary or secondary	7	2	4		1
	36	8	19	4	5

Renal function

Serum creatinine exceeding 1.5mg/dl were found in 17 patients (Table II). In this group of patients four deaths followed renal revascularisation. Excluding these patients an improvement of function was found in nine of the remaining 13 patients, in two of whom a primary nephrectomy was performed. In another two patients a long-lasting stabilisation was achieved.

Discussion

Total occlusion as the end point of progression in chronic renal artery stenosis is reported to affect approximately five per cent of all patients with stenotic disease [4], but in our experience this was 9.6 per cent [5]. Renal viability usually is maintained in cases of total renal artery occlusion by collateral perfusion. Many factors that influence the appropriateness of revascularisation versus nephrectomy have been examined, including renal length, histologic features and split renal function studies [3]. Surgical therapy is recommended by the experience reported by Whitehouse et al [4], who found frequent progression of renal failure and blood pressure control in 10 patients with non-operative treatment.

589

TABLE II. Outcome of 17 patients with pre-operative azotemia

Pat.	Age (yr)	Sex	Serum creatinine (mg/dl) pre-op	Serum creatinine (mg/dl) follow-up	Blood pressure cured or improved	Contralateral stenosis or disease	Perioperative death	Follow-up interval (months)	Comment
MC	33	f	1.5	2.0	+			72	patient lost
JK	39	m	1.5	1.3	+			36	kidney without function
WH	48	m	1.5	1.9 prim. nephr.	+			28	
RF	34	m	1.5	1.1	+			15	
WW	63	m	1.6	-		+	+	2 days	
AJ	58	m	1.6	1.7	+	+		43	patient lost
HL	51	m	1.7	1.4				24	
SS	46	f	1.8	1.5	+			13	
GF	54	m	2.0	-		+	+	7 days	
WD	58	m	2.4	-		+	+	6 days	
AL	45	f	2.7	3.2				18	
JW	38	m	3.2	2.8	+			11	thrombosis
MH	27	m	3.4	2.9 prim. nephr.	+	+		131	patient lost
JC	48	m	4.0	1.0	+	single kidney		30	death
FB	58	m	4.5	3.2	+	+		7.5	death
KS	51	f	5.9	-		+	+	4 days	
JW	47	f	7.9	7.1	+	no function		25	

The significant incidence of bilateral disease with progression of stenosis in the contralateral kidney makes preservation of renal tissue desirable. Our experience shows, that in a high percentage a long-lasting influence on renal function and blood pressure can be achieved by salvage of the kidney, but that there was a high perioperative mortality. In 17 of the 36 patients preservation of renal function was the main indication for reconstructive intervention, and with four of five deaths, mortality is nearly confined to this group. Factors of assumed possible influence on this are analysed in Table III. Sex, generalised arteriosclerosis and local complications were of no importance for survival, whereas age, bilateral involvement and serum creatinine elevation were significantly greater in the patients who died. Out of 19 patients with normal renal function only one patient died (5.3%) in contrast to four out of 17 patients with impaired renal function (23.5%).

Table IV analyses the possible influence of the operative method on death

TABLE III. Influence of clinical factors on perioperative mortality

		mean age (yr)	male	female	bilateral procedure	Manifestations of gen. arterioscl.	creatinine elevations	local complications
Perioperative death	5	53.4 (41−63)	3	2	4	2	1	1
Survival	31	46.4 (27−58)	18	13	1	9	13	5

TABLE IV. Influence of operative method on death and complication rates

Operative procedure on the occluded artery	n	n deaths	n thromboses
Primary nephrectomy	3		
Thromboendarterectomy	11	2	1
Thromboendarterectomy and patch plasty	7		2
Aortorenal reimplantation	10	1	
Aortorenal bypass	5	2	2
Bilateral procedures*	5	4	1

* Operative procedures included

and complication rate. Aortorenal bypass was accompanied by a significantly higher rate of fatal and nonfatal complications than other procedures, but it is demonstrated again, that bilateral procedures carry the highest risk. In regard to hypertension, nephrectomy may be the most reliable cure, but in cases where contralateral renal function is bad and preservation of renal function is critical, indication for revascularisation is important.

In conclusion this review clearly demonstrates benefits from surgical management of renovascular hypertension caused by chronically occluded renal arteries. The cured or improved status of hypertension in 85 per cent of survivors is comparable to the experience of others. Improved renal function in patients with total renal artery occlusion treated by revascularisation was achieved in 11 of 13 surviving patients. These results, obtained in a group of high risk patients indicate the difficult problem of the correct selection of patients for operation.

References

1   Flye MW, Anderson RW, Fish JC, Silver D. *Ann Surgery 1982; 195:* 346
2   Lawrie GM, Morris GC, De Bakey ME. *Surgery 1980; 88:* 753
3   Schefft P, Novick AC, Stewart BH, Straffon RA. *J Urol 1980; 124:* 184
4   Whitehouse WM, Kazmers A, Zelenock GB et al. *Surgery 1981; 89:* 753
5   Eigler FW, Dostal G, Montag H, Jakubowski HD. *Thorac Cardiovasc Surg 1983; 31:* 45

RENAL INVOLVEMENT IN SYSTEMIC AMYLOIDOSIS

M Browning, R Banks, C Tribe, P Bacon, P Hollingworth, C Kingswood, J Poulding, P Harrison, J C Mackenzie

Southmead Hospital, Bristol, United Kingdom

Summary

In a study of 124 patients with systemic amyloidosis, renal involvement was the major presenting feature in 68 per cent of patients with AA and 42 per cent with AL disease. Renal failure contributed to the deaths of 72 per cent and 33 per cent of patients respectively. In 23 renal biopsies from patients with AA disease, quantitative glomerular amyloid infiltration correlated with urinary protein excretion and with serum creatinine. Seven of these patients had repeat biopsies; change in glomerular amyloid correlated with changes in both renal function and proteinuria. Four patients with end-stage renal amyloidosis have been successfully managed on CAPD for 37 patient months.

Introduction

Amyloidosis is an uncommon disease which is characterised by the widespread deposition of homogeneous protein fibrils. Renal involvement frequently occurs and is a major cause of morbidity and mortality [1]. Characterisation of the chemical nature of the protein fibrils has led to a new system of classification of human amyloidosis [2]. Two types predominate. AA amyloidosis, which includes reactive systemic (secondary) amyloidosis, is characterised by fibrils of amyloid protein A. AL amyloidosis, which includes primary and myeloma-related amyloidosis, is characterised by fibrils derived from the light chains of the immunoglobulin molecule. We report a retrospective study of systemic amyloidosis and compare renal involvement in the clinical and pathological courses of AA and AL disease. A simple technique for the quantitation of glomerular amyloid deposition is described and its clinical relevance discussed. We also present our experience in the management of end-stage renal disease in patients with systemic amyloidosis.

Patients and methods

From 1971 to 1982 , 103 patients with systemic amyloidosis were referred to an amyloid clinic run jointly by the departments of nephrology, rheumatology and pathology. Tissue diagnosis of amyloidosis had been made prior to referral. Rectal (56%) and renal (23%) biopsies accounted for tissue diagnosis in the majority of cases, the remainder comprising liver, tongue, spleen, nerve and lymph node biopsies. Blood urea, serum creatinine, creatinine clearance and urinary protein excretion were monitored in these patients using a sequential, computerised auto-analyser (Technicon Co Ltd). An additional 21 cases were diagnosed at necropsy.

The distribution of amyloid in biopsy and necropsy material and its staining characteristics, including the potassium permanganate reaction of Wright [3], together with the presence or absence of recognised associated diseases, enabled the cases to be divided into AA and AL systemic amyloidosis.

Per cent glomerular amyloid was estimated on renal biopsy specimens stained with Sirius Red dye. The glomeruli were copied by a single, experienced technician on to a magnetised drawing board linked to a computerised planimeter (MOP Reichert-Jung). The areas of amyloid deposition were summated and expressed as a percentage of the total area within Bowman's capsule. The average of at least five glomeruli was used as an estimate of the degree of amyloid deposition within the glomeruli. The reproducibility of the technique has been reported elsewhere [4].

Results

Clinical Course

Of the 124 patients studied, AA amyloidosis accounted for 76, of which 33 were male and 43 female. Fifty-five cases were associated with rheumatoid disease, 13 with chronic infections and three with Crohn's disease. The average age at diagnosis was 57.9 (range 18–81) years.

AL amyloidosis comprised 48 cases, of which 25 were male and 23 female. Thirteen cases were associated with myelomatosis, and 11 with benign immuno-globulin dyscrasias. In the remaining 24 cases no underlying immunocyte abnormality was identified. The average age at diagnosis in AL amyloidosis was 61.7 (range 29–88) years.

The major features at the time of diagnosis of amyloidosis are shown in Table I. Renal involvement was the dominant feature at presentation in both AA and AL amyloidosis. The prognosis was poorer at all stages in the course of the disease in AL compared with AA amyloidosis. One year survival from the time of diagnosis was 67 per cent for AA and 27 per cent for AL disease (p <0.001, Logrank test), falling to 55 per cent and seven per cent respectively at two years (p < 0.001, Logrank test). All patients with AL amyloidosis had died within three years of diagnosis. In AA amyloidosis eight patients survived five years or more, with a maximum survival of 11 years.

Eighty-two (of the original 124) patients are known to have died. Necropsy was performed in 66 cases. Amyloid infiltration of the kidney was found at necropsy in all of the 36 cases of AA and in 24 of the 30 cases of AL amyloidosis. Renal failure contributed to the deaths of 26 patients with AA and 10 patients with AL disease. Non-renal amyloid involvement contributed to

TABLE I. Major presenting features at tissue diagnosis of amyloid in patients with AA and AL amyloidosis

Presenting Features	AA	AL
Renal		
proteinuria, nephrotic syndrome	44	16
renal failure	8	4
Gastrointestinal disturbance	9	13
Neuropathy	1	7
Congestive heart failure	-	7
Other	14	5
Total No of patients	76	48*

*In AL amyloidosis, two patients presented with congestive heart failure and carpal tunnel syndrome, and two with congestive heart failure and gastrointestinal distrubance

the death of only one patient with AA amyloidosis. In AL disease, however, cardiac and gastrointestinal amyloid contributed to the deaths of 13 and seven cases respectively.

Various drugs (D-penicillamine, chlorambucil, colchicine and dimethyl-sulphoxide) were used singly or in combination in the treatment of amyloidosis without consistent benefit. Details of our experience of drug treatment in AA amyloidosis is reported elsewhere [5,6].

Of six patients with end-stage renal disease and systemic amyloidosis, two patients were treated with haemodialysis, in both cases for periods of four months. One committed suicide and the other was withdrawn after intractable hypotension on dialysis. Four patients (2 with AA and 2 with AL amyloidosis) have been treated with continuous ambulatory peritoneal dialysis (CAPD) for 16, 12, 8 and 1 months. In all cases adequate control of uraemia and fluid balance has been achieved. The incidence of peritonitis in these patients (one episode per 6 months) is the same as for all other patients on CAPD in our unit (one episode per 5.7 months).

Renal biopsy

Forty-eight renal biopsies have been obtained from 40 patients. Quantitation of glomerular amyloid has been performed on 28 biopsies from 21 patients. Clinical data from patients at the time of these biopsies are given in Table II.

The degree of glomerular amyloid infiltration at initial renal biopsy was compared in the 16 cases of AA and five cases of AL amyloidosis shown in Table II. Patients with AL amyloidosis presented with a significantly greater degree of glomerular amyloid deposition than patients with AA amyloidosis (p <0.01, Wilcoxon rank sum test).

TABLE II. Data from 28 renal biopsies. Per cent glomerular amyloid is compared with serum creatinine and urinary protein at the time of biopsy

Patient	Type of Amyloid	Per cent Glomerular Amyloid	Serum Creatinine (μmol/L)	Urinary Protein Excretion (g/24 hours)
1	AA	29	–	5.0
2	AA	57	150	6.8
3	AA	55	1325	–
4 (a)	AA	13.8	84	2.2
(b)	AA	21.0	64	1.6
5 (a)	AA	25	67	7.2
(b)	AA	38	267	11.0
6 (a)	AA	26.7	359	4.0
(b)	AA	19.1	154	0.1
7 (a)	AA	10	150	0.6
(b)	AA	13.7	57	0.9
8 (a)	AA	6.7	95	0.4
(b)	AA	16.4	146	1.8
9 (a)	AA	35.3	620	19.0
(b)	AA	17.1	355	0.6
10	AA	12	61	9.5
11 (a)	AA	19.6	105	9.5
(b)	AA	38.5	78	6.6
12	AA	5.5	559	1.9
13	AA	27	112	3.0
14	AA	12	95	7.0
15	AA	9.2	60	3.6
16	AA	32	188	–
17	AL	53	155	13.0
18	AL	38	737	–
19	AL	42	127	10.7
20	AL	79	484	9.1
21	AL	65	500	2.0

In 16 initial and seven repeat biopsies that showed AA amyloid infiltration, the relationship between per cent glomerular amyloid and urinary protein excretion was studied. A significant correlation was found ($r=0.5$, $p < 0.05$). A similar correlation ($r=0.5$, $p < 0.05$) was seen between glomerular amyloid and serum creatinine in these cases. Of the seven patients with AA amyloidosis who had repeat renal biopsies performed 13–20 months after initial biopsy, five showed an increase in glomerular amyloid deposition and two a decrease. Strong correlations were found between the change in per cent glomerular amyloid and both the change in serum creatinine ($r=0.8$, $p \simeq 0.02$) and the change in urinary protein excretion ($r=0.8$, $p < 0.05$) in these patients.

Discussion

Amyloid involvement in the kidney is common in both AA and AL amyloidosis. Over two-thirds of the patients with AA and almost one half of patients with AL amyloidosis presented with the features of renal involvement. In both types of disease the majority manifested as the nephrotic syndrome or as proteinuria detected on routine testing. Relatively few patients presented with features of overt renal failure.

Progressive renal impairment however was the dominant feature in the clinical courses of both AA and AL amyloidosis, and contributed to the deaths of two-thirds of patients with AA and one-third of patients with AL amyloid disease.

The prognosis in both types of amyloidosis was poor. Our patients with AL amyloidosis fared significantly less well than those with AA disease. Several factors account this. Involvement of organs other than the kidney contributed to the deaths of the majority of patients with AL amyloidosis, but was not a factor in AA amyloidosis. Similarly, the per cent glomerular amyloid at renal biopsy was significantly greater in AL amyloidosis, but this may simply reflect presentation at a more advanced stage of the disease.

A relationship has previously been reported between the degree of glomerular amyloid deposition, estimated by semiquantitative techniques, and the severity of proteinuria [7]. Mackensen et al [8] also reported a correlation between semiquantitative glomerular amyloid and renal function. Other studies, however, have found no such association [7]. The present study has shown correlation between quantitative glomerular amyloid and both urinary protein excretion and serum creatinine in AA amyloidosis. Insufficient renal biopsies have been performed in AL amyloidosis to draw similar conclusions.

Little is known about the histological progression of amyloid deposition in the kidney. Regression of renal amyloid infiltration together with clinical improvement has been reported [9]. In the present study renal biopsy was repeated in seven patients receiving treatment for AA amyloidosis. Five showed an increase in glomerular amyloid and two a decrease. It is impossible to say whether the changes in per cent glomerular amyloid reflect progression and regression of amyloid infiltration. Changes in per cent glomerular amyloid, however, correlated well with changes in urinary protein and serum creatinine over the same period in these patients, suggesting that the histological changes reflect the clinical course of the renal disease in this condition.

For those with end-stage renal disease and systemic amyloidosis both haemo-dialysis and renal transplantation are established methods of treatment [10]. The role of long-term peritoneal dialysis has still to be determined. After 37 patient months, CAPD has provided satisfactory control of uraemia and fluid balance in four of our patients, suggesting adequate dialysis and ultrafiltration across a peritoneum potentially infiltrated with amyloid. We suggest that CAPD is the treatment of choice in selected patients with end-stage renal disease and systemic amyloidosis.

Acknowledgment

The authors are most grateful to Miss Kathryn Edmonds for her invaluable assistance in the preparation of the manuscript and Tables.

References

1   Cohen AS. *N Engl J Med 1967; 277:* 628
2   Glenner GG. *N Engl J Med 1980; 302:* 1283
3   Wright JR, Calkins E, Humphrey RL. *Lab Invest 1977; 36:* 274
4   Tribe CR, Poulding JM, Harrison P, Bacon PA. *Proc Eur Amyloid Res Symp.* Chertsey, England: Reed Books. In press
5   Bacon PA, Tribe CR, Harrison P, Mackenzie JC. *Eur J Rheumatol Inflamm 1979; 3:* 70
6   Bacon PA, Cadge B, Harrison P, Tribe CR. *Proc Eur Amyloid Res Symp.* Chertsey, England: Reed Books. In press
7   Tornroth T, Falck HM, Watin F, Wegelius O. In Glenner GG, e Costa PP, de Freitas F, eds. *Amyloid and Amyloidosis.* Amsterdam: Excerpta Medica. 1980: 191–199
8   Mackensen S, Grund KE, Bader R, Bohle A. *Virchows Arch (Pathol Anat) 1977; 375:* 159
9   Falck HM, Tornroth T, Skrifvars B, Wegelius O. *Acta Med Scand 1979; 205:* 651
10 Leading Article. *Lancet 1980; i:* 1062

Open Discussion

NICHOLLS (Sheffield) I should like to comment on your use of a linear regression for change in glomerular amyloid versus change in serum creatinine, because creatinine is not a linear quantity, and a change of 200μmol/L for instance from 100 to 300μmol/L is of greatly different significance from a change from 700 to 900μmol/L.

BROWNING Are you suggesting that we should have plotted our results as a reciprocal?

NICHOLLS You should have made some attempt to look at glomerular filtration rate by whatever method you chose.

BROWNING We found that looking at creatinine clearance there was not a correlation between glomerular amyloid and the creatinine clearance in these patients.

ROBINSON (Birmingham) I would like to ask two questions. Firstly, in the two patients in whom there appeared to be a regression of amyloid on biopsy findings, was this due to a sampling variation or did it correlate with proteinuria and creatinine in the way you suggested in the overall group? Secondly, I would like to congratulate you on your results of CAPD in these patients. We have rather similar experiences on fewer patients. One wonders whether this is comparable to the results achieved in early days with diabetics. This is an important point as many people appear to discard patients with amyloid as being unsuitable for treatment. I hesitate, however, to draw a conclusion that CAPD is better than haemodialysis as we have treated a patient with AA amyloidosis very successfully for several years on haemodialysis until he developed a septicaemia from an abscess which lay in his osteomyelitis, which unbeknown to us was still active.

BROWNING In answer to the first question, there was very good correlation between the decrease in percentage of glomerular amyloid and the clinical parameters in those patients. We do not have further biopsies as these patients have creatinines which have reduced in one case from over 600 to 150μmol/L and in the second patient from 350 to 150μmol/L associated with satisfactory decreases in their urinary protein excretion. There is, therefore, good correlation between changes in glomerular amyloid and the clinical changes in the patients. With respect to the second point, I do not think that we are necessarily saying that CAPD is better than haemodialysis. Our experience of haemodialysis, however, has not been a very happy one, but this was only in two patients, and I think we must be careful about drawing any conclusions from this. I think there are, however, theoretical practical advantages to using CAPD in patients with amyloid, particularly in patients with AL amyloidosis who tend to get cardiomyopathies and in whom the circulatory stress of haemodialysis perhaps is a little bit risky. Drawing an analogy to the diabetics is a very valid thing to do. In as much as diabetes is a systemic condition with involvement of other organs. We would say that in our experience patients do well on CAPD and we would now think it unreasonable not to treat such patients.

GABRIEL (London) You implied that the peritoneal membrane might become infiltrated with amyloid protein. Is this theoretical or have you seen it at autopsy?

BROWNING We have seen it in AL amyloidosis.

GABRIEL What percentage please.

BROWNING I cannot give you an exact figure as we have not done enough biopsies.

OGG (London) I was interested in the patients you had on haemodialysis and peritoneal dialysis. I wondered whether you had excluded the possibility of adrenal insufficiency in your patient who died of intractable hypotension. We have had two such patients, one with AA and one with AL amyloidosis and it is an easy diagnosis to miss, as one tends to attribute cardiovascular disturbance to myocardial amyloid. It is, however, a very nice condition to treat if you make the diagnosis.

BROWNING There is an association described in the literature, but I do not know in that particular case, as we did not get an autopsy.

DAL CANTON (Naples) I suppose that you carried out autopsies on the patients that died, and if so did you find any difference in amyloid deposition between cortical renal areas and medullary zones? This would be important because the only defect in renal function may be a defect of urinary concentration and dilution.

BROWNING I do not know the answer to that problem. Other people, however, have implicated the interstitium more than the glomerular deposition in renal insufficiency, but we have not studied this particular point.

MERY (Paris) Going back to patients in whom renal amyloidosis seemed to diminish, I would like to know what was the associated disease with the amyloidosis in these patients? I would also like to make a comment. One should not be too optimistic about the prognosis in such patients treated by peritoneal or haemodialysis, because from the experience one gets from patients with familial mediterranean fever treated by haemodialysis, it appears that four years after the patient has reached terminal renal failure there appears to be a turning point and many patients die at about that time from cardiac or gastrointestinal involvement. The follow up of your patients was for less than four years, and so I think that one should not be too optimistic with respect to the very long term.

BROWNING Yes, I would agree with that, but on the other hand without treatment the patients would have been dead anyway.

MERY Of course one has to treat these patients, but I feel that four years later is an important time.

BROWNING I agree that the follow up of our patients has not been long enough yet. With respect to your question on underlying disease there was a mixture: one patient had Crohn's disease, one had pulmonary tuberculosis and the rest I believe were all patients with rheumatoid arthritis.

WATER EXCRETION IN NEPHROTIC SYNDROME. RELATIONSHIP BETWEEN BLOOD VOLUME AND PLASMA VASOPRESSIN

M Usberti, S Federico, B Cianciaruso, C Pecoraro, V E Andreucci

University of Naples, Naples, Italy

Summary

In order to verify whether or not an increased secretion of ADH may cause the water retention commonly observed in nephrotic syndrome, 12 nephrotic patients and 11 normal subjects were studied in basal conditions and following a water load or iso-osmotic blood volume expansion. A significant direct correlation was observed between plasma ADH and Posm in controls but not in nephrotics . Plasma ADH was inversely correlated with BV in nephrotics but not in controls. Blood volume expansion in nephrotic patients was effective in reducing plasma ADH and promoting a water diuresis.

These results demonstrate a sustained volume mediated secretion of ADH in nephrotic syndrome, which is responsible for the impairment in water excretion.

Introduction

An impairment in renal water excretion resulting in hyponatraemia and hypo-osmolality occurs in most nephrotic patients. The mechanism responsible for this water retention has not been fully clarified. Recent studies in patients with nephrotic syndrome [1,2], cirrhosis [3] or congestive heart failure [4] have given some evidence in favour of a key role of a reduction in effective blood volume on the abnormal water retention.

The present study was undertaken to verify if an increased secretion of ADH may account for water retention in nephrotic syndrome and, if it does, to characterise its relationship with blood volume.

Methods

The study was performed in 12 patients with nephrotic syndrome and 11 normal subjects; all were normotensive with normal renal function.

After three hours of bed rest plasma volume and total blood volume were measured by calculating the distribution space of ^{125}I labelled albumin, as previously described [5]. Then a one-hour clearance period (basal clearance period) was performed with collection of urine by spontaneous voiding. Blood samples for creatinine, osmolality, sodium, potassium, albumin, ADH and renin activity (PRA) were withdrawn at the middle-point of the clearance period.

Water load study

After the basal clearance period five nephrotics and five controls underwent a water load study. After drinking 20ml/kg BW of water in 20 minutes, clearance periods were then carried out hourly until U/P osm ratio, after an initial decrease, rose to one or more; at this time it was presumed that all the ingested water had been excreted. Plasma osmolality was measured at 30, 60, 90, 150 and 210 minutes after water ingestion. Glomerular filtration rate (GFR) was measured as inulin clearance, renal plasma flow (RPF) as PAH clearance.

Expansion study

The effect of blood volume expansion on plasma ADH and water excretion was studied in four nephrotic patients and four control subjects. After basal clearance period 3.3ml/kg BW of 20 per cent human albumin solution were infused i.v. in 15 minutes. Plasma osmolality and ADH concentrations were measured before and at 10, 20, 60 minutes after the completion of the infusion. Blood volume, GFR, PRA, plasma albumin, urine output, urinary sodium and osmolality were determined before and one hour after the infusion.

Results

No difference was found in basal condition and after the water load between nephrotics and controls for GFR and RPF, whereas plasma osmolality, serum sodium, blood volume and serum albumin were significantly lower in nephrotics than in controls. Basal values of ADH were similar in nephrotics and controls, being 3.6 ± 0.5pg/ml and 2.7 ± 0.6pg/ml respectively.

The values of Posm obtained before and after the water load were plotted against the respective values of plasma ADH. A highly significant correlation was observed in controls, $y=0.28 (x-279.5)$, $r=0.910$, $p<0.001$, (Figure 1) but not in nephrotics. In these patients in spite of very low values of plasma osmolality ADH secretion was never inhibited. Normal subjects diluted maximally the urines 60 minutes after the water load and the ingested water was completely eliminated in 150 minutes. Nephrotics reached a minimal Uosm after 120 minutes. The ingested water was completely eliminated in 240 minutes. One nephrotic patient was unable to produce free water after the water load.

Figure 2 shows an inverse correlation, $y=18.47 (x-0.21)$, $r=0.755$, $p<0.001$ between blood volume and ADH values in nephrotics. The data were obtained from all nephrotics in basal condition and after blood volume expansion. No

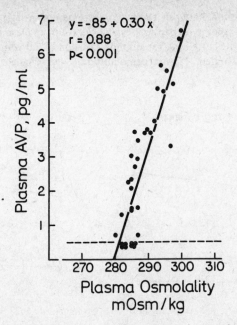

Figure 1. Relationship between ADH and Posm in normal subjects

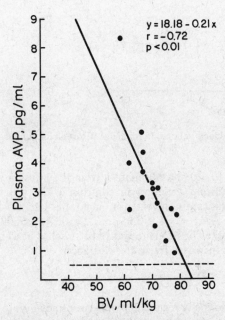

Figure 2. Relationship between ADH and blood volume in nephrotic patients

605

correlation was found between these two parameters in normal subjects. The effects of blood volume expansion on blood volume, plasma osmolality and ADH are shown in Figure 3. After albumin infusion blood volume was increased in both groups studied. Plasma osmolality did not change. ADH decreased

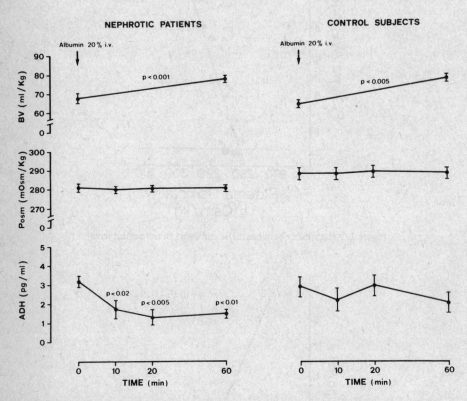

Figure 3. Effects on blood volume, Posm and ADH of albumin infusion in normal subjects and nephrotic patients ($\overline{x} \pm SD$)

significantly after 10, 20 and 60 minutes from the infusion only in nephrotics; there was no significant variation in controls. Urine volume and free water clearance were significantly increased in nephrotics (from 0.43 ± 0.04 to 5.0 ± 7.0, $p < 0.025$ and from -0.64 ± 0.05 to 3.2 ± 0.64, $p < 0.005$ respectively). In controls, on the other hand, there was only a slight but significant increase of diuresis without an increased free water clearance.

Discussion

ADH secretion is normally regulated by plasma osmolality. In nephrotic patients ADH secretion was not inhibited by a water load, despite very low values of plasma osmolality. Taken together our results demonstrate that it is the reduced blood volume which stimulates ADH secretion in nephrotic syndrome; an inverse correlation between blood volume and plasma ADH was, in fact, observed in nephrotics (Figure 2) but not in non-nephrotic controls.

The iso-osmotic expansion of blood volume was followed by a sustained inhibition of ADH and by a water diuresis in those nephrotic patients who exhibited a severe reduction in blood volume. After 20 per cent albumin infusion urine output rose also in two nephrotics with normal blood volume and in non-nephrotic controls but these subjects remained unable to produce free water, since their plasma concentrations of ADH were only slightly reduced.

In conclusion, our study has given the first demonstration that impaired water excretion in the nephrotic syndrome is due to a sustained, volume mediated secretion of ADH secondary to a severe reduction of blood volume.

References

1   Berlyne GM, Braun C, Adler A et al. *Arch Intern Med 1981; 141:* 1275
2   Krishna GG, Danovitch GM. *Kidney Int 1982; 21:* 395
3   Bichet D, Szatalowicz V, Chaimovitz C et al. *Ann Intern Med 1982; 96:* 413
4   Szatalowicz VL, Arnold PE, Chaimovitz C et al. *N Engl J Med 1981; 305:* 263
5   Cannella G, Castellani A, Mioni G et al. *Clin Sci Med 1977; 52:* 19

Open Discussion

MALLICK (Chairman)   Can I ask you how you would associate your results with the recent suggestion of Berlyne and his colleagues* that if you immerse nephrotics up to the neck and no higher in water they have a change in urine output both of sodium and water?

CIANCIARUSO   Well, they have the same effect and they have an increase in diuresis and an increase in natriuresis. In our studies sodium excretion increases more significantly in normals than in nephrotics, in other words there was a natriuresis in normal subjects but a water diuresis in nephrotic patients.

DORHOUT MEES (Utrecht)   We and many others have found that in a significant proportion of nephrotic syndrome patients there is no decrease in blood volume†. We have also studied free water clearance and found it decreased but not in all patients to the same extent. Your mean osmolarity was only down to 160mOsm/L while it waa down to 80mOsm/L in normals. We found it much lower in nephrotic patients, although there was still a decrease in free water clearance. How sure are you that ADH was indeed involved here? I gather from the standard variation that some of your patients indeed had a very low urine osmolarity as a proof of the suppression of ADH and that they may have significant water excretion. You calculated a correlation between ADH and plasma

*   Berlyne GM, Sutton J, Bronn C et al. *Clin Sci 1981; 61:* 605
†   Dorhout Mees EJ, Roos JC, Boer P. *Am J Med 1979; 67:* 378

osmolarity; was there also a correlation between ADH and minimal urine osmolarity reached during expansion?

CIANCIARUSO Well you know the plasma volume measurement in nephrotic syndrome is still a matter of controversy. We have low values of blood volume and we think that this may be explained by the fact that we correct blood volume with wet weight. Other studies have either not corrected for body weight or they use dry weight. I think that our measure of blood volume is more correct for several reasons. First of all we think that it is very hard to establish dry weight: if you measure the blood volume and then shrink the patient with diuretic therapy, you then take the dry weight. Also because there may be an effect of extracellular pressure on blood volume itself. Our data on blood volume are supported by the relationship between plasma albumin and blood volume in our nephrotic patients and in our controls. This kind of correlation was not found by others.

DORHOUT MEES We did of course correct our blood volume measurements but this is not the point of discussion at the moment. I just wanted to know whether your decrease in urine osmolarity in some of your nephrotic patients down to say about 60mOsm/L and whether this correlated with your ADH measurements?

CIANCIARUSO Yes, it does.

BROWN (London) Two questions: first of all you gave us very little information about your group of nephrotics: have they been treated with diuretics and if so at what stage have these been stopped, because obviously these are going to have a huge influence on both ADH, plasma sodium and on blood volume?

CIANCIARUSO Any treatment was stopped three weeks before the study.

BROWN The other question is: were your patients actually retaining sodium at the time that they were being studied? Do you have any information on the urinary sodium excretion?

CIANCIARUSO Yes, the patients have five days of urinary excretion studies before the study and they had a normal sodium diet and the urinary excretion was between 35 and 50mEq/24 hours. We gave them the same amount of sodium they lost in the urine and after three days that they maintained the same body weight we assumed that they were in sodium balance and then we studied them.

BAKIR (Chicago) How long after you injected albumin did you measure the blood volume in the nephrotics? The reason I am asking is that there are a few studies that suggest that injected albumin leaks out of the vascular space, you know after 15 minutes.

CIANCIARUSO Yes, after 10 minutes leakage of albumin overestimates the blood volume. On the other hand the correction which we made with wet weight will underestimate blood volume. So there are two possible errors which may counterbalance each other.

CATTELL (London) I am a little unclear; if I understood you correctly, you gave the same challenge in terms of water loading to your controls and your nephrotics and similarly you gave the same albumin loading to the two groups. I would suggest that these are probably not comparable: in the case of water ingestion because of low plasma oncotic pressure you will not have the same effect in the vascular compartment, depending on how you think ADH is activated, because of the low oncotic pressure and the leakage of water. Similarly in the administration of albumin you have the two separate problems of albumin leakage and water reabsorption into the vascular compartment by virtue of a rise in plasma oncotic pressure. How did you cope with these two possible differences in the two groups?

CIANCIARUSO Even if a transcapillary leakage of infused albumin was present, the blood volume increased in the same way in nephrotics and controls. In the same way with acute water load we obtained a significant decrease of plasma osmolarity in nephrotics, which was not followed by any variation of ADH levels.

Proc EDTA (1983) Vol 20

INTERACTION BETWEEN THE MACROPHAGE SYSTEM AND IgA IMMUNE COMPLEXES IN IgA NEPHROPATHY

D Roccatello, **R Coppo**, B Basolo, G Martina, C Rollino, D Cordonnier*, G Busquet*, G Picciotto, L M Sena†, G Piccoli

*Osp S Giovanni, Torino, *Centre Hospitalier Regional et Universitaire de Grenoble, †III Cattedra Patologia Generale dell'Università di Torino, Italy*

Summary

In nine patients with IgA nephropathy, the function of the mononuclear phagocyte system was assessed by measuring in vivo clearance of anti-D coated red blood cells (RBC) and in vitro phagocytosis of sensitised RBC by monocytes.

A strict correlation was found between in vivo macrophage function and in vitro monocyte phagocytosis. Statistical correlations were also found between in vivo clearance values and IgAIC and C_{3d} values.

A defective macrophage and monocyte function affects patients with major signs of clinical activity, highest IgAIC values, signs of complement activation and the most unfavourable clinical course.

Introduction

Experimental and immunological data suggest that circulating IgA immune complexes (IgAIC) are involved in the pathogenesis of two nephropathies characterised by mesangial deposits of IgA: primary IgA nephropathy (pIgAGN) and Henoch-Schönlein nephritis (HSGN) [1,2]. The mononuclear phagocyte system is assumed to play a protective role by removing circulating immune complexes (IC), and defective clearance might theoretically lead to prolonged circulation and possibly increased tissue deposition [3]. Increased circulating IC seems to impair the Fc receptor function of macrophages [4]. In some circumstances it is unclear whether macrophage dysfunction is due primarily to impaired expression of the cell-surface membrane receptor or due to receptor blockade by blocking factors [5].

We have measured immunospecific in vivo and in vitro clearance by the macrophage-monocyte system and the amounts of circulating IC in nine patients with IgA nephropathies to investigate whether the possible interaction between circulating IC and the macrophage system influences the course of this disease.

Materials and methods

Patients

Six patients with pIgAN (all males, mean age 39.6, range 16.7 years) and three patients with HSGN (two males, mean age 22.3, range 10.4 years) were studied. Each had a Rh-positive blood type. The diagnosis of pIgAGN was made on the presence of mesangial proliferative lesions with IgA (100%) and C_3 (82%) deposits. The diagnosis of HSGN was made in the presence of glomerulonephritis with IgA (100%) and C_3 (100%) deposits and three signs of systemic disease (skin rash, arthralgia and abdominal pain). Four patients (three pIgAGN and one HSGN) were considered to have an active disease because of recently increased serum creatinine concentrations, a haematuria (25 RBC/high power microscopic field) and/or protein loss >3g/day.

Control subjects

Ten normal volunteers from the hospital staff were examined as controls for the clearance of ^{51}Cr-labelled sensitised red blood cells and for the in vitro phagocytosis assay. Sera from 55 apparently healthy laboratory personnel were tested as controls for the detection of IgAIC and C_{3d}.

Clearance of ^{51}Cr-labelled sensitised red blood cells [6]

Fifteen millilitres of citrated blood was collected. Three times washed erythrocytes were incubated with $100\mu Ci$ of ^{51}Cr and then with an appropriate amount of purified anti-RhD serum (Centre de Transfusion Sanguine, Lyon). After several washes 1ml of packed red blood cells (RBC) resuspended in 10ml 0.15M NaCl was reinjected. Blood samples were taken at 10, 20, 30, 60, 90 min. The half-life clearance (T_{50}) was calculated as recommended by the International Committee for Standardization in Hematology.

In vitro phagocytosis assay

Isolation of monocytes from patients was performed by a modified Seljelid and Pertoft's method [7]. Briefly monocytes were separated from peripheral blood collected in EDTA (ethylene-diamine-tetracetate), using two different gradients of Percoll (density solution I: 1.085g/ml, solution II: 1.064g/ml). Three suspensions of 0.3×10^6 monocytes in RPMI medium (DIFCO Laboratories) containing 3% bovine serum albumin were mixed with three 0.5ml aliquots of a 0.5% suspension of autologous RBC sensitised with purified anti-RhD serum and incubated at 37°C respectively for 15, 30, 45 min. After staining with Acridine orange, the percentage values of ingested RBC/100 monocytes from each sample were plotted on a linear scale against time. The linear slope (obtained in all cases) subtended an angle assumed as 'index of phagocytosis'. The results were expressed as angular coefficient.

IC assays

The detection of circulating IgAIC and IgGIC was performed employing a modified conglutinin solid phase assay as previously described [2].

C_{3d} evaluation

This complement breakdown product was measured as previously described [2].

Results were expressed as the percentage of the C_{3d} measured after complete activation induced by inulin (NHS – 1%).

Results

^{51}Cr labelled sensitised RBC clearance studies

The half-life in normal volunteers was 30.1 ± 6.4min. The corresponding values obtained in patients were 45.8 ± 23min (pIgAGN) and 48.5 ± 19 min (HSGN) (Table I). One of three patients with HSGN had moderate prolongation of clearance half-time (60min). Two of six patients with pIgAGN displayed a marked reduction of the clearance (80min and 69min), and one patient had a T_{50} value at the upper limit of normal.

TABLE I. In vivo (T_{50}) and in vitro (phagocytosis index) macrophage function in nine patients with IgA nephropathy

	T_{50} (min)	Phagocytosis index (angular coefficient)
Healthy people	30.1 ± 6.4	1.08 ± 0.17
Primary IgA GN	45.8 ± 23	0.96 ± 0.34
Henoch-Schönlein GN	48.5 ± 19	0.71 ± 0.31

In vitro phagocytosis assay

The results of kinetic analyses of the ability of monocytes derived from pIgAGN and HSGN patients to promote ingestion via their Fc receptors are shown in Table I. Normal values range from 0.84 to 1.33 (mean value 1.08 ± 0.17 tgα). All three patients with delayed clearance of sensitised RBC also displayed a reduced 'index of phagocytosis'.

IC assays

The mean values of IgAIC in the patients were significantly higher than those of the control group (p<0.001) (Table II). Five of six patients with pIgAGN and

612

TABLE II

	IgAIC $\mu g/ml$ ΔIgA	IgGIC $\mu g/ml$ ΔIgG	C3d %NHS-I inulin
Healthy people	28.8 ± 65	6.5 ± 14	4.2 ± 1.3
Primary IgAGN and			
Henoch-Schönlein GN	891.6 ± 823	16.2 ± 12	7.1 ± 2.4
Student's t test p value	<0.001	<0.1	<0.01

one of three patients with HSGN had circulating IgAIC. Mean values of IgGIC of the patients were not significantly different from those of healthy people.

C_{3d} detection

One patient with HSGN and two patients with pIgAGN displayed high plasma values of C_{3d}.

Correlations between in vivo clearance, in vitro phagocytosis, IgAIC, C_{3d} and clinical activity

A good correlation was found between sensitised RBC in vivo clearance and in vitro phagocytosis of monocytes (r= -0.7, p<0.02). A statistical correlation was also found between C_{3d} values and data on RBC clearance (r= 0.7, p<0.05). A good correlation was observed between IgAIC and half-life clearance values of anti-D coated RBC (r= 0.68). All four clinically active patients had detectable IgAIC in serum, while only two of four active patients displayed macrophage and monocyte Fc receptor dysfunction. However these two patients (pIgAGN) were found to have a marked reduction in the rate of clearance, reduced index of phagocytosis, increased serum creatinine, signs of urinary activity, increased values of C_{3d}, the highest values of IgAIC (not only at the time of clearance studies but also in the previous follow-up) and the most unfavourable clinical course. In addition a patient with pIgAGN with moderate increase in creatinine (considered inactive at the time of study) who displayed a relatively recent reduction of clinical activity and had still detectable IgAIC in the serum, had T_{50} and C_{3d} values at the upper limits and an index of phagocytosis at the lower limit of normal.

Discussion

The macrophage system is thought to have a critical role in the removal of immune complexes (IC) from the circulation through their interaction with cell-surface receptors for the Fc component and C_{3b}. It has been demonstrated that the uptake of IgG-labelled RBC by splenic macrophage is reduced in patients with Systemic Lupus Erythematosus and other diseases [8,9] and was thought to result from blockade of the macrophage Fc receptors by IC [7]. Delay in the clearance of IC might result in their continued circulation thereby enhancing deposition in organs.

We studied the clearance of anti-D sensitised autologous erythrocytes from the circulation and the phagocytosis of anti-D coated RBC by peripheral monocytes in nine patients with IgA nephropathies. We observed high values of IgAIC in these patients, particularly during active phases and we found there was a defective macrophage and monocyte Fc receptor function in the cases with major signs of clinical activity, highest IgAIC values at the time of study as well as in the previous follow-up, signs of complement activation and the most unfavourable course.

The apparent combination of clinical and laboratory findings of active disease with a defective macrophage function is consistent with the hypothesis that persistently high values of IgAIC, associated with an impaired immune clearance might increase the renal load of immunologically active materials, thus influencing the course of the disease.

References

1 Rifai A, Small PA, Ayoub EM. *Clin Immunol Immunopathol 1981; 20:* 419
2 Coppo R, Basolo B, Martina G et al. *Clin Nephrol 1982; 5:* 230
3 Mannik M, Arend WP, Hall AP et al. *J Exp Med 1971; 133:* 713
4 Haakenstad AO, Mannik M. *J Immunol 1974; 112:* 1939
5 Lawley TJ, Russel PH, Fauci AS et al. *N Engl J Med 1981; 304:* 185
6 Crome P, Mollison PL. *Br J Haemat 1964; 10:* 137
7 Seljelid R, Pertoft H. *Methods for Studying Mononuclear Phagocytes.* New York; Academic Press 1981: 201
8 Frank MM, Hamburger MI, Lawley TJ et al. *N Engl J Med 1979; 300:* 518
9 Jaffe CJ, Vierling JM, Jones EA. *J Clin Invest 1978; 62:* 1069

Open Discussion

FEEHALLY (Manchester, UK) The sort of red cell clearance study you use has been widely used in investigating immune mechanisms, but clearly a red cell with immunoglobulin on its surface is very big and an antigen-antibody complex is very small. I wonder how certain you are that the coated red cell is really a good model for investigating clearance of small antigen-antibody complexes?

COPPO The levels of IgA containing circulating immune complexes were sometimes very high and the degree of FC receptor dysfunction was sometimes important, but I think that probably there is not a strict correlation between the quantitative amount of circulating immune complexes and the dysfunction of FC receptors. As you know, probably qualitative differences are more important than quantitative ones.

RITZ (Heidelberg) Dr Coppo, you mentioned among other findings that you found in the circulating immune complexes both IgA1 and IgA2. Could you give us some details of the methods used and specifically the antibody used to clarify whether this finding is in agreement or disagreement with reports in the literature?

COPPO The antibodies we used were kindly provided by Professor J P Vaerman of Brussels and they were highly purified. He presented the quality of these antibodies in a recently published paper*. The amount of cross reactivity between anti-IgA2 and IgA1 immunoglobulin is very low and that is very different from the commercially available antibody. As you know it is very difficult to find an anti-IgA2 antibody to react only with IgA2 and that is the most important problem when you evaluate the IgA subclasses.

SCHREIBER (Cleveland, Ohio, USA) Do you feel that your data represents an inherited defect in macrophages for phagocytosis 'lazy macrophage', or do you feel that there is some inhibitory substance which you are apparently removing with plasmapheresis affecting phagocytosis? A correlate to that would be to activate your macrophages in culture with BCG or some other type of antigen and then re-attempt your assay.

COPPO No we did not culture monocytes. I think that there are some substances that can in some way be involved in the dysfunction of gamma FC receptor. We suppose that IgAIC are these kind of substances, even though, as you know, the interaction between FC alpha or FC gamma receptors is still under study. The fact that after we used plasmapheresis we got normal function with both these tests for investigating FC receptor function, is suggestive of the hypothesis of both high levels of circulating IgA containing immune complexes or some other kind of inhibitor like anti-monocyte antibody.

BAKIR (Chicago, USA) Were the serum C_3 values in your patients normal, and did you exclude post-streptococcal glomerulonephritis in these patients? Would you like to comment on the glomerular immune deposits by immunofluorescence?

COPPO All these cases had been biopsied in one to four years previously. In all these cases the diagnosis was made by biopsy. The renal deposits were in all cases IgA and in about five or six cases of primary IgA nephropathy C_3 deposits were also present. We excluded a diagnosis of post-streptococcal glomerulo-nephritis from both the clinical and the pathological point of view.

BAKIR Was the serum C_3 normal in all those patients?

COPPO C_3 and C_4 were normal but we found that some cases, as you have seen before, presented an activation of the complement system detected by increased amounts of C_3. As you know you can have a normal amount of C_3 and C_4 with high levels of C_{3d}, probably because the consumption is accompanied by an increased synthesis.

CLARKSON (Adelaide, Australia) Our results are very similar to yours with this type of study. I would like to ask you whether you did HLA typing on all of the patients you studied? As you mentioned in your talk there is a prolonged red cell half-life in patients who have B8-DR3 haplotype and it is important that this is excluded.

* Delacroix D, Dehennin JP, Vaerman JP. *J Immunol Methods 1982; 51:* 49

COPPO Yes we performed HLA typing in the case who had very high levels of IgA containing immune complexes and an important FC receptor dysfunction. This patient did not show any improvement from the clinical point of view or from the immunological point of view with plasmapheresis; we looked for HLA and we found this kind of haplotype, therefore I think that our observations are similar to those of others who found a defective FC receptor function in patients with B8-DR3 haplotype.

CLARKSON Did you type the other patients you studied?

COPPO We did it only for the positive ones at the moment, I mean the cases with a prolonged half-life clearance of sensitised RBC. The other patient I showed previously had a BW 35 locus.

Proc EDTA (1983) Vol 20

DELAYED CLEARANCE OF SPECIFIC POLYMERIC IgA IMMUNE COMPLEXES IN PATIENTS WITH IgA NEPHROPATHY

J Sancho, J Egido, F Rivera, L Hernando

Fundacion Jimenez Diaz, Madrid, Spain

Summary

The presence of multimeric (polymeric and monomeric) IgA immune complexes (IC), detected by Raji cell assay and by the inhibition binding assay, as well as the specific polymeric IgA-IC were examined before and after the ingestion of 100g protein. A rise in multimeric IgA-IC occurred in three out of seven controls with a peak at two to four hours after the meal, being cleared thereafter. The amount of multimeric IC present at fasting in four of six patients diminished at two to four hours after food challenge reaching a new peak around six hours. In both controls and patients, IC containing antibodies against diet antigens (e.g. ovalbumin) paralleled those of multimeric IgA-IC. In controls the specific polymeric IgA-IC presented a maximal peak with distribution similar to multimeric IgA-IC, but with a faster disappearance from the circulation. By contrast, polymeric IgA-IC remained elevated 24 hours after food ingestion in most patients. These results suggest that a defect in the hepatic clearance of circulating polymeric IgA-IC exists in patients with IgA nephropathy.

Introduction

The existence of high serum IgA values in a large proportion of patients with IgA nephropathy [1] and the increased proportion of polymeric serum IgA in patients with primary IgA nephropathy [2] suggests that, together with an increased production of IgA by peripheral lymphocytes after polyclonal stimulation in vitro [3], a defect in the hepatic clearance of IgA, similar to that observed in certain liver disease [4], might occur. In this paper we examine the hypothesis that the clearance of specific polymeric IgA immune complexes is delayed in patients with primary IgA nephropathy.

617

Materials and methods

Human sera

Seven healthy non atopic adults and six patients with IgA nephropathy were subjected to an oral challenge of 100g protein. Sequential blood samples were collected and stored at −70°C in aliquots until analysis.

Isolation of proteins

Human secretory component (SC), human IgG and human IgM were isolated as previously described [5].

Immune complexes containing antibodies against food antigens

Antibodies to bovine serum albumin (BSA) or ovalbumin (OA) were quantified according to the methods of Paganelli et al [6].

IgA and IgG-containing immune complexes

IgG-IC were measured by the Raji cell radioimmunoassay [7]. IgA-IC were determined by the Raji cell radioimmunoassay modified by Hall et al [8] and by an anti-IgA inhibition binding assay [9]. Specific polymeric IgA-IC were detected by the Raji SC binding assay previously described [4].

Results

After food ingestion a rise in IgA Raji IC occurred in five out of seven controls but, only in three of these subjects values greater than $T_i/U_i = 1$ were found

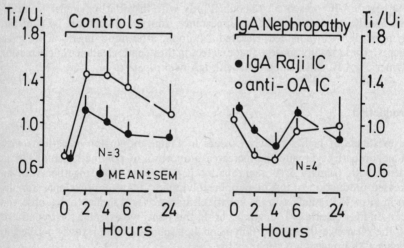

Figure 1

with a peak at two to four hours after the meal (Figure 1). Interestingly, a similar peak distribution of anti-OA-IC was observed with a maximum at two to six hours after eating (Figure 1). In all patients with IgA-Raji-IC at fasting (n=4) the IC fell to normal levels at two to four hours. Later IgA-IC in all these patients rose again to reach a new peak, which occurred six hours after the meal. The other two patients had no IgA-IC at any time. In patients with IgA nephropathy a similar distribution of anti-OA-IC was seen; that is, a fall at two to four hours and a rise six to 24 hours after protein challenge (Figure 1), suggesting high mean values of anti-OA specific IgA-IC.

By contrast, there was no correlation between the rise of IgA-IC (detected by the anti-IgA inhibition binding assay), observed in three controls and patients with the anti-OA or anti-BSA containing IC. Although a rise of IgG complexes was seen in three patients there was no correlation with the distribution of anti-BSA or anti-OA-IC. The seven normal individuals had normal IgG-IC values before and after the meal (data not shown).

After the meal the three normal controls with positive Raji IgA-IC and anti-OA-IC (Figure 1) had a similar distribution of polymeric IgA-IC (Figure 2) with a peak at two hours and a rapid rate of clearance after that time.

In contrast, a continuing rise in polymeric IgA-IC was observed in five out of six patients (Figure 2) with a significantly higher mean value than controls between six and 24 hours. These data suggest the existence of a specific defect in the clearance of polymeric IgA-IC in patients with IgA nephropathy.

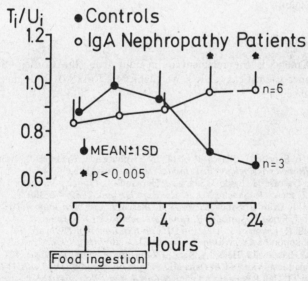

Figure 2

Discussion

The results presented here suggest a different behaviour of specific polymeric IC in normal subjects and in patients with IgA nephropathy after food ingestion. The three controls who presented Raji IgA-IC and anti-OA-IC after the meal, also showed an increase in the amount of polymeric IgA-IC. These complexes disappeared faster from the circulation than multimeric (polymeric and/or monomeric) IgA complexes detected by the classic Raji cell assay. Although the presence of secretory component on human hepatocytes remains controversial these results are in favour of the existence of a specific hepatobiliary transport of polymeric IgA-IC in humans.

The continuing rise of polymeric IgA-IC in patients with IgA nephropathy is in favour of a defect in the selective transport of polymeric IgA-IC, as probably may occur in patients with alcoholic cirrhosis [4]. Since in other disease linked to IgA, such as dermatitis herpetiformis, abnormal immunospecific splenic mononuclear phagocyte system clearance has also been demonstrated [10], our results do not preclude other clearance defects on the Fc or C3 receptors of the mononuclear phagocyte system and an enhancement of glomerular IgA deposition. The basis for this defective immunospecific mononuclear phagocyte system clearance is speculative, but pathologic states which interfere with hepatic clearance of serum IgA, such as cirrhosis, result in accumulation of polymeric serum IgA, which inhibits chemotaxis, phagocytosis and prevents complement mediated clearance.

A similar inhibition of serum IgA has been demonstrated in patients with IgA nephropathy. It is conceivable that these facts, together with the IgA-specific immune regulatory abnormalities found in these patients, might favour the prolonged circulation of immune complexes and their subsequent deposition in the mesangium.

Acknowledgments

Dr Jaime Sancho is the recipient of a grant from the Consejo Superior de Investigaciones Cientificas (CSIC). We thank Mrs Rosa Mª Rodriguez for secretarial assistance.

References

1 Egido J, Sancho J, Blasco R et al. In Hamburger J, Crosnier J, Grunfeld J, eds. *Actualités Nephrologiques de l'Hopital Necker.* Paris. 1982: 174
2 Lopez Trascasa M, Egido J, Sancho J, Hernando L. *Clin Exp Immunol 1980; 42:* 247
3 Egido J, Blasco R, Sancho J et al. *Clin Exp Immunol 1982; 47:* 309
4 Sancho J, Egido J, Sanchez Crespo M, Blasco R. *Clin Exp Immunol 1982; 47:* 327
5 Sancho J, Egido J, Gonzalez E. *J Immunol Methods 1983.* In press
6 Paganelli R, Levinsky J, Atherton DJ. *Clin Exp Immunol 1981; 46:* 44
7 Theophilopoulos AW, Wilson CB, Dixon FJ. *J Clin Invest 1976; 57:* 169
8 Hall RP, Lawley TJ, Heck JA, Katz SI. *Clin Exp Immunol 1980; 40:* 431
9 Kauffman RM, Van Es LA, Daha MR. *J Immunol Methods 1982; 40:* 117
10 Lawley TJ, Hall RP, Fauci AS et al. *N Engl J Med 1981; 304:* 185

Open Discussion

RITZ (Heidelberg) I would like to congratulate you on your superb methodology. My comment relates not to your data but rather to your conclusion that a defect of hepatocyte secretory component is involved in the genesis of delayed immune complex clearance. You are certainly aware of the large species differences especially between rodents and humans with respect to hepatocyte IgA polymer elimination. Indeed a recent paper* gave cogent arguments against a role of hepatocyte as opposed to biliary duct epithelium in IgA polymer elimination in humans.

EGIDO I know this work very well, effectively it's in the rodents that the secretory component at hepatocyte level is very important, and so these animals clear up very quickly polymeric IgA immune complexes. However even polymeric IgA immune complexes could be eliminated either through the secretory component receptor in the hepatocytes or in the sinusoids or through the biliary secretions. At the moment I would only like to remark that it is probably the liver which is the organ involved in the elimination of polymeric IgA immune complexes.

FEEHALLY (Manchester) As you may know Cairns† from our department has also shown that the clearance of immune complexes after food is delayed in a variety of glomerular diseases. This variation in complex levels with regard to food leads us to believe that it is mandatory that all immune complex serum samples should be taken in the fasting state, and secondly presumably makes it difficult to interpret the literature where immune complexes containing IgA are related to disease activity. No mention is made in the literature as to whether patients have recently eaten or not. Would you like to comment on this?

EGIDO The samples obtained from our patients were obtained in a fasting state and the patients had not eaten protein in the previous 24 hours. In addition the IgA is probably specific for diet antigens. By contrast the IgG immune complexes and also the IgA immune complexes measured by the inhibition-binding technique had no close correlation to the antibodies against albumin or BCA.

CLARKSON (Adelaide) As you know our group in Adelaide has been working on hepatic clearance of autologous IgA containing immune complexes in patients with IgA nephropathy, and the results lead us to the same conclusions as your group. What worries us, however, is that in most patients it seems that exacerbations of the disease are related to upper respiratory or pulmonary infections where hepatic clearance may not be relevant.

EGIDO At the moment there are two models of IgA nephropathy, one after oral ingestion and one after intravenous administration. I don't want to say

* Delacroix DL, Hodgson MJF, McPherson A et al. *J Clin Invest 1982; 70:* 230
† Cairns SA, London A, Mallick NP. *J Clin Lab Immunol 1981; 6:* 121

from the results of our study that the oral antigens are important in the pathogenesis of the disease. Probably they may only indirectly suggest either an increased permeability as in dermatitis hepatiformus and some coeliac-like diseases or that they only represent an immunological abnormality or derangement in immune regulation, in that these patients have an abnormal response against common antigens. I agree with your paper in which you have found antibodies against intestinal bacterial antigens.

ACUTE AND CHRONIC NEPHRITIDES: TWO DIFFERENT DISEASES?

A M El Nahas, R Lechler, S Zoob, A J Rees

Royal Postgraduate Medical School, Hammersmith Hospital, London, United Kingdom

Summary

The role of the immune system in the progression of experimental nephrotoxic serum nephritis (NTN) in rats has been evaluated. Proteinuria and renal functional impairment during the sub-acute phase of the disease determined the long-term prognosis of the nephritis regardless of the humoral autologous antibody levels. In contrast to the acute, immune mediated glomerulonephritis, chronic glomerular scarring in NTN proceeds independently of the host immune response.

Introduction

Glomerulonephritis remains the largest single cause of chronic renal failure in the developed world. The progression of chronic glomerulonephritis is often a relentless process with end-stage renal failure occurring many years after the onset of the disease [1]. Acute glomerulonephritis, although often of unknown aetiology, is characterised by an underlying immune mediated inflammatory response. It is not known, however, whether the persistence of the original immunological cause of inflammation is necessary for progressive scarring or whether it can evolve independently; perhaps as a direct consequence of the reduction in functional renal mass analogous to the glomerulosclerosis occurring after experimental sub-total nephrectomy [2]. We have studied the role of the persistent immune response in the progression of nephrotoxic nephritis (NTN) in rats. In these animals the acute nephritis is mediated by the rats' autologous antibody response [3], but the role of such humoral immune response in the progression of the nephritis to chronicity remains to be determined.

Material and methods

We used inbred, male, Sprague-Dawley rats weighing 200g at the beginning of the study. The nephrotoxic nephritis was induced according to the telescoped model; rats were pre-immunised with rabbit gamma globulin (RγG) on day five, and injected on day zero with the rabbit nephrotoxic serum containing a high titre of anti-rat glomerular basement membrane (GBM) antibodies. To determine the role of the autologous antibody response on the nephritis, we designed a novel experimental approach whereby by day 30 after the induction of the nephritis we transplanted the chronic nephritic kidneys into two groups of syngeneic recipients; the first, pre-immunised against rabbit gamma globulin and recreating the donor's immune environment (group I) and the second, naive, non-immunised, rats (group II). Kidneys from nephritic donors were simultaneously transplanted into group I and II rats, and the course of the disease, in the two recipients, compared.

Progression of nephritis was assessed by serial measurement of proteinuria, renal function, autologous antibody production and renal morphology at time of death.

Results

Nephritis progressed in the recipients as 11 of our 14 rats died from chronic renal failure. The course of the nephritis was identical for each pair of transplanted nephritic kidneys as judged by the strong correlations between the serum creatinine (r=0.962), proteinuria (r=0.938) and survival (r=0.982) for each pair. This progression occurred in spite of significant differences in the

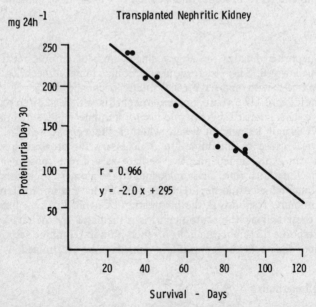

Figure 1. Correlation between nephritic kidney functional survival (days) and 24-hour urine protein excretion (mg/24 hours) at time of transplantation

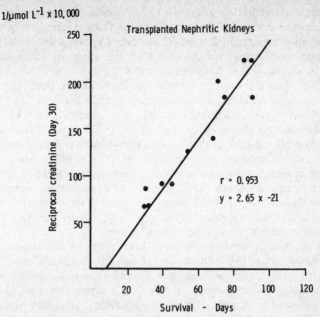

Figure 2. Correlation between nephritic kidney functional survival (days) and reciprocal of
serum creatinine (μmol/L) at time of transplantation

amount of circulating autologous antibodies between the two recipient groups.
The course of the transplanted nephritic rats was predetermined by the degree
of proteinuria (r=0.966) and serum creatinine (r=0.953) at time of transplantation (Figures 1 and 2).

In our model, the only important influence on the rate of glomerular scarring
was the type and extent of injury to donor kidneys at the time of transplantation.
This is evidenced by exceptionally close correlations between donor proteinuria
as well as reciprocal serum creatinine and graft survival with more than 90 per
cent of the variability we observed being accounted for in this way.

Discussion

Typically, patients with chronic glomerulonephritis develop renal failure years
or decades after the onset of their disease [1]. Although the mechanisms underlying the immune mediated injury of acute glomerulonephritis are currently
better understood, little is known about the factors involved in the progressive
scarring of chronic renal diseases.

Nephrotoxic serum nephritis, in the rat, is an experimental model of immune
mediated glomerulonephritis that bears some similarities to human diffuse
proliferative nephritis. In this model the acute injury depends entirely on the
host autologous antibody response [3]. We have demonstrated, using a novel
experimental approach, that in contrast to acute injury, the titre of autologous
antibody has no influence on progressive glomerular scarring after NTN. Using

625

a double transplantation approach, we observed that right and left kidneys from the same donors behaved in an identical fashion regardless of the recipients immune environment. In this model, the only important determinant of the rate of glomerular scarring was the extent of the injury to donor kidneys at the time of transplantation. Both proteinuria and serum creatinine at time of transplantation, during the sub-acute phase of the nephritis, predicted the outcome of the nephritic kidneys. Sub-acute phase proteinuria could be the marker of the severity of the underlying nephritis, but equally it could be the reflection of compensatory glomerular hyperperfusion and hyperfiltration, thought to be nephrotoxic in other models of experimental chronic renal failure [4].

Our data demonstrate the feasibility of using double renal transplantation between syngeneic rats as a method of achieving controlled experiments on the factors that influence the progression of experimental nephritis. Similarly, we have shown that in the nephrotoxic model of immune mediated nephritis, in rats, glomerular sclerosis and chronic renal failure develop independently of the persistence of the original cause of injury.

In man, similar observations have been made in acute post streptococcal glomerulonephritis [5] and in anti-glomerular basement membrane disease [6], where the nephritis progressed to end-stage renal failure well after the acute immune mediated injury has subsided. It seems, therefore, in experimental animals as well as in man, that acute and chronic glomerulonephritis differ in their pathogenesis and while immunosuppression remains the cornerstone of therapy of acute nephritis its role in the later chronic phases of the disease needs to be re-evaluated.

References

1   Cameron JS. In Black DAK, Jones DR, eds. *Renal Disease.* Oxford: Blackwell Scientific Publications. 1979: 329–345
2   Morrison AB. *Lab Invest 1962; 11:* 321
3   Unanue ER, Dixon FJ. *J Exp Med 1965; 121:* 715
4   Brenner BM, Meyer TW, Hostetter TH. *N Engl J Med 1982; 307:* 652
5   Schacht RC, Gluck MC, Gallo GR, Baldwin DS. *N Engl J Med 1976; 295:* 977
6   Rees AJ, Lockwood CM. Peters DK. In Kincaid-Smith P, D'Apice AG, Atkins RC, eds. *Progress in Glomerulonephritis.* New York: Wiley Medical Publications. 1979

Open Discussion

D'AMICO (Chairman) Did you study at autopsy the degree of sclerosis?

EL NAHAS We looked at glomerular sclerosis and tubular atrophy and it correlated very well between right and left kidney.

ADU (Birmingham) I think this is a very elegant study. I was not happy about the conclusion you reached because, if I understood your results correctly, the non-immunised animals also had some circulating antibodies to rabbit IgG and I don't think one can presume more antibody necessarily means worse disease.

626

EL NAHAS Yes, but from the very strong correlation between the proteinuria and survival and renal function and survival it leaves very little for other variables to determine the overall prognosis. So all that the antibody might have had is a permissive additional effect. It's very likely to be a minimal one.

FEEHALLY (Manchester) I may have missed this point but was there any difference in blood pressure between any of the groups which might have skewed the results?

EL NAHAS We did not measure blood pressure, but there was no difference in the vascular sclerosis or periglomerular fibrosis between the right and left kidneys.

MOORHEAD (London) We have developed a hypothesis of lipid nephrotoxicity in nephrotic syndrome, which proposes that initiating immune mediated events giving rise to proteinuria induce profound abnormalities of lipid metabolism which are capable of inducing self perpetuating renal glomerular and interstitial disease. However Edwards* has shown that nephrotoxic serum nephritis rats may be improved by lipid reduced diets and deteriorate with high lipid diets. These experiments and yours fit well with our suggestions. Are you in retrospect able to say whether abnormalities of lipid/lipoprotein metabolism were different in the two groups of transplanted rats? Were they comparably hyperlipidaemic?

EL NAHAS Nephrotic rats have very lipaemic serum although we have not measured total cholesterol or triglycerides but retrospectively we stained the kidneys for fat and we found some glomerular fat as well as a great deal of tubular fat deposition, but again it seems that for each pair of kidneys the glomerular and tubular deposition was similar. Although I have no data it seems likely that the proteinuria at day 30 reflects to some extent the hyperlipidaemia and there might have been a correlation between hyperlipidaemia and survival.

ALLISON (Glasgow) I also found that a very elegant study which enables you to do lots of interesting little things. You ended your presentation by speculating that the management of the acute heterologous mediated anti-GBM response disease would be different from the management of the end-stage chronic renal failure and so I think I know where you are going. Are you going on to talk about the work hypothesis and Brenner's† thoughts on protein load? Here we have a model to look at dietary protein content of these rats, the group that have the autologous antibody present and the group that don't.

EL NAHAS Yes, as you probably know we did further experiments on this model and we studied the effect of low protein diet introduced after day 30 on the progression. Those on a low protein diet, with no difference in the antibody

* Edwards KDS. In Schreiner GE, ed. *Controversies in Nephrology*. Masson Publications 1982; *3*: 3
† Brenner BM, Meyer TW, Hostetter TM. *N Engl J Med 1982; 307*: 625

titres, did well whereas those left on a normal protein diet died from renal failure. That's why I said damage or compensation, because proteinuria for all I know might reflect some compensation not just glomerular damage.

ALLISON Did you study carefully the histology of those animals that died and those that didn't?

EL NAHAS Yes and glomerulosclerosis was decreased and tubular atrophy almost absent in the low protein diet although tubular calcification was similar in the two groups.

D'AMICO (Milan) In spite of proteinuria remaining or proteinuria reversing with this diet?

EL NAHAS Proteinuria is very variable. If you put rats on a low protein diet the proteinuria decreases within a few hours whereas if you put them on a high protein diet proteinuria increases four-fold within 24 hours. Thus during a dietary protein experiment proteinuria becomes almost of no value.

ALLISON It's a very variable model as there are big inter-animal differences. Some animals develop massive proteinuria quickly while some won't. It is not an easy model to work with.

EL NAHAS That's precisely why we designed this double transplant model.

Proc EDTA (1983) Vol 20

CHRONIC PLASMA EXCHANGE IN SYSTEMIC LUPUS ERYTHEMATOSUS NEPHRITIS

W F Clark, D C Cattran*, J W Balfe*, W Williams†, R M Lindsay, A L Linton

*University of Western Ontario, London, Ontario, *University of Toronto, Ontario, Canada, †University of the West Indies, Kingston, Jamaica*

Summary

Thirty-nine patients with systemic lupus erythematosus (SLE) and diffuse proliferative glomerulonephritis have been enrolled in a multi-centre randomised controlled prospective study of chronic 4L plasma exchange therapy performed every three to four weeks. In the patients randomised to the pheresis (P) group and who received either albumin or plasma as replacement, there was a difference of 33 per cent better renal function at this time in the study. This difference did not achieve a significance with a p value of <0.05. However, the 30 patients randomised into the P group to receive albumin replacement did demonstrate a 50 per cent difference from the C group which was significant at a p value of <0.045. This also correlated with a statistically significant reduction in immune complex titres in the P versus the C groups. Chronic 4L plasma exchange with albumin replacement may be a useful therapeutic adjunct in patients with SLE and diffuse proliferative glomerulonephritis.

Introduction

Over the past seven years there has been a proliferation of clinical reports outlining the benefits of plasma exchange therapy in patients with systemic lupus erythematosus (SLE) [1-9]. Dermatological, rheumatological, neurological, pulmonary and renal manifestations of SLE have been reported to benefit from acute plasma exchange therapy. It is difficult to interpret the published non-randomised series due to the variability of SLE itself and some of the end-point measurements employed. To reduce these confounding factors, we have attempted to study in a randomised controlled prospective fashion chronic 4L plasma exchange therapy in a well-defined renal subgroup of patients with SLE, in whom serial biochemical determinations of renal function have been made.

Methods

Patients

Patients were selected from the teaching hospitals of the Universities of Western Ontario, Toronto and the West Indies. All met a minimum of four of the ARA criteria for the diagnosis of SLE and had at least one episode of ANA positivity, elevated DNA binding and complement depression. All had a renal biopsy with the diagnosis of diffuse proliferative glomerulonephritis. Patients were excluded from entry to the study if their creatinine clearance was less than 30ml/min, or if their serum creatinine was greater than 3mg/100ml. Each patient gave his/her informed consent according to the guidelines of the Human Ethics Committees at the participating universities, prior to entry and randomisation.

Plasmapheresis

Patients randomised into the plasmapheresis (P) group received five 4L plasma exchanges in the first two weeks of trial entry, if considered to have active disease by a previously published scale [10]. Otherwise, the patients received 4L plasma exchange every three to four weeks. In London and Toronto the patients received replacement with five per cent human serum albumin, whereas patients in Kingston, Jamaica received replacement with plasma. In London all procedures were performed on the IBM 2997 or Haemonetics Model 30; in Toronto all procedures were performed on the Haemonetics or the CS 3000; and patients in Kingston, Jamaica underwent plasma exchange on the Haemonetics Model 30 cell separator. Almost all procedures were performed on an outpatient basis and access to the circulation was gained by venepuncture of the medial cubital fossae.

Study design

At each Centre, after patients had given their informed consent, they were randomised by process of split equal randomisation. This was carried out by a designated non-medical person at each Centre who removed a pre-folded slip of paper from a bowl. At each Centre the number of patients projected to be involved in the study (London: 18, Toronto: 12, Kingston: 12) provided the basis for the number of slips of paper which were divided equally into P and control (C) groups. The slips were then folded and placed in a bowl until the time of patient entry when a designated non-medical person removed the pre-folded slip. Patients in the P and C group received conventional therapy of steroids ± cytotoxics and the management of these medications was under the control of their referring physicians. All referring physicians agreed to increase the dose of steroids if patients showed disease activity and to reduce steroids when the disease was quiescent. Determination of disease activity and quiescence was based on the judgment of the referring physicians after assessing immunological, biochemical and clinical factors in each patient. The monthly quantity of steroids and cytotoxic medication was recorded for each patient in the P and C groups. Patients were seen every three to four weeks at which time blood was withdrawn for determination of serum creatinine, albumin, Clq binding, DNA binding, C_3, C_4 and C_{H50} determinations. In addition, a 24-hour urine for protein was collected at these outpatient visits and the frequency and duration of hospitalisation, if any, during the interval time period was recorded. All blood samples in the P group were performed prior to the plasma exchange.

The mean serum creatinine, albumin and 24-hour protein excretion at trial entry was compared with the mean value up to the point of this report, using the Student t test. The frequency of abnormal immunological tests, e.g. DNA or Clq binding elevation or C_3, C_4 and C_{H50} depression was compared between P and C patients. In view of the fact that two Centres were using albumin replacement, it was thought reasonable to compare pheresis employing serum albumin replacement and if the numbers were adequate, to compare this with the pheresis where plasma was used as a replacement.

Patients were dropped from the study if there was a doubling in their entry serum creatinine value and this value was repeated in a minimum of one week, following more intensive therapy, and was still doubled or greater. A doubled value was considered as their last determination. After drop-out the study patients could undergo any form of therapy which their referring physician considered appropriate for their management and their follow-up was maintained.

Results

Eighteen patients were enrolled in the study from London; 12 from Toronto and nine from Kingston, Jamaica. Twenty of the patients were randomised into the P group and 19 into the C group. Both P and C patients had an average of six of the ARA criteria at time of entry to the study. Sixteen of 20 P patients were female and 18 of 19 C patients. The mean age of the P group was 26 and the C group 25. Nine of 20 P patients at entry had greater than 3.5gm protein in the urine versus six of 19 C patients. Nine of the 20 P patients had hypertension and 10 of the 19 C patients at entry. There were no obvious differences in major risk factors between the two groups at trial entry. Of the 20 P patients, eight have completed three years of the study; one is lost to follow-up; one has deceased and 10 others are still enrolled in the study. In the C group, three patients have completed three years of the study; three have been dropped out due to a doubling, or greater, in their serum creatinine level; two have been lost to follow-up and 11 remain in the study.

Renal function

At the time of entry into the study, there was no significant difference between the serum creatinine values of the P and C groups (P: 1.2mg/100ml, C: 1.1mg/100ml). At this time in the study the P group's serum creatinine has declined to 1.1mg/100ml, whereas the C group's has risen to 1.4mg/100ml. The confidence that this difference is due to chance is less than 0.085 (Student t test). If one

631

assesses the 30 patients who were randomised to receive albumin as their exchange fluid, the entry creatinine for the P group is 1.2mg/100ml and in the C group is 1.1mg/100ml, but the serum creatinine drops to 1.0 for the P patients and rises to 1.5 in the C group. The confidence that this 50 per cent change difference in renal function is due to chance is less than 0.045. No significant differences were noted between the P and C groups in terms of their serum albumin levels or in the 24-hour urine protein excretion at entry, or to date.

Immunological tests

No major differences were noted between P and C groups in terms of the frequency of elevated DNA binding or complement depression. However, P patients did experience significantly less episodes of elevated immune complex titres as measured by Clq binding.

Medication

There was a slight but significantly greater reduction in prednisone in the P versus the C groups, otherwise there was no apparent difference in the steroid medication at the time of trial entry or in the number of patients receiving cytotoxic therapy, or the dose of cytotoxic therapy. In both P and C groups, seven patients each did not receive cytotoxic therapy.

Drop-outs

Three patients in the C group were dropped out because of a doubling in their serum creatinine which was not reversed within one week. Two of the three patients received intensive plasma exchange schedules with creatinines returning to the normal range over a one to two month schedule. Both patients have remained with stable renal function. One patient refused the addition of plasma exchange and was treated for several weeks with intensive cytotoxic and steroid therapy. When this patient's creatinine reached 10mg/100ml she agreed to undergo plasma exchange, but following her second treatment refused any further procedures. This patient has been on haemodialysis therapy for the past three years for treatment of her end-stage renal failure.

Deaths

One patient in the P group developed bronchopneumonia in the interval between her plasma exchanges and underwent a deterioration in renal function associated with lupus disease activity. She was treated with antibiotic therapy for bronchopneumonia and given high dose steroids for treatment of her SLE and succumbed from a septicaemia. A post-mortem was available.

Lost to follow-up

One patient in the P group was lost to follow-up, having been involved in the study for greater than one year and this was due to transportation difficulties in that the patient had to fly to the pheresis Centre. Two patients in the C group were lost to follow-up: one after completing two years in the study moved to a different country; the other was lost to physician follow-up, having moved from the city of her treatment without the knowledge of her physician.

Discussion

Although the study is small, there appears to be no obvious difference between P and C groups in age or prognostic factors at the time of study entry. We conclude that plasma exchange with five per cent human serum albumin or plasma replacement solution performed every three to four weeks in patients with SLE and diffuse proliferative glomerulonephritis is associated with a preservation in renal function in patients in the P versus the C group. The confidence that this observation is not due to chance is a $p < 0.085$ (Student t test) in comparison of means.

The size of the study may have precluded us detecting the benefits of plasma exchange at a p value of <0.05. The difference in serum creatinine between the P and C groups at last assessment would represent an approximate difference of 33 per cent. If these data are representative of a true difference between the procedures, then 140 patients, 70 in each group (two-sided t test $\alpha_2 = 0.05, \beta = 0.20$) would be required to demonstrate the clinical efficacy of plasma exchange in SLE and diffuse proliferative glomerulonephritis. However, in the 30 patients randomised to albumin replacement versus conventional therapy, a 50 per cent difference in renal function is noted between plasma exchange and control patients which is significant at a p value of <0.045. This finding, which also correlates with the significantly lower serum immune complex titre in pheresed versus controls, suggests that 4L plasma exchange performed every three to four weeks and replacing with five per cent serum albumin may be valuable adjunctive therapy in a well-defined subgroup of patients with renal systemic lupus erythematosus. Due to the nature of this study the long-term efficacy and safety of the regimen we have employed will require careful clinical trial from several centres with prolonged follow-up periods, before this form of therapy can be advocated.

Acknowledgments

This work was supported by a grant from the Physician's Services Incorporated Foundation. We gratefully acknowledge the efforts of John J Koval and Mary Arnett for computation and statistical evaluation. We thank Mrs Patti Stevens and Miss Vikkie McCallum for their expert technical assistance.

References

1   Verrier-Jones J, Bucknall RC, Cumming RH et al. *Lancet 1976; i:*709
2   Pinching AJ. *Br J Hosp Med 1978; 20:* 552
3   McKenzie PE, Taylor AE, Woodroffe AJ et al. *Clin Nephrol 1979; 12:* 97
4   Clark WF, Lindsay RM, Ulan RA et al. *Clin Nephrol 1981; 16:* 20

5   Clark WF, Lindsay RM, Cattran DC et al. *Can Med Assoc J 1981; 125:* 171
6   Wysenbeck AJ, Smith JW, Krakauer LS. *Plasma Ther 1981; 2:* 61
7   Verrier-Jones J, Cumming RH, Bacon PA et al. *Q J Med 1979; 48:* 555
8   Isbister JP, Ralston M, Wright R. *Arch Intern Med 1981; 141:* 1081
9   Gipstein RM, Adams DA, Grobie MT et al. *Am J Med Sci 1982; 284:* 37
10   Clark WF, Linton AL, Cordy PE et al. *Can Med Assoc J 1978; 118:* 1391

Open Discussion

SCHREIBER (Cleveland, USA) Considering the baseline creatinines of the starting groups, which were quite low, I wondered what percentage of patients had increasing creatinines prior to your treatment and how soon after the diagnosis was treatment instituted in each of the groups?

CLARK I think the mean time would have been less than three months from the time of the renal biopsy. Timing in patients with lupus is a problem, as you know, and you can lengthen the prognosis considerably by going back to the first symptom.

SCHREIBER Was the creatinine increasing proportionately in both groups?

CLARK I think it was approximately the same: about half were considered to have active disease at the time of entry to the study in both groups.

SCHREIBER I guess I feel uncomfortable looking at serological data and then trying to decide whether the renal disease is active or not. Some of the patients we see who appear, from a nephrological point of view, to be stable may have high serological values and so I am not sure what to do with them. I would hesitate to start therapy with two drugs and plasma pheresis in an individual who appears to have a stable creatinine of 100μmol/litre, even though they had indicative high serological data.

RITZ (Heidelberg) Were any of the patients on diuretics? I am asking this question because the plasmapheresis group had nephrotic range proteinuria (4 grams per day) whereas the control group did not (2 grams per day). Could these minor differences of serum creatinine not have resulted from changes in hydration status and diuretic use?

CLARK Some of the patients were on diuretics and some on antihypertensives. I think, though, that if you are talking about a shift in creatinine of 50μmol/litre I would be surprised if you could produce that with diuretics unless you severely dehydrated your patient. You are talking about a difference in renal function of 33 to 50 per cent.

RITZ Well, I would not have difficulty in having a nephrotic patient change the serum creatinine from 110 to 140μmol/litre by altering hydration status and administrating diuretics. I think this is a severe shortcome of your study.

CLARK Well, that's interesting.

DE VECCHI (Milan) You did not mention the social or financial cost of such a long-term plasmapheresis. Did you consider hospitalisation on the day of plasmapheresis? Secondly, what is the survival from the point of view of renal function in your lupus patients before this study?

CLARK No, we did not consider the cost: this varies very much from country to country. Before assessing the cost we wanted to find out if the technique works and this was our initial concern. This issue of cost is a social one and not a medical issue.

D'AMICO (Chairman) Is it your opinion that in some way plasma plus albumin is any different from albumin alone as a replacement fluid?

CLARK There has been a suggestion of a difference, but I feel this is purely a suggestion.

ULTRASTRUCTURAL APPEARANCES OF NEPHRON DAMAGE IN ACUTE POISONING WITH ETHYLENE GLYCOL

L Cieciura, Z Kidawa, S Orkisz, K Trznadel

2nd Clinic of Internal Diseases, Military Medical Academy, Łódź, Poland

Summary

Renal biopsy material from five patients with acute ethylene glycol poisoning was taken five, 10, 16 and 22 days following poisoning and examined by electron microscopy. We found extensive crystal deposits in glomerular interloop spaces. In some of the tubules crystal accumulation seemed independent of time following poisoning. No morphological markers of reabsorption were found in the tubules tightly filled with crystals, while tubules with empty lumen had signs of enhanced reabsorption. In the early period of poisoning there were signs of epithelial damage while in the late periods, signs of epithelial regeneration prevailed. The results provide new information on the pathogenesis of anuria in acute poisoning with ethylene glycol.

Introduction

Recent investigations on renal structural changes induced by ethylene glycol poisoning have revealed renal tubular injuries appearing mainly as hydropic and vacuolar degeneration in the convoluted tubules [1–6]. Large numbers of calcium oxalate crystals were also found within the tubule lumen, leading to partial or total obstruction [1–6]. Renal glomeruli were either unchanged [1,2,4] or insignificantly so [3,5], although Siew [6] described substantial changes. Observations on the renal interstitium were equivocal, some investigators found no changes [1,2,4], while others observed oedema [3] and inflammatory foci [5,6]. Most investigations of the kidney in acute poisoning by ethylene glycol (APEG) have been primarily concerned with its histology [1–5] and only few reports on renal ultrastructure have appeared.

We evaluated ultrastructural changes in the kidney in patients who survived APEG. Renal biopsy was performed at various times following the poisoning, enabling us to assess changes in early periods as well as late.

Material and methods

Renal biopsy specimens were taken once from each of five patients at five, 10, 16 and 22 days following APEG. Biopsy material was fixed in 0.2M cacodylate buffer with 2.5 per cent glutaraldehyde and two per cent paraformaldehyde (pH 7.4) for three hours then, postfixed in two per cent osmium tetroxide for two hours. After dehydration the tissue specimens were embedded in Araldite, cut into ultra-thin sections and examined with a Philips EM 300 transmission electron microscope.

Results

Renal glomeruli

Electron microscopy revealed clearly encapsulated flocculent deposits of amorphous material of low electron density within the mesangium. The podocyte cytoplasm was thinned with a substance of similar consistency. The glomerular basement membrane was formed into layers filled with the same homogenous flocculent material. The parietal lamina of the Bowman's capsule was thickened in most cases (Figure 1).

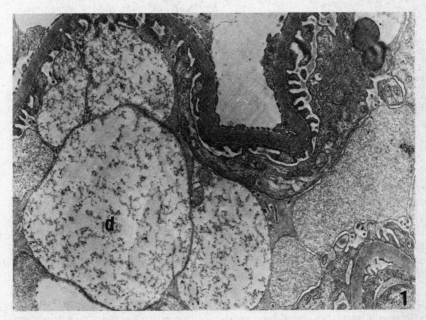

Figure 1. The encapsulated flocculent deposits (d) of amorphous material within the mesangium, x 6300 (reduced for publication)

Renal tubules

The lumina of the proximal and distal tubules were tightly filled with deposits; they were observed at all times, five to 22 days (Figure 2). On day five cytoplasmic vacuolisation was noted on the luminal side of the tubular cells. The cytoplasm formed thick spike-shaped protrusions devoid of microvilli, which subsequently became detached into the lumen. The tubular lumen was filled, sometimes tightly, with desquamated cell fragments or whole cells (Figure 3).

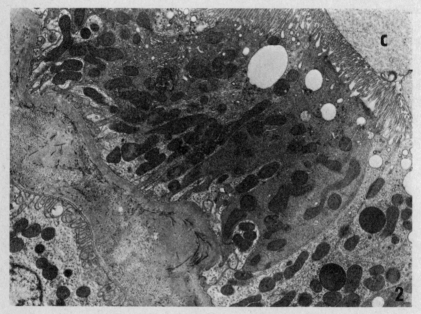

Figure 2. The lumina of the proximal tubules are tightly filled with crystals (c). The basement membrane is formed into layers filled with the same flocculent material, x 5000 (Reduced for publication)

As in the glomeruli, deposits of amorphous material, consisting of several separate encapsulated units, were also noted within the proximal and distal tubular lumina.

In the interstitial tissue the deposits were found in the intercellular exudate and were not encapsulated. Sometimes they were located within the tubular basement membrane, rendering it thickened and formed into many layers. Similar amorphous deposits were also found within vascular lumina.

Varying degrees of distension of intervillous and intercellular spaces, as well as in spaces between parabasal invaginations, occurred. In tubules with the lumen or intercellular spaces closed by crystals, the spaces were reduced to a minimum. On the other hand, in the unchanged areas they were markedly distended and

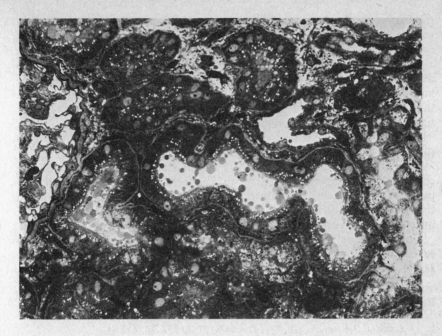

Figure 3. The cytoplasmic vacuolisation at the luminal side of the tubular cells. The cytoplasm formed thick spike-shaped protrusions devoid of microvillae, which subsequently became detached into the lumen, x 125 (reduced for publication)

vacuolisation was increased, particularly in the proximal tubules. The renal glomeruli as well as the interstitial tissue between the renal tubules contained blood cells and plasma cells.

In the distal and proximal tubular cells and to a less extent, in the podocytes, lysosomal activity was increased as manifest by increased vacuolisation of the Golgi apparatus and formation of primary lysosomes. Also numbers of secondary lysosomes, phagolysosomes and multivesicular and residual bodies were increased. The tubular epithelial cells were injured to varying degrees.

In biopsy material taken later in the course of APEG numbers of patent renal tubules, cleared from deposits, were increased. They were accompanied by epithelial cell desquamation and replacement by regenerated cells.

Amorphous deposits were removed from the interstitial tissue earlier than from the tubular lumen. In the intercellular spaces of the connective tissue electron-lucent exudate with flocculent suspension appeared at the beginning and increased in the course of time, replacing encapsulated homogenous deposits. The lysosomal activity started increasing from day 10 and continued to the end of the observation.

Discussion

Renal biopsy material taken from five to 22 days following APEG enabled evaluation of acute as well as late ultrastructural changes accompanying acute

639

renal failure. Amorphous deposits observed on electron microscopy corresponded with reported calcium oxalate and carbonate crystals [6]. Also the location of calcium oxalate deposits was similar to those reported with other techniques [6].

Calcium oxalate crystals exerted mechanical and toxic effects on the surrounding tissue. Extensive glomerular interloop oxalate deposits compressed the podocytes and reduced their intervillous spaces. Of importance is the fact that the crystals persisted until 22 days following APEG. In the tubules tightly filled with crystals, no morphological evidence of reabsorption was found, while the distension of parabasal and intercellular spaces in the uninjured areas suggested a compensatory increase in tubular reabsorption.

In the early period of APEB, there predominated compression of tubular cell microvilli by crystals, and their toxic effects on tubular cells, leading to pathologic protrusions, desquamation and necrosis of the epithelial cells. In the later period, regeneration of the tubular epithelium and disappearance of interstitial exudates prevailed.

These electron microscopic observations throw new light on the pathogenesis of anuria in APEG while the presence of crystal deposits in renal tissue as late as after 22 days must have therapeutic implications.

References

1   Berman LB, Schreiner GE, Feys J. *Ann Int Med 1957; 46:* 611
2   Bove KE. *Am J Clin Path 1966; 45:* 46
3   Collins JM, Hennes DM, Holzgang CR et al. *Arch Intern Med 1970; 125:* 1059
4   Flanagan P, Libcke JH. *Am J Clin Path 1964; 41:* 171
5   Parry MF, Wallach R. *Am J Med 1974; 57:* 143
6   Siew S. *Israel J Med Sci 1979; 15:* 698

THE PREDICTIVE VALUE OF HIPPURAN UPTAKE IN ACUTE RENAL FAILURE

G J Abels-Fransen, H Y Oei, E J Dorhout Mees, H A Koomans

University Hospital Utrecht, Utrecht, The Netherlands

Summary

In this study the hippuran uptake capacity (HUC) in 32 patients with an acute deterioration of renal function was measured. The HUC_2 is the ratio between the activity accumulated in the kidneys in the first two minutes, divided by the injected dose, which was measured by the gammacamera, during standardised renography. Thirteen patients had an acute glomerular disease (AGD) and 19 patients had acute tubular necrosis (ATN). During the acute deterioration of renal function, the HUC_2 values ranged between 0 and 3.0 in the AGD group and between 1.9 and 8.7 in the ATN group. In only one patient of this latter group was the HUC_2 value below three. Measurement of HUC_2 is useful in the differential diagnosis of acute renal failure. It can be performed in the absence of urine production and indicates renal blood perfusion despite complete absence of filtration. When the HUC_2 value is higher than three, ATN is the most probable aetiology of the acute renal failure and recovery of renal function can be expected. Values below this limit most probably indicate AGD.

Introduction

Differential diagnosis of the underlying pathology in patients with acute renal failure (ARF), especially in the presence of anuria or oliguria, by urine and blood analysis is not always conclusive. It has been reported, that in patients with acute tubular necrosis the kidneys show sufficient accumulation of ^{131}I-orthoiodohippurate (^{131}I-OIH) even although glomerular filtration is almost nil. Good visualisation of the kidneys, during gammacamera renography with ^{131}I-OIH may predict the recovery of renal function [1,2]. However, visual interpretation of uptake on a scintigram is inaccurate. In this study, the uptake of ^{131}I-OIH in patients with ARF was measured and the method used was similar to the previously described measurements of hippuran uptake capacity in renal transplant patients [3].

641

Patients and method

The present analysis is based on 32 patients, 18 male and 14 female, showing rapidly progressive renal failure, characterised by an increasing serum creatinine. None of the patients had a history of renal disease. On the day of examination, anuria or oliguria was present in 14 patients. For 14 patients haemodialysis was necessary just before or after the study. During the ^{131}I-OIH study, their serum creatinine values ranged between 365μmol/L and 1545μmol/L. The creatinine clearance was in all cases less than 12ml/min. The 32 patients were divided into two groups: 13 patients, aged 27–79 yrs (59 ± 13), had an acute glomerular disease (AGD), and 19 patients, aged 26–80 yrs (53 ± 18), had acute tubular necrosis (ATN).The diagnosis in eight AGD patients was established by biopsy. The diagnosis in the remaining five AGD patients and the 19 ATN patients was based on clinical signs and subsequent course. Patients with urinary tract obstruction were excluded. Table I shows the pathology in the 13 AGD patients.

TABLE I. Values of serum creatinine in μmol/L and the diagnosis of the AGD patients

Last known serum creatinine (months before ARF)	max serum creatinine	ultimate serum creatinine*	diagnosis**
188 (2)	1200	500	cholesterol emboli
140 (1)	520	317	cholesterol emboli
?	1445	700	RPGN (b)
130 (14)	1200	374	RPGN (b)
?	1465	CHD	RPGN (b)
?	1460	430	RPGN (b)
100 (12)	1187	500	RPGN (b)
?	800	CHD	cortical necrosis
134 (1)	1161	CHD	Goodpasture's syndrome
78 (24)	1435	CHD	scleroderma
103 (2)	1550	CHD	metastases in kidneys (b)
107 (6)	1405	301	RPGN (b)
?	866	148	RPGN (b)

*   CHD = chronic haemodialysis
** RPGN = rapidly progressive glomerulonephritis; b = biopsy proven

Renography was performed by means of a gammacamera (Siemens LFOV) with a high energy parallel-hole collimator, and a mini-computer system. The actual injected dose (11Mbq) of ^{131}I-OIH was measured exactly with a gamma-camera by counting the syringe before and after administration at a distance of 10cm from the collimator. The examination was performed in supine position with the detector of the gammacamera underneath the patient. Data acquisition in list mode was started at least two minutes before the bolus injection of hippuran for the subtraction of activity from previous administration of radio-nuclides in some cases. The regions of interest were chosen with a lightpen on a CRT-display. The time of entry of radioactivity into the kidneys was determined on the time-activity curve, at 4-sec intervals. For the correction of blood-background activity, the activity caudal to the kidneys was used. The HUC_2 is the activity accumulated in the kidneys in the first two minutes, corrected for background, divided by the dose in counts per second.

Results

In Figure 1, the HUC_2 values of the ATN patients and the AGD patients are plotted against the serum creatinine measured on the same day. As shown in this figure, there is no correlation between the two values. Thus, the HUC_2 value does not depend on glomerular filtration.

In the AGD group the HUC_2 value, measured during ARF, ranged between 0 and 3.0 (2.0 ± 0.8), and in the ATN group between 1.9 and 8.7 (4.8 ± 1.8). Only one patient of this latter group had a HUC_2 value lower than three (Figure 2). This data suggests that ATN is the most probable aetiology in patients having HUC_2 values higher than three.

In Figure 3 the HUC_2 values, measured during the acute deterioration, are

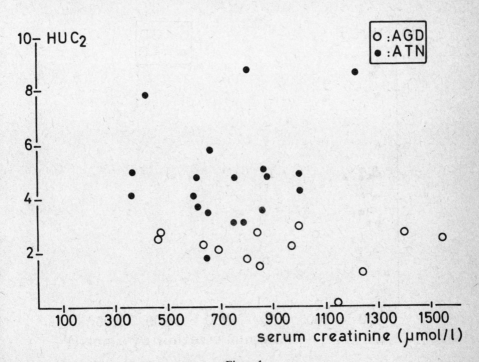

Figure 1

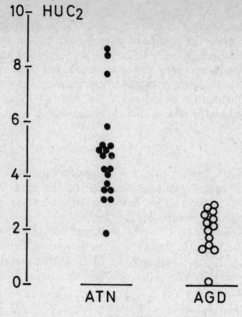

Figure 2

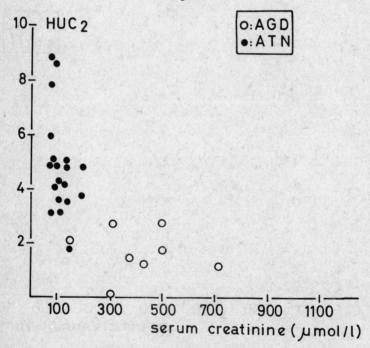

Figure 3

plotted against the ultimate serum creatinine. The ultimate serum creatinine is the serum creatinine measured two to 12 months after the acute phase. As shown in this figure, the ultimate serum creatinine values, found in the 19 ATN patients, varied between 70 and 200μmol/L (normal 50 to 120μmol/L; 14 of these patients returned completely to normal. In five patients of the AGD group, the renal function did not recover. In the remaining eight AGD patients, the renal function recovered partially; their ultimate serum creatinine values ranged between 148 and 700μmol/L (Table I).

Discussion

HUC_2 is a semiquantitative measurement of hippuran trapped by the kidneys after a bolus injection. This value depends on renal cortical perfusion and the capacity of the proximal tubule to extract hippuran from the blood. In our previous paper [4], a significant correlation was demonstrated between effective renal plasma flow and the hippuran uptake value. This supports the contention that the HUC_2 value is an indirect measure of renal blood flow.

This observation confirms the impression that a good visualisation of the kidneys, during a ^{131}I-OIH study in patients with ARF, predicts recovery of renal function.

As shown in this study, quantification of renal hippuran uptake capacity clearly divides the two groups of patients. In all AGD patients the HUC_2 value was lower than three; the renal function of these patients did not improve (n = 5) or recovered only partially (n = 8). On the contrary, almost all ATN patients had a HUC_2 value greater than three, and the renal function of these patients recovered completely (n = 14) or almost completely (n = 5).

The HUC_2 values, presented in this study, are not corrected for tissue attenuation. The thickness of the tissue between the kidneys and the gamma-camera can vary between two and seven centimetres. Thus, the individual variation in tissue attenuation is not small and should not be neglected.

In conclusion the measurement of HUC_2 in patients with acute renal failure is useful for differential diagnosis of the renal disease. It can be performed in the absence of urine production and indicates renal blood perfusion, despite complete absence of filtration. When the HUC_2 value is greater than three, ATN is the most probably cause of the ARF and recovery of the renal function can be expected. Values below three, indicate most probably AGD.

References

1   Harwood TH, Hiesterman DR, Robinson RG et al. *Arch Intern Med 1976; 136:* 916
2   Staab EV, Hopkins J, Patton DD et al. *Radiology 1973; 106:* 141
3   Oei HY, Ephraim KH, Jessurun RFM et al. In Joekes AM, ed. *Radionuclides in Nephrology.* New York: Grune & Stratton. 1982:283
4   Oei HY, Ephraim KH, Jessurum RFM et al. *Proc EDTA 1975; 12:* 441

Proc EDTA (1983) Vol 20

DRUG-INDUCED GRANULOMATOUS INTERSTITIAL NEPHRITIS

Ph Vanhille, D Kleinknecht*, L Morel-Maroger, A Kanfer†, V Lemaitre, J Ph Mery†, P Callard, M Dracon, J Laederich*

*Centre Hospitalier de Valenciennes, *Hôpital de Montreuil, and †Hospital Bichat, Paris, France*

Summary

Among 22 cases of drug-induced acute interstitial nephritis (AIN), noncaseating interstitial granulomas were found in eight cases (36%). Acute renal failure (ARF), oliguric in three patients, appeared within 1—20 days after the beginning of therapy. Clinical symptoms suggesting a hypersensitivity reaction were unusual, marked blood eosinophilia was absent, and immunologic tests were inconstantly positive. The discovery of interstitial granulomas may be a clue to the diagnosis of drug-induced AIN, especially when the inflammatory infiltrates do not contain eosinophils. Since significant residual renal impairment may be observed the benefit of early steroid therapy must be debated.

Introduction

Since the work of Baldwin et al in 1968 [1], acute interstitial nephritis (AIN) due to drug hypersensitivity is a well-recognised entity. The incidence of this peculiar form of acute renal failure (ARF) may account for up to eight per cent of all ARF seen in some studies [2]. Frequently, the onset of ARF is associated with haematuria, sometimes macroscopic, and the existence of an immunologic basis is suggested by the occurrence of extra-renal clinical manifestations such as fever, skin rash, arthralgia and blood and/or urinary eosinophilia [2, 3]. In the absence of these symptoms, an early renal biopsy is very helpful in the identification of drug-induced AIN showing focal or diffuse interstitial infiltrates composed of lymphocytes, plasma cells and eosinophils [4]. In some patients, epithelioid cell granulomas with giant cells are observed and this pathological feature may be a clue to the diagnosis of AIN due to drug hypersensitivity [5].

Patients

Among 22 patients with drug-induced AIN, interstitial noncaseating granulomas were found in eight cases (36%, group I). Their disease patterns were compared with those of patients with drug-induced AIN without granulomas (14 cases, group II).

In group I, the offending drugs were cotrimoxazole (two cases), penicillin, hydrochlorothiazide + triamterene, glafenin, floctafenin, noraminopyrine and paracetamol. None of the patients in group I was known to have sarcoidosis or an infection such as toxoplasmosis or typhoid fever.

In group II, the drugs involved were cotrimoxazole (two cases), penicillin + oxacillin, ampicillin, amoxicillin, cephalothin, rifampicin (two cases), tienilic acid, glafenin (two cases), niflumic acid, indomethacin + acetylsalicyclic acid and ajmaline. None of the patients in groups I and II had known pre-existing renal disease.

Results

The frequency of the main clinical, biological and immunological features diagnostic of AIN in patients with and without granulomas is outlined in Tables I and II.

TABLE I. Frequency of the main clinical and biological features in patients with (Group I) and without (Group II) interstitial granulomas

	Group I (n = 8)	Group II (n = 14)
Age (years)	20–79	18–80
M/F ratio	1.7/1	1.3/1
Fever	2 (25%)	9 (64%)
Skin rash	1 (12.5%)	5 (36%)
Arthralgia	0	1 (7%)
Haematuria (micro or macroscopic)	1 (12.5%)	6 (44%)
Oliguria	3 (37.5%)	5 (36%)
Blood eosinophilia ($>500/mm^3$)	0	5 (36%)

TABLE II. Immunological data in Group I (with granulomas) and Group II (without granulomas)

	Group I (n = 8)	Group II (n = 14)
Increased serum IgE	4/6	3/9
Circulating immune complexes (PEG or Clq binding-assay)	1/7	6/13
IF* negative	6/7	13/14
IF* positive	1/7 C3 focal, TBM	1/14 C3 focal, TBM

* Immunofluorescent findings on renal biopsy

ARF appeared within 1–20 days in group I and one day to six weeks in group II after the beginning of therapy. The frequency of oliguria was similar in patients of both groups. In group I there was a lower incidence of clinical and biological symptoms when compared with group II. Haematuria was observed in one patient and systemic manifestations indicative of an immune response were very unusual: fever, skin rash, and arthralgia were present in only three patients, without marked blood eosinophilia. A rise in serum IgE was found in 4/6 patients in group I and in 3/9 patients in group II. Circulating antibodies to the drug, detected by the antiglobulin test, were found in two patients of group II and one patient of group I. Immunofluorescence studies of renal tissue were negative in both groups, except in two cases – one in each group – where faint and focal deposits of C3 were observed along the tubular basement membrane.

On light microscopy (Table III), in group I, the noncaseating granulomas with epithelioid cells were numerous in six cases and moderate or rare in two cases. Multinucleated giant cells were noted in two patients. In all patients of both groups, there were focal or diffuse cortical interstitial infiltrates mainly composed of lymphocytes and plasma cells. Interstitial eosinophils were noted in approximately 50 per cent of patients in each group. Nearly all biopsy specimens showed interstitial oedema and tubular epithelial damage.

TABLE III. Renal histology in Group I (with granulomas) and Group II (without granulomas)

	Group I (n = 8)	Group II (n = 14)
Interstitial granulomas		
extensive	6/8	0
focal	2/8	0
Interstitial eosinophils	4/8	6/14
Interstitial inflammation		
diffuse	5/8	9/14
focal	3/8	5/14
Tubular damage	8/8	13/14
Acute arteriolar necrosis	0/8	2/14

TABLE IV. Outcome in Group I (with granulomas) and Group II (without granulomas)

	Group I (n = 7)	Group II (n = 14)
Dead	0/7	2/14†
Remission	4/7	11/14
Uraemia	3/7*	1/14

* One patient treated with prednisolone
† One patient treated with prednisolone + cyclophosphamide

All patients survived in group I, but this group appeared to fare rather worse than patients in group II because of a higher incidence of significant residual renal impairment (Table IV).

Discussion

The finding of noncaseating granulomas with epithelioid cells within the renal interstitium is an unusual and peculiar feature in drug-induced AIN [5]. The difficulty in differentiating this type of AIN from other types of ARF is strongly emphasised in our series, especially in group I: systemic clinical manifestations are frequently absent, blood eosinophilia is rare, immunological tests are inconstantly positive and other factors may be often considered as the precipitating causes for the observed ARF.

Therefore, the diagnosis of drug-induced AIN should be considered in any patients with ARF of unknown origin; in such cases, the finding of noncaseating granulomas on renal biopsy is an important feature for diagnosing AIN due to drug hypersensitivity [5, 6].

The precise mechanism responsible for this pathologic disturbance is not yet well elucidated. The available data strongly suggest the participation of cell-mediated immunity. It may be postulated that renal interstitial accumulation of the drug induces a delayed hypersensitivity response which will bring about the invasion of the interstitium with activated T lymhpocytes. These T cells release a variety of lymphokines that modulate granuloma formation and polyclonally activate B lymphocytes to secrete immunoglobulins [7, 8]. This immuno-pathogenetic hypothesis does not exclude the possibility of antibody mediated mechanisms since granulomatous interstitial lesions have been found in experimental anti-TBM disease [9].

Incomplete recovery of renal function may be observed in granulomatous AIN and justifies prompt and definitive withdrawal of the offending drug and all chemically-related drugs. The beneficial effect of early steroid therapy on renal function needs further assessment in this kind of nephritis, especially when granulomas are extensive.

References

1 Baldwin DS, Levine BB, McCluskey RT et al. *N Engl J Med 1968; 279:* 1245
2 Linton AL, Clark WF, Driedger AA et al. *Ann Intern Med 1980; 93:* 735
3 Mery J Ph, Morel-Maroger L. In Giovanetti S, Bonomini V, d'Amico G, eds. *Proc 6th Int Congress of Nephrology.* Basel: Karger. 1976: 524–529
4 Ooi BS, Wellington J, First MR et al. *Am J Med 1975; 59:* 614
5 Kleinknecht D, Vanhille Ph, Morel-Maroger L et al. In Hamburger J, Crosnier J, Funck-Brentano JL, eds. *Actualités Néphrologiques de l'Hôpital Necker.* Paris: Flammarion. 1982: 111–145
6 Mignon F, Mery J Ph, Morel-Maroger L et al. In Crosnier J, Funck-Brentano JL, Bach JF, Grunfeld JP, eds. *Actualités Néphrologiques de l'Hôpital Necker.* Paris: Flammarion. 1983: 200
7 Van Ypersele De Strihou C. *Kidney Int 1979; 16:* 751
8 Finkelstein A, Fraley DS, Stachura I et al. *Am J Med 1982; 72:* 81
9 Magil AB. *Hum Pathol 1983; 14:* 36

Proc EDTA (1983) Vol 20

THE EFFECT OF PREVENTIVE ADMINISTRATION OF VERAPAMIL ON ACUTE ISCHAEMIC RENAL FAILURE IN DOGS

M Papadimitriou, E Alexopoulos, V Vargemezis, G Sakellariou, I Kosmidou, P Metaxas

Aristotelian University of Thessaloniki, 'Aghia Sophia' Hospital, Thessaloniki, Greece

Summary

In 15 healthy mongrel dogs the kidneys were exposed bilaterally, the renal pedicle was clamped on one side (control kidneys) and verapamil, 0.5mg/kg body weight, was given intravenously. Ten minutes later the renal pedicle on the other side was clamped (verapamil group). At the end of a 60-minute ischaemic period, blood flow was re-established. The mean time to initiation of diuresis was shorter in the verapamil group and creatinine clearance was significantly higher. At the end of the two-hour experiment the mean fractional excretion of sodium and the mean urinary excretion of LDH were higher in the control group. C_{Na}, C_K, C_{osm} and C_{urea} were significantly higher in the verapamil group during the two-hour period of study after revascularisation. On a statistical basis 60 minute acute ischaemic renal failure is significantly modified by the administration of verapamil.

Introduction

Acute ischaemic renal failure (AIRF) remains a problem in clinical renal transplantation. Forced diuresis before nephrectomy, the use of Collins solution for flushing the kidney and cooling are the mainstays of cadaveric kidney preservation. On the other hand, when the warm ischaemic time is prolonged, the results are not encouraging. Interest has recently been focused on the prevention of acute renal failure by certain agents having an influence at the mitochondrial level [1, 2]. For instance, the role of calcium on ischaemic cell damage and the effect of preventive administration of calcium antagonists in experimental models of acute renal failure produced by continuous infusion of norepinephrine into the renal artery of the dog has been reported [3]. In this study, we investigated the effect of preventive administration of verapamil on the course of experimental AIRF induced by clamping the renal pedicle for 60 minutes.

Materials and methods

Fifteen healthy mongrel dogs were used. After anaesthesia with sodium thiopental and mannitol diuresis, both kidneys were exposed by bilateral flank incisions. The renal pedicle was clamped on one side (control group) and 0.5mg/kg of body weight of verapamil was given intravenously. Ten minutes later, the renal pedicle of the other kidney was clamped (verapamil group). The ischaemic period for both kidneys was 60 minutes at the end of which clamps were removed and blood flow was re-established. Blood and urine samples were collected before the clamping (baseline values) and after revascularisation for two hours. The time of initiation of diuresis, the urine flow rate, the endogenous creatinine clearance (C_{Cr}), the clearance of urea (C_{urea}), sodium (C_{Na}), potassium (C_K) and osmolality (C_{osm}), the excretion fraction of sodium (FE_{Na}) and the urinary excretion of lactic dehydrogenase (LDH) were measured. The Student's t-test for paired data was used for the statistical analysis.

Results

The mean time to initiation of diuresis after revascularisation was 7.2 min in the verapamil group and 20.3 min in the control group of kidneys (p<0.001) (Figure 1).

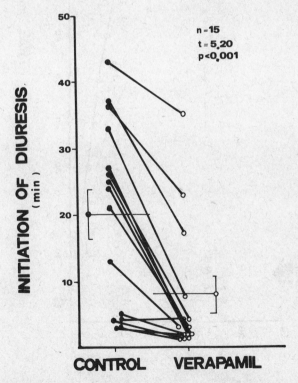

Figure 1. Time of initiation of diuresis after revascularisation

651

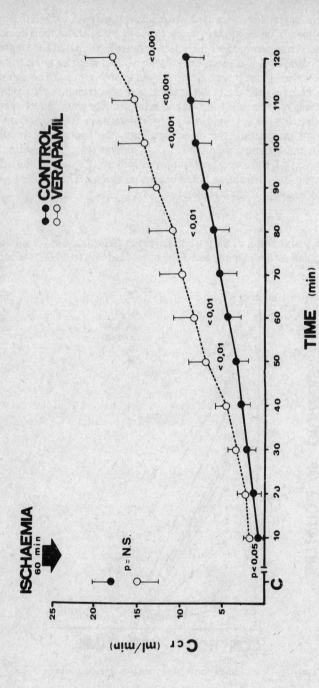

Figure 2. Schematic presentation of C_{Cr} (mean ± SE) changes after the 60 minute ischaemia

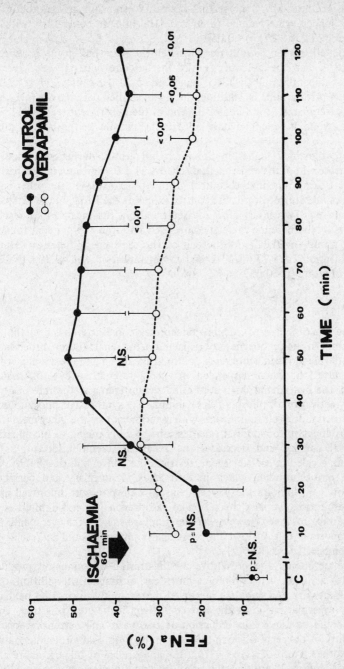

Figure 3. Schematic presentation of FE$_{Na}$ (mean ± SE) during the two-hour period after revascularisation

In addition, at the end of the second hour the verapamil group produced a significantly higher urine volume (3.80 ± 0.41ml/min) in comparison with the control group (2.62 ± 0.32) ($p < 0.05$).

C_{Cr} during all studied periods was higher in the verapamil group (Figure 2). Thus, finally C_{Cr} reached 115 per cent of the baseline value (17.63 ± 3.03ml/min) in the verapamil group, while it remained at 50 per cent (8.94 ± 1.71ml/min) in the control group. In addition, during all studied periods, the C_{urea} was higher in the verapamil group and at the end of the experiment reached 11.54 ± 2.39ml/min, while it remained only 5.92 ± 1.13ml/min in the control group ($p < 0.01$).

The C_{osm} remained higher in the verapamil group, during all periods of study and at the end of the experiment reached 4.21 ± 0.48ml/min in comparison with 2.42 ± 0.26ml/min in the control group ($p < 0.001$). On the other hand, there was a rapid return towards the control values of the FE_{Na} in the verapamil group (Figure 3). Two hours after revascularisation, the mean FE_{Na} reached 283 per cent of the baseline value in comparison with the 489 per cent found in the control group ($p < 0.01$). At the end of the experiment the mean urinary LDH concentration was 5.77 ± 3.42 IU in the verapamil group and 49.30 ± 17.22 IU in the control group ($p < 0.05$).

Discussion

Recently the role of increased calcium concentration in cytosol has been thought to be important in the pathogenesis of ischaemic acute renal failure. Mitochondria of norepinephrine-induced acute renal failure in the dog maintained a higher free Ca^{++} concentration, when suspended in media resembling cytosol, than in controls. On the other hand, high cytosolic calcium increases the rate of glycogenolysis by activation of phosphorylase, inhibits the synthesis of phospholipids, activates mitochondrial phospholipases with deterioration of the inner membrane function, produces mitochondrial calcification, possibly owing to incompatible mitochondrial damage and decreases the renal citrate oxidation [4, 5, 6].

Verapamil, a calcium blocker agent, restricts the conversion of ATP to ADP in vascular smooth muscle, which in turn leads to coronary and peripheral vasodilatation [7], inhibits the oxygen consumption rate with improved mitochondrial respiration, impairs the action of vasopressin [8] and diminishes the tubuloglomerular balance. However, recent findings suggest that verapamil also plays an important role in lowering mesangial contraction and increasing the ultrafiltration coefficient (Kf) [9].

In our experiments the preventive administration of verapamil produced together with a higher urine volume a much earlier diuresis. In addition, renal function (glomerular and tubular) improved more rapidly during the next two hours after revascularisation in the verapamil than in the control group. These differences could be due to the reduction of vasospasm and better preservation of the viability of the renal tissue in the verapamil group. Mannitol alone did not protect the other group of kidneys from the appearance of oliguric acute renal failure. It is therefore likely that the preventive administration of verapamil has a favourable influence on the course of AIRF in dogs. It seems that a milder non-oliguric form of acute renal failure is produced. This is important in cadaveric kidney transplantation, where the severity of ischaemic damage and the time of initiation of diuresis play a critical role in the survival of the renal graft. For this reason we have already been using an intracellular type of perfusate containing verapamil in kidney transplantation and up to now the results do seem encouraging (unpublished observations).

References

1 Schrier RW, Arnold PE, Burke TJ. In Eliahou HE, ed. *Acute Renal Failure.* London: John Libbey. 1982: 21
2 Schrier RW, Arnold PE, Gordon JA et al. *Kidney Int 1983; 23:* 427 (Abstract)
3 Burke TJ, Arnold PE, Grossfeld PD et al. In Eliahou HE, ed. *Acute Renal Failure.* London: John Libbey. 1982: 239
4 Carafoli E. In Smellie RMS ed. *Calcium and Cell Regulation.* London: The Biochemical Society. 1974: 89
5 Trump BF, Berezesky IK, Smith MW et al. In Kaizer H, ed. *Neoplasms: Comparative Pathology of Growth in Animals, Plants and Man.* London: Williams and Wilkins. 1981: 217
6 Simpson DP. *Biochem Med 1967; 1:* 168
7 Schamroth L. *Am Heart J 1980; 100:* 1070
8 Berl T. *Kidney Int 1981; 19:* 15
9 Ishikawa I, Miele JF, Brenner BM. *Kidney Int 1979; 16:* 137

STUDIES ON THE GLOMERULAR FILTRATION BARRIER AND ON THE URINARY EXCRETION OF BASEMENT MEMBRANE GLYCOPROTEINS DURING THE ACCELERATED MODEL OF NEPHROTOXIC SERUM NEPHRITIS

J C Davin, M Davies*, J M Foidart, C H Dubois, C Dechenne, P Mahieu

State University of Liège, Liège, Belgium and *The Welsh National School of Medicine, Cardiff, United Kingdom

Summary

A proliferative glomerulonephritis was induced in rats preimmunised with rabbit IgG by injecting a sub-nephrotoxic dose of rabbit anti-rat GBM IgG. All the rats developed a severe proteinuria within 2—5 days after the injection of anti-GBM IgG. At the same time, many mononuclear phagocytes infiltrated the glomeruli, the colloidal iron staining of the glomerular filtration barrier was altered, and the urinary excretion of laminin and of neutral proteinase strongly increased. However, the pattern and intensity of staining of different collagenous and non-collagenous BM glycoproteins were not modified, as shown by indirect immunofluorescence microscopy. The existence of a direct significant correlation between the proteinuria and the laminin urinary excretion, and between the latter and the urinary neutral proteinase activity suggests that lysosomal proteinase of mononuclear phagocytes may be involved in the damage of the GBM during the course of this experimental glomerulonephritis.

Introduction

A number of cellular and humoral factors have been investigated as possible mediators of glomerular damage in experimental glomerulonephritis. Fibrin [1,2], complement [3] and polymorphonuclear leucocytes [4] are involved in the development of glomerular injury. More recently, Schreiner et al [5], using an accelerated model of nephrotoxic nephritis (NTN), have shown that mononuclear phagocytes of predominantly extra-renal origin, infiltrate the kidneys and may contribute to some functional abnormalities. Davies et al [6] have shown that neutrophil and monocyte neutral proteinases are able to degrade GBM in vitro. In this work, an accelerated model of NTN has been induced in rats in order to determine: (1) whether some anionic charges of the GBM are altered during the course of this disease; (2) whether these eventual alterations might be correlated with the proteinuria, the urinary excretion of some anionic BM glycoproteins and the urinary excretion of neutral proteinases.

Materials and methods

The accelerated model of NTN

The model of Schreiner et al [5] was used. Sprague-Dawley (female) rats weighing 100–120g were preimmunised with 1mg of rabbit IgG in 0.5ml of complete Freund's adjuvant injected intraperitoneally. One week later, the rats received 1mg of rabbit anti-rat GBM IgG intravenously. This dose was chosen on the basis of preliminary experiments demonstrating that 1–2mg of rabbit anti-GBM IgG did not induce a significant proteinuria in non-immunised rats. Proteinuria was determined by the method of Kingsbury and Clarck [7].

Morphological studies of kidney sections

Rats were killed at various periods of time, from one to 21 days after the injection of anti-GBM IgG and the kidneys were examined by light and immunofluorescence microscopy. For light microscopy, portions of rat kidneys were fixed in Bouin's renal fixative, sectioned at 4μm and stained with haematoxylin and eosin or with the periodic acid-Schiff and the colloidal iron reagents. For immunofluorescence microscopy, kidney specimens were snap frozen in liquid nitrogen, sectioned at 2μm on a cryostat, and stained with fluorescein isothiocyanate (FITC) conjugated antisera to rabbit IgG, rat Ig and rat C_3. Commercial FITC-antisera were used (Behring-Werke AG, Marburg/Lahn, West Germany). The kidney sections were also incubated with various antibodies directed against basement membrane components i.e. laminin, fibronectin, type IV and V collagens. The specificity of these antibodies has been previously demonstrated [8].

Measurement of urinary laminin excretion and of urinary neutral proteinase activity

Twenty four hour urine collections were used. After dialysis against distilled water, urinary laminin excretion was determined by a solid phase radioimmunoassay [8]. Results are expressed in μg/24 hours. The urinary neutral proteinase activity was measured by a previously described method [8,9], using (^{3}H)-acetyl-casein and (^{3}H) azocasein as substrates. Results are expressed in units/24 hours. One unit is equal to the quantity of the neutral proteinase degrading 1mg of substrate/hour.

Results

Morphological aspect of glomeruli

Microscopic examination of the kidney within 2–5 days after the injection of anti-GBM IgG revealed a glomerular hypercellularity. This hypercellularity was the consequence of: (a) an infiltration by mononuclear, esterase positive, cells [10]; (b) a proliferation of intrinsic glomerular cells [10]. No crescents were

657

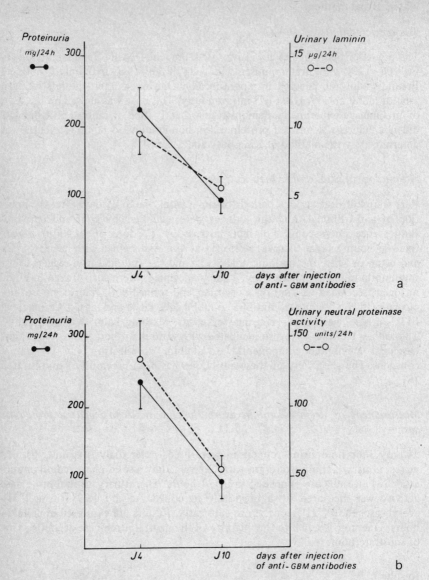

Figure 1.
  (a) Evolution of the urinary laminin excretion and of the proteinuria in rats injected with anti-GBM IgG. Results are the means (± SEM) of 26 determinations on day 4 and of 14 determinations on day 10
  (b) Evolution of the urinary neutral proteinase activity and of the proteinuria in the same rats. Results are the means (± SEM) of 22 determinations on day 4 and of 10 determinations on day 10

658

seen. Immunofluorescence study of the kidneys demonstrated the presence of linear deposits of rat Ig, rat C_3 and rabbit IgG along the GBM. No fixation was detectable on other kidney structures. All animals injected exhibited the same appearances. The pattern of staining and the intensity of binding to glomerular structures of antibodies directed against laminin, fibronectin, type IV and type V collagens remained unchanged as shown by indirect fluorescence. However, the colloidal iron staining of the glomerular capillary walls was focally altered in most glomeruli.

Urinary excretion of laminin and of neutral proteinases

All the rats presented a severe proteinuria reaching about 200mg/24 hours four days after the injection of anti-GBM IgG. The proteinuria decreased thereafter reaching about 100mg/24 hours on day 10 (Figure 1). The urinary laminin excretion and the urinary neutral proteinase activity followed the same evolution as the proteinuria (Figures 1a and 1b). Furthermore, a significant direct correlation was observed: (a) between the proteinuria and the urinary neutral proteinase activity (Figure 2); (b) between the proteinuria and the urinary laminin excretion (Figure 3); (c) between the urinary laminin excretion and the urinary neutral proteinase activity (Figure 4).

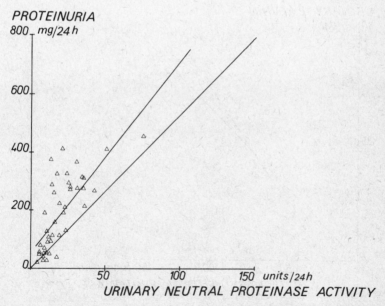

Figure 2. Correlation between the proteinuria and the urinary neutral proteinase activity (r=0.83; p<0.001)

659

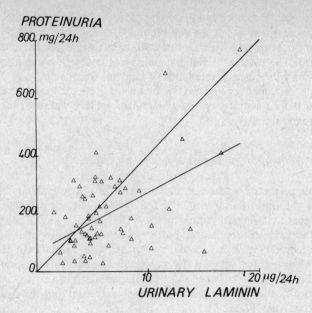

Figure 3. Correlation between the proteinuria and the urinary laminin excretion (r = 0.51; p < 0.01)

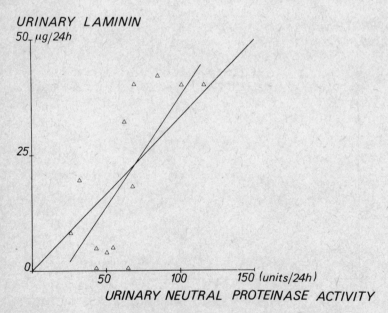

Figure 4. Correlation between the urinary laminin excretion and the urinary neutral proteinase activity (r = 0.73; 0.01 > p > 0.001)

Conclusions

It has been shown that human polymorphonuclear neutrophils and mononuclear phagocytes contain proteinases that degrade GBM at neutral and acid PH values in vitro. In the accelerated model of NTN, mononuclear phagocytes infiltrate most glomeruli within two to five days after the injection of anti-GBM IgG. A close temporal relationship is observed between this infiltration and: (a) the loss of some anionic sites from the glomerular filtration barrier; (b) the increase of the urinary excretion of an anionic BM glycoprotein, i.e. laminin; (c) the increase of the urinary neutral proteinase activity. We therefore suggest that, in this model of glomerulonephritis, neutral proteinases, some of which being of macrophagic origin, may contribute to the functional alterations of the glomerular filtration barrier.

References

1 Naish PF, Penn GB, Evans DJ, Peters DK. *Clin Sci 1972; 42:* 643
2 Thomson NM, Simpson IJ, Peters DK. *Clin Exp Immunol 1975; 19:* 301
3 Cochrane CG, Unanue ER, Dixon FJ. *J Exp Med 1965; 122:* 99
4 Cochrane CG. *Adv Immunol 1968; 9:* 97
5 Schreiner GF, Cotran RS, Pardo V, Unanue ER. *J Exp Med 1978; 147:* 369
6 Davies M, Hughes KT, Thomas GJ. *Renal Physiol 1980; 3:* 116
7 Kingsbury FB, Clarck CP. *J Lab Clin Med 1926; 11:* 981
8 Foidart JM, Berman JJ, Paglia L et al. *Lab Invest 1980; 42:* 525
9 Starkey PM. In Barrett J, ed. *Proteinases in Mammalian Cells and Tissues.* Amsterdam: North Holland. 1977: 57–84
10 Dubois CH, Foidart JM, Hautier MB et al. *Europ J Clin Invest 1981; 11:* 91

CORTICAL INFARCTION IN RABBITS WITH SERUM SICKNESS FOLLOWING CYCLOSPORIN A THERAPY

G H Neild, K Ivory, D G Williams

Guy's Hospital, London, United Kingdom

Summary

Rabbits given acute serum sickness (ASS) and treated with Cyclosporin A (CyA) developed glomerular capillary thrombosis and cortical infarction. These lesions were associated with severe endothelial injury and platelet-fibrin-leucocyte thrombi. They were not seen in untreated rabbits with ASS, nor in normal rabbits given CyA alone in equivalent doses. A similar renal lesion has been reported in patients receiving CyA following bone marrow transplantation.

Introduction

Nephrotoxicity is an important complication of CyA which usually causes tubular damage and reversible renal failure in a dose-dependent manner [1, 2]. Another renal complication has been recently described in CyA-treated bone marrow recipients who developed a haemolytic-uraemic syndrome (HUS) with thrombocytopenia and fragmented red cells, associated with glomerular capillary thrombosis [2]. During experiments in which we examined the effect of CyA on ASS (immune complex) nephritis in rabbits [3], we noted that with a high dose of 25mg/kg/day of CyA some rabbits became oliguric. The most severely oliguric had macroscopic infarction of the renal cortex. In this paper we describe the glomerular and tubular lesions which are very similar to those seen in bone marrow recipients treated with CyA.

Materials and methods

Experimental model of ASS

Female NZW rabbits (1.8–2.5kg) were injected i.v. with 250mg/kg crystallised bovine serum albumin (BSA). BSA was radiolabelled with Na^{125}I by the chloramine-T method. BSA was given either alone or together with 5µg/kg of E. coli endotoxin (Difco Labs, LPS.W, E. coli 0111:B4). BSA elimination was followed, as previously described [3, 4]. Antigen elimination was considered complete when less than one per cent of the initial activity remained.

Serology

Precipitating antibody was measured by radial immunodiffusion of neat serum into agarose containing BSA. An enzyme-linked immunosorbent assay (ELISA) method was used to measure total immunoglobulin antibody activity (Ig) to BSA, and the IgM antibody fraction [4]. The amount of circulating immune complexes was measured by precipitation of serum globulin bound to BSA ^{125}I, and their size was measured by ultracentrifugation of serum in 12–40 per cent sucrose gradients for 18 hours at 175,000g. Serum C_3 concentrations were measured by radial immunodiffusion.

Proteinuria

Proteinuria was measured by the Lowry method after TCA precipitation. Proteinuria greater than 150mg/100ml in a 24-hour volume was considered abnormal. An episode of 'significant proteinuria' was defined as two or more consecutive days of abnormal proteinuria.

Haematuria, glycosuria and oliguria

Haematuria and glycosuria were measured in fresh urine samples using 'Labstix' dip sticks (Ames, UK). A significant period of haematuria was defined as two or more days of 1+ or more haematuria. Oliguria was defined as a two day period (or longer) during which the mean daily urine volume was 50 per cent less than the mean of the previous four days.

Histology

Rabbits were killed on day 12 after BSA injection, or two to three days after immune elimination when elimination occurred after day 10. Whole sections of kidneys were fixed in 10 per cent buffered formal-saline. Sections were stained by the periodic acid-Schiff (PAS) reaction and with Martius Scarlet blue (MSB). Glomerular proliferation was scored on a scale of 0, ±, 1 to 4+ and was considered present when the score was 1+. Cryostat sections were examined with immunofluorescence (IF) using fluorescein conjugated antisera to BSA, rabbit whole immunoglobulin (Ig), IgG, IgM, C_3, fibrinogen and albumin (Nordic Pharmaceuticals). Paraffin-embedded tissue sections were dewaxed, pronase-digested and examined for fibrinogen using a peroxidase-anti-peroxidase (PAP) technique. Renal tissue was processed for electron microscopy.

Cyclosporin

Cyclosporin A was dissolved in a solvent vehicle of Miglyol 812 and 100 per cent ethanol at a concentration of 100mg/ml and given by deep intramuscular injection.

Experimental protocol

Twenty-three rabbits were given BSA plus endotoxin but received no other parenteral treatment (untreated animals). Groups of rabbits receiving CyA (15 or 25mg/kg/day) were given BSA plus endotoxin or BSA alone (see Table I). Two groups of animals were used as controls. Twenty-one with ASS received equivalent volumes of solvent alone for the same period as the treated groups. Six normal rabbits were given CyA 25mg/kg for five days: in addition on day 0 three were given i.v. saline plus $5\mu g/kg$ endotoxin, three were given saline alone.

TABLE I. Histopathological data of rabbits with ASS treated with Cyclosporin A

Rabbits (numbers)	Treatment Dose mg/kg/day	Days	Glomerular proliferation (% numbers)	Glomerular thrombi (% numbers)	Cortical infarction (% numbers)
BSA with endotoxin					
CyA-treated					
1) 12	15	−2 to +8	8	42	25
2) 5	25	−2 to +3	0	20	20
Control					
3) 32	−	−	84	0	0
BSA no endotoxin					
CyA-treated					
4) 5	15	−2 to +8	0	40	20
5) 6	25	−2 to +3	0	83	67
6) 5	25	0 to 5	0	80	40
Control					
7) 12	−	−	42	0	0

Results

Clinical data

CyA inhibited the proteinuria normally occurring with ASS, but did not inhibit the haematuria (see [3]). Rabbits also became oliguric (30%) and developed glycosuria (44%), two features which do not normally occur in ASS. Using BSA *alone* the nephritis was usually mild, with slight proteinuria and haematuria but when such rabbits were given BSA and CyA the disease produced was as severe as in those which received BSA and endotoxin.

664

CyA had no significant inhibitory effect on the humoral response as measured by (i) the time to BSA elimination; (ii) the magnitude or character of the antibody response; (iii) the amount or size of circulating immune complexes; (iv) the fall in C_3 at the time of immune elimination [3].

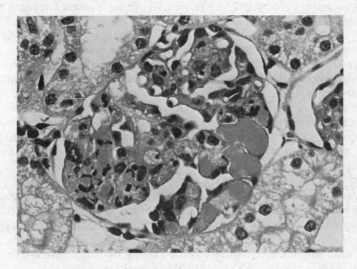

Figure 1. Glomerulus with multiple capillary thrombi, some of which are associated with polymorph infiltration (H & E x 25)

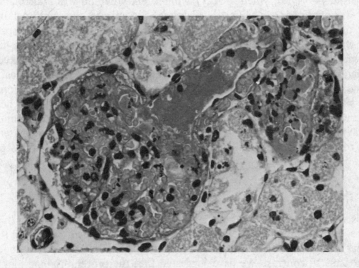

Figure 2. Necrotic glomerulus with thrombosis of afferent arteriole. Some of the surrounding tubules are also infarcted (H & E x 25)

Histology

Eighty-seven per cent of rabbits given BSA and endotoxin developed glomerular proliferation. Proliferation was less common in those given BSA alone. Treatment with CyA significantly reduced glomerular proliferation [3] but was associated with several new histological features which were more diffuse and severe in rabbits receiving 25mg/kg of CyA. These changes were not seen in untreated ASS or rabbits given CyA alone.

a) Glomerular capillary thrombi: Capillary loops were partially or totally occluded by amorphous, eosinophilic material and these areas were often infiltrated with polymorphs (Figure 1). In some cases capillary thrombi were associated with focal and segmental glomerular infarction (Figure 2) and necrosis of the afferent arterioles. The thrombi were PAS positive, and stained scarlet with MSB. IF examination showed strongly positive staining for BSA, but weak and equal staining for Igs, IgG, IgM, C_3 and albumin. Fresh thrombi (one to two days old) stained strongly positive for fibrinogen by both IF and immunoperoxidase.

b) Tubular and interstitial injury: Rabbits developed foci of dilated tubules, in which the height of the tubular epithelium was greatly reduced, or tubular cells appeared to be entirely absent. Amorphous eosinophilic casts which appeared to consist of the shed tubular epithelium were often seen in the tubules. At its most severe there was total tubular necrosis. Severe macroscopic infarction was associated with interstitial haemorrhage.

Electron microscopy showed swelling and disruption of the endothelial cytoplasm. At times, when grossly swollen, endothelium was indistinguishable from degranulated ('exhausted') platelets. Sometimes the endothelium was raised off the basement membrane, and the expanded subendothelial space was filled with a loose amorphous material or occasionally electron dense material with the periodicity of fibrin. At times capillary loops were packed with degenerating cells including platelets, polymorphs, and mononuclear cells. Strands of fibrin ran through this cellular mass. At later stages, the loops were filled with an electron dense mass of amorphous material, which did not have the periodicity of fibrin. Glomerular infarction was associated with accumulation of polymorphs in the capillary lumen phagocytosing amorphous material. In areas of tubular infarction peritubular capillaries were occluded by platelet thrombi.

Discussion

In this new model of glomerular and tubular infarction the vascular injury is initiated when immune complexes are being rapidly formed, suggesting that the vascular damage and haematuria are initiated by an immune complex dependent mechanism. In contrast, we have suggested that the proteinuria and glomerular proliferation in unmodified ASS may be T-cell mediated [3]. Vascular damage and endothelial injury are features of ASS although the mechanism [3] causing damage [6, 7] remains unknown. Vascular permeability increases and immune complexes are deposited in the vessel walls [5]. Arterial injury may progress to a proliferative and necrotic arteritis. However, severe endothelial injury is not a feature of ASS, and capillary thrombosis and glomerular infarction do not occur.

What is the pathogenetic mechanism of the new lesion that we have observed? There are several conditions with a similar appearance. Glomerular capillary thrombosis and cortical infarction may occur in rabbits following the Shwartzman reaction. The classic generalised Shwartzman reaction (GSR) follows two i.v. injections of endotoxin [6]. The first, or 'priming' dose, prepares the animal so that the intravascular coagulation triggered by the second dose initiates wide-spread thrombosis. Rabbits may be primed in other ways (e.g. pregnancy, pre-treatment with steroids), so that a single dose of endotoxin causes a GSR. Furthermore, if rabbits are primed for a GSR, then an infusion of immune complexes can replace endotoxin and trigger the reaction [7]. Although the pathogenesis of GSR has remained elusive, experiments suggest that the priming dose of endotoxin has a direct effect on the vascular endothelium.

It has been reported that some bone marrow recipients treated with CyA develop an HUS-like illness with glomerular and tubular infarction [2] similar to that described in our rabbits with CyA-treated ASS. Little is known of the pathogenesis of HUS, but recently Remuzzi et al [8] showed that in patients with HUS vascular synthesis of PGI_2 was reduced. Moreover, many of these patients lacked a prostacyclin stimulating factor (PSF) in their plasma which was necessary for synthesis of PGI_2 by vascular tissue. We have subsequently found that CyA therapy profoundly reduces PSF activity in plasma [9], but has no effect on platelets, or PGI_2 synthesis by aorta taken from CyA-treated animals.

From our observations and those in HUS and marrow transplantation, a unifying hypothesis can be made. Local production by vascular endothelium of PGI_2 limits excessive platelet aggregation and thrombus formation at sites of endothelial injury. In the absence of PSF, synthesis of PGI_2 is impaired and vascular injury can progress to capillary thrombosis and necrosis of the vessel wall. We suggest that ASS, graft-versus-host disease after marrow transplantation and HUS are three examples of different mechanisms of endothelial injury which, when they occur in the absence of PSF, result in the same final vascular injury.

Acknowledgments

We are grateful to the Medical Research Council who supported this work.

References

1 Klintmalm GBG, Iwatsuki S, Starzl TE. *Lancet 1981; i:* 470
2 Shulman H, Striker G, Deeg JH et al. *N Engl J Med 1981; 305:* 1392
3 Neild GH, Ivory K, Hiramatsu M, Williams DG. *Clin Exp Immunol 1983:* In press
4 Neild GH, Ivory K, Williams DG. *Br J Exp Pathol 1982; 63:* 605

5 Kniker WT, Cochrane CG. *J Exp Med 1968; 127:* 119
6 Thomas L, Good RA. *J Exp Med 1952; 96:* 605
7 Lee L. *Exp Med 1963; 117:* 365
8 Remuzzi G, Misiani R, Marchesi D et al. *Lancet 1978; ii:* 871
9 Neild GH, Rocchi G, Remuzzi G et al. *Transplant Proc 1983:* In press

ULTRASONIC FINDINGS IN ANALGESIC NEPHROPATHY

M Weber, B Braun, H Köhler

University of Mainz, Mainz, FRG

Summary

Thirty-four patients with analgesic nephropathy (AN) were investigated by real-time ultrasonography. In 11 of 14 dialysis patients and in 16 of 20 patients with renal insufficiency calcified renal papillae were documented surrounding the internal echo in a typical garland pattern. Incomplete garland pattern of papillary calcifications or development of hydronephrosis occurred in patients with a history of renal colic due to detachment of necrotic papillae. Moreover, AN was assumed in 10 patients with renal insufficiency of unknown origin after detection of typical ultrasonic signs of AN and confirmed by a hitherto unknown history of analgesic abuse.

Introduction

Analgesic nephropathy represents a common cause of renal insufficiency in certain geographic areas [1–3]. Diagnosis is complicated because analgesic abuse is often not admitted, thus being unknown to the physicians in about 50 per cent of the cases [3]. In the present study we investigated patients with an established diagnosis of analgesic nephropathy by ultrasonography in order to describe the scanning pattern of the kidneys. In a second group of patients with renal insufficiency of unknown origin we tested whether ultrasonography was able to identify analgesic nephropathy.

Methods

Thirty-four patients with analgesic nephropathy, 14 on chronic intermittent haemodialysis and 20 patients with renal insufficiency (serum creatinine 1.5–9.5mg/100ml) were investigated by ultrasonography. The average phenacetin ingestion amounted to 17.5kg and 8.5kg respectively. A second group of patients consisted of all in- and outpatients with renal insufficiency of unknown origin.

669

In this group ultrasonography was applied as an early step in diagnostic procedure.

Commercially available real-time sector scanners with 3.5 MHz transducers were used.

Results

Calcifications of the renal papillae were documented in 11 of 14 dialysis patients and in 16 of 20 patients with renal insufficiency due to analgesic nephropathy. The calcification always surrounded the internal echo in a typical garland pattern (Figure 1). Calcification began at the tip of the papilla with still perceptible low sonodense pattern of unchanged renal pyramids (Figures 1–3). In dialysis patients the papillary calcifications sometimes involved whole renal pyramids (Figure 4). Thirteen patients with a history of renal colic showed an incomplete garland pattern of papillary calcifications due to detachment of necrotic papillae (Figure 3). This incomplete garland pattern of calcification also occurred in six cases with only patchy calcification of the papillae and no history of renal colic. In two cases combination of garland calcification

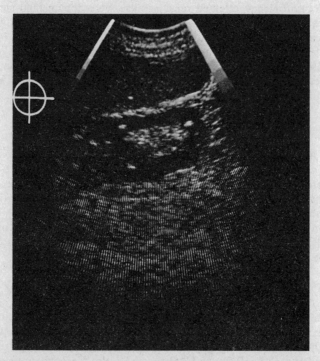

Figure 1. Typical garland pattern of papillary calcifications in analgesic nephropathy, with only a few calcifications showing distal shadowing in this section plane

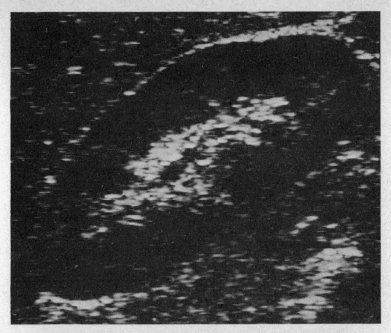

Figure 2. Normal human kidney showing low level echoes corresponding to renal pyramids forming a typical garland pattern around the internal echo

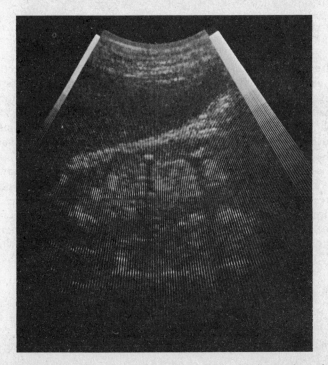

Figure 3. Incomplete garland pattern of papillary calcification in a patient with analgesic nephropathy and a history of renal colic (creatinine 5mg/100ml). The calcification starts at the tip of the papillae with less echogenic renal pyramids still perceptible

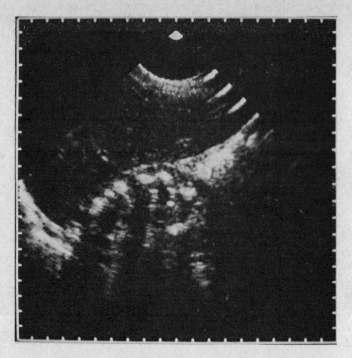

Figure 4. End-stage renal insufficiency due to analgesic nephropathy. Note the garland pattern of pyramidal calcifications in a shrunken kidney with similar echogenicity between cortex and internal echo

with hydronephrosis occurred as a consequence of ureteric obstruction by a detached papilla. Reduction of kidney size and shrunken cortex was detected in severe cases of renal insufficiency and in patients treated by chronic intermittent haemodialysis. In patients with moderate renal insufficiency, however, kidneys showed a normal size for many years with only a slight thinning of the cortex. In dialysis patients a similar echogenicity between cortex and internal echo of the shrunken kidney was usually documented.

In the second group of patients with renal insufficiency of unknown origin scanning revealed the typical ultrasonic signs of analgesic nephropathy in 10 cases, three of them complicated by hydronephrosis. The tentative diagnosis was confirmed by obtaining a hitherto unknown history of analgesic abuse. Three other patients showing similar ultrasonic findings suffered from nephrocalcinosis due to primary hyperparathyroidism (1) and sarcoidosis with hypercalciuria (2) (Figure 5).

Discussion

Pathologists describe early, intermittent and advanced changes in analgesic nephropathy with papillary and medullary alterations appearing first [4,5]. The advanced changes are characterised by total necrosis of the inner medulla

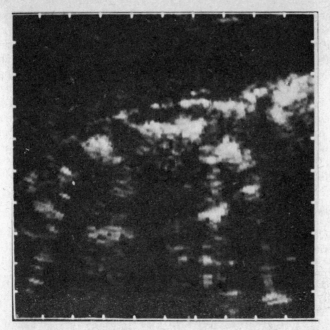

Figure 5. Calcified renal pyramids in a patient with nephrocalcinosis due to sarcoidosis (creatinine 5.2mg/100ml)

and papillae, as well as cortical scarring. Small fragments of these necrotic papillae may crumble away or entire papillae may be detached. However, many papillae remain in situ and calcify.

Radiological changes in analgesic nephropathy have been well described by Lindvall [6]. Our present study indicates that ultrasonography may also be able to document typical signs in analgesic nephropathy. In about 80 per cent of patients with a known history of analgesic abuse, a complete or incomplete garland pattern of papillary or even pyramidal calcifications was documented (Figures 1,3,4). Some other diseases may show similar ultrasonic signs, such as nephrocalcinosis (Figure 5), which favours medullary calcium deposition as well as formation of renal stones. In contrast calcification in analgesic nephropathy starts at the tip of the papilla whereas pyramidal calcification takes place only in severe renal insufficiency (Figures 3 and 4). In renal calculi, which are often solitary, a typical garland pattern is uncommon. Diabetes mellitus may also be associated with renal papillary necrosis and consecutive calcification. However, in 21 patients with chronic renal insufficiency due to diabetic nephropathy, we were not able to demonstrate any papillary calcification. Diseases known to be associated with renal papillary necrosis or calcification such as medullary sponge kidney, sickle cell disease or chronic liver disease [7,8] may possibly show similar ultrasonic findings. After exclusion of these diseases, we believe the scanning pattern to be typical for analgesic nephropathy.

The possibility of establishing a tentative diagnosis by non-invasive and

673

routinely performed ultrasonography seems to be of great importance as physicians may be able to detect a hitherto unknown analgesic abuse by observing typical ultrasonic findings as in 10 of our own patients. In patients with moderate renal insufficiency, the long term prognosis is good provided that total abstinence from analgesics is achieved. In dialysis patients, the basic diagnosis of end-stage renal failure is unknown in about 10 per cent of the cases [9]. In some of these patients, typical ultrasonic signs may possibly detect an unknown abuse of analgesic mixtures. Although kidney function has already been damaged irreversibly in this group of patients, knowledge of analgesic abuse is important because of the increased risk of developing uroepithelial carcinoma in these patients [10]. We believe that ultrasonography might be helpful in establishing the sometimes difficult diagnosis of analgesic nephropathy.

References

1   Brynger H, Brunner RP, Chantler C et al. *Proc EDTA 1980; 17:* 4
2   Kincaid-Smith P. *Kidney Int 1980; 17:* 250
3   Mihatsch MJ, Hofer HO, Gutzeiler F et al. *Schweiz Med Wschr 1980; 110:* 108
4   Burry A. *Kidney Int 1978; 13:* 34
5   Gloor FJ. *Kidney Int 1978; 13:* 27
6   Lindvall N. *Kidney Int 1978; 13:* 93
7   Edmondson HA, Reynold TB, Jacobson HG. *Arch Intern Med 1966; 118:* 255
8   Harrow BR, Sloane JA, Liebmann NC. *N Engl J Med 1963; 268:* 269
9   Wing AJ, Brunner FP, Brynger H et al. *Proc EDTA 1978; 15:* 3
10 Mihatsch MJ, Manz T, Knüsli C et al. *Schweiz Med Wschr 1980; 110:* 255

Proc EDTA (1983) Vol 20

INCIDENCE, DIAGNOSIS AND EVOLUTION OF 'NON A–NON B' HEPATITIS IN HAEMODIALYSIS UNITS

R Matesanz, J L Teruel, J González Sainz, R Bueno, R Marcén, C Quereda, J Ortuno

Centro Ramón y Cajal, Madrid, Spain

Summary

Over a four year period, 34 patients on chronic haemodialysis with non A–non B hepatitis were studied. Although clinical symptoms were mild or absent in most patients, biochemical evolution seemed to be serious as more than 70 per cent became chronic or showed a relapsing pattern. Blood transfusions play an important role in the spread of this disease; on the other hand in our experience patient to patient transmission was less relevant.

Introduction

Non A–non B hepatitis is the most frequently occurring type of hepatitis in those haemodialysis (HD) units where virus B prophylaxis is effective [1]. Diagnosis can only be made by exclusion of known aetiological factors as specific tests are not presently available. This paper describes our experience of non A–non B hepatitis.

Patient details

From 1977 to 1981, 154 patients were dialysed in our unit: 85 at home after a training period, 84 at the hospital, 18 in both places and three HBs Ag positive patients who from the start of their treatment were dialysed in an isolated hospital room. HBs Ag (RIA) and serum alanine-transferases (SMAC-20) were determined monthly in hospital patients and every three months in home patients. Anti-core antibodies (HBc Ab) and HBs Ab were tested yearly. Whenever an enzymatic elevation was detected (after ruling out technical mistakes, congestive cardiac failure and systemic bacterial infection), a virological screen was performed: Epstein-Barr virus (Paul Bunnell-Davidson Test), cytomegalovirus (a four-fold increase in specific antibody titre and/or cell culture isolation from urine), virus A (specific HVA-Ab, IgM and IgG by RIA) and virus B (HBs Ag, HBs Ab and HBc Ab by RIA). No isolation measures were taken after the diagnosis of any 'non B' hepatitis.

Results

Non A–non B hepatitis was diagnosed by the presence of confirmed enzymatic elevation, and the absence of: congestive cardiac failure, bacterial infection, hepatotoxic drugs, and no seroconversion for CMV, EBV, virus A, and virus B. According to these criteria, during the period of study, 43 enzymatic elevations were detected and classified as follows:

Virus A	1
Virus B	1 (in chronic carrier)
CMV	1
EBV	2
Drugs	4
Non A–non B	34 (79%)

There were no cases of HBs Ag seroconversion. The only HBs Ag positive patient with enzymatic elevation was a chronic carrier with biopsy-proven chronic active hepatitis before the start of HD treatment.

The distribution of the 34 non A–non B hepatitis cases throughout the four years was rather uniform, lacking clear epidemic outbreaks. There was a history of blood transfusion in the three month period prior to enzymatic abnormalities in 16 patients (47 per cent, and this reached 64 per cent when the hypothetical incubation period was extended to eight months [2]. There was no difference between hospital and home patients (10.7 vs 19.6 hepatitis/100 patients/year).

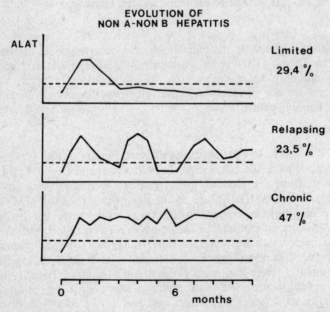

Figure 1. Patterns of sequential serum alanine aminotransferase (ALAT) values in patients with non A–non B hepatitis

Both groups received a similar number of units of blood: 1.41 vs 1.40 units/patient/year (no systematic pre-transplant transfusions were given). Clinical symtomatology was mild or absent (usually asthenia, anorexia and weight loss). Bilirubin was slightly elevated (4.6mg/dl) in only one patient. Long-term evolution, however, was by no means trivial, as only 10 patients had a self-limited course (29%), while 16 (47%) had a chronic evolution (more than 6 months) and eight (23%) showed relapsing enzyme elevations (Figure 1). No routine biopsy was performed in these patients.

Discussion

The key role of blood transfusion in the spread of this disease can be supported by the following facts: a high incidence of blood transfusion prior to onset, similarity between hospital and home dialysis patients with respect to frequency of transfusions and hepatitis, and the uniform temporal distribution of cases lacking any clear epidemic outbreak. Thus, in haemodialysis units, blood transfusions seem to be more important than other mechanisms such as patient to patient transmission. Although home dialysis patients sporadically dialyse in hospital (in the training room, separated from hospital patients) for medical or other reasons (3% of HD sessions during period of study), the chance of patient to patient transmission is actually much greater in those patients always dialysed in the hospital. Besides, three home HD patients were not transfused nor dialysed in hospital during the eight month period before the onset of hepatitis and therefore, it is necessary to attribute these cases to other mechanisms.

The existence of at least two poorly identified agents responsible for non A–non B hepatitis [3] makes it difficult to come to any conclusion. The situation is even more complicated in haemodialysis patients by the administration of multiple drugs, the existence of a dialysis related pathology, such as the accumulation of silicone refractile particles in the liver [4], and perhaps other still poorly understood factors. The relatively high incidence of non A–non B hepatitis and its evolution to chronicity [5] in up to 70 per cent of our cases, although the prognosis seems to be better than for other forms of chronic hepatitis [6], are worrisome aspects of dialysis therapy. These facts should be kept in mind when considering the risks of pre-transplant blood transfusions.

References

1   Simon N, Mery JP, Trepo C et al. *Proc EDTA 1980; 17:* 173
2   Tateda A, Kikuchi K, Numazaki Y et al. *J Infect Dis 1979; 139:* 511
3   Yoshizawa H, Itoch Y, Iwakiri S et al. *Gastroenterology 1981; 81:* 107
4   Morales JM, Colina F, Arteaga J et al. *Proc EDTA 1982; 19:* 265
5   Galbraith RM, Dienstag JL, Purcell RH et al. *Lancet 1979; i:* 951
6   Robinson WS. *J Infect Dis 1982; 145:* 287

PART XIX

DIABETES MELLITUS

Chairmen: C Jacobs
          J F Moorhead

Proc EDTA (1983) Vol 20

IS RENAL GLYCOSURIA A BENIGN CONDITION?

S De Marchi, E Cecchin*, A Basile, G Proto, W Donadon*,
D Schinella*, A Lengo, P De Paoli*, A Jus*, D Villalta*,
F Tesio*, G Santini*

*Stabilimento Ospedaliero di Codroipo (Udine), and
Stabilimento Ospedaliero di Pordenone, Italy

Summary

HLA typing and a range of autoantibodies were evaluated in five families affected
with type A renal glycosuria. HLA typing demonstrates that this inherited
disease is controlled by an autosomal dominant gene located on chromosome six
in close genetic linkage with the HLA complex. All affected family members
have significant titres of autoantibodies to nuclear antigens, native DNA, smooth
muscle, mitochondria, liver antigens, thyroglobulin, thyroid microsomes and
renal tubule brush border with variable association. This suggests that renal
glycosuria is a complex HLA-linked disease with increased susceptibility to
multiple autoantibody production and this urges caution with respect to its
classical definition as a benign condition.

Introduction

Primary renal glycosuria (RG) is an inherited disorder of renal tubule function in
which significant amounts of glucose are excreted in the urine in the simultaneous
presence of normal blood glucose concentration. It is generally considered to be
benign [1]. The fortuitous discovery of significant titres of autoantibodies to
thyroglobulin and thyroid microsomes in a 27 year old woman with RG prompted
us to evaluate both a large range of autoantibodies and HLA typing in this
interesting 'freak of nature'.

Materials and methods

We studied five unrelated families affected with RG (25 patients) and 40 healthy
relatives. No consanguinity was reported. Control group consisted of 100 subjects:
50 women and 50 men (mean age 38 years; range 16–60 years) with normal
renal function.

The diagnosis of RG was determined by measuring fasting glycosuria, 24-hour
urinary glucose and by performing a renal glucose titration as previously described

by Elsas and Rosemberg [2]. The specificity of the tubule defect for glucose reabsorption was confirmed by evaluation of urinary pH, 24 hour protein and bicarbonate excretion, urinary free amino acid pattern, clearances of creatinine, uric acid, calcium and β-2-microglobulin, and tubular phosphate reabsorption ($T_p = (C_{Cr} \times P_p) - U_p \times V$). Each subject was submitted to an ammonium chloride load test and to a fluid deprivation test.

HLA typing was performed on peripheral blood lymphocytes by the Standard National Institutes of Health two stage microcytotoxicity test. One hundred and four selected antisera were used to determine 37 specificities: 12 in the A locus, 19 in the B locus and six in the C locus. We investigated a large variety of auto-antibodies including antibodies to nuclear antigens (standard fluorescent antibody technique), native DNA (Farr's technique), smooth muscle (indirect immuno-fluorescent technique (IIT)), mitochondria (IIT), gastric parietal cells (IIT on cryostat sections of human gastric mucosa), pancreatic islets (IIT on cryostat sections of human group O pancreatic gland), thyroglobulin (IIT and tanned red cells haemoagglutination technique) thyroid microsomes (IIT on cryostat sections of thyrotoxic thyroid gland), liver antigens (IIT) and renal tubule brush border (IIT).

Results

Renal glucose titration studies in our patients demonstrated a reduction of both the minimal threshold (TminG) and the maximal reabsorptive capacity (TmG) for glucose reabsorption delineating a type A RG as proposed by Reubi [3]. Endogenous clearances of creatinine, tubular phosphate reabsorption, daily proteinuria and bicarbonaturia and urinary free amino acids were in the normal range. Endogenous clearances of uric acid, calcium and β-2-microglobulin corrected for the creatinine clearance were also normal. This range of investigations excluded other inherited or acquired renal tubular dysfunction. In each family all the affected members carried a haplotype which was not present in the healthy relatives demonstrating that the gene responsible for RG segregates with the HLA complex. The HLA haplotypes linked to RG trait in our families are summarised in Table I. The HLA-A, -B and -C locus antigen frequencies of one affected patient of each family were calculated and compared with the antigen frequencies of 120 normal blood donors. No significant difference was observed between the

TABLE I. HLA haplotypes linked to renal glycosuria trait in five families

Families	Affected members	Unaffected members	HLA haplotypes
Family 1	5	3	A1, B5
Family 2	2	2	A11, BW44, CW4
Family 3	6	12	BW16
Family 4	3	6	A2, B15, CW3
Family 5	9	17	A9, B27

patients and the normal population for any of the antigens studied.

Table II summarises the frequencies of autoantibodies in our families with RG and in controls. All the affected members had significant titres of auto-antibodies to nuclear antigens, native DNA, smooth muscle, mitochondria, liver antigens, thyroglobulin, thyroid microsomes and renal tubule brush border in variable association. These autoantibody titres were significantly higher than those of healthy controls but lower than those of patients with symptoms of overt autoimmune disease.

TABLE II. Frequencies of autoantibodies in five families affected with renal glycosuria and in controls

Autoantibodies	Affected members (n = 25)	Unaffected members (n = 40)	Controls (n = 100)
Nuclear antigens	42	3	4
Native DNA	16	0	0
Mitochondria	5	0	0
Smooth Muscle	47	6	5
Liver antigens	21	3	3
Thyroglobulin	32	3	4
Thyroid microsomal	32	3	4
Pancreatic islets	0	0	0
Gastric parietal cells	0	0	0
Renal tubule brush border	42	0	0

All values are expressed as %

Discussion

The presence of autoantibodies in RG has never been reported and its significance is unclear. Many autoantibodies, such as antinuclear antibodies and thyroid antibodies occur more frequently and in higher titres in certain immune diseases than in healthy subjects and there is some evidence that seroreactions may precede the development of clinical disease [4]. On the other hand extensive population surveys have confirmed that in most instances autoantibodies do not have any obvious relation to the diseases [5]. Although none of our patients have clinical evidence of autoimmune diseases, this association with autoantibodies urges caution against the classical definition of RG as a benign condition. The question must be asked whether such predisposition to multiple autoantibody production increases the susceptibility to autoimmune diseases or whether these immunological abnormalities might represent early manifestation of an under-lying autoimmune disease in patients at present clinically healthy. In fact autoimmunity has a late and variable age of onset [6] and the mean age of our patients is relatively low (34 years). It will be most interesting to see whether or not they will develop symptoms. Moreover there is circumstantial evidence from cross-sectional studies and a limited amount of more straightforward evidence from longitudinal studies that autoantibodies act as risk factors. They appear to be associated with excess mortality from vascular causes and cancer [7]. The presence of autoantibodies in all the affected members of our families suggests a role of genetic factors in predisposing patients with RG to produce autoantibodies. Recently a great deal of information has been obtained about the function of the HLA system in regulating the immune response [8]. In more than 40 conditions it has been found that the susceptibility to disease is associated with a particular HLA-A, -B or -D locus type. The mechanism of this association is as yet unknown but most of these diseases have a definite or suspected autoimmune pathogenesis [9]. On the basis of extensive study on the related H_2 system in the mouse it has been postulated that the HLA-D locus is closely linked to other, yet undefined immune related genes. Persons with certain non-specific D alleles may carry a closely linked immune related gene that makes them more likely to produce autoantibodies when challenged by autologous antigens [10].

HLA typing in our families demonstrates that RG trait segregates with HLA and suggests that the inherited disease is controlled by an autosomal dominant gene located on the sixth pair of human chromosomes in a close genetic linkage with the Major Histocompatibility Complex. One interpretation suggests that the location of the abnormal gene near the HLA complex might have a role in explaining the immunological findings in our patients. Alternatively such predisposition to autoantibody production might be due to an, as yet unidentified, metabolic impairment related to RG. In summary, our data suggest that RG is a complex HLA linked disease with an increased susceptibility to multiple autoantibody production. Most of the possible mechanisms for the association of HLA, autoantibodies and RG as well as the probability that such predisposition to autoantibody production may favour a susceptibility to autoimmune diseases remains a matter for future research which will depend on better knowledge of this interesting inherited disease, perhaps too easily considered a 'freak of nature'.

References

1   Brenner BM, Rector FC. *The Kidney*. Philadelphia: Saunders. 1981
2   Elsas LJ, Rosemberg LE. *J Clin Invest 1969; 48:* 1845
3   Reubi FC. *Ciba Foundation Symposium on the Kidney*. Boston: Little Brown. 1954
4   Aho K, Sistonen P, Takala J et al. *Acta Med Scand 1982; 211:* 213
5   Irvine WJ. *Proc Roy Soc Med 1971; 67:* 548
6   Rowley MJ, Buchanan H, Mackay IR. *Lancet 1968; ii:* 24
7   Aho K. *Med Biol 1980; 58:* 8
8   Bodmer WF, Bodmer JG. *Br Med Bull 1978; 34:* 309
9   Motulsky AG. *N Engl J Med 1979; 300:* 918
10   McDevitt HO. *N Engl J Med 1980; 303:* 1514

Open Discussion

MOORHEAD (Chairman) Have you performed any twin studies looking for concordance?

De MARCHI No, we have no twins in our families.

PARSONS (London) One of the interesting things is that when you follow-up renal glycosuria patients over years a proportion of them develop diabetes mellitus and I wonder if you find more pancreatic autoantibodies at this stage? Is this one autoimmune problem you didn't see? You seem to have a lot of families and some of them must be quite old patients with renal glycosuria. Renal glycosuria in the old patients is uncommon, they don't present in their middle age and beyond. You were describing patients who were quite old, is that true?

De MARCHI In our patients we have no autoantibodies to pancreatic islets but the question of the association of renal glycosuria and diabetes mellitus is very interesting. However, since the biochemical aetiology of renal glycosuria is not fully understood it is not reasonable, in our opinion, to make a definite statement concerning the linkage of the two clinical entities. Nevertheless our findings could contribute to a better knowledge of the question. We have known for several years that type I diabetes mellitus is a disease with a probable autoimmune pathogenesis and in which different types of autoantibodies occur more frequently and in higher titres than in other subjects, exactly as we have found in renal glycosuria. Moreover we have investigated the glycaemic and the insulinaemic curve during glucose tolerance test in patients with renal glycosuria and in controls. The glycaemic curves were normal or greater than those of controls but contrary to what we would have expected the insulin values during the glucose tolerance test were not lower. In fact the insulinaemic curve of patients with renal glycosuria and an ideal body weight were higher than those of controls. These findings suggest that renal glycosuria is a complex metabolic derangement with a disruption of the normal glycaemia insulin feedback. We have to remember that the hyperinsulinaemia could play a role in predisposing patients with renal glycosuria to develop diabetes mellitus because of the failure of the beta cell. Of course this is only a hypothesis and more longitudinal studies are needed to confirm the association between the two clinical entities.

Proc EDTA (1983) Vol 20

INSULIN RESISTANCE IN URAEMIA. AN INSULIN RECEPTOR OR AN INTRACELLULAR DEFECT?

O Schmitz, C Hasling*, E Hjøllund*, H E Hansen,
V Posborg Petersen, H Beck-Nielsen*

*Aarhus Kommunehospital, *Aarhus Amtssygehus, Aarhus, Denmark*

Summary

The present study was designed to determine the participation of a decreased insulin binding versus that of a post-binding defect in uraemic insulin resistance and to examine the possible effect of dialysis treatment. This was done by constructing an in vivo insulin dose-response curve using the euglycaemic clamp technique. We found that the maximal responsiveness to insulin was decreased in uraemic patients. Long-term dialysis treatment improved the maximum glucose metabolism significantly (7.7. ± 0.7mg/kg/min versus 10.7 ± 0.6mg/kg/min, $p < 0.01$). On the contrary we found no clearcut alteration of the half-maximal insulin concentrations in relation to dialysis. In conclusion, this report indicates that the insulin resistance in uraemia is primarily due to post-binding defects, i.e. an impaired intracellular glucose metabolism or an abnormal glucose transport system.

Introduction

Insulin resistance, defined as a state in which insulin infusion elicits a less than normal response [1], is widely prevalent in uraemic patients [2]. The mechanisms behind this abnormality, i.e. an insulin receptor versus a postreceptor defect, are still debated. Experiments on insulin binding to monocytes, erythrocytes and rat adipocytes have given conflicting results [2–4]. The aim of the present study was to determine the participation of a decreased insulin binding versus a post-binding defect in the uraemic insulin resistance and to examine a possible influence of long-term dialysis treatment. This was done by constructing an in vivo insulin dose-response curve using the euglycaemic clamp technique [5]. Using this technique, insulin resistance may be classified as being due to either a decreased *sensitivity* or a decreased *responsiveness* to insulin. These two abnormalities are manifest by a shift to the right of the insulin dose-response curve and a reduced maximum response to insulin respectively [1]. The spare receptor concept indicates that a reduced insulin receptor binding usually results in insulin insensitivity while a postreceptor defect results in insulin unresponsiveness.

Materials and methods

Subjects

Eight patients with end-stage renal failure participated in the study. The underlying renal disease was chronic glomerulonephritis (n=4), chronic interstitial nephritis (n=2), diabetic nephropathy (n=1) and polycystic disease (n=1). Ideal body weight was within 15 per cent of normal in all patients. The mean age was 46 years, range 30—65 years. The patients were studied twice, namely within four weeks prior to commencement of dialysis treatment (serum creatinine: 1093 ± 89μmol/litre and serum urea 42.5 ± 1.9mmol/litre) and again after several weeks on chronic dialysis, which consisted of haemodialysis five hours thrice weekly (n=4) or CAPD (n=4). No patient received any medication known to affect glucose tolerance. The study was approved by the local Ethical Committee and informed consent obtained from all subjects.

Protocol

The patients were admitted to the hospital the day before the study. On the morning after an overnight fast the subjects were connected to the artificial pancreas (Biostator GCIIS, Life Science Instruments, Elkart, Indiana, USA). In addition, a cannula for intermittent blood sampling was inserted. The following Biostator constants were used: BD was set at fasting glucose minus 3mg/dl, QD 20, and RD 1mg/min/kg body weight. In addition, a background infusion of glucose was given. To conduct the glucose clamp, mode 7 of the preprogrammed algorithms was used. The subjects were infused with soluble insulin in three doses over a 120 min period each. The doses given were 0.5, 2.0 and 4.0mU/kg body weight/min.

Methods

Plasma insulin was determined by wick-chromotography [6]. Free insulin was measured after serum had been incubated at 37°C for 150 min and subsequently precipitated with polyethylene glycol [7]. Insulin binding to monocytes was assayed as described previously [8].

Calculations

The amount of glucose infused to maintain euglycaemia was calculated at 10-min intervals throughout the experiments and expressed as the amount infused per kg per min. It is established that equilibrium between insulin concentrations in plasma and in the extravascular compartment takes about 90 min [9] so only glucose infusion rates over the last 30 min were used for determining

687

the insulin dose response curve. Hepatic glucose production was assumed to be suppressed to insignificant values [10]. Therefore the steady state glucose infusion rate (SSGIR) was taken as a measure of the amount of glucose metabolised.

Data are given as means ± SEM. Statistical analysis was performed using a two tailed paired and unpaired t-test.

Results

The steady state values of plasma insulin concentrations and glucose infusions of the seven non-diabetic uraemics pre- and post-dialysis are given in Table I. Although the insulin concentrations were similar, SSGIR was in all three situations

TABLE I. Plasma insulin concentrations[1] and SSGIR[2] during the euglycaemic clamps in seven uraemic patients before and after commencement of dialysis

	0.5mU/kg/min		2.0mU/kg/min		4.0mU/kg/min	
	I μU/ml	SSGIR mg/kg/min	I μU/ml	SSGIR mg/kg/min	I μU/ml	SSGIR mg/kg/min
Predialysis	39 ± 5	1.9 ± 0.4	140 ± 12	6.2 ± 0.5	321 ± 23	7.7 ± 0.7
Postdialysis	40 ± 5	3.1 ± 0.6 *	127 ± 12	8.5 ± 0.6 **	315 ± 33	10.7 ± 0.6 **

1 Steady state plasma insulin concentrations during the 90–120 min period.
2 Steady state glucose infusion rates during the 90–120 min period.
* p<0.05 compared to predialysis values.
** p<0.01 compared to predialysis values.
All values are given as mean ± SEM.

significantly higher postdialysis compared to predialysis. However, the plasma insulin concentrations required to achieve half-maximal stimulation of glucose metabolism were almost identical in the two situations (66 ± 7μU/ml versus 65 ± 7μU/ml). Nevertheless a few of the patients exhibited a clearcut shift of the dose-response curve to the left after initiation of dialysis treatment. ^{125}I-binding to monocytes did not increase significantly after dialysis treatment in any of the subjects. (The specific cell binding fraction at tracer concentration was 2.50 ± 0.29 x 10^{-2} versus 2.40 ± 0.28 x 10^{-2} per 5 x 10^6 monocyte per ml.)

Figure 1 shows the blood glucose, plasma free insulin concentrations and glucose infusion rates in one uraemic type 1 diabetic patient studied the day prior to dialysis treatment, i.e. with a severe degree of azotaemia and again after 16 days on CAPD. Blood glucose was brought into steady state at about 90mg/dl by the artificial pancreas before the euglycaemic clamp study. As can be seen blood glucose and plasma free insulin were similar in the two experiments. However, postdialysis SSGIR was increased by 70 per cent, 53 per cent and 38 per cent compared to predialysis after infusion of insulin in doses of 0.5, 2.0 and 4.0mU/kg/min, respectively. Figure 2 demonstrates that dialysis

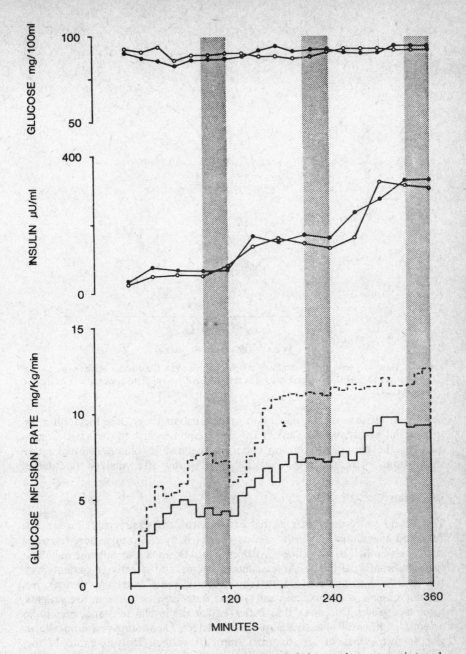

Figure 1. Blood glucose, plasma free insulin and glucose infusion rate in one uraemic type 1 diabetic patient studied by the euglycaemic clamp method when uraemic prior to the institution of CAPD o–o, and after 16 days of CAPD ●–●. Glucose infusion rate predialysis —, post CAPD - - - -

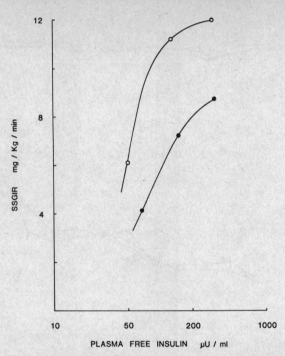

Figure 2. Dose response curve obtained in one uraemic type 1 diabetic patient prior to the institution of CAPD o—o, and after 16 days of CAPD ●—●. (The same patient as shown in Figure 1)

besides an increase of the maximum or near-maximum glucose metabolism in this patient also induced a shift of the dose response curve towards left. Consequently, the plasma insulin concentration required to obtain half-maximum stimulation decreased from $78\mu U/ml$ to $47\mu U/ml$ after dialysis treatment.

Discussion

The present study demonstrates that patients with end-stage renal failure have a decreased maximum responsiveness as evaluated by the insulin dose-response curve. Haemodialysis as well as CAPD improved the maximum glucose metabolism significantly, although the maximum response in the dialysed patients was still decreased compared to a matched control group (data not shown). We did not observe any significant shift of the dose-response curve in the patients taken as a group. Our study thus indicates that the insulin resistance present in uraemia is primarily due to a post-binding defect, i.e. an impaired intracellular glucose metabolism or an abnormal transport system. Dialysis improved the abnormal intracellular process, although a complete return to normal was not obtained. The insulin binding capacity of monocytes confirmed the results of the insulin dose-response curve by confirming that insulin receptor defects are only of minor importance for the insulin resistance in uraemia. This is, of course,

690

accepting the condition that insulin binding to monocytes reflects binding to target tissues.

Acknowledgments

The expert assistance of Annette Lorentzen and Anni Bundesen is gratefully acknowledged.
The study was supported by the Danish Research Council.

References

1   Kahn CR. *Metabolism 1978; 27 (Suppl 2):* 1893
2   Smith D, DeFronzo RA. *Kidney Int 1982; 22:* 54
3   Gambhir KK, Archer JA, Nerurkar SG et al. *Nephron 1981; 28:* 4
4   Maloff B, Lockwood D. *Diabetes 1981; 30 (Suppl 1):* 28A
5   DeFronzo RA, Tobin JD, Andres R. *Am J Physiol 1979; 237:* E214
6   Ørskov H, Thomsen AG, Yde H. *Nature 1968; 219:* 193
7   Nakagawa S, Nakagawa H, Sasuki T et al. *Diabetes 1973; 22:* 590
8   Beck-Nielsen H, Pedersen O, Kragballe K et al. *Diabetologi 1977; 13:* 563
9   Scherwin RS, Kramer KJ, Tobin JD et al. *J Clin Invest 1974; 53:* 1481
10 Rizza RA, Mandarino LJ, Gerich JE. *Am J Physiol 1981; 240:* E630

Open Discussion

MOORHEAD (Chairman)   Do you know what it is about uraemia that prevents intracellular glucose metabolism from being normal?

SCHMITZ   No, we don't know at the moment because it may be some of the uraemic toxins. One may try to find out by incubating, for example, adipocytes and uraemic serum. This may provide some answers.

INTRAPERITONEAL INSULIN REGIMENS AND DIABETIC NEPHROPATHY

R L Stephen, J G Maxwell, C Kablitz, S C Jacobsen, B Hanover, F Tyler

University of Utah, Salt Lake City, Utah, USA

Summary

Five patients with severe diabetic nephropathy (SN) and six patients with moderate diabetic nephropathy (MN) have been treated with intraperitoneal (i.p.) insulin administered by multiple injections. The five SN patients progressed to end-stage kidney disease. The six MN patients (five of whom are described) show stabilisation (and in two cases possibly some improvement) of renal function over time intervals ranging from eight to 23 months.

Introduction

The onset of persistent, clinically detectable ($\geqslant$ 500mg/24 hr) proteinuria and commencing decline of glomerular filtration rate (GFR) in patients with insulin-dependent diabetes mellitus (IDDM) reportedly herald continuing inevitable decline in renal function [1–5]. Mogensen has reported that strict control of blood pressure could retard, but not arrest, this rate of decline [6].

At the University of Utah, we have implanted subcutaneous peritoneal access devices in 21 patients with IDDM for the purpose of administering intraperitoneal (i.p.) insulin, using multiple injection techniques (3–4 times daily). The design and fabrication of the device and its operative implantation have been described [7] as have some preliminary results in patients afflicted with nephropathy due to IDDM [8,9]. This report deals primarily with the continuing nephrological evaluation of these latter patients.

Methods

Eleven patients with diabetic nephropathy at the time of entry into the trial were arbitrarily classified into two groups: five patients with severe nephropathy (SN) demonstrating serum creatinines ranging from 4.2–6.4mg/dl, creatinine clearances $<$ 20ml/min/1.73m^2 and proteinuria varying from 3.6–12.9g/24 hr; six patients with moderate nephropathy (MN) with serum creatinines ranging from 1.1–2.7mg/dl, creatinine clearances ranging from 25–71ml/min/1.73m^2 and proteinuria varying from 0.5–6.3g/24 hr. All 11 patients were afflicted by retinopathy, the duration of diabetes in the SN group ranged from 17–30 (mean, 22.6) years and that in the MN group ranged from 14–33 (mean, 23.8) years.

Following operative implantation, we allowed approximately one month stabilisation time for wound healing and adjustment of insulin dosage, then the renal status of each individual patient was followed by serial measurements of serum creatinine, creatinine clearance and 24 hr proteinuria, each of these assessments being performed approximately once each calendar month. Because proteinuria in individual patients fluctuated widely from month to month (sometimes by 100 per cent or more), this data is transformed to proteinuria (mg/24 hr)/urinary creatinine (mg/24 hr) (P/C), so that at least patients' errors in urine collection techniques are nullified. Linear regression analysis was performed for reciprocal serum creatinine values, creatinine clearance values and P/C. In addition to home blood glucose monitoring (HBG) records, the patients' glycaemic status was assessed by glycosylated haemoglobin values (HbA$_1$), also performed approximately once per month.

All patients were supplied with sphygmomanometers and were requested to record blood pressures 2–3 times daily. Consistent blood pressure readings $\geqslant$ 135/$\geqslant$ 85mmHg on two consecutive days required consultations and remedial measures.

Results

Patients with severe nephropathy

Although all patients in the SN group demonstrated HbA$_1$ levels consistently within the normal range and they also maintained reasonable blood pressure control, they progressed inexorably to end-stage renal failure within one year. Three are now treated by haemodialysis and two have received successfully functioning renal transplants.

Patients with moderate nephropathy

The first patient (Patient No 1) in the MN group showed a significant reversal of the decline in renal function and the disappearance of proteinuria, then withdrew from the programme after five months because of an obstructed access device [9]. The remaining five patients (patients 2–6) have been treated with multiple dose i.p. insulin over time periods ranging from 8–23 (mean, 18.6) months for a total of 93 patient-months.

Glycaemic control HbA$_1$ results (n=40) have not yet been assessed beyond 12 months for any patient but over this period of time, the mean value for all patients was 8.27 per cent with a range of 7.32–9.43 per cent (normal range 4.2–9.1 per cent).

Serum creatinine values Regression lines for reciprocal serum creatinine values

693

(n=81) in the five patients are shown in Figure 1. Patients No 2 and 3 demonstrate a very slight and insignificant decrease in the slopes of reciprocal creatinine values (10/CRE α -0.015t and -0.007t respectively). Patients No 4, 5 and 6 show an equally insignificant increase in the slopes. What is significant (p<0.01) is that patient No 3 demonstrated an arrest in the decline of reciprocal creatinine values (10/CRE α -0.073t: r=0.937) which had been followed for five years prior to commencing an i.p. insulin regimen.

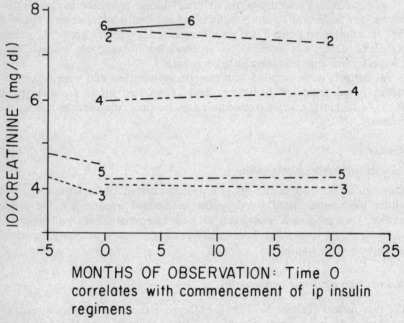

RECIPROCAL SERUM CREATININES VS. TIME IN 5 PATIENTS

Figure 1

Figure 2, which also demonstrates the regression lines for reciprocal serum creatinine values in the five patients, supplies perspective in relation to the studies of two other groups of investigators. The lines K-K-K and K^1-K^1-K^1 bound an area which is a facsimile of that reported by Kjellstrand et al (10). These authors describe the decline in renal function observed in 12 diabetic patients, with 90 per cent of their reciprocal creatinine values falling within the bounded area. The lines J^0-J^1 and J^0-J^2 are derived from the studies of Jones et al [1] and represent the two extremes in the rates of decline in renal function (as measured by reciprocal creatinine values) in nine patients.

694

RECIPROCAL SERUM CREATININE TRENDS IN 5 (IP) PATIENTS VS "TRADITIONAL" TRENDS

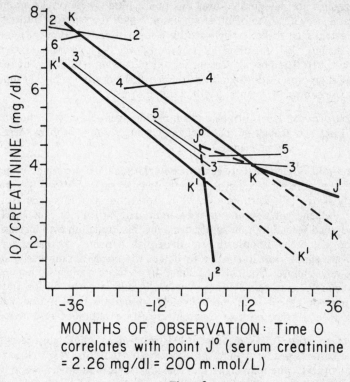

MONTHS OF OBSERVATION: Time O
correlates with point J^o (serum creatinine
= 2.26 mg/dl = 200 m.mol/L)

Figure 2

Creatinine clearance The regression lines of creatinine clearance values (n=58) with respect to time (t=months) for patients 2–6 are respectively: −0.47t +93.3; 0.57t +25.7; −0.43t +66.2; −0.03t +25.9; 0.87t + 48.6. With the exception of Patient No 3 where r=0.604, all correlation coefficients are < 0.50.

P/C The regression lines for 24 hr proteinuria (n=57) as transformed to P/C for patients 2–6 are respectively: −0.005t +0.38; 0.063t +3.7; 0.053t +1.2 (r=0.566); −0.022t + 1.87; −0.47t +4.91 (r=0.784).Correlation coefficients for Patients No 2, 3 and 5 are < 0.30. Note that Patient No 6 entered the study with uncontrolled hypertension (160/110) which was corrected concomitant with commencing his i.p. insulin regimen.

Discussion

The five patients with severe nephropathy progressed to end-stage renal failure, a logical sequel for persons afflicted by a severe glomerulopathy and with less than 20 per cent residual renal function. In contradistinction, the five patients with moderate nephropathy have maintained stable renal function for a total of 93 patient-months. Furthermore glomerular damage, as assessed by 24 hr proteinuria, has not deteriorated over this time period. These results are markedly at variance with those of other studies in which the reported outlook for clinically established diabetic nephropathy is unanimously one of 'progressive, relentless decline' [4] occurring 'in an orderly way' [1] which is 'extremely predictable' [10]. The possible reasons for our discordant results may be related to: 1) too short observation periods; 2) insensitive measurements; 3) superior blood glucose control; 4) chance; 5) the route of insulin delivery.

Observation periods Times of observation ranging from eight to 23 months are relatively brief and it may be that over the ensuing months or years, declining renal function will become manifest.

Measurements Correlations between inverse creatinine and creatinine clearance values and the more sensitive measurements of GFR such as ^{51}CrEDTA are not particularly strong [4]. Furthermore, 24 hr proteinuria values vary substantially under the influence of several external conditions, particularly exercise. Thus, it can be argued forcefully that subtly declining renal function with increasingly severe glomerulopathy is occurring in these five patients: the measurements employed are simply too insensitive to detect the changes. Conversely, serum creatinine values above $200\mu mol/L$ (2.26mg/dl) correlate strongly with a decreasing GFR and Patients Nos 3 and 5, who are in this category, demonstrate no decrease over time periods of approximately 21 months each. Indeed, Patient No 3 shows a distinct positive trend in creatinine clearance measurements.

Blood glucose control As recorded by HbA_1 values, blood glucose control in the five patients has been good, probably better than that reported in other publications [4,5]. One may argue that this slight overall improvement in blood glucose control is responsible for the stabilisation of renal function: an unconvincing hypothesis.

Chance All five patients reported in this article plus two others (unpublished data) just happened to enter a period of temporary stabilisation of renal function following commencement of i.p. insulin regimens!

Insulin delivery route There are indications that good glycaemic control will reverse microalbuminuria and thus possibly prevent or delay renal failure in susceptible patients with IDDM. It also appears that good glycaemic control, per se, will not prevent established diabetic nephropathy progressing to end-stage renal disease.

Certainly in animals and probably in humans, a significant proportion of insulin injected intraperitoneally enters directly into the portal circulation, thus primarily insulinising the liver as in the physiological state. It is possible that insulin directed into the portal, rather than the systemic, circulation more effectively modulates certain metabolic factors other than glucose. Such metabolic effects may stabilise declining renal function whose precise pathogenesis is still totally unclear in patients with IDDM.

References

1   Jones RH, Mackay JD, Hayakawa H et al. *Lancet 1979; i:* 1105
2   Mauer SM, Steffes MW, Brown DM. *Am J Med 1981; 70:* 603
3   Parving H-H, Smidt UM, Friisberg B et al. *Diabetologia 1981; 20:* 457
4   Viberti GC, Bilous RW, Mackintosh D et al. *Am J Med 1983; 74:* 256
5   Viberti GC, Bilous RW, Mackintosh D et al. *Br Med J 1983; 286:* 598
6   Mogensen CE. *Diabetes 1976; 25:* 872
7   Jacobsen SC, Hanover BK, Stephen RL et al. *Proc Int Symp on Hemoperfusion and Artif Organs, ISAO, Ankara, Turkey 1982.* In press
8   Stephen RL, Jacobsen SC, Maxwell JG et al. In Friedman EA, L'Esperance FA, eds. *Diabetic Renal-Retinal Syndrome.* New York: Grune & Stratton Inc. 1982: 447–461
9   Stephen RL, Maddock RK, Kablitz C et al. *Diabetic Nephropathy 1982; 1:* 8
10 Kjellstrand CM, Whitley K, Comty C et al. *Diabetic Nephropathy 1982; 1:* 5

Open discussion

ULDALL (Toronto) I think we should all be encouraged by the results Dr Stephen appears to have obtained with this ingenious device. They come as a happy relief after the discouraging reports which claim that once proteinuria is persistent in Type I diabetes mellitus the progress of the downhill course is inevitable. We in Toronto as a result of an ongoing controlled trial of continuous subcutaneous insulin infusion compared with conventional therapy have, in some preliminary unpublished data, some results which support Dr Stephen's findings. Briefly we have found that proteinuria after the institution of 'tight' nomoglycaemia becomes very selective compared with the non selective proteinuria that is known to be present in established and advanced diabetic glomerulosclerosis. Secondly in patients with renal failure not too far advanced there is a tendency for some patients to stabilise and we have patients who two years after starting insulin infusion have renal function which is slightly better than when they started their infusion. We also have four patients in the infusion group whose proteinuria has disappeared after variable periods of time. These are people who had modest proteinuria in the region of 1–1.5g/24 hr. This has not happened in patients with proteinuria in excess of 10g/24 hr.

JACOBS (Chairman) Have you any comment on this Dr Stephen?

STEPHEN I know of Dr Uldall's work and I feel everybody has to work at this as much as they can.

JACOBS I would like to ask Dr Uldall whether the patients you have just been talking about were all normotensive or did you have some with persistent hypertension? You know of the debate between the relative control of blood pressure and control of glycaemia in slowing the evolution of diabetic nephropathy.

ULDALL You are absolutely right that the control of hypertension is so far the only outside intervention that has been proven to change the course of this otherwise downhill disease, but even from homogenous results we have not been able to flatten out the downhill course completely. So we have controlled blood pressure equally well in the control and treatment groups and there is still a difference between the two groups with respect to the effect on renal function and proteinuria. Could I ask Dr Stephen how he managed to maintain such good normoglycaemia overnight with an intraperitoneal device which can only be injected in the evening before going to bed?

STEPHEN The device holds a certain quantity of insulin and especially now that we have narrowed the conduit into the peritoneal cavity it is obvious the insulin can diffuse in over a period of time. We note that the duration of action of insulin has extended from six to seven hours to nine to 10 hours and in one case to 12 hours. Presumably the device is holding insulin and slowing diffusion to the peritoneal cavity over time.

PARSONS (London) These are very interesting results and really report for the first time the holding of reciprocal creatinine over 24 months. One of the interesting things when you biopsy these patients they all have advanced lesions and it seems difficult to understand how you can undo diabetic glomerulosclerosis although Mauer* has done this in the rat. When the creatinine reaches this value there is a widespread lesion and I think all one can look for is an increase in function of the remaining remnant kidney. One of the interesting hormones that will increase the GFR and perhaps hold the creatinine is growth hormone. I wonder whether these patients to whom you are giving insulin rather suddenly into the portal circulation are really having much more normoglycaemia and perhaps more hypoglycaemia and therefore their growth hormones are going to be very much higher? Can you give us any information about the incidence of hypoglycaemia over a 20 month period compared with the previous few years?

STEPHEN I would say it was increased not by much and in most cases not very severely. In something like sixteen patient years there have been four episodes of hypoglycaemia that followed the manipulative release of an obstruction and there have been four episodes of hypoglycaemia requiring assistance by another person without any preceding obstruction. In three of those cases it was because the patient took a meal time dose of insulin and for a variety of reasons, including a Parisien restauranteur not serving one patient, the meal was not eaten and they were in trouble and they knew it. The incidence of severe hypoglycaemia was very low. When one considers those eleven patients, if we count the first five, nine have consistently maintained their haemoglobin A_1 values in the normal range for periods of time up to two years and that is not a bad track record.

BILOUS (London) I would like to make a few points. Firstly there was one patient in the series reported by Viberti† whose renal function tended to stabilise

---

* Mauer SM, Steffes MW, Sutherland DER. *Diabetes 1975; 24:* 280
† Viberti GC, Bilous RW, Mackintosh D et al. *Br Med J 1983; 1:* 598

after a period of continuous subcutaneous insulin infusions and as far as I know this girl still has exactly the same renal function two years from starting her infusions and maybe there is a sub-group of patients in whom it is possible to stabilise the decline with improving glycaemic control despite the fact that a biopsy performed on this girl did confirm extensive diabetic change. The other point I would like to make is again in the patients we studied at Guys there was a differing rate of decline in different patients although the average of the decline of GFR was 1ml/min/month. It think it is important that in studies like this there is a long-term follow-up before therapeutic intervention with changing glycaemic control before we can draw conclusions as to the effect of this over the decline in renal function.

STEPHEN I have not drawn any conclusions except that the game isn't over — that's the only conclusion. The second thing was there may be a sub-group of these patients in which case we were extraordinarily lucky because the first six stumbled over our front door and entered our programme. Nobody knows how to identify this hypothetical sub-group and we certainly made no effort to. The third comment, and I thoroughly agree with it, is that one would like to follow these patients for months or years before and also after one has intervened in some way or other and at times this is possible and at times it is not. I remember that case you reported and she was Number 4, I think, in your report in the British Medical Journal but that was only one of six. In our series we have six of six and so I feel this is worthy of further investigation.

LONG-TERM CONTINUOUS AMBULATORY PERITONEAL DIALYSIS

C T Flynn

Iowa Lutheran Hospital, Des Moines, Iowa, USA

Summary

This paper reports experience with 65 patients treated by continuous ambulatory peritoneal dialysis (CAPD) during the past five years. The patients are divided into 33 non-diabetic and 32 diabetic and the latter are subdivided into blind and sighted. Cumulative actuarial survival on CAPD calculated at five years was highest for blind diabetics, intermediate for non-diabetic and lowest for sighted diabetics. Blind diabetics had the lowest rate of drop-out from CAPD. Many patients, especially in the non-diabetic and sighted diabetic groups required temporary haemodialysis which allowed them to return to CAPD.

Introduction

The advent of CAPD [1] coincided with an increasing number of diabetic patients with end-stage renal disease presenting for treatment. The opportunity for diabetic control by intraperitoneal insulin [2], the control of volume overload and hypertension by osmotic ultrafiltration and the steady haemodynamics together suggested a special role for CAPD in the treatment of diabetic patients. Another merit of CAPD is that it can be a home self-care therapy, although this requires detailed training and follow-up and, most importantly, motivated patients.

This paper reports the results of a five year CAPD experience with emphasis on self-care in blind patients, actuarial survival, peritonitis and haemodialysis back-up support.

Patients and methods

Some 65 patients were treated by CAPD between May 1978 and April 1983. Of these, 33 were non-diabetic and 32 were diabetic, 23 either legally [3] or totally blind. The first six patients were treated using dialysate in bottles and without an organised CAPD clinic. The remaining patients all used dialysate

700

in plastic bags and were trained in CAPD by specialised nurses. Procedures for training non-diabetic, diabetic and blind patients were developed, but were fundamentally similar. The nurses each taught all groups of patients. Detailed evaluation was carried out each month, including laboratory studies in the fasting state, details of which are published elsewhere [4].

Intraperitoneal insulin was used exclusively in all diabetic patients and the blind were taught how to perform the administration. Special guides for insulin administration by the blind were used. The cause, duration, treatment and outcome of all episodes of peritonitis, catheter related problems, hospitalisations and other significant medical events were recorded. A medical social worker and renal dietician were available to all patients and took part in each monthly evaluation. Cumulative actuarial life tables were constructed at five years [5]. In addition, cumulative actuarial life tables of patient survival, as distinct from survival on CAPD were constructed. Patients who required temporary haemodialysis but who returned to CAPD were not withdrawn from the survival on CAPD life table.

Results

Of the 65 patients, 31 are still receiving treatment by CAPD. The remainder either died, were transferred to haemodialysis or received a transplant.

Survival

The cumulative actuarial survival on CAPD at the five year point is 60 per cent for blind patients, 40 per cent for sighted diabetics and 45 per cent for non-diabetics. Actual patient survival was better for non-diabetic and sighted diabetics than survival on CAPD but the small numbers prevent statistical analysis. Patient survival and survival on CAPD for blind patients was identical.

Peritonitis

There were a total of 115 episodes of peritonitis among the 65 patients. Eighteen patients have never had peritonitis, 19 have had only one episode and one patient has had seven episodes with the remainder intermediate. The rate of peritonitis steadily fell over the five years and is lower in all current patients than the overall rates in each group of patients. The current blind patients have a rate of one episode of peritonitis every 99 weeks, the current sighted diabetics one every 43 weeks and the current non-diabetics one every 56 weeks.

Support haemodialysis

Only 12 patients received CAPD as their only form of treatment, eight are alive and four dead. Of the remaining 23 current patients, 14 received prior haemodialysis and nine have received temporary haemodialysis and returned to CAPD.

Discussion

The actuarial or life table is a method for statistically projecting survival rates on a particular treatment for a particular length of time. The chosen length of time may not exceed the longest single patient exposure time to the risk of dying. In these results the longest exposure time for blind patients is three-and-a-half years, for sighted diabetics four years, and for non-diabetics four years. These variations, along with relatively small numbers in each group make conclusions somewhat tentative even though the life tables were meticulously constructed.

In plain numbers, of 23 blind diabetics 13 are alive (one with sight following vitrectomy), and 10 are dead. Of the latter, nine died on CAPD and one returned to haemodialysis. At all times the blind patients have had the least rate of peritonitis and consequently have had the least rate of drop-out because of this complication and needed the least haemodialysis back-up support in order to restart CAPD. Before drawing conclusions from these findings it is important to make the following observations:

1. All patients were managed in a consistent fashion by the same team of nurses, doctors and social workers once the CAPD clinic was established. The commitment to success was thus the same for all patients.

2. Most of the patients were classed as at high risk and with a relatively poor prognosis compared to transplanted patients or patients not offered CAPD. In these circumstances comparison of survival rates between groups of CAPD patients without a detailed knowledge of the individual patients is difficult and statistical analysis is hampered by small numbers.

3. Blind patients seemed not to find the exchange procedure burdensome. After the multiple problems associated with declining renal function, fluid retention, hypertension and poor diabetic control, they welcomed CAPD with relief and were motivated to succeed. Having in most cases learned to cope with blindness they incorporated the exchange procedure in their daily routine without difficulty.

In conclusion it would appear that, as a group, the blind patients who chose CAPD were more motivated than a heterogeneous group of sighted patients who also chose CAPD. This may be relevant in view of the reported high drop-out rates from CAPD in Europe [6]. The other conclusion is that haemodialysis is required to support a CAPD programme.

References

1 Popovich RP, Moncrief JW, Decherd JB et al. *ASAIO 1976; 5:* 64
2 Flynn CT, Nanson J. *Trans ASAIO 1979; 25:* 114
3 Havener WH. *Synopsis of Ophthalmology.* St Louis: CV Mosby Co. 1975: 567
4 Flynn CT, Shadur CA. *Am J Kid Dis 1983; 1:* 15
5 Cutler SJ, Ederer F. *J Ch Dis 1958; 8:* 699
6 Kramer P, Broyer M, Brunner FP et al. *Proc EDTA 1982; 19:* 34

Open Discussion

JACOBS (Chairman) First I would like to congratulate you on the superb work of you and your team. These results are certainly due to a highly motivated medical and nursing team. I was wondering if it was also a consequence of a degree of super-selection. Can you tell us how many blind diabetic patients you have rejected from CAPD treatment during the period of your study?

FLYNN None: everybody who has come for treatment has been treated. These are not patients who have been put on a training programme and selected out because they were unable to do it. Of the 23 patients, 22 were trained to carry out the procedure themselves, one was not and the CAPD was performed by his wife.

RONCO (Vicenza) Which system did your blind patients use?

FLYNN They use 2L bags, the majority use a 2.5% Dextrose solution and only occasionally a 4.25% solution (Travenol, Dianeal) in a single bag.

RONCO Did they use the system called Travexchange, which has been developed for blind patients?

FLYNN No, I don't think that system is specifically for the blind.

ULDALL (Toronto) Have you any data on the degree of blood glucose control which was achieved in your patients and whether this was different in the blind and sighted diabetic patients?

FLYNN The control of blood glucose is satisfactory and providing the patient performs the exchange on time and eats appropriately, hypoglycaemia is uncommon and hyperglycaemia is rare. A comparison between the diabetic and non-diabetic patients reveals that the non-diabetics are slightly diabetic in view of the fact that they are uraemic and receiving a glucose load. The average glycosylated haemoglobin in the diabetic patients, both blind and sighted, in our group is 9.4, the average for the non-diabetics is 8.7. Both these results are marginally elevated. The triglyceride concentration of the diabetic patients using intraperitoneal insulin tended to be normal, although they had low HDL. The majority of the non-diabetic patients not using insulin had elevated triglycerides and low HDL.

BARTOVA (Prague) How long did it take you to evaluate the exact amount of insulin required when you changed from subcutaneous to the intraperitoneal route?

FLYNN All diabetic patients start on intraperitoneal insulin in hospital and we do not use any long-acting insulin for the two days prior to catheter insertion. On the morning the exchange starts we guess the insulin dose and measure

703

the blood glucose hourly and adjust the dose as required. It is not difficult although one must recognise that after the patient has gone home the insulin requirement may change: they usually fall.

WING (London) You have emphasised the importance of back-up haemodialysis for these patients. Have you analysed the total amount of dialysis time and could you tell us the proportion of time which was haemodialysis as opposed to CAPD?

FLYNN I do have the data but not with me. The longest period was of three weeks with the majority in the region of 10 days.

Proc EDTA (1983) Vol 20

PROGRESS IN SEGMENTAL NEOPRENE-INJECTED PANCREAS TRANSPLANTATION. ADVANTAGES AND DISADVANTAGES OF USING CYCLOSPORIN A

J Traeger, J M Dubernard*, E Bosi†, A Gelet*, S El Yafi, A Secchi†, C Cardozo, J L Touraine

Clinique de Néphrologie, INSERM U 80, *Service d'urologie, Hôpital Ed Herriot, Lyon, France, †Clinica Medica VIII, San Raffaele University Hospital, Milan, Italy

Summary

We performed 39 neoprene-injected pancreatic transplants (38 segmental and 1 total) in 37 insulin-dependent diabetic recipients from October 1976 to May 1983. The best results were obtained when the pancreas was transplanted simultaneously with the kidney (25 cases). The use of Cyclosporin A (CyA) for immunosuppression did not reduce the early pancreatic failures, but it seems to have slightly improved the long-term survival. The glycaemic control was better in patients treated by CyA alone than in those receiving steroids. The main side effects of CyA were nephrotoxicity and some immunoglobulin abnormalities with or without lymphoproliferative disorders occurring after treatment with CyA and ALG.

Introduction

Pancreas transplantation in insulin-dependent diabetics is intended as a means of restoring the insulin secretion. At the Herriot Hospital of Lyon, 39 pancreatic transplants from cadaveric donors were performed in 37 patients between October 1976 and May 1983. The pancreas was grafted alone in 11 cases, before the kidney in two cases, after the kidney in one case, and simultaneously in 25 cases. We report here some aspects of our clinical experience.

Patients

The 37 recipients of pancreatic transplants were insulin-dependent (Type 1) diabetic patients, aged 34.9 ± 8.6 years with a duration of diabetes of 20.4 ± 6.1 years (mean $\pm$ SD). All the patients were affected by severe long-term diabetic complications, at the end-stage degree in most cases. The recipients of combined pancreatic and renal transplants were affected by end-stage renal failure due to diabetic nephropathy, and they were maintained on a haemo- or peritoneal dialysis prior to transplantation.

705

Transplant technique

Thirty-eight of the 39 pancreatic transplants were segmental, while one of the most recent was total. In all the cases, the exocrine pancreatic secretion was handled by injecting neoprene into the ductal system. This polymer floculates on contact with the pancreatic juice leading to an extended fibrosis of the exocrine parenchyma without affecting the endocrine tissue [1]. An omento-plasty around the pancreatic graft was performed starting from case 7, to provide a mechanism of reabsorption of the residual exocrine secretion.

The pancreatic graft was placed in the iliac fossa of the recipient, and vascu-larised by anastomosis to iliac artery and vein. When a kidney transplant was associated, it was placed in the opposite iliac fossa. Donors were heart-beating cadavers selected on ABO compatibility and negative cross-match; HLA and DR typing were performed in all cases, but not considered for matching donors and recipients.

Immunosuppression

Three protocols of immunosuppression were successively employed [9].

Protocol A (conventional) included azathioprine, anti-lymphocyte-globulin (ALG) and steroids.

Protocol B consisted of Cyclosporin A (CyA) from the day of transplantation, ALG, plus steroids during rejection.

Protocol C (combined) consisted of an initial course of conventional treatment, and a subsequent switch to CyA some weeks or months later, after stabilisation of renal function.

Results

Survival

The survival rate of the 37 patients undergoing primary pancreatic transplanta-tion was 75 per cent at six months, 65 per cent at one year and 49 per cent at two years. The overall survival of the 39 pancreatic grafts was 49 per cent at three months, 36 per cent at six months, 21 per cent at one year and 13 per cent at two years.

Different rates of survival were obtained in the different transplant series, with regard to the association of pancreatic with renal transplants: indeed, while only two single pancreatic transplants survived more than three months, in the 25 simultaneous combined transplants the pancreatic graft survival improved, attaining the 67 per cent at three months, 50 per cent at six months, 38 per cent at one year and 24 per cent at two years. In the same series, the patient and renal graft survival were 70 per cent and 59 per cent at six months, 64 per cent and 47 per cent at one year and 48 per cent and 30 per cent at two years,

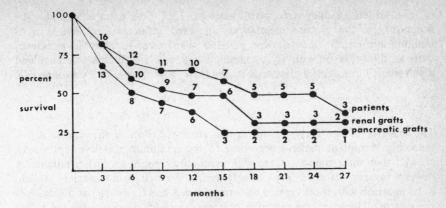

Figure 1. Patient, renal graft and pancreatic graft survival after combined simultaneous pancreas plus kidney transplantation (n:25)

respectively (Figure 1). Of those 25 transplants eight were treated according to protocol A, seven to protocol B and 10 to protocol C. In the latter group, seven recent cases have not yet been switched to CyA. The use of CyA from the day of transplantation (protocol B), did not greatly improve the short-term survival of the pancreatic grafts (71% at three months vs 62% and 69% for protocols A and C respectively).

However, on a long-term basis, treatment with CyA seems to be beneficial for the pancreatic graft, attaining 30 per cent at two years (protocols B and C), in comparison with 12 per cent of the conventional therapy (protocol A).

The pancreatic grafts lost for immunological reasons were four (50%) with protocol A and two (29%) with protocol B. None of the patients treated with protocol C lost the pancreatic graft by rejection, but since this group includes all the most recent transplants, a correct estimation and comparison with the two previous protocols is not yet possible. In addition to rejection, which accounted for six failures, the other causes of loss of pancreatic function in the simultaneous pancreatico-renal transplant series were vascular thromboses (two cases), and death of the patients from cardiovascular complications (three cases), malignancies (two cases), chronic hepatitis (one case) and disseminated intravascular coagulation subsequent to irreversible kidney rejection (one case). Currently (30 May 1983), 10 patients have pancreatic grafts functioning and are insulin independent, three of them for more than one year.

Pancreatic endocrine function

When successful, pancreatic transplantation led to the disappearance of the clinical signs of diabetes and to insulin-independence within some days after transplantation. The ability of the pancreatic graft to respond to either a glucose load or to non-glucose dependent stimuli was preserved, although some differences characterised these patients with respect to a properly matched population

707

of non-diabetic kidney transplant patients [2]. The pancreatic endocrine function and the glucose metabolism appeared influenced by the type of immunosuppression: indeed, the patients who received steroids associated with azathioprine or with CyA exhibited a degree of glucose tolerance and a pattern of insulin release less satisfactory than those treated by CyA alone [3].

Cyclosporin toxicity

The analysis of the early post-operative renal function in the double simultaneously transplant patients according to the immunosuppressive treatments, showed that the patients treated with protocol B required a higher number of dialyses (average of seven per patient) during the first post-transplant month, in comparison with those treated with protocols A and C (average of 0.7 dialyses per patient). Moreover, the rate of the plasma creatinine decrease after transplantation was lower with protocol B than with protocols A and C, achieving eight days after transplantation values of 535 ± 103 and 193 ± 39μmol/litre, respectively.

Besides the effects of the CyA on the renal function, we observed two mild episodes of hepatotoxicity, which resolved after dose reduction of the drug.

In addition, among the 10 patients who received CyA and ALG at the same time, we observed one case of restriction of immunoglobulin (Ig) heterogeneity, two cases of monoclonal peaks, and three cases of fatal infectious and lymphoproliferative syndromes [4].

Discussion

After the first unsuccessful attempts performed during the sixties, pancreatic transplantation has been reconsidered as an alternative approach in the management of insulin-dependent diabetes following the description of new and safer transplant techniques [1,5]. Since then, the number of pancreatic transplants performed worldwide and the number of institutions involved in such activity have steadily increased [6]. The progressive improvement in techniques, the accumulation of experience and the association of pancreas with kidney transplantation have allowed a continuous improvement in results. However, even in experienced hands pancreatic graft survival is still relatively poor [7.8]. The reasons rest on the technical problems which have not yet been completely solved, on the mechanisms of rejection which are still unclear, and on the poor condition of the patients at the time of transplantation due to advanced diabetic complications.

The introduction of CyA for immunosuppressive therapy allowed a dose reduction and in some cases the abolition of steroid treatment, which therefore improved the pancreatic endocrine function and the glycaemic control in such pancreatic transplant recipients [3].

On the other hand, the nephrotoxicity of CyA represented a major problem, especially when the drug was administered during the immediate post-operative period. For that reason, and as CyA was not able to reduce the rate of the early pancreatic failure, we now prefer to employ conventional treatment initially, giving CyA after stabilisation of renal function [9]. Moreover, the serious immunoglobulin abnormalities and the lymphoproliferative disorders occurring after combined CyA and ALG therapy dramatically indicates the potential risk of such combinations [4].

References

1   Dubernard JM, Traeger J, Neyra P et al. *Surgery 1978; 84:* 633
2   Pozza G, Traeger J, Dubernard JM et al. *Diabetologia 1983; 24:* 244
3   Traeger J, Dubernard JM, Pozza G et al. *Transplant Proc 1983; 15:* 1326
4   Touraine JL, El Yafi S, Bosi E et al. *Transplant Proc 1983; 15:* in press
5   Sutherland DER. *Diabetologia 1981; 20:* 435
6   Sutherland DER. *Transplant Proc 1983; 15:* 1303
7   Dubernard JM, Traeger J, Pozza G et al. *Transplant Proc 1983; 15:* 1318
8   Sutherland DER, Goetz CG, Elick BA et al. *Transplantation 1982; 34:* 330
9   Traeger J, Dubernard JM, Bosi E et al. *Transplant Proc 1983; 15:* in press

Open Discussion

ULDALL (Toronto) Do you have any patients in the long-term survivors with renal and pancreas transplants who have developed a recurrence of glucose intolerance or have they all remained non-diabetic?

TRAEGER Normally they remain with normal glucose tolerance tests and good graft function until rejection appears. Rejection is usually a rapid process and within a few days there is hyperglycaemia with recurrence of diabetes mellitus and the patients have to be restarted on insulin. The treatment of these acute rejections is difficult and up until now only a few rejection episodes have been successfully treated.

JACOBS (Chairman) Have the patients with solely pancreatic transplants (without kidney transplantation) the same degree of renal failure?

TRAEGER No, the patients receiving a pancreatic transplant alone were in chronic renal failure, but not yet on dialysis.

BOSKOVICJ (Sarajevo) Is there a characteristic clinical picture after pancreatic transplant rejection or is there only a loss of insulin action? How do you diagnose an acute rejection?

TRAEGER This is a problem as it is very difficult to diagnose the rejection early. The patient has clinical signs of diabetes mellitus, and by this time it is usually too late to treat the rejection. We lack a marker of acute rejection.

BOSKOVICJ Is it necessary to remove the transplanted pancreas after rejection?

TRAEGER This is not necessary.

KERR (Newcastle upon Tyne) You showed one patient who rejected his kidney while his pancreas remained. Do you often see the reverse, that is where the pancreas is rejected while the kidney is retained? Is it practicable to teach your patients to check their own blood glucose daily?

TRAEGER Usually the kidney is rejected first and this is an advantage for the pancreatic transplanter because it is easier to recognise kidney rejection. We then treat this rejection and so protect the pancreas. This is probably the reason why our pancreatic transplant results are better when both renal and pancreatic transplants are done together.

RENAL AND PANCREATIC TRANSPLANTATION IN THE TREATMENT OF DIABETIC RENAL FAILURE

J Michael, P McMaster, D Adu, O M Gibby, J H Turney

Queen Elizabeth Hospital, Birmingham, United Kingdom

Summary

Twenty-two diabetic patients with renal failure have entered an integrated dialysis and transplant programme in 30 months. Ten have subsequently undergone combined renal and segmental pancreatic transplantation, and have been followed for between one month and 25 months. Currently 80 per cent of the kidneys and 40 per cent of the pancreatic grafts are functioning. Four of the 22 patients have died from myocardial disease. Pancreatic transplantation at the time of renal grafting in diabetics does not significantly increase morbidity, and currently offers a 40 per cent chance of freedom from exogenous insulin. The successful treatment of diabetic renal failure is not compromised by the addition of this developmental procedure.

Introduction

The diabetic in renal failure is less likely to be accepted for dialysis or transplantation in the United Kingdom than in many European countries or in North America [1]. Diabetics form less than two per cent of all patients alive on treatment in the UK compared with four per cent in the Federal Republic of Germany and 13 per cent in Sweden [2]. The difference is mirrored in annual acceptance rates, diabetic patients now accounting for 25–30 per cent of new patients in the USA [3], 22 per cent in Sweden, 8.8 per cent in the Federal Republic of Germany and only 5.5 per cent in the UK [2].

Clinical pancreatic transplantation in diabetic patients initiated by Lillehei and colleagues [4] was limited by technical complications associated with exocrine leakage until ductal occlusion techniques were introduced [5]. The introduction of these newer surgical techniques and the use of Cyclosporin A as an immunosuppressive agent has resulted in an increased interest in the use of combined renal and segmental pancreatic transplantation. This paper reviews our experience of this technique in the context of an integrated treatment programme for diabetic patients with renal failure.

711

Patients

Between January, 1981, and June, 1983, 22 diabetic patients with renal failure were enrolled in an integrated dialysis and transplant programme. The 16 patients starting dialysis, at our unit representing 13 per cent of all patients accepted for dialysis during this period. A further four patients have been accepted for treatment but are currently receiving conservative management. During this period four patients were referred for consideration but not accepted for treatment because of extensive coronary and peripheral vascular disease. One patient was offered treatment but declined. The remaining six patients were started on dialysis in other units and referred for transplantation. There were nine females and 13 males, ages ranged from 13–62 at the onset of dialysis. The youngest patient had renal failure secondary to focal segmental glomerulosclerosis and had diabetes diagnosed two years before the onset of renal failure. With this exception all patients had biopsy proven diabetic nephrosclerosis or a long history of diabetes with microvascular complications preceding the onset of proteinuria and uraemia. All but two patients were insulin dependent. At the start of dialysis all patients except the youngest had diabetic retinopathy with varying degrees of visual impairment, three patients being completely blind. The majority had other diabetic complications with evidence of hypertension, ischaemic heart disease, peripheral vascular disease and peripheral and autonomic neuropathy.

Dialysis

All patients were commenced on continuous ambulatory peritoneal dialysis (CAPD) with serum creatinines in the range 800–1600μmol/litre. Intraperitoneal insulin administration was used in the majority. The decision to use CAPD was influenced by the advantages of this technique for patients with myocardial and vascular disease but also by a shortage of haemodialysis facilities. The incidence of peritonitis in this group of patients did not differ from that seen in the non-diabetic group in our unit. One patient had to be transferred to haemodialysis after 26 months on CAPD due to loss of dialysis and ultrafiltration capacity of the peritoneal cavity, this patient having suffered several episodes of peritonitis. Two patients on CAPD underwent single toe amputation for ischaemic complications and one patient was treated for tuberculosis. Three patients died while on CAPD all from acute myocardial infarction within three months of starting treatment.

Transplantation

Ten patients have undergone combined cadaveric renal and segmental pancreatic transplantation. Following a standard renal transplant operation the pancreatic segment was anastomosed to the iliac vessels in the opposite iliac fossa according to standard tecnhiques [6]. All pancreatic grafts have undergone ductal injection with polyisoprene latex, distal arteriovenous fistulae have not been formed. Post-operative heparinisation has been continued for ten days controlled with

712

whole blood clotting times (Hemachron). Intravenous aprotinin (Trasylol) was given for 48 hours post-operatively. Immunosuppression was with Cyclosporin A (15mg/kg/d) starting pre-operatively and Prednisolone 20mg/d. Insulin administration by intravenous infusion pre-operatively was discontinued post-operatively once normoglycaemia was achieved.

Results

One patient died following a cardiac arrest on the 10th post-operative day with normal kidney and pancreas function. This was associated with myocardial ischaemia possibly exacerbated by hyperkalaemia in association with Cyclosporin A treatment. The remaining patients are alive two to 25 months following transplantation (Table I).

TABLE I. Renal and segmental pancreatic transplant: graft survival

	Tx Date	Age	Patient	Kidney	Pancreas
1	23.5.81	15	Alive	+	+
2	15.6.81	30	Alive	+	– (Rejection day 15)
3	23.9.81	43	Alive	+	+
4	3.1.82	51	Died – day 10	+	+
5	18.2.82	36	Alive	+	+
6	2.3.82	28	Alive	+ (Vasc. Rej.)	– (? 13 months)
7	18.10.82	28	Alive	– (Day 20 – Vasc. Rej.)	– (Day 10 – Thrombosis)
8	17.1.83	32	Alive	+	– (Week 4 – Rejection)
9	23.3.83	25	Alive	+	– (Week 6 – Thrombosis)
10	23.4.83	47	Alive	+	+

(+ = Functioning graft; - = Non-functioning graft)

One renal allograft was lost to irreversible vascular rejection after one month. The remaining eight renal grafts are functioning satisfactorily although two have histological evidence of chronic vascular rejection. The overall renal allograft survival is 80 per cent. Of the seven patients with more than one year's follow-up the one year kidney graft survival rate is 71 per cent. Two patients have been converted to Prednisolone and Azathioprine for chronic Cyclosporin nephrotoxicity.

The overall pancreas graft survival is 40 per cent with an actual graft survival from two to 25 months. Apart from the one graft functioning at the time of the patient's death five other pancreatic grafts have been lost. Two pancreatic grafts were lost within two weeks, one from rejection in association with a reversible rejection episode in the kidney and one from thrombosis, anticoagulants

713

having been discontinued because of an intraperitoneal haemorrhage. One pancreas was lost at four weeks probably from rejection at the time of a renal rejection episode which was reversed. The remaining two pancreas losses occurred at six weeks and 13 months respectively, probably from thrombosis. Both graft losses occured suddenly, the later one being in a patient with hypotension and heart failure due to ischaemic heart disease. A one year actuarial pancreatic graft survival rate of 40 per cent needs cautious interpretation because of the small numbers involved.

Post-operative complications due to the addition of a pancreatic graft to the standard renal transplant operation have consisted of brief episodes of abdominal discomfort associated with hyperamylasaemia and two episodes of intraperitoneal haemorrhage in association with anticoagulation. In both cases the blood drained via the Tenkhoff CAPD catheter which had been left in situ as an intraperitoneal drain. One patient subsequently had an intraperitoneal abscess drained. There was no mortality attributable to the addition of the pancreatic transplant to the operation.

Glycaemic control

All patients discontinued exogenous insulin within 24 hours of the operation, although insulin was occasionally reintroduced at the time of steroid treatment of renal rejection episodes. Mean glycosylated haemoglobin values were 8.3 per cent in the patients with functioning pancreatic grafts compared with 12 per cent in the group treated by CAPD. Part of this difference results from the improved renal function. In keeping with previous reports [7] although fasting and post-prandial glucose concentration may be normal in patients whose pancreas graft function allows them to remain off exogenous insulin, glucose tolerance tests reveal an abnormal pattern of glycaemic control following a 75g oral glucose load (Figure 1). The pattern of glucose response compares with that previously reported from denervated pancreatic grafts secreting insulin into the systemic circulation.

Discussion

Although the mortality of diabetic patients on dialysis and transplant programmes is higher than that of non-diabetics (18% overall mortality in our patients) we have shown that with a flexible multidisciplinary team offering an integrated treatment programme, diabetic renal failure can be managed successfully. The fact that so few diabetics are treated in the United Kingdom results from the overall limited resources available to the nephrologist and the limited expectations of diabetic physicians.

The role of pancreatic transplantation as an adjunct to renal allografting is less clear. We have shown that using current techniques the addition of a pancreas to a renal transplant operation does not significantly add to the morbidity or increase mortality and does not jeopardise the successful treatment of diabetic renal failure. The ultimate aim of providing long-term normal glycaemic metabolism from a procedure that is safe enough to be offered to diabetic patients

714

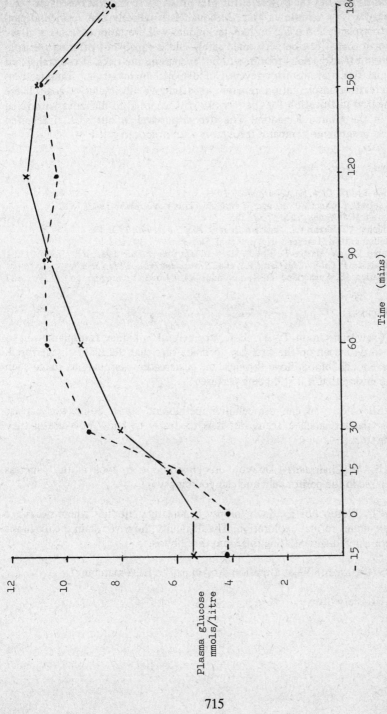

Figure 1. 75g oral glucose tolerance test 3 months (x) and 12 months (•) after combined renal and segmental pancreatic transplant (Cyclosporin A)

on diagnosis and has the potential for preventing the complications of diabetes over decades is as remote as ever. Although it is unlikely that segmental pancreatic transplantation using current techniques will ever approach this goal, we have shown that it can be performed safely and is capable of offering a reasonable period off exogenous insulin without increasing the risks of the transplant operation. The prevention or reversal of diabetic microvascular complications by pancreatic transplantation remains an attractive albeit elusive goal. There is no medical justification for the low priority accorded to diabetics with renal failure in the United Kingdom. The overall survival in our small integrated treatment programme compares favourably with other series [8].

References

1   Cameron JS. *Diabetic Nephropathy 1983; 2:* 1
2   Jacobs C, Brunner FP, Brynger H et al. *Diabetic Nephropathy 1983; 2:* 12
3   Avram MM. *Nephron 1982; 32:* 285
4   Lillehei RC, Simon RL, Najarian JS et al. *Ann Surg 1970; 172:* 405
5   Dubernard JM, Traeger J, Neyra P et al. *Surgery 1978; 84:* 633
6   Calne RY, McMaster P, Rolles K et al. *Transplant Proc 1980; 13 (Suppl 2):* 51
7   McMaster P, Gibby OM, Calne RY et al. *Transplant Proc 1981; 13:* 371
8   Najarian JS, Sutherland DER, Simmons RL. *Annals of Surgery 1979; 190:* 487

Open Discussion

KERR (Newcastle upon Tyne) It is very helpful in kidney transplantation to be able to do a scan on the first day to make sure that the kidney is perfused. Is there enough blood flow through the pancreatic transplant to make such a scan to ensure that it is still being perfused?

MICHAEL Yes, you can use selinium-methionine scans. Some workers are studying platelet labelled scans but it is too early to know how useful they are going to be.

MOORHEAD (Chairman) Do you use laparoscopy to look at the pancreas which is free in the peritoneum and can you biopsy it?

MICHAEL We do not routinely biopsy pancreatic grafts but where necessary it is done under formal exploration. The difficulty, however, is in the diagnosis of rejection and differentiating this from thrombosis.

JACOBS (Chairman) What attention do you pay to HLA matching?

MICHAEL Very little.

PART XX

BONE DISEASE AND PARATHYROID HORMONE

Chairmen: A Fournier
G R D Catto

Proc EDTA (1983) Vol 20

INFLUENCE OF ALUMINIUM HYDROXIDE INTAKE ON HAEMOGLOBIN CONCENTRATIONS AND BLOOD TRANSFUSION REQUIREMENTS IN HAEMODIALYSIS PATIENTS

J B Cannata, P Ruiz Alegria, M V Cuesta, J Herrera, V Peral

Hospital General de Asturias, Universidad de Oviedo, Oviedo, Spain

Summary

To investigate the likely influence of aluminium hydroxide intake ($Al(OH)_3$) on haemoglobin concentrations and blood transfusion requirements we studied 27 long-term haemodialysis patients for 24 months divided in two equal periods: (P I and P II). All patients received oral iron as a fasting single dose, intravenous iron being used only occasionally. During P I $Al(OH)_3$ was given thrice daily, during P II $Al(OH)_3$ was reduced significantly by stopping the breakfast dose, thereby separating the oral iron from the influence of the binder.

After $Al(OH)_3$ reduction haemoglobin increased, the requirement for blood transfusion decreased, and the need for intravenous iron also decreased. Serum phosphorous did not change. This suggests that $Al(OH)_3$ might interfere with erythropoiesis and we consider it advisable to avoid the morning dose of $Al(OH)_3$ which in many cases is not necessary.

Introduction

Aluminium hydroxide ($Al(OH)_3$) has been widely used as a harmless phosphate binder. However, there is convincing evidence about its absorption [1–4] and toxicity [5–8].

Many haemodialysis patients take $Al(OH)_3$ thrice daily with meals. In many cases ferrous sulphate is taken in a similar schedule without taking into account: a) the likely action of phosphate binders as iron binders; b) that ferrous sulphate is better absorbed in acid medium; c) not every meal has enough phosphorous to make it necessary to use phosphate binders. Many populations have two main and one light meal daily, which might be a good reason for using binders only twice daily.

The aim of this study was to evaluate the likely influence of $Al(OH)_3$ intake on haemoglobin (Hb) concentrations and blood transfusion requirements in patients on long-term haemodialysis.

Patients and methods

Twenty-seven patients were followed for 24 months, dialysis was thrice weekly (13.5hr/week) using dialysers $1.0-1.3m^2$, and employing deionised water with an aluminium (Al) content of less than $0.6\mu mol/L$. The daily protein intake was between $1.2-1.5g/kg/day$. All patients received water soluble vitamin supplements and oral ferrous sulphate in a single fasting dose of $150-300mg/day$. Intravenous (i.v.) iron was used only occasionally for short periods, without stopping the oral iron, in those patients who had iron deficiency and who did not increase either the serum iron or Hb with oral supplements. The i.v. dose used was iron dextran 0.5g every fortnight for a maximum of three months.

The follow-up was divided in two periods of 12 months, P I and P II (Figure 1).

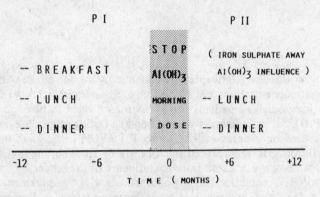

Figure 1. Protocol of study

During P I the patients received $Al(OH)_3$ (233mg tablets) with meals thrice daily, during P II we reduced significantly the $Al(OH)_3$ intake ($p<0.025$) by stopping the breakfast dose, thereby keeping the morning dose of iron away from the influence of $Al(OH)_3$ (Figure 1). At the end of P I the mean time on haemo-dialysis was 37.8 ± 17 months.

During both periods at monthly intervals we checked the daily intake of $Al(OH)_3$ tablets and measured the serum phosphorous (P), Hb, the number of units of blood transfused, the i.v. iron infused and the serum iron. Throughout the study we transfused patients only when symptoms of anaemia became unacceptable. Two of the 27 patients received, as a planned procedure (one in P I and the other during P II), four units each without following the above mentioned criteria as a part of a transplant protocol.

Statistical details

All values are expressed as a mean $\pm$ SD and they were compared using a paired t-test.

720

Results

The number of $Al(OH)_3$ tablets remained stable throughout P I and P II. During P II, in spite of the significant $Al(OH)_3$ reduction, the serum P did not change, Hb slightly increased, the number of units of blood transfused decreased and the need for i.v. iron decreased (Table I).

Other monthly values, which are not displayed in Table I, showed a similar trend.

TABLE I. Results from P I and P II

	P I			$Al(OH)_3$ reduction	P II		
$Al(OH)_3$ (tablets/day)	8.4±4	8.4±4	8.2±4	⌐— ** —⌐ 7.9±4 5.6±3	5.8±3	5.9±3	5.8±4
Serum phosphorous (mmol/L)	1.7±0.3	1.5±0.3	1.5±0.3	1.5±0.3	1.6±0.3	1.6±0.3	1.5±0.2
Haemoglobin (g/100ml)	8.0±2	8.0±2	8.3±3	8.3±2	8.7±3	8.6±3	8.8±3
Blood transfusion† (units/patient/ year)	⊢------------ 3.19 -----------⊣			⌐— * —⌐	⊢------------ 1.50 ---------------⊣		
i.v. iron (g/year)	⊢------------- 15 --------------⊣				⊢----------- 9 -----------------⊣		
Serum iron (µg/100ml)	103±53	80±42		93±44		99±52	93±45
Time (months)	−12	−6	−3	0	+3	+6	+12

* $p<0.05$; ** $p<0.025$

† One blood transfusion = 300ml of packed red cells or 500ml of whole blood

Discussion

Recently several studies have been carried out showing that $Al(OH)_3$ intake leads to significant Al absorption with the risk of toxicity for haemodialysis patients [1–4]. Most studies have been of bone and brain in which Al toxicity has been well established [5–8]. Other studies have suggested that high-Al dialysate may induce anaemia which can be reversed using low-Al dialysate [9, 10].

To our knowledge nothing has been published about the role of $Al(OH)_3$ on erythropoiesis either by its absorption and direct toxic effect on bone marrow, by its action as an iron binder in the gastrointestinal tract, or by reducing the iron absorption through gastroduodenal pH elevations.

We believe the necessity for phosphate binders must be reassessed as in many countries the daily phosphorous intake is divided between two rather than three meals. In our study we found no change in serum P after stopping the morning dose of $Al(OH)_3$ presumably due to the fact of a low phosphorous content of our patients' breakfasts. This demonstrates the lack of need for binders with light meals.

In many Latin countries the lightest meal is breakfast, while in others it is lunch or dinner. This makes it necessary to tailor the dose of $Al(OH)_3$ for each patient depending on the dietary habits.

At the time we performed our study we did not have facilities for measuring serum ferritin and Al concentrations which could have given us more precise data about iron stores and Al absorption. However, we believe our results suggest that $Al(OH)_3$ might interfere with erythropoiesis either by a direct toxic effect through its absorption, by its probable action as an iron binder, or as an agent increasing the gastroduodenal pH impairing iron absorption.

On this basis we consider it advisable to give, whenever possible, ferrous sulphate as a single fasting dose keeping it away from the influence of $Al(OH)_3$. We also recommend dividing the $Al(OH)_3$ intake with the main meals, avoiding unnecessary therapy which could be toxic rather than beneficial.

References

1   Marsden SNE, Parkinson IS, Ward MK et al. *Proc EDTA 1979; 16:* 588
2   Gorsky JE, Dietz AA, Spencer H, Osis D. *Clin Chem 1979; 25:* 1739
3   Fleming LW, Stewart WK, Fell GS, Halls DJ. *Clin Nephrol 1982; 17:* 222
4   Cannata JB, Briggs JD, Junor BJR, Fell GS. *Br Med J 1983.* In press
5   Elliot HL, Dryburgh F, Fell GS et al. *Br Med J 1978; 1:* 1101
6   Parkinson IS, Ward MK, Feest TG et al. *Lancet 1979; i:* 406
7   Cournot-Witmer G, Zingraff J, Plachot JJ et al. *Kidney Int 1981; 20:* 375
8   Hodsman AB, Sherrard DJ, Alfrey AC et al. *J Clin Endocrinol Metab 1982; 54:* 539
9   Short AIK, Winney RJ, Robson JS. *Proc EDTA 1980; 17:* 226
10 O'Hare JA, Murnaghan DJ. *N Engl J Med 1982; 306:* 654

Open Discussion

VERBEELEN (Brussels) Did you measure serum aluminium in your patients in order to see if the reduction of aluminium hydroxide intake results in a decrease of serum aluminium?

CANNATA No, as I said, unfortunately we didn't measure serum aluminium.

DRUEKE (Paris) I don't know if I missed it, what was the erythrocyte mean corpuscular volume in your patients and did it increase after the supposed increased iron absorption in your patients?

CANNATA We don't have mean corpuscular volume for all our patients and this is the reason why I didn't include the data. Some of them had a normocytic and others microcytic anaemia.

PARSONS (London) Can you explain why in the second period the phosphate decreased on average when you were giving less aluminium hydroxide? Where was the phosphate going that previously the patients received? With less aluminium hydroxide you had lower or similar values of serum phosphate.

CANNATA Well, I wouldn't say that the serum phosphate decreased, I think it remained similar and the explanation I think, as I said, is that in our country breakfast is very light and phosphorus intake at breakfast time is minimal. There is no reason at all to give two or three aluminium hydroxide tablets with breakfast. This is one message which comes from the paper, we use three times a day a drug that we should use, I think, twice with main meals.

PARSONS What was your criteria for transfusion? One of the most impressive results was the reduction in the number of units of blood you transfused. Can you tell us when you decide to transfuse as you might have been less enthusiastic in the second period unless you had strict criteria?

CANNATA The criteria was when symptoms of anaemia became unacceptable. We didn't use haemoglobin as a guide. If I have to give you a figure I would say that we never transfused our patients unless the PCV was less than 14 or 15 per cent. We had a very restrictive policy about transfusion.

FROEHLING (Potsdam) Which kind of aluminium hydroxide do you administer to your patients? It's well known that different drugs of aluminium hydroxide have different resorption of aluminium. In my opinion your doses of aluminium hydroxide in the first period of your study is too high. The mean dose of aluminium hydroxide in our patients agrees with your dose in the second period.

CANNATA We use aluminium hydroxide as a simple preparation such as Alu Cap or Aludrox. The aluminium hydroxide content for each tablet is less than other countries, that is 233mg each tablet, nearly half that of other countries. We give six daily which is nearly 1g.

DRATWA (Brussels) To reinforce your first hypothesis about direct aluminium toxicity and erythropoiesis, we had the opportunity to treat six patients with high serum aluminium values and we treated them with desferrioxamine; these patients didn't get any iron supplements. By treating them with desferrioxamine we removed some aluminium and decreased the serum values, and we saw that haemoglobin increased dramatically and that blood transfusions were dramatically reduced. I think this reinforces your first proposition.

CANNATA You are quite right but as I said our aim was really to test other unknown factors apart from the aluminium absorption as a cause of altered erythropoiesis.

723

MAK (London) Is there any difference in the dietary intake of phosphate between the first and second period of your study? Have you measured PTH values during the first and second period?

CANNATA This is very difficult to answer. All patients had the same kind of diet, about 1.2–1.5g protein per kilogram body weight. It is difficult to know if some patients ate more phosphorus than others. I don't think you can say anything more about the diet in regular patients unless you do specialised balanced studies. Regarding your second question unfortunately I have PTH results from only the first period and so I can't answer that point.

HIGH-EFFECTIVE ALUMINIUM FREE PHOSPHATE BINDER. IN VITRO AND IN VIVO STUDIES

H Schneider, K D Kulbe*, H Weber*, E Streicher

*Katharinenhospital, and *Fraunhofer Institute, Stuttgart, FRG*

Summary

For the purpose of intestinal phosphate binding we have developed aluminium free natural polymers consisting of heteropolyuronic acid charged with different cations. The in vitro experiments showed an efficacy two to three times greater than Aludrox®. During up to six months of clinical application no serious side effects have been detected, constipation ceased and serum phosphate was maintained in an acceptable range.

Introduction

Aluminium accumulation and its sequelae in chronic renal failure patients [1–4] is possibly a consequence of aluminium hydroxide medication, providing correct water preparation for dialysis is achieved. For the purpose of intestinal phosphate binding we have developed aluminium free substances which have been tested in vitro and in vivo.

Methods

The substances under investigation are natural polymers consisting of hetero-polyuronides charged with calcium or a combination of calcium and iron (Fe^{++} and Fe^{+++}). These natural polymers are non-toxic, licensed food additives and do not cause constipation. The substance is produced in small particles 1–2mm in size.

We have studied the capacity for phosphate removal by differently charged heteropolyuronides in vitro in Tris buffer solution under different pH conditions and compared the results with commonly available aluminium phosphate binders. Furthermore the calcium charged substance has been incubated with human duodenal juice, which has been enriched with 2g sodium phosphate imitating the phosphate load of an average meal. During the two-hour incubation period the phosphate binding capacity has been determined. Ten chronic renal failure patients with continuous problems in controlling their serum phosphate by conventional aluminium hydroxide therapy were treated with the calcium charged substance for up to six months and four additional patients received the calcium-iron charged product for up to three months.

Results

The polymer charged with calcium or a combination of calcium and iron contains little sodium (20mg/g) or potassium (7.8mg/g). The calcium content was found to be 140–160mg/g, the iron content of the calcium-iron charged product was 40mg/g (Figure 1).

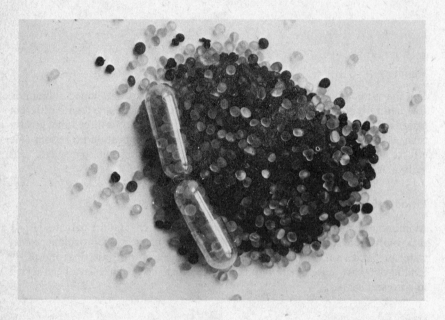

Figure 1. Mixture of the polymeric substance. Fair particles are calcium-charged, dark particles are charged with a combination of calcium and iron

In the first study 1g of the charged polymers were incubated in 200ml Tris buffered solution containing 0.4g phosphorus at 37°C (Figure 2). The calcium charged substance failed to work under acidotic pH conditions (pH 2), whereas the calcium-iron charged product was capable of binding 0.05g phosphate (16% of total binding capacity) under acidotic condition. Coming to neutral and alkalotic pH values, the particles swell in the presence of phosphate and the charged cations are released gradually allowing phosphate to be entrapped. The calcium charged substance was capable of binding 0.2g phosphorus (50%), whereas the calcium-iron charged product neutralised 0.29g phosphorus (72.5%)

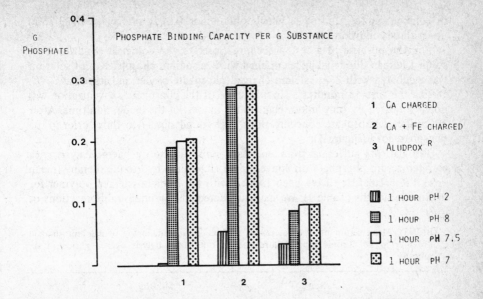

Figure 2. Phosphate binding capacity of the calcium charged product (1) and the calcium-iron charged polymer (2) in comparison to Aludrox® (3) under different pH conditions

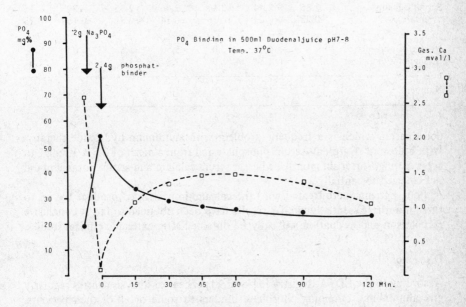

Figure 3. Phosphate binding effect of 2.4g calcium charged polymer in human duodenal juice at 37°C enriched with 2g sodium phosphate over a 120 minute incubation period

in comparison to Aludrox®, which only binds 0.095g phosphorus (23.75%) under these conditions.

For the purpose of a test procedure closer to physiological conditions we studied human duodenal juice enriched with 2g sodium phosphate. This solution was incubated with 2.4g calcium charged phosphate binder and stirred at 37°C. During the first 45 minutes a sharp decline of the phosphate concentration was noted followed by only minor changes for the rest of the incubation time. After 120 minutes phosphate concentrations were found similar to those prior to the phosphate load (Figure 3).

Ten patients suffering from end-stage renal failure on haemodialysis with elevated serum phosphate on conventional aluminium hydroxide therapy (mean dose 2.8 ± 1.8g/day) have been treated with the calcium charged polymer for up to six months (Table I). We have not detected any undesirable reactions or

TABLE I. Mean serum phosphate, serum calcium levels and dosage of calcium charged polymer in 10 chronic renal failure patients on haemodialysis over a period of six months

| | Start | Months | | | | | |
		1	2	3	4	5	6
Serum phosphate mg%	8.5 ±1.7	6.0 ±2.2	5.5 ±1.1	5.6 ±1.5	5.8 ±1.2	6.0 ±1.3	6.1 ±1.0
Serum calcium mmol/L	2.35 ±0.23	2.44 ±0.21	2.41 ±0.16	2.46 ±0.14	2.35 ±0.10	2.29 ±0.16	2.15 ±0.13
Dosage of phosphate binder g/day		4.6 ±1.8	5.0 ±1.9	5.5 ±1.9	5.6 ±1.8	6.0 ±1.7	5.4 ±1.8
Number	10	10	10	10	7	6	5

constipation which is a frequent problem with aluminium hydroxide therapy. With a dose of 4–7g/day serum phosphate fell from a mean of 8.5 ± 1.7mg% to 6.1 ± 1.0mg% after six months, whereas serum calcium and serum potassium did not change substantially.

Four patients were treated with the calcium-iron charged product for up to three months. Essentially similar results have been obtained so far. A conclusive comparison and evaluation will only be obtained after extended clinical studies.

Discussion

According to the EDTA Registry [5] over 90 per cent of dialysis centres regularly give aluminium containing phosphate binders to some or all of their patients. Only a few centres (16%) regularly monitor aluminium concentrations in water and dialysis fluid and in patients' serum [5], so the question about the cause of aluminium accumulation cannot be answered reliably at the moment. But there is consistent data [6–10] that aluminium is resorbed enterally, so its use should be abandoned if possible.

The new substances tested for their phosphate binding capacity are natural polymers consisting of heteropolyuronides and charged with calcium and iron cations. The iron containing preparation trapped phosphate under acidotic pH conditions, whereas under neutral and alkalotic pH values the particles swell and dissolve in the presence of phosphate. Calcium is release gradually and calcium-phosphate is formed which partially remains in the polymeric matrix. Depending from the polymers' calcium load and the phosphate ingestion there might be some calcium available for absorption, as serum calcium values rose in some patients. Possibly a cation exchange between calcium and sodium or potassium may take place, as we have noticed decreasing serum potassium concentration in particular cases. As far as the in vitro experiments are concerned, the phosphate binding efficacy per g substance is two to three times greater than that of Aludrox®. This polymer system can be used for controlled release of other ions (e.g. zinc, magnesium) and of water soluble drugs avoiding undesired high substance concentrations.

References

1 Alfrey AC, Mishell JM, Burks J et al. *Trans ASAIO 1972; XVIII:* 257
2 Pierides AM, Edwards WG, Cullum UX et al. *Kidney Int 1980; 18:* 115
3 Cournot-Witmer G, Zingraff J, Plachot J et al. *Kidney Int 1981; 20:* 375
4 Drueke T. *Nephron 1980; 26:* 207
5 Wing AJ. *Report of EDTA Registry on Water Preparation, Dialysis Practice and Encephalopathy in Dialysis Patients in the European Community 1981*
6 Cam JM, Luck VA, Eastwood JB et al. *Clin Sci Mol Med 1976; 51:* 407
7 Kaehny WD, Hegg AP, Alfrey AC. *N Engl J Med 1977; 296:* 1389
8 Mayor GH, Keiser JA, Ku PK. *Science 1977; 197:* 1187
9 Recker RR, Blotcky AJ, Leffler JA et al. *J Lab Clin Med 1977; 90:* 810
10 Fleming LW, Stewart WK, Fell GS et al. *Clin Neph 1982; 17:* 222

Open Discussion

SLATOPOLSKY (St Louis, USA) I want to congratulate you on this excellent paper, there is hope that one day we will be able to get rid of aluminium. I am concerned about the values you obtain after six months' treatment, phosphate 6mg% and calcium 2.2mmol/L, the phosphate is too high and the calcium too low. I suspect that the amount of binders you have used is too small and I strongly suggest that you increase the dose to correct the serum phosphate.

SCHNEIDER You are quite correct, the amount of phosphate binder has to be increased. The decreasing serum calcium may not be a real effect as the number of patients are small.

KERR (Newcastle-upon-Tyne) Congratulations on what could be a very important advance for all of us. I am pleased to hear that these are naturally occurring substances which are believed to be non-toxic. Can you tell us how they occur naturally? Are they licensed food additives only in their natural form or in their combined form? How far have you got with getting them on the market?

SCHNEIDER   The natural polymers are 'natural' in as much as they are not charged. Once they are charged they become medications and have to go through the Regional Drugs and Medicines Authorities.

RITZ (Heidelberg)   If your claims are confirmed you may have found, as we say in German, "Sie haben das Ei des Colombus gefund". I have one difficulty with your data, on the ordinate you plotted phosphate, and you claimed that 1g of the compound binds 0.2–0.3g phosphate, are you referring to phosphorus or phosphate?

SCHNEIDER   It's phosphate.

RITZ   Therefore the efficacy is quite low?

SCHNEIDER   We have compared the efficacy to other aluminium containing phosphate binders currently available and from this point of view the efficacy is quite high, for example three times as high as Aludrox®.

BOMMER (Munich)   Our problem is the amount of phosphate binders the patients have to take. We can confirm that, in the few patients we have studied, the plasma phosphate falls as much as or even more than with aluminium hydroxide. We find that we need only 70 per cent of the new binder compared with aluminium hydroxide, is this your experience?

SCHNEIDER   I have the same experience. There are some patients maintained with 2–3g daily with the natural polymer while others require up to 8–9g daily to maintain adequate serum phosphate concentrations. Up to 10g daily may be taken without problems.

FOURNIER (Chairman)   This represents, for me, a breakthrough in the treatment of uraemic hyperparathyroidism. It would be interesting to undertake a metabolic balance study of phosphate and calcium with this new preparation. I don't know if the fall in plasma calcium represents a negative calcium balance.

SCHNEIDER   We have some studies underway on this problem, but I can't give any results as yet.

Proc EDTA (1983) Vol 20

SECONDARY HYPERPARATHYROIDISM IN CHRONIC HAEMODIALYSIS PATIENTS: A CLINICO—PATHOLOGICAL STUDY

V Mendes, V Jorgetti, J Nemeth*, A Lavergne*, Y Lecharpentier*, C Dubost†, C Cournot-Witmer, R Bourdon†, A Bourdeau, J Zingraff, T Drüeke

*INSERM U90, Hôpital Necker-Enfants Malades, *Hôpital Lariboisiere, †Hôpital Widal, Paris, France*

Summary

Fifty-eight patients on intermittent haemodialysis underwent parathyroidectomy because of severe secondary hyperparathyroidism. Mean individual parathyroid gland weight was 689 ± 62 (SEM) mg. Mean total gland weight per patient was between two and three grams. Increasing nodule formation within hyperplastic glands appeared to develop with increasing time of duration of hyperparathyroidism. Patients with chronic pyelonephritis had a higher gland weight than those with chronic glomerulonephritis. A direct relationship was found between gland weight and circulating immunoreactive parathyroid hormone, but an inverse relationship between gland weight and plasma aluminium concentration. The higher the parathyroid gland aluminium, the higher was the bone aluminium concentration.

Introduction

Decreased plasma ionised calcium due to increased plasma phosphorus and/or diminished $1,25(OH)_2D_3$ is the principal cause implicated in the secondary hyperparathyroidism of chronic renal failure. The progression and severity of hyperparathyroidism is, however, quite variable from one uraemic patient to another and is not readily explained solely by the decrease in ionised calcium. Several additional factors have been recognised in recent years which may also play a role in the pathogenesis of this type of hyperparathyroidism [1]. Acute [2] or chronic [3] exposure to aluminium (Al) may also interfere with parathyroid hormone (PTH) secretion.

Patients and methods

Fifty-eight uraemic patients aged 18–70 years (31 males and 27 females) were included in the study. Their mean estimated duration of chronic renal failure

731

was between one and 19 years and their time on intermittent haemodialysis treatment between one and 10 years. Eighteen patients had chronic glomerulonephritis, 18 chronic pyelonephritis, and 11 polycystic kidney disease. In the remaining 11 patients, the precise nature of the nephropathy was unknown. All the patients underwent parathyroidectomy between 1976 and 1982 based on the diagnosis of severe secondary hyperparathyroidism. In fact, three to four of these patients were misdiagnosed between 1976 and 1978. They had predominant dialysis osteomalacia [3], a new pathological entity not yet well recognised at that time.

In some patients, an additional biopsy of the thyroid gland and of bone was performed in order to determine tissue Al concentrations. For the sake of comparison, parathyroid and thyroid tissue samples were also removed from non-uraemic patients with primary hyperparathyroidism.

Biochemical determinations comprised plasma calcium (atomic absorption spectrometry), phosphorus (colorimetric method), alkaline phosphatase (enzymatic method), plasma and tissue Al (atomic absorption spectrometry with graphite furnace), and plasma immunoreactive iPTH (radioimmunoassay with an anti-COOH terminal antibody). Tissue weight was always determined as fresh wet weight. Light microscopic analysis of 222 parathyroid glands was undertaken using haematoxylin-eosin-safran stained paraffin sections according to a previously described technique [4].

Statistical methods

Statistical analysis was performed using Student's paired or unpaired t test where appropriate.

Results

Mean ± SEM values before parathyroidectomy were respectively 2.72 ± 0.049 mmol/litre for plasma calcium, 2.20 ± 0.010mmol/litre for plasma phosphorus, 6679 ± 2094nKat/litre for plasma alkaline phosphatases (normal, 500–1500 nKat/litre), 3.56 ± 0.49μmol/litre for plasma Al (normal, <0.7μmol/litre), and 2.86 ± 0.36ng/ml for iPTH (normal, ≤0.5ng/ml).

Individual parathyroid gland weight was between 22 and 3880mg (mean ± SEM, 689 ± 62mg) for a total of 222 removed glands. The total gland weight removed per patient was between 104 and 9775mg. The majority of patients had a total parathyroid mass weighing between 250 and 2500mg. The gland weight histogram is shown in Figure 1.

When comparing patient groups with different types of nephropathy, a difference in total parathyroid gland weight became apparent between subjects having chronic pyelonephritis (n=18) and those having chronic glomerulonephritis (3308 ± 498 versus 1824 ± 358mg, p<0.01). The estimated time of progression of chronic renal failure in both groups was comparable (4.7 versus 5.3 years).

The light microscope analysis of parathyroid glands revealed the presence

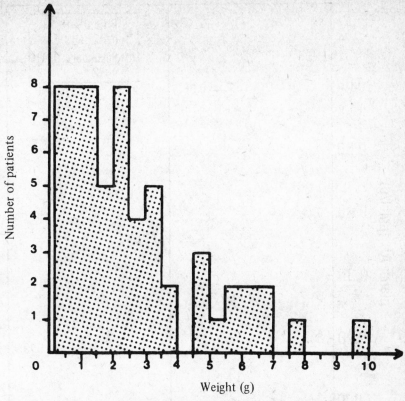

Figure 1. Histogram of parathyroid gland weight per patient

of principal cells and oncocytes with a varying incidence from one patient to the other and even within different sections of the same gland. Four types of gland architecture were defined: 30 glands had a pure nodular appearance (mean gland weight, 1301 ± 243mg); 62 glands showed diffuse hyperplasia with clearcut nodule formations (mean gland weight 730 ± 97mg); 38 glands showed diffuse hyperplasia with only scarce nodule formation (mean gland weight, 492 ± 93mg), and 92 glands were purely hyperplastic (mean gland weight, 543 ± 96mg). In only 12 patients were all three or more respective glands of the same type. Seven out of the 58 patients had a duration of chronic renal failure exceeding 10 years. They had all parathyroid glands with a clearcut nodular appearance. No relationship existed between parathyroid gland weight and plasma calcium, phosphorus, or alkaline phosphatase. However, a positive correlation was found between gland weight and plasma iPTH concentration (n=31, r=0.41, p<0.05). Moreover, a negative correlation existed between gland weight and plasma Al concentration (n=20, r=0.45, p<0.05) when considering only patients with a total gland weight of 2000mg or less and their highest plasma Al concentration during the months before parathyroidectomy.

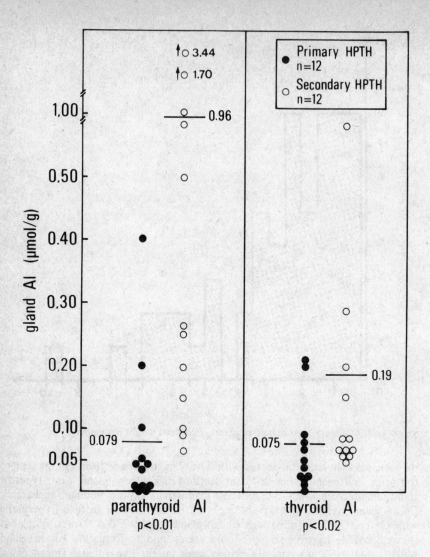

Figure 2. Al concentration of parathyroid and thyroid glands per gram wet tissue weight in haemodialysis patients with secondary hyperparathyroidism and in non-uraemic patients with primary hyperparathyroidism

Figure 2 shows Al concentrations in parathyroid and thyroid tissue of dialysed patients with secondary hyperparathyroidism as compared to non-uraemic patients with primary hyperparathyroidism. Whereas the Al content of the parathyroid and thyroid tissue was comparable for the latter, it was higher in the parathyroid glands than in the thyroid glands for the former. When comparing the Al concentration of parathyroid glands to that of bone, a significant correlation between both parameters could be demonstrated (n=9, r=0.74, p<0.01).

Discussion

The clinical and pathological presentation of secondary hyperparathyroidism in chronically uraemic patients shows a strikingly variable pattern from one subject to another. The present study was designed to help clarify some of the questions concerning the heterogeneity of expression of this formidable complication of chronic renal failure.

It shows that increasing nodule formation within the parathyroid glands of haemodialysis patients occurs probably as a function of the time during which hyperparathyroidism develops. This does not explain the often important heterogeneity of individual gland weight and light microscopic appearances as already noted by others [5,6]. It indicates, however, that nodule formation within the parathyroid glands represents a rather continuous transformation from initially diffuse hyperplasia to more and more nodular structures.

Our study shows further that the severity of hyperparathyroidism, at least in terms of gland weight, appears also to depend on the type of the underlying kidney disease: patients with chronic pyelonephritis developed a greater mean parathyroid gland mass than those with chronic glomerulonephritis, for a comparable time of progression of documented chronic renal failure. It is possible that a relationship exists with the finding that vitamin D deficient osteomalacia is also more frequently observed in the former than in the latter [7].

The positive, though weak relationship, between parathyroid gland weight and plasma iPTH concentration using an anti-carboxyl terminal antibody points to the usefulness of PTH determinations, at least for the majority of patients. This does, of course, not exclude the possibility of apparently inconsistent, unexplained hormone values in some patients.

Finally, our study underlines the almost certain interference of aluminium with parathyroid function. In addition to its inhibitory effect on the mineralisation process in bone [3,8,9], aluminium could inhibit parathyroid hormone secretion and thereby lead to a reduction in parathyroid gland size, either by a direct action [10] or indirectly via an increase in plasma calcium [2]. The observed negative relationship between gland mass and Al concentration of the present study points in this direction.

Acknowledgments

The authors wish to thank the numerous medical teams of the Paris area who referred patients included in the present study (Centres of AURA home dialysis, AURA "Bessin", Edouard Rist, St Maurice, St Cloud, Alma). They further express their gratitude to Ms F Prouillet for valuable technical help and Ms A Kennedy for excellent secretarial assistance.

References

1   Brown EM, Wilson RE, Eastman RC et al. *J Clin Endocrinol Metab 1982; 54:* 172
2   Cannata JB, Briggs JD, Bunor BJR et al. *Lancet 1983; i:* 501
3   Drüeke T. *Nephron 1980; 26:* 207
4   Lecharpentier Y, Dubost Cl, Ferrand J et al. *Arch Anat Cytol Path 1983; 31:* 49

5   Katz AD, Kaplan L. *Arch Surg 1973; 107:* 51
6   Hasleton PS, Ali HH. *J Pathol 1980; 132:* 307
7   Mora-Palma F, Ellis HA, Cook DB et al. *Proc EDTA 1982; 19:* 188
8   Cournot-Witmer G, Zingraff J, Plachot JJ et al. *Kidney Internat 1981; 20:* 375
9   Ott S, Maloney NA, Coburn JW et al. *N Engl J Med 1982; 307:* 709
10   Morrissey J, Rothstein M, Mayor G, Slatopolsky E. *Kidney Internat 1983; 23:* 699

Open Discussion

RITZ (Heidelberg)   The appearance of nodules certainly indicates that parathyroid cells somehow escaped local mechanisms of growth control. As you are aware from work in primary hyperparathyroidism, nodule formation may or may not reflect monoclonal proliferation. Do you by any chance have glucose-6-phosphate dehydrogenase data to confirm or refute this possibility?

DRÜEKE   Unfortunately we were not able to do that study in the present patients. I am very aware of that study. There are also in vitro studies with dispersed parathyroid cells from patients with secondary hyperparathyroidism. They show that the calcium suppressibility of parathyroid hormone secretion in vitro is quite different from one patient to the other, indicating the occurrence of escape at least in some of them. However, I am not aware of a distinction of the presence or not of nodule formation within the glands which have been tested.

RITZ   The second question related to the difference between patients with glomerulonephritis as opposed to patients with pyelonephritis, the latter had more severe hyperparathyroidism. Did the group with pyelonephritis have a greater proportion of women? The reason I am asking this is that I found more than a decade ago that uraemic women tended to have a greater prevalence and severity of hyperparathyroidism than men. This was confirmed in a number of subsequent reports. This is not completely surprising since primary hyperparathyroidism is also more common in women. Consequently, may the difference between glomerulonephritis and pyelonephritis in your study not be due to the fact that women tend to have pyelonephritis more frequently than men?

DRÜEKE   If I remember well, we checked whether there was a difference in sex and whether this could explain the observation gland weight. We did not find any difference.

WAUTERS (Lausanne)   In patients with analgesic nephropathy we have observed lower calcium, higher alkaline phosphatase and high PTH serum levels when compared to patients with interstitial nephritis of other causes. What was the number of patients in this group having analgesic nephropathy?

DRÜEKE   I cannot give you the precise answer, but I can assure you that it was only a minority of patients, if any.

PARSONS (London) If I understand what you are saying correctly, the patients with the largest glands have pyelonephritis, and therefore have probably had renal failure longer than the patients with glomerulonephritis, but you are also saying that the smallest glands have the highest aluminium content. Does that mean that the patients with chronic pyelonephritis have not been given aluminium, or are their levels lower than the patients with glomerulonephritis? There are some reports, particularly in animal work, that hyperparathyroidism is associated with an increased transfer of aluminium across the gut. Now this would be self-limiting if the bigger the gland the higher the parathyroid hormone, in theory the higher the aluminium should be in the plasma, but this is not borne out by your findings. Is that so?

DRÜEKE As to your first question, I did point out that the estimated duration of renal failure in pyelonephritis was the same as that in patients with chronic glomerulonephritis, but as you know, the estimation might be erroneous. It is so difficult to know the very beginning of chronic renal failure. We have no exact data on the administration of aluminium to these patients before they were regularly dialysed, so I cannot answer the second part of your first question. As to your second question, it has not been shown, to my knowledge that parathyroid overfunction increases absorption of aluminium. What has been shown is that increased body retention of aluminium occurred in the hyperparathyroid rats in which these studies have been done, which is not quite the same thing. Up to now there is no precise way, to my knowledge, of studying intestinal aluminium absorption.

KERR (Newcastle upon Tyne) Going back to Professor Ritz's question, it could be, of course, that he has observed more hyperparathyroidism in women because more women have pyelonephritis and not vice versa. We have also observed, the last time we analysed it, that parathyroids are larger in patients with pyelonephritis. Last year we presented a paper here* showing that patients with pyelonephritis develop more osteomalacia and they were more hypocalcaemic, which might explain why they have more stimulated parathyroids. Did you look at the serum calcium in your groups to see whether those with pyelonephritis are lower than those with glomerulonephritis?

DRÜEKE At the time of dialysis there was clearly no difference in serum calcium. I cannot assure you whether in the long-standing evolution before haemodialysis there has been at some moments some difference.

SLATOPOLSKY (St Louis) I am glad to hear you found a higher concentration of aluminium specifically in the parathyroid glands than in other tissues. We have also found an inverse correlation between aluminium and PTH in the serum. We found that aluminium per se suppresses the release of PTH in dispersed isolated cells in vitro. Aluminium does not produce a toxic effect, we can wash the aluminium and incubate the cells in a lower medium of calcium

* Mora-Palma FJ, Sellares VL, Ellis HA et al. *Proc EDTA 1982; 19:* 188

there is a remarkable secretion of PTH. Aluminium does not interfere with the biosynthesis of conversion of PTH, but interferes with the secretion of PTH. This may be important as you are aware, due to the fact that the patients with aluminium induced osteomalacia has very low parathyroid hormone and PTH has been shown to play a role in the genesis of this osteomalacic component.

DRÜEKE Thank you for your remark. I am well aware of your studies. The problem is, however, to know whether chronic aluminium intoxication could not lead to some pathological alteration of the cells. We have now some electron microscope findings which clearly show that there might be some morphological alterations of the cell structure, not only in bone but also in parathyroid glands.

FROEHLING (Potsdam) At what aluminium concentrations are toxic effects in parathyroid glands observed? In our investigations we have found a positive correlation between PTH and serum aluminium above a limit of about $115\mu g/$ml.

DRÜEKE Do I understand a positive relation?

FROEHLING Yes.

DRÜEKE This is interesting. It is quite the opposite to Dr Slatopolsky's findings. I would expect that with increasing long-standing aluminium intoxication the plasma parathyroid hormone level would diminish so it might be a biphasic phenomenon. Initially there could be some increased aluminium retention in the organism due to hyperparathyroidism, but with long-standing aluminium intoxication very clearly parathyroid function diminishes. I would not, of course, say that aluminium intoxication is a good means of treating hyperparathyroidism.

EFFECT OF SECONDARY HYPERPARATHYROIDISM ON THE ANAEMIA OF END-STAGE RENAL FAILURE: IN VIVO AND IN VITRO STUDIES

P Grützmacher, H W Radtke, W Fassbinder, K-M Koch, W Schoeppe

University Hospital, Frankfurt/Main, FRG

Summary

Changes in haematocrit of 29 haemodialysis patients were followed 12 months before, close to and 12 months after parathyroidectomy. Mean haematocrit decreased significantly from 31.6 ± 8.6 per cent to 29.1 ± 8.4 per cent and increased to 33.3 ± 7.9 per cent after PTX. Serum erythropoietin concentration, investigated pre and 6–12 months post PTX, at a time, when an increase of haematocrit values had been observed, did not significantly change (63 ± 58 vs 67 ± 37mU/ml). The effect of 1–84 bovine parathyroid hormone on erythropoiesis was studied in vitro. A dose-related inhibition of colony formation of both fetal mouse liver and human bone marrow erythroid cells was observed in the presence of two to 8U parathyroid hormone/ml, suggesting direct bone marrow toxicity by excessive parathyroid hormone concentrations.

Introduction

Hyperparathyroidism (HPTH) is a common complication in end-stage renal failure which frequently requires surgical intervention to prevent progression of renal osteodystrophy. Furthermore, multiple interactions of parathyroid hormone (PTH) with other complications of chronic renal disease have been reported [1]. A beneficial effect of parathyroidectomy (PTX) on anaemia has been reported [2], but this has not been confirmed by others [3]. However, anaemia is a known finding even in primary hyperparathyroidism [4], and inhibition of erythropoiesis by bone marrow fibrosis [2], direct inhibition of RNA synthesis [5] and erythroid precursor cell proliferation [6] have been suggested as pathogenetic mechanisms.

Patients and methods

Between 1975 and 1982 severe HPTH with advanced renal osteodystrophy, hypercalcaemia and progressively increasing PTH concentrations made parathyroidectomy (PTX) necessary in 29 of 160 of our home dialysis patients. The influence of hyperparathyroidism on renal anaemia and the effect of PTX was studied. The mean of three sequential haematocrit readings 12 months before, close to and 12 months following PTX were compared.

In addition, serum erythropoietin (EP) concentrations were determined in six patients immediately before and six to 12 months following PTX, at a time when anaemia had already improved. Erythropoietin measurement was by a sensitive in vitro bioassay (fetal mouse liver cell assay and direct microscopic observation of colony forming units) as described in detail [7]. To exclude a possible effect of PTH and uraemic toxins on EP measurement, molecules below 15,000 daltons were removed using an Amicon filter.

To investigate the direct effect of PTH on in vitro erythropoiesis 1—84 bovine PTH at a concentration of 0—8U/ml was tested in murine fetal liver and human bone marrow cell cultures in the presence of sufficient amounts of EP (32mU/ml).

Statistical analysis was performed using Student's paired t-test. Values are given as mean values ± SD.

Results and discussion

The influence of hyperparathyroidism on haematocrit is shown in Figure 1. During the 12 months prior to surgery, anaemia deteriorated markedly in almost every patient (mean haematocrit decreased from 31.6 ± 8.6% to 29.1 ± 8.4%, $p < 0.01$).

However the individual response of severe HPTH on anaemia varies widely. Four of twenty-nine patients had an increase of haematocrit, probably due to the correction of iron deficiency (1), recovery from pericarditis (1) and reversion of uraemia after the onset of regular dialysis (2). After parathyroidectomy the response is more uniform; mean haematocrit increased from 29.1 ± 8.4 per cent to 33.3 ± 7.9 per cent ($p < 0.001$), some patients increasing 10 per cent in 12 months.

When the haematocrit profiles were studied over a longer period a comparatively slow recovery from anaemia, which was not complete even after 12 months, was observed in some patients, indicating the complex nature of this disease.

Figure 2 shows the changes in haematocrit of a 28 year old patient on haemodialysis since September 1969, followed up three years pre and post PTX. Dialysis was performed six to eight hours three times/week using a $1m^2$ Kiil dialyser. Therapy with androgens, vitamin B12 and folic acid, heparin and iron changed only slightly. Three years before PTX, when PTH concentrations were normal, the haematocrit had stabilised at 30 per cent. With progression of HPTH a marked decrease could be observed, which was completely reversed following PTX. However, recovery from anaemia took nearly two years. MCV and erythrocyte haemogloblin did not change significantly.

To evaluate possible factors involved in the improvement of anaemia, changes in EP production were investigated. In six patients direct comparison could be made since corresponding serum samples immediately before and six to 12 months after PTX were available. Whereas haematocrit values had increased in

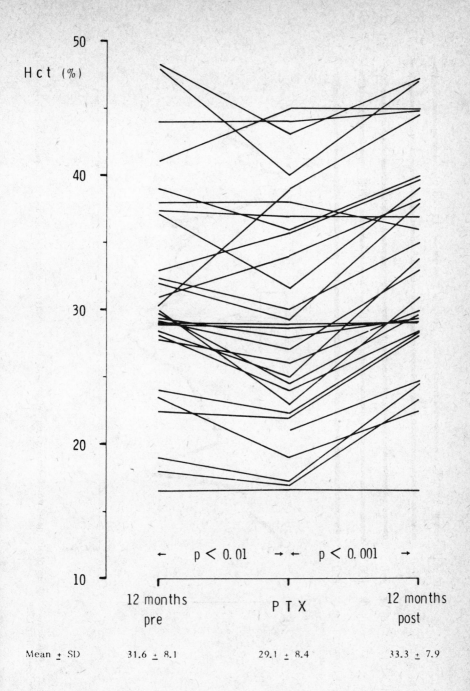

Figure 1. Effect of parathyroidectomy on haematocrit in haemodialysis patients (n=29)

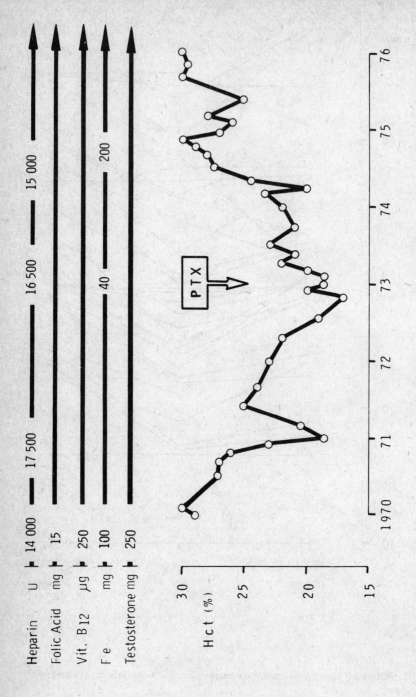

Figure 2. Long-term follow up of the haematocrit three years before and after parathyroidectomy in a 28 year old patient on haemodialysis since September 1969

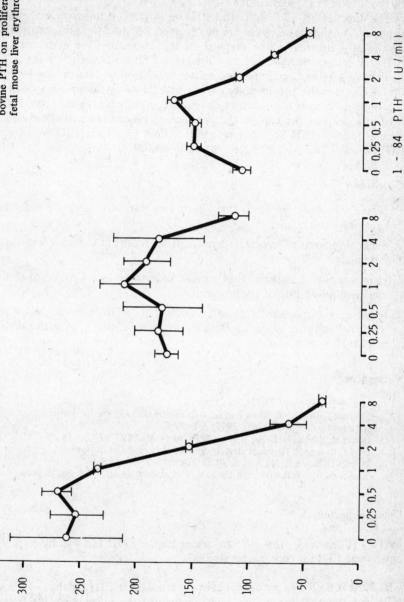

Figure 3. In vitro effect of 1–84 bovine PTH on proliferation of fetal mouse liver erythroid cells

743

each case (29.3 ± 5.2 vs 33.7 ± 5.7%, p<0.001), serum EP concentration did not show a consistent change (63 ± 58 vs 67 ± 37mU/ml), thus excluding increase in EP production as a causative factor.

The direct effect of 1–84 bovine PTH on in vitro erythropoiesis is shown in Figure 3. A biphasic response can be observed: whereas CFU-E formation was significantly elevated in the presence of 0.25 to 1.0U PTH/ml compared to PTH free culture medium, a further increase in PTH concentration in the culture resulted in a pronounced and dose-related inhibition of fetal mouse liver erythroid cell growth. The inhibitory effect of PTH on erythroid cell growth was confirmed in human bone marrow cell cultures prepared in the same way. Human erythroid colonies per cm^2 in the presence of various concentrations of PTH were as follows: PTH 8U/ml: 4 ± 1; PTH 4U/ml: 11 ± 1; PTH 2U/ml: 18 ± 1.4; PTH 1U/ml: 33 ± 3; and PTH free: 40 ± 2 (p < 0.001).

Conclusion

1 Severe secondary hyperparathyroidism can markedly aggravate anaemia in haemodialysis patients.

2 Surgical removal of hyperparathyroid glands results in improvement of renal anaemia.

3 Improvement of anaemia after parathyroidectomy is not mediated through increased production of erythropoietin.

4 In vitro erythropoiesis is directly inhibited by PTH in murine and human erythroid cultures, suggesting bone marrow intoxication by excessive amounts of PTH.

References

1   Massry SG. Nephron 1977; 19: 125
2   Zingraff J, Drüeke T, Marie P et al. Arch Intern Med 1978; 138: 1650
3   Barbour G. Arch Intern Med 1979; 139: 889
4   Boxer M, Ellman L, Geller R et al. Arch Intern Med 1977; 137: 588
5   Levi J, Bessler H, Hirsch et al. Acta Haematol 1979; 61: 125
6   Meytes D, Bogin E, Ma A et al. J Clin Invest 1981; 67: 1263
7   Thevenod F, Radtke HW, Grützmacher P et al. Kidney Int 1983; 24: In press

Open Discussion

CATTO (Chairman) Why did you choose bovine PTH? Did you have access to any human PTH for your culture studies?

GRÜTZMACHER No, we did not have access to human PTH and the 1–84 bovine PTH was the only preparation which contained the intact molecule fraction.

CATTO Do you think there could be any direct toxic effect from the bovine PTH, which would not be seen if you used human PTH?

GRÜTZMACHER I think that this is very unlikely. We excluded artificial effects which could interfere with the results by use of heat inactivation and found no inhibition when the PTH was inactivated. With human PTH up to now we did only preliminary studies with fragments. We have no preparation of the whole PTH of human origin.

LAMPERI (Genoa) Did you study the human BFU-E formation in culture with the PTH? I studied this cell in similar conditions without having any significant modification.

GRÜTZMACHER Up to now we have only performed experiments using CFU-E formation and we plan to repeat these experiments measuring BFU-E. I think in the literature there is some contradiction about the sensitivity of these different erythroid cells to erythropoietin and also to PTH, at least in vitro.

SALTISSI (London) I would like to congratulate you firstly on the foresight of this study. I too have a specific interest in this subject and have been studying patients at Charing Cross Hospital both on haemodialysis and CAPD. As regards stable haemodialysis patients I so far have results on 20 patients, divided into 10 with hyperparathyroidism and 10 without. In them I concur with you and can confirm that there is no difference between the groups as regards erythropoietin. I have also found that patients without hyperparathyroidism are significantly less anaemic based on red cell mass rather than haematocrit measurements which can, of course, be misleading. I may also suggest that from your data it is possible that the patients with hyperparathyroidism may be more thirsty and have higher plasma volumes than post-parathyroidectomy. However, the most remarkable difference between the groups I have found both in the comparable studies and post-parathyroidectomy is in terms of ^{51}Cr red cell survival. With recent work on the mechanisms of action of PTH there are good theoretical reasons why this may be so and I wonder if you have any comments on this?

GRÜTZMACHER Well we have no evidence that patients with manifest hyperparathyroidism have more thirst leading to haemodilution which may contribute to a lower haematocrit. Moreover actual blood pressure, body weight as well as weight gains did not differ significantly during the study period.

SALTISSI Have you any comments on the effect hyperparathyroidism may have on red cell survival?

GRÜTZMACHER Yes, if hyperparathyroidism markedly shortens red cell survival I would expect an increase in reticulocytes and we have measured reticulocytes and did not see significant changes. However we did not measure red cell survival to check this possibility.

MEMBERSHIP OF
THE EUROPEAN DIALYSIS AND TRANSPLANT ASSOCIATION
EUROPEAN RENAL ASSOCIATION

Membership of the European Dialysis and Transplant Association (EDTA) — European Renal Association (ERA) is open to qualified workers in fields that are of interest to the Association (haemodialysis, peritoneal dialysis, continuous ambulatory peritoneal dialysis, renal transplantation and the broad field of nephrology, including clinical nephrology, renal physiology, renal pathology, etc). Full membership is limited to scientists who reside in Europe and adjacent countries: associate membership is available to scientists from other countries.

Candidates for full or associate membership must be proposed by two full or associate members on a form provided by the Secretary-Treasurer. This proposal, accompanied by a letter of recommendation from one of the proposers, should be sent to the Secretary-Treasurer for consideration by the Council.

All members are entitled to:

1   Receive information about the annual Congress and all General Assemblies of the Association;

2   Participate in the annual Congress, and

3   Receive an annual copy of the Proceedings of the EDTA—ERA.

For further information, write to:

Dr S T Boen
Department of Nephrology and Dialysis
Sint Lucas Hospital, Jan Tooropstraat 164
1061 AE Amsterdam, The Netherlands

SUBJECT INDEX

Calcium Metabolism, *continued*
  effect of glycine and methionine
    supplements on urinary excretion,
    407
  effect of pyridoxine therapy on
    urinary excretion, 417
  effect of Verapamil in preventing
    ischaemic injury in an experimental
    model, 650
  effects of increased sodium intake on
    urinary saturation, 384
  hypercalciuria, 374
  in idiopathic calcium nephrolithiasis,
    450
  in stone formers during dietary
    calcium and oxalate restriction,
    401
  phosphate therapy in absorptive
    hypercalciuria, 384
  relationship of parathyroid hormone
    to hypertension in experimental
    animals, 220
  relationship of urinary excretion to
    dietary protein, 411
  relationship to Vitamin D after
    transplantation, 213
  urine saturation in stone formers,
    445
Calcium Oxalate stone formers, 440
Calcium Oxalate stones, thiazide prophylaxis, 477
Calcium Phosphate, in urinary stone
  formation, 386
Calcium Stone Disease,
  bone mineral content relationship to
    urinary calcium excretion, 460
  treatment by high fluid intake, 438
  tubular function and relationship to
    sodium intake, 455
Captopril
  causing acute renal failure, 536
  dosage required in CRF, 530
  effect on cell membrane transport,
    493
  haematological toxicity, 536
  induced deterioration in transplant
    function in patients with arterial
    stenosis, 325
  side effects, 530
Cardiac Function, during haemodialysis
  in patients with coronary heart disease,
  181
Cardiovascular
  complications on short dialysis, 114
  coronary vessel angioplasty, 175
  low incidence of disease with long
    dialysis schedules, 122

Cardiovascular, *continued*
  no difference in complication rate
    between long and short dialysis,
    139
  stability during short dialysis, 143
Carpal Tunnel Syndrome
  as a complication of long-term
    haemodialysis, 122, 130
Catecholamines, in pregnancy induced
  hypertension, 520
Cation exchange, using polymers charged
  with calcium or iron, 725
Cefoxitime, in the treatment of infected
  stone disease, 469
Cell Mediated Immunity
  in haemodialysis and CAPD patients,
    190
  in haemodialysis patients, 338
Cell membrane, inhibition of ATP
  activity in hypertension, 489
Children
  aseptic bone necrosis, 99
  causes of death on renal replacement
    therapy, 91
  causes of graft failure, 98
  epidemiology of hypertension in
    Neapolitan school children, 551
  experience with CAPD, 93
  growth on renal replacement therapy,
    101
  modes of treatment in selected
    countries, 82
  nitrogen balance and nutritional
    status during haemofiltration, 201
  nutritional status change after
    switching to haemofiltration from
    haemodialysis, 207
  survival on renal replacement therapy
    programmes, 84
Cholecalciferol, *see* Vitamin D
Chronic Renal Failure, *see* Renal Failure,
  Chronic
Citrate
  differing effects of the sodium and
    potassium salt on urinary calcium
    excretion, 382
  effect in calcium nephrolithiasis,
    373, 375
  renal stone formation, 382
Coagulation, during dialysis with heparin
  and MD-805, 144
Conn's Syndrome
  relationship of blood pressure to
    renal function following surgical
    removal, 487
  sodium metabolism and hyperten-
    sion, 484

751

Oxalate, *continued*
    effect of calcium and oxalate
      restriction on probability of stone
      formation, 401
    effect of diet, thiazides and allo-
      purinol on urinary excretion, 434
    effect of glycine and methionine
      supplements on urinary excretion,
      407
    excretion and calcium nephro-
      lithiasis, 373, 375
    in relation to hypercalciuria, 372
    possibility that subclinical pyridoxine
      deficiency may lead to stone
      formation, 410
    response of urinary excretion to
      pyridoxine therapy in calcium
      oxalate stone formers, 417

Paediatric Patients, *see* children
Pancreas
    recognition of rejection in
      transplants, 709, 716
    transplantation in patients with
      diabetes mellitus, 705, 711
Parathyroid, histology in haemodialysis
  patients with severe secondary hyper-
  parathyroidism, 731
Parathyroid Hormone
    effect on erythrocyte sodium
      potassium co-transport, 512
    in idiopathic calcium nephrolithiasis,
      450
    no change in plasma concentration
      with amino acid supplements,
      407
    no effect on stopping oral aluminium
      hydroxide, 207
    relationship to parathyroid weight
      in haemodialysis patients, 731
    relationship to serum calcium after
      transplantation, 213
    role in the development of hyper-
      tension in experimental animals,
      220
Parathyroidectomy
    effect on blood pressure in experi-
      mental animals, 220
    incidence in patients on long and
      short dialysis schedules, 129
    in haemodialysis patients with severe
      secondary hyperparathyroidism,
      731
    response of anaemia, 739
Percutaneous angioplasty, in the treatment of renovascular hypertension,
  582

Perforation, bowel, as a complication of
  CAPD, 236
Pericarditis, incidence during long and
  short haemodialysis, 132
Peritoneal absorption, glucose, 195
Peritoneal Dialysis, *see also* CAPD
    treatment for acute renal failure,
      Registry details, 64
Peritonitis
    during CAPD, 700
    endogenous in CAPD, 228
    in CAPD patients, 236
    incidence in CAPD patients in the
      USA, 243
    incidence in CAPD patients with
      diabetes mellitus, 700
    reduction in incidence with new
      connector system, 223
    relationship to patient's age, 248
    relationship to patient's sex, 248
    sclerosing in CAPD, 241
pH, relationship to renal stone formation, 374, 376
Phagocytosis, macrophage and monocyte
  in IgA nephropathy, 610
Phosphate
    changes following reduction of oral
      aluminium hydroxide, 723
    effect of reduced aluminium
      hydroxide intake in haemodialysis
      patients, 719
    effective control with aluminium free
      binder, 725
    efficacy of **natural** polymers in
      controlling plasma concentration,
      730
    relationship of urinary excretion to
      dietary protein, 411
    relationship to $1,25(OH)_2$ chole-
      calciferol after transplantation, 213
    renal threshold in patients with
      idiopathic nephrolithiasis, 450
    studies with aluminium free binder,
      725
    therapy in absorptive hypercalciuria,
      384
    therapy for stone disease in patients
      with renal tubular acidosis, 473
Phosphorus, urine saturation in stone
  formers, 445
Plasma Volume, in pregnancy induced
  hypertension, 520
Plasmapheresis
    in the treatment of SLE, 629
    in the treatment of steroid resistant
      transplant rejection, 362
Platelets, binding sites for angiotensin, 562

762

AUTHOR INDEX

Page numbers in brackets

763

Beck-Nielsen H, Medical Department III, Aarhus Amtssygehus, DK-8000 Aarhus C, Denmark (686)

Beretta-Piccoli C, Ospedale Italiano di Lugano, CH-6962 Viganello, Switzerland (483)

Bergrem H, Medical Department B, Rikshospitalet University Hospital, Oslo, Norway (286)

Beroniade V, Faculté de Médecine Université de Montréal et Hotel-Dieu de Montréal, Québec, Canada (530)

Bettinelli A, Pediatric Dialysis Unit, University of Milan, Milan, Italy (201)

Billiouw JM, Renal Division of the Department of Medicine, University Hospital, De Pintelaan 185, B-9000 Gent, Belgium (176)

Bing RF, Department of Medicine, University of Leicester, Leicester, England (546)

Bloodworth L, Department of Renal Medicine, Welsh National School of Medicine, Cardiff, Wales (213)

Bommer G, Department of Internal Medicine and Virology, Pettenkofer Institut, University of München, FRG (161)

Bommer J, Department of Internal Medicine and Virology, Pettenkofer Institut, University of München, FRG (161)

Bono F, Department of Internal Medicine and Nephrology, University of Parma, Parma, Italy (111)

Bonomini V, Institute of Nephrology, St Orsola University Hospital, Via Massarenti 9, 40130 Bologna, Italy (315)

Bosi E, Clinica Medica VIII, San Raffaele University Hospital, Milan, Italy (705)

Boulanger JC, Service de Gynécologie-Obstétrique, Hôpital Nord, 8000 Amiens, France (520)

Bourdeau A, Département de Physiologie, Hôpital Necker Enfants Malades, 161 rue de Sevres, 75743 Paris, France (731)

Bourdon R, Laboratoire de Biochimie, Hôpital Fernand Widal, Paris, France (731)

Bourke E, Allegheny Professional Building, Suite 200, 490 E North Avenue, Pittsburgh, PA 15212, USA (243)

Bournerias F, Centre d'Hémodialyse, Centre Hospitalier, 3 place Silly, 92211 Saint-Cloud, France (207)

Bradley JA, Western Infirmary, Glasgow, Scotland (320)

Brando B, Renal Unit, Niguarda-Ca'Granda Hospital, Piazza Ospedale Maggiore 3, Milan, Italy (265, 455)

Brasa S, Divisione Nefrologia, Spedali Civili, Brescia, Italy (223)

Braun B, II Department of Internal Medicine, University of Mainz, Langenbeckstr. 1, D-6500 Mainz, FRG (669)

Briggs JD, Western Infirmary, Glasgow, Scotland (320)

Brisson E, Laboratoire d'Immunologie Néphrologique et de Transplantation, U.E.R. Pitié-Salpétrière, 83 bd de l'Hôpital, F75651 Paris, Cedex 13, France (349)

Brocks P, Department of Urology, Hvidovre University Hospital, DK-2650 Hvidovre, Denmark (477)

Broggi ML, Renal Unit, Niguarda-Ca'Granda Hospital, Piazza Ospedale Maggiore 3, Milan, Italy (265)

Brown CB, Royal Hallamshire Hospital, Sheffield, England (271)

Brown JJ, MRC Blood Pressure Unit, Western Infirmary, Glasgow, G11 6NT, Scotland (483)

Brown RC, Department of Medical Biochemistry, Welsh National School of Medicine, Cardiff, Wales (213)

Browning M, Department of Renal Medicine, Southmead Hospital, Westbury-on-Trym, Bristol, BS10 5ND, England (595)

Broyer M, Hôpital Necker Enfants Malades, Paris, France (1, 76)

Brunner FP, Department für Innere Medizin, Universität Basel, Basel, Switzerland (1, 76)

Bruno M, Divisione de Nefrologia e Dialisi, Ospedale Regionale, Mauriziano Umberto I, Torino 10128, Italy (434)

Brynger H, Department of Surgery I, Sahlgrenska Sjukhuset, Göteborg, Sweden (1, 76, 280)

Bueno R, Nephrology Department and Virology Laboratory, Centro Ramon y Cajal, Madrid 34, Spain (675)

Bunch TW, Division of Nephrology, Mayo Clinic, Rochester, MN 55905, USA (473)

Busnach G, Renal Unit, Niguarda-Ca'Granda Hospital, Piazza Ospedale Maggiore 3, Milan, Italy (265)

Cosci P, Renal Unit, Maggiore Hospital, Lodi, Italy (455)
Cournot-Witmer C, Laboratoire des Tissus Calcifiés et INSERM U30, Hôpital Necker Enfants Malades, 161 rue de Sevres, 75743 Paris, France (731)
Cuesta MV, Servicio de Nefrologia, Hospital General de Asturias, Apartado 243, Oviedo, Spain (719)
Cumming AMM, MRC Blood Pressure Unit, Western Infirmary, Glasgow, G11 6NT, Scotland (483)
Cuthbertson B, Protein Fractionation Centre, Ellen's Glen Road, Edinburgh, Scotland (271)

D'Amico G, Divisione de Nefrologia, Ospedale S Carlo and Istituto, Clinica Medica IV, Universita di Milano, Milan, Italy (514)
D'Anna F, Department of Nephrology, Second Faculty of Medicine, University of Naples, Naples, Italy (551, 582)
D'Avanzo L, Department of Nephrology, Second Faculty of Medicine, University of Naples, Naples, Italy (551)
Dahl C, Department of Urology, Hvidovre University Hospital, DK-2650 Hvidovre, Denmark (477)
Dal Canton A, Department of Nephrology, Second Faculty of Medicine, University of Naples, Naples, Italy (499, 551, 582)
Daniele PG, 1st Analisi Chimica Strumentale, Universita di Torino, Torino, Italy (434)
Danielson BG, Department of Internal Medicine, University Hospital, 3-751 85 Uppsala, Sweden (411)
Darai G, Department of Virology, University of Heidelberg, FRG (161)
Dathe G, Department of Urology, University Hospital, Frankfurt/Main, FRG (291)
David S, Department of Internal Medicine and Nephrology, University of Parma, Parma, Italy (111)
Davies DL, Department of Medicine, Western Infirmary, Glasgow, G11 6NT, Scotland (483)
Davies M, The Welsh National School of Medicine, KRUF Institute, Cardiff, Wales (656)
Davin JC, University of Liege, Department of Pediatrics, Hôpital de Baviere, 66 bd de la Constitution, 4020 Liege, Belgium (656)
Davison AM, Department of Renal Medicine, St James's University Hospital, Leeds, LS9 7TF, England (566)
De Ferrari, ME, Renal Unit, Niguarda-Ca'Granda Hospital, Piazza Ospedale Maggiore 3, Milan, Italy (455)
de Fremont JF, Service de Néphrologie, Hôpital Nord, 8000 Amiens, France (401, 520)
de Jong PE, Department of Medicine, State University Hospital, 9713 E2 Groningen, The Netherlands (538, 577)
de March A, Endocrinological Gynaecology Department, S Orsola Hospital, Bologna, Italy (156)
De Marchi S, Department of Internal Medicine, Stabilimento, Ospedaliero di Codroipo, Udine, Italy (681)
De Paoli P, Department of Immunology, Ospedaliero de Pordenone, Pordenone, Italy (681)
De The H, Department of Pharmacology, Hôpital Necker, 161 rue de Sevres, 75015 Paris, France (489)
de Zeeuw D, Department of Medicine, Division of Nephrology, State University Hospital, 9713 EZ Groningen, The Netherlands (507, 538, 577)
Dechenne C, University of Liege, Department of Pediatrics, Hôpital de Baviere, 66 bd de la Constitution, 4020 Liege, Belgium (656)
Degli Esposti E, Division of Nephrology and Dialysis, Malpighi Hospital, Bologna, Italy (156)
Deinhardt F, Department of Virology, Pettenkofer Institut, University of München, FRG (161)
Demory JE, Service de Gynécologie-Obstétrique, Hôpital Nord, 8000 Amiens, France (520)
Denneberg T, Department of Nephrology, University Hospital, Malmoe, Sweden (427)
Desailly I, Laboratoire de Biochimie, Hôpital Nord, 8000 Amiens, France (520)
Devynck MA, Department of Pharmacology, Hôpital Necker, 161 rue de Sevres, 75015 Paris, France (489)

766

Di Nucci GD, Department of Haematology, University of Rome, Rome, Italy (150)
Dodd NJ, King's College Hospital Renal Unit, Dulwich Hospital, London, England (186)
Donadon W, Cardiorheumatological Center, Ospedaliero de Pordenone, Pordenone, Italy (681)
Donckerwolcke RA, Het Wilhelmina Kinderziekenhuis, University of Utrecht, Utrecht, The Netherlands (1, 76)
Donker AJM, Renal Transplantation Unit, State University Hospital, Groningen, The Netherlands (325, 577)
Donnelly PK, University Department of Surgery, Royal Victoria Infirmary, Newcastle upon Tyne, England (297)
Dorhout Mees EJ, Department of Nephrology, University Hospital Utrecht, Catharijnesingel 101, 3511 GV Utrecht, The Netherlands (641)
Dostal G, Department of General Surgery, University Clinic, Essen, FRG (587)
Dracon M, Department of Nephrology, Centre Hospitalier de Valenciennes, 59322 Valenciennes, France (646)
Dratwa M, Department of Nephrology, Brugmann University Hospital, Brussels, Belgium (190)
Drueke T, Department de Néphrologie and INSERM U90, Hôpital Necker Enfants Malades, 161 rue de Sevres, 75743 Paris, France (731)
Dubernard JM, Service d'urologie, Hôpital Ed. Herriot, 69374 Lyon, Cedex 08, France (705)
Dubois CH, University of Liege, Department of Pediatrics, Hôpital de Baviere, 66 bd de la Constitution, 4020 Liege, Belgium (656)
Dubost C, Service de Chirurgie Viscerale, Hôpital Fernand Widal, Paris, France (731)
Dupont E, Department of Immunology, Erasme University Hospital, Brussels, Belgium (190)
Duranti E, Div. di Nefrologia, Ospedale de Arezzo, Arezzo, Italy (445)

Edefonti A, Pediatric Dialysis Unit, University of Milan, Milan, Italy (201)
Edward N, Aberdeen Royal Infirmary, Aberdeen, Scotland (271, 305)
Egido J, Servicio de Nefrologia, Fundacion Jimenez Diaz (Universidad Autonoma), Madrid, Spain (617)
Eigler FW, Department of General Surgery, University Clinic, Essen, FRG (587)
El Nahas AM, Royal Postgraduate Medical School, Hammersmith Hospital, London, England (623)
El Yafi S, Clinique de Néphrologie, Hôpital Ed. Herriot, 69374 Lyon, Cedex 08, France (705)
Elli M, V Surgical Pathology, University of Rome, Rome, Italy (150)
Ernst W, Department of Nephrology, University Hospital, D-6000 Frankfurt/Main 70, FRG (362)
Esposito C, Department of Nephrology, Second Faculty of Medicine, University of Naples, Naples, Italy (499)

Fassbinder W, Klinikum d. Johann Wolfgang Goethe-Universitat, Zentrum Innere Medizin, Abteilung Nephrologie, Theodor-Stern-Kai 7, D-6000 Frankfurt/Main 70, FRG (291, 362, 739)
Federico S, Department of Nephrology, Second Faculty of Medicine, University of Naples, Naples, Italy (603)
Fellström B, Department of Internal Medicine, University Hospital, S-751 85 Uppsala, Sweden (411)
Fievet P, Service de Néphrologie, Hôpital Nord, 8000 Amiens, France (520)
Flamigni G, Endocrinological Gynaecology Department, S Orsola Hospital, Bologna, Italy (156)
Flatmark A, Medical Department B, Rikshospitalet University Hospital, Oslo, Norway (286)
Flynn CT, Iowa Lutheran Hospital, Des Moines, Iowa, USA (700)
Foidart JM, University of Liege, Department of Pediatrics, Hôpital de Baviere, 66 bd de la Constitution, 4020 Liege, Belgium (656)
Foucault C, Laboratoire d'Hémobiologie, U.E.R. Pitié-Salpétrière, 83 bd de l'Hôpital, F75651 Paris, Cedex 13, France (349)
Fournier A, Service de Néphrologie, Hôpital Nord, 8000 Amiens, France (401, 520)

Mendes V, Department de Néphrologie and INSERM U90, Hôpital Necker Enfants Malades, 161 rude de Sevres, 75743 Paris, France (731)

Mertani E, Department of Nephrology, Groupe Hospitalier Pitié-Salpétrière, 83 bd de l'Hôpital, 75651 Paris, Cedex 13, France (236)

Mery JPh, Department of Nephrology, Hôpital Bichat, 46 rue Henri Huchard, 75018 Paris, France (646)

Metaxas P, 2nd Propedeutic Department of Medicine, Aristotelian University of Thessaloniki, 'Aghia Sophia' Hospital, Thessaloniki, Greece (650)

Metivier F, Clinique Medicale, Hôpital Broussais, Paris, France (349)

Meyer P, Clinique Néphrologique, Hôpital Necker, 161 rue de Sevres, 75015 Paris, France (489)

Michael J, Queen Elizabeth Hospital, Birmingham, England (711)

Minar E, 1st Medical Clinic, University of Vienna, Vienna, Austria (417)

Minetti L, Renal Unit, Niguarda-Ca'Granda Hospital, Piazza Ospedale Maggiore 3, Milan, Italy (265, 455)

Monnier N, Centre d'Hémodialyse, Centre Hospitalier, 3 place Silly, 92211, Saint-Cloud, France (207)

Montoliu J, Nephrology Service, Hospital Clinic i Provincial, c/Casanova 143, Barcelona 36, Spain (572)

Morel-Maroger L, Department of Nephrology, Hôpital Bichat, 46 rue Henri Huchard, 75018, Paris, France (646)

Morganti A, Centro di Fisiologia Clinica, e Ipertensione, Via F. Sforza 35, 20122 Milan, Italy (514)

Morley P, Western Infirmary, Glasgow, Scotland (320)

Mrochen H, Department of Intensive Medicine, Humboldt University, Berlin, GDR (331)

Mussat T, Service de Néphrologie, Hôpital de la Pitié, 83 bd de l'Hôpital, 74013 Paris, France (169)

Myking OL, The Hormone Laboratory, University of Bergen, School of Medicine, Bergen, Norway (195)

Nakagawa S, Tokyo Medical and Dental University, Tokyo, Japan (144)

Nancollas GH, Chemistry Department, State University of New York at Buffalo, Buffalo, New York, 14214, USA (386)

Nanni-Costa, A, Institute of Nephrology, St Orsola University Hospital, Via Massarenti 9, 40130 Bologna, Italy (315)

Navis GJ, Department of Medicine, Nephrology Unit, State University Hospital, 9713 EZ Groningen, The Netherlands (577)

Neild GH, Renal Unit, Guy's Hospital, London, England (662)

Nemeth J, Service Central d'Anatomie et Cytologie Pathologiques, Hôpital Lariboisiere, Paris, France (731)

Nicholls AJ, Royal Hallamshire Hospital, Sheffield, England (271)

Oei HY, Department of Nuclear Medicine, University Hospital Utrecht, Catharijnesingel 101, 3511 GV Utrecht, The Netherlands (641)

Olivas E, Servicio de Nefrologia, Hospital Provincial de Madrid, Madrid, Spain (338)

Orkisz S, Department of Histology, Military Medical Academy, Zeromskiejo 113, 90–549 Lodz, Poland (636)

Ortuno J, Nephrology Department and Virology Laboratory, Centro Ramon y Cajal, Madrid 34, Spain (675)

Ota K, Tokyo Women's Medical College, Tokyo, Japan (144)

Pabico RC, Nephrology Unit, Department of Medicine, University of Rochester Medical Center, Rochester, New York 14642, USA (450)

Pagano A, Istituto di Igiene, dell'Universita de Milano, Milan, Italy (469)

Pak CYC, Section on Mineral Metabolism, Department of Internal Medicine, University of Texas Health Science Centre, 5323 Harry Hines Boulevard, Dallas, Texas 75235, USA (371)

Pansiot S, Division of Nephrology, University Hospital, Lausanne, Switzerland (139)

Papa A, Department of Nephrology, Second Faculty of Medicine, University of Naples, Naples, Italy (551)

Papadimitriou M, 2nd Propedeutic Department of Medicine, Aristotelian University of Thessaloniki, 'Aghia Sophia' Hospital, Thessaloniki, Greece (650)

Parsons V, King's College Hospital Renal Unit, Dulwich Hospital, London, England (186)

Pazardjiklian I, Istituto di Igiene, dell'Universita de Milano, Milan, Italy (469)

Pecoraro C, Department of Nephrology, Second Faculty of Medicine, University of Naples, Naples, Italy (603)

Peral V, Servicio de Nefrologia, Hospital General de Asturias, Apartado 243, Oviedo, Spain (719)

Perdue ST, UCLA Tissue Typing Laboratory, 15–22 Rehabilitation Center, 1000 Veteran Avenue, Los Angeles, CA 90024, USA (253)

Perez-Garcia R, Servicio de Nefrologia, Hospital Provincial de Madrid, Madrid, Spain (338)

Pernollet MG, Department of Pharmacology, Hôpital Necker, 161 rue de Sevres, 75015 Paris, France (489)

Picca M, Pediatric Dialysis Unit, University of Milan, Milan, Italy (201)

Picciotto G, Servizio de Medicina Nucleare, Ospedale S Giovanni, Torino, Italy (610)

Piccoli G, Div. di Nefrologia e Dialisi, Nuova Astanteria Martini, Largo Gottardo 143, Torino 10154, Italy (610)

Pierides AM, Division of Nephrology, Mayo Clinic, Rochester, MN 55905, USA (473)

Piron M, Renal Division of the Department of Medicine, University Hospital, De Pintelaan 185, B-9000 Gent, Belgium (176)

Pleskov L, Service de Néphrologie, Hôpital Nord, 8000 Amiens, France (520)

Poignet JL, Service de Néphrologie, Hôpital de la Pitié, 83 bd de l'Hôpital, 74013 Paris, France (236)

Ponticelli C, Divisione Nefrologia, Ospedale Maggiore Policlinico, Via Commenda 15, 20122 Milan, Italy (223, 469)

Pontoriero G, Renal Unit, Niguarda-Ca'Granda Hospital, Piazza Ospedale Maggiore 3, Milan, Italy (455)

Posborg Petersen V, Medical Department C, Aarhus Kommunehospital, DK-8000 Aarhus C, Denmark (686)

Poulding J, Department of Histopathology, Southmead Hospital, Westbury-on-Trym, Bristol, BS10 5NB, England (595)

Power DA, University of Aberdeen and Blood Transfusion Service, Aberdeen Royal Infirmary, Aberdeen, Scotland (305)

Proto G, Department of Internal Medicine, Stabilimento, Ospedaliero de Codroipo, Udine, Italy (681)

Proud G, University Department of Surgery, Royal Victoria Infirmary, Newcastle upon Tyne, England (297)

Pruna A, Service de Néphrologie, Hôpital Nord, 8000 Amiens, France (401)

Quereda C, Nephrology Department and Virology Laboratory, Centro Ramon y Cajal, Madrid 34, Spain (675)

Raab R, Department of Nephrology, University Hospital, Frankfurt/Main, FRG (291)

Rademark C, Department of Urology, University Hospital, Lund, Sweden (460)

Radtke HW, Klinikum d. Johann Wolfgang Goethe-Universitat, Zentrum Innere Medizin, Abteilung Nephrologie, Theodor-Stern-Kai 7, D-6000 Frankfurt/Main 70, FRG (739)

Rees AJ, Royal Postgraduate Medical School, Hammersmith Hospital, London, England (623)

Reveillaud RJ, Centre d'Hémodialyse, Centre Hospitalier, 3 place Silly, 92211 Saint-Cloud, France (207)

Revert L, Nephrology Service, Hospital Clinic i Provincial, c/Casanova 143, Barcelona 36, Spain (572)

Ringoir S, Renal Division of the Department of Medicine, University Hospital, De Pintelaan 185, B-9000 Gent, Belgium (176)

Ritz E, Sektion Nephrologie, Medizinische Klinik, Universität Heidelberg, 69 Heidelberg, FRG (161, 220, 407, 562)

Rivera F, Servicio de Nefrologia Fundacion Jimenez Diaz, (Universidad Autonoma), Madrid, Spain (617)

Robertson JIS, MRC Blood Pressure Unit, Western Infirmary, Glasgow, G11 6NT, Scotland (483)

Robertson WG, MRC Mineral Metabolism Unit, The General Infirmary, Leeds, LS1 3EX, England (440)

Roccatello D, Divisione di Nefrologia e Dialisi, Nuova Astanteria Martini, Largo Gottardo 143, Torino 10154, Italy (610)

Rogland B, Department of Nephrology, University Hospital, Lund, Sweden (460)

Rollino C, Divisione de Nefrologia e Dialisi, Nuova Astanteria Martini, Largo Gottardo 143, Torino 10154, Italy (610)

Romano G, Department of Nephrology, Second Faculty of Medicine, University of Naples, Naples, Italy (499)

Rombola G, Renal Unit, Niguarda-Ca'Granda Hospital, Piazza Ospedale Maggiore 3, Milan, Italy (455)

Ronzani M, Divisione di Nefrologia e Dialisi Ospedale Regionale, Mauriziano Umberto I, Torino 10128, Italy (434)

Rosenfeld JB, Department of Pharmacology, Hôpital Necker, 161 rue de Sevres, 75015 Paris, France (489)

Rottembourg J, Service de Néphrologie, U.E.R. Pitié-Salpétrière, 83 bd de l'Hôpital, 75651 Paris, Cedex 13, France (169, 236, 349)

Ruiz Alegria P, Servicio de Nefrologia, Hospital General de Asturias, Apartado 243, Oviedo, Spain (719)

Russell GI, Area Renal Unit, Leicester General Hospital, Leicester, England (546)

Russo D, Department of Nephrology, Second Faculty of Medicine, University of Naples, Naples, Italy (499, 582)

Sabbatini M, Department of Nephrology, Second Faculty of Medicine, University of Naples, Naples, Italy (499)

Saccaggi A, Pediatric Dialysis Unit, University of Milan, Milan, Italy (201)

Sakellariou G, 2nd Propedeutic Department of Medicine, Aristotelian University of Thessaloniki, 'Aghia Sophia' Hospital, Thessaloniki, Greece (650)

Sala C, Centro di Fisiologia Clinica, e Ipertensione, Via F. Sforza 35, 20122 Milan, Italy (514)

Sancho J, Servicio de Nefrologia, Fundacion Jimenez Diaz, (Universidad Autonoma), Madrid, Spain (617)

Sandberg L, Blood Centre, Sahlgrenska Sjukhuset, Göteborg, Sweden (280)

Santini G, Department of Immunology, Ospedaliero de Pordenone, Pordenone, Italy (681)

Santoro A, Division of Nephrology and Dialysis, Malpighi Hospital, Bologna, Italy (156)

Sasaoka T, Yokosuka Kyosai Hospital, Japan (144)

Sasdelli M, Div. di Nefrologia, Ospedale de Arezzo, Arezzo, Italy (445)

Savazzi L, Department of Internal Medicine and Nephrology, University of Parma, Parma, Italy (111)

Scalamogna A, Divisione Nefrologia, Ospedale Maggiore Policlinico, Via Commenda 15, 20122 Milan, Italy (223)

Scalia A, Divisione de Nefrologia, Ospedale S. Carlo and Istituto, Clinica Medica IV, Universita di Milano, Milan, Italy (514)

Schandene L, Department of Immunology, Erasme University Hospital, Brussels, Belgium (190)

Scheuermann EH, Department of Nephrology, University Hospital, D-6000 Frankfurt/Main 70, FRG (291, 362)

Schinella D, Unit of Nephrology and Dialysis, Ospedaliero de Pordenone, Pordenone, Italy (681)

Schlepper M, Kerckhoff-Klinik, Bad Nauheim, FRG (181)

Schmidt P, 1st Medical Clinic, University of Vienna, Vienna, Austria (417)

Schmidt-Gayk H, Department of Nephrology, Universität Heidelberg, 69 Heidelberg, FRG (407)

Schmitz O, Medical Department C, Aarhus Kommunehospital, DK-8000 Aarhus C, Denmark (686)

Schneider H, Katharinenhospital, Stuttgart, FRG (725)

Schoeppe W, Klinikum d. Johann Wolfgang Goethe-Universitat, Zentrum Innere Medizin, Abteilung Nephrologie, Theodor-Stern-Kai 7, D-6000 Frankfurt/Main 70, FRG (291, 362, 739)

Scholz D, Department of Urology, Humboldt-University, Berlin, GDR (331)

Scholze J, Department of Medicine, Humboldt-University, Berlin, GDR (331)

Schütterle G, Zentrum für Innere Medizin, 6300 Giessen, FRG (181)

Schuur KH, Department of Medicine, State University Hospital, Groningen, The Netherlands (538)

Scurr DS, MRC Mineral Metabolism Unit, The General Infirmary, Leeds, LS1 3EX, England (440)

Secchi A, Clinica Medica VIII, San Raffaele University Hospital, Milan, Italy (705)

Selwood NH, UK Transplant, Bristol, England (1, 76)

Semple PF, MRC Blood Pressure Unit, Western Infirmary, Glasgow, G11 6NT, Scotland (483)

Sena LM, III Cattedra Patologia Generale dell'Universita de Torino, Torino, Italy (610)

Sergeant V, MRC Mineral Metabolism Unit, The General Infirmary, Leeds, LS1 3EX, England (440)

Shenton BK, University Department of Surgery, Royal Victoria Infirmary, Newcastle upon Tyne, England (297)

Shewan G, University of Aberdeen and Blood Transfusion Service, Aberdeen Royal Infirmary, Aberdeen, Scotland (305)

Sis JM, Medizinische Klinik, Sektion Nephrologie, Universität Heidelberg, 69 Heidelberg, FRG (562)

Slooff MJH, Department of Internal Medicine and Surgery, State University Hospital, Groningen, The Netherlands (325)

Smeby LC, Institute of Biophysics, University of Trondheim, Trondheim, Norway (195)

Smith L, Department of Surgery I, Sahlgrenska Sjukhuset, Göteborg, Sweden (280)

Smith MJV, Division of Urology, Medical College of Virginia, Richmond, Virginia 23298, USA (422, 466)

Sonego S, Divisione de Nefrologia e Dialisi, Ospedale Regionale, Mauriziano Umberto I, Torino 10128, Italy (434)

Stenberg P, Department of Pharmacology, University Hospital, Malmoe, Sweden (427)

Stephen RL, University of Utah, Salt Lake City, Utah, USA (692)

Stewart KN, University of Aberdeen and Blood Transfusion Service, Aberdeen Royal Infirmary, Aberdeen, Scotland (305)

Strada A, Divisione Nefrologia, Spedali Civili, Brescia, Italy (223)

Streicher E, Katharinenhospital, Stuttgart, FRG (725)

Strippoli P, Service de Néphrologie, Hôpital de la Pitié, 83 bd de l'Hôpital, 75013 Paris, France (236)

Sturani A, Division of Nephrology and Dialysis, Malpighi Hospital, Bologna, Italy (156)

Stutte HJ, Department of Pathology, University Hospital, D-6000 Frankfurt/Main 70, FRG (362)

Surian M, Divisione di Nefrologia e Dialisi, Niguarda-Ca'Granda Hospital, Piazza Ospedale Maggiore 3, Milan, Italy (455, 469)

Swales JD, Department of Medicine, University of Leicester, Leicester, England (546)

Taccone-Gallucci M, V Surgical Pathology, University of Rome, Rome, Italy (150)

Tarrant J, King's College Hospital Renal Unit, Dulwich Hospital, London, England (186)

Taube D, Renal and Tissue Typing Laboratoreis, Guy's Hospital, London, England (309)
Taverner D, Department of Medicine, University of Leicester, Leicester, England (546)
Taylor RMR, University Department of Surgery, Royal Victoria Infirmary, Newcastle
upon Tyne, England (297)
Tegzess AM, Renal Transplantation Unit, State University Hospital, Groningen,
The Netherlands (325)
Teotino N, Pediatric Dialysis Unit, University of Milan, Milan, Italy (201)
Tepper T, Department of Medicine, Division of Nephrology, State University Hospital,
Groningen, The Netherlands (507)
Terasaki PI, Department of Surgery, UCLA School of Medicine, Center for the Health
Sciences, Los Angeles, California 90024, USA (253)
Teruel JL, Nephrology Department and Virology Laboratory, Centro Ramon y Cajal,
Madrid 34, Spain (675)
Tesio F, Unit of Nephrology and Dialysis, Stabilimento, Ospedaliero de Pordenone,
Pordenone, Italy (681)
Thormann J, Kerckhoff-Klinik, Bad Nauheim, FRG (181)
Thurston H, Department of Medicine, University of Leicester, Leicester, England (546)
Tielemans C, Department of Nephrology, Brugmann University Hospital, Brussels,
Belgium (190)
Toledano D, Service de Néphrologie, Hôpital de la Pitié, 83 bd de l'Hôpital, 75013 Paris,
France (169)
Topelmann I, Department of Radiology, Humboldt-University, Berlin, GDR (331)
Touraine JL, Clinique de Néphrologie, Hôpital Ed. Herriot, 69374 Lyon, Cedex 08, France
(705)
Traeger J, Clinique de Néphrologie, Hôpital Ed. Herriot, 69374 Lyon, Cedex 08, France
(705)
Tranbaloc P, Department of Pathology, Groupe Hospitalier Pitié-Salpétrière, 83 bd de
l'Hôpital, 75651 Paris, Cedex 13, France (236)
Tribe C, Department of Histopathology, Southmead Hospital, Westbury-on-Trym, Bristol,
BS10 5NB (595)
Tricerri A, Divisione de Nefrologia e Dialisi, Ospedale Regionale, Mauriziano Umberto I,
Torino 10128, Italy (434)
Triebel F, Laboratoire d'Immunologie Néphrologique et de Transplantation, U.E.R. Pitié-
Salpétrière, 83 bd de l'Hôpital, F75651 Paris, Cedex 13, France (349)
Trznadel K, 2nd Clinic of Internal Diseases, Military Medical Academy, Zeromskiego 113,
90–549 Lodz, Poland (636)
Tschöpe W, Department of Nephrology, Universität Heidelberg, 69 Heidelberg, FRG (407)
Turney JH, Queen Elizabeth Hospital, Birmingham, England (711)
Turolo L, Centro di Fisiologia Clinica, e Ipertensione, Via F. Sforza 35, 20122 Milan, Italy
(514)
Tyler F, University of Utah, Salt Lake City, Utah, USA (692)

Uccello F, Department of Nephrology, Second Faculty of Medicine, University of Naples,
Naples, Italy (499)
Ulman J, Silesian School of Medicine, Katowice, Poland (557)
Usberti M, Department of Nephrology, Second Faculty of Medicine, University of Naples,
Naples, Italy (603)

Valderrabano F, Servicio de Nefrologia, Hospital Provincial de Madrid, Madrid, Spain (338)
Valeri M, V Surgical Pathology, University of Rome, Rome, Italy (150)
Van Den Berg CJ, Division of Nephrology, Mayo Clinic, Rochester, MN 55905, USA (473)
van der Hem GK, Department of Medicine, State University Hospital, Groningen,
The Netherlands (538)
van der Slikke LB, Renal Transplantation Unit, State University Hospital, Groningen,
The Netherlands (325)

van der Woude F, Renal Transplantation Unit, State University Hospital, Groningen, The Netherlands (325)

van Son WJ, Renal Transplantation Unit, State University Hospital, Groningen, The Netherlands (325)

Vangelista A, Institute of Nephrology, St Orsola University Hospital, Via Massarenti 9, 40130 Bologna, Italy (315)

Vanhille Ph, Department of Nephrology, Centre Hospitalier de Valenciennes, 59522 Valenciennes, France (646)

Vanholder R, Renal Division of the Department of Medicine, University Hospital, De Pintelaan 185, B-9000 Gent, Belgium (176)

Vargemezis V, 2nd Propedeutic Department of Medicine, Aristotelian University of Thessaloniki, 'Aghia Sophia' Hospital, Thessaloniki, Greece (650)

Vasconez F, Servicio de Nefrologia, Hospital Provincial de Madrid, Madrid, Spain (338)

Vendemia F, Divisione de Nefrologia, Ospedale S Carlo and Istituto, Clinica Medica IV, Universita di Milano, Milan, Italy (514)

Verhoest P, Service de Gynécologie-Obstétrique, Hôpital Nord, 8000 Amiens, France (520)

Vessby B, Department of Geriatrics, University Hospital, Uppsala, 5751 85 Uppsala, Sweden (411)

Villalta D, Department of Immunology, Ospedaliero de Pordenone, Pordenone, Italy (681)

Von Bloch L, Allegheny Professional Building, 490 E North Avenue, Pittsburgh, PA 15212, USA (243)

Wauters JP, Division of Nephrology, University Hospital, Lausanne, Switzerland (139)

Weber H, Fraunhofer Institute, Stuttgart, FRG (725)

Weber M, 1st Department of Internal Medicine, University of Mainz, Langenbeckstr. 1, D-6500 Mainz, FRG (669)

Welsh K, Renal and Tissue Typing Laboratories, Guy's Hospital, London, England (309)

Wessel-Aas T, Department of Nephrology, University of Trondheim, Trondheim, Norway (195)

Weston MJ, King's College Hospital Renal Unit, Dulwich Hospital, London, England (186)

Wideröe, T-E, Department of Nephrology, University of Trondheim, Trondheim, Norway (195)

Willebrand E von, Transplantation Laboratory, Fourth Department of Surgery, University of Helsinki, Haartmaninkatu 3A, SF 00290 Helsinki 29, Finland (356)

Williams DG, Renal Unit, Guy's Hospital, London, England (662)

Williams W, Department of Medicine, University of the West Indies, Kingston, Jamaica (629)

Wing AJ, St Thomas' Hospital, London, England (1, 76)

Wizemann V, Zentrum für Innere Medizin, 6300 Giessen, FRG (181)

Wolf H, Department of Urology, Hvidovre University Hospital, DK-2650 Hvidovre, Denmark (477)

Woodhead JS, Department of Medical Biochemistry, Welsh National School of Medicine, Cardiff, Wales (213)

Wybran J, Department of Immunology, Erasme University Hospital, Brussels, Belgium (190)

Yap PL, Edinburgh and South East Scotland Blood Transfusion Service, Edinburgh, Scotland (271)

Zanelli P, Department of Internal Medicine and Nephrology, University of Parma, Parma, Italy (111)

Zazgornik J, 1st Medical Clinic, University of Vienna, Vienna, Austria (417)

Zingraff J, Department de Néphrologie and INSERM U90, Hôpital Necker Enfants Malades, 161 rue de Sevres, 75743 Paris, France (731)

Zoob S, Royal Postgraduate Medical School, Hammersmith Hospital, London, England (623)

Zuccala A, Division of Nephrology and Dialysis, Malpighi Hospital, Bologna, Italy (156)

Zucchelli P, Division of Nephrology and Dialysis, Malpighi Hospital, Bologna, Italy (156)

TECHNOLOGY FOR HAEMODIALYSIS

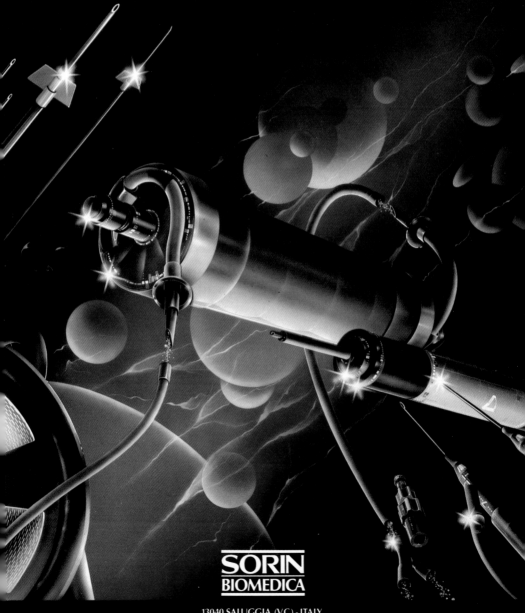

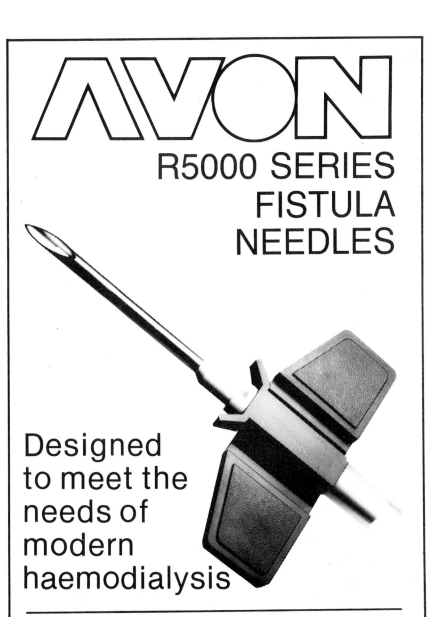
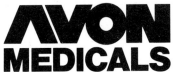

Portalysis 101®

The portable haemodialysis system

☆ Water treatment
☆ Dialysing fluid mixing
☆ Dialysing fluid flow and control
☆ Blood flow and control
☆ Heparin infusion
☆ Conventional dialysis procedure
☆ In a suitcase for ease of travel

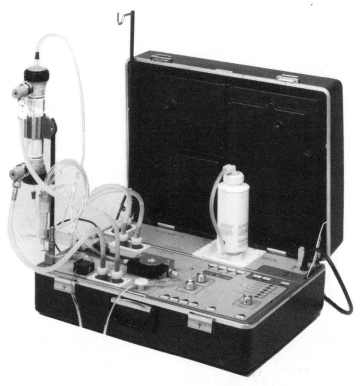

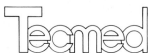

TECMED LIMITED
9 Little Ridge, Welwyn Garden City
Hertfordshire AL7 2BH, England
Telephone: (07073) 22307   Telex: 299327

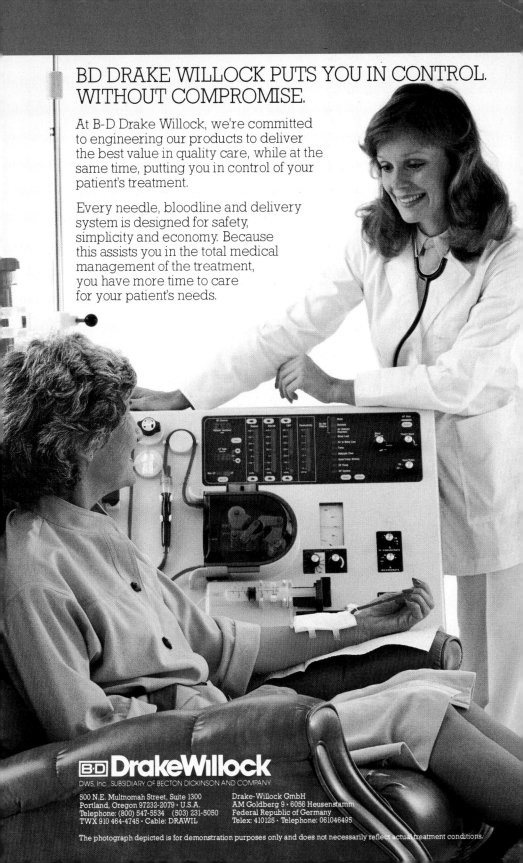

BD DRAKE WILLOCK PUTS YOU IN CONTROL. WITHOUT COMPROMISE.

At B-D Drake Willock, we're committed to engineering our products to deliver the best value in quality care, while at the same time, putting you in control of your patient's treatment.

Every needle, bloodline and delivery system is designed for safety, simplicity and economy. Because this assists you in the total medical management of the treatment, you have more time to care for your patient's needs.

B·D DrakeWillock

DWS, Inc., SUBSIDIARY OF BECTON DICKINSON AND COMPANY

500 N.E. Multnomah Street, Suite 1300
Portland, Oregon 97232-2079 · U.S.A.
Telephone: (800) 547-5534   (503) 231-5050
TWX 910 464-4748 · Cable: DRAWIL

Drake-Willock GmbH
AM Goldberg 9 · 6056 Heusenstamm
Federal Republic of Germany
Telex: 410125 · Telephone: 061046495

The photograph depicted is for demonstration purposes only and does not necessarily reflect actual treatment conditions.

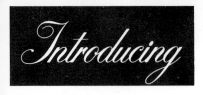

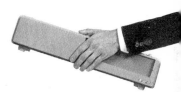
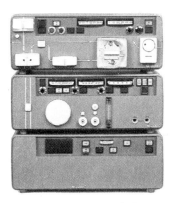
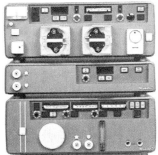
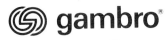

RENALYTE

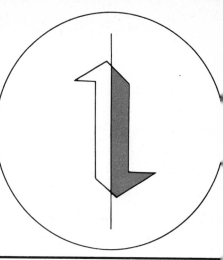

HAEMODIALYSIS FLUIDS

* Complete formulation service.
* Guaranteed deliveries.
* Manufactured under close pharmaceutical supervision.
* Quality guaranteed.

* Kompletter Formeldienst.
* Garantierte Lieferungen.
* Herstellung strengstens von Apothekerin überwacht.
* Garantierte Qualität.

* Service complet de formulation.
* Delais de livraison garantis.
* Fabriqué sous la surveillance sévère des pharmaciens.
* Qualité Garantie.

Macarthys
laboratories
limited

COPPEN ROAD SELINAS LANE
DAGENHAM, ESSEX RM8 1HR
Telephone 01-593 7581   RENALYTE is a Registered Trademark

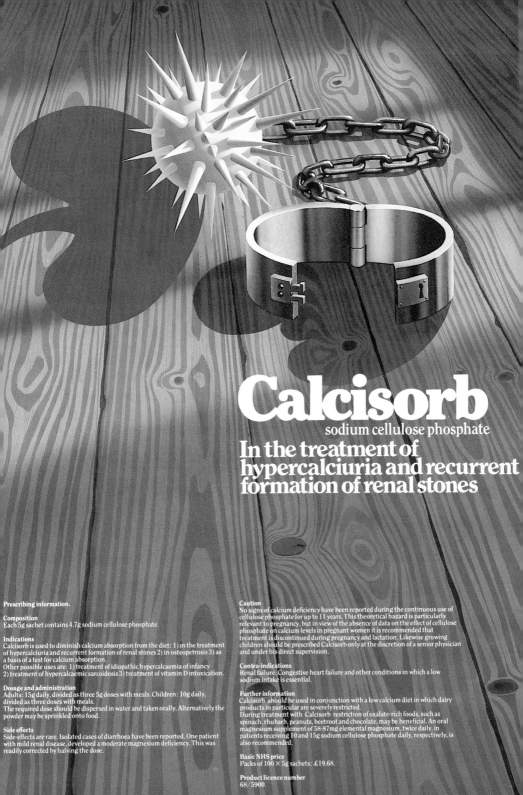

Calcisorb

sodium cellulose phosphate

In the treatment of hypercalciuria and recurrent formation of renal stones

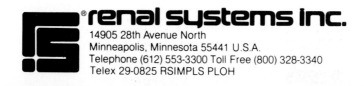

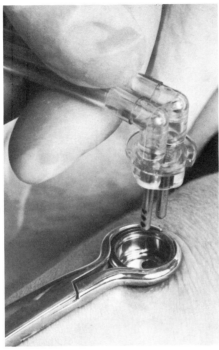

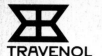

TRAVENOL

THE COMPLETE SPECTRUM OF PRODUCTS AND SERVICES TO MEET THE NEEDS OF THE DIALYSIS COMMUNITY

- Comprehensive product range for CAPD and Haemodialysis

- Training and educational support

- Home care services

- Scientific services

- Product innovation and state-of-the-art technology:

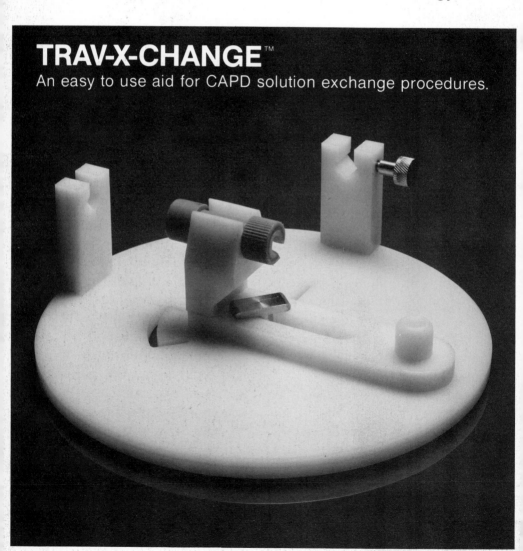

TRAV-X-CHANGE™

An easy to use aid for CAPD solution exchange procedures.

TRAVENOL U.V. SYSTEM:
THE CLOSED SYSTEM THAT OPENS THE WAY TO BETTER CAPD

INNOVATING FOR LIFE

THIS IS THE TWENTIETH VOLUME OF
THE PROCEEDINGS OF THE EUROPEAN DIALYSIS
AND TRANSPLANT ASSOCIATION
– EUROPEAN RENAL ASSOCIATION

The following volumes are still in print, and are available from Booksellers

Volume 19	£37.50 net
Volume 18	£35.00 net
Volume 17	£30.00 net
Volume 16	£25.00 net
Volume 14	£6.00 net
Volume 13	£6.00 net
Volume 12	£5.50 net
Volume 11	£4.50 net

PITMAN PUBLISHING LTD